FUNDAMENTALS OF
DIAGNOSTIC RADIOLOGY

FOURTH EDITION

EDITORS

William E. Brant, MD, FACR

Professor of Radiology
Director, ThoracoAbdominal Imaging Division
Department of Radiology and Medical Imaging
University of Virginia
Charlottesville, Virginia

Clyde A. Helms, MD

Professor of Radiology and Orthopaedic Surgery
Chief, Division of Musculoskeletal Radiology
Department of Radiology
Duke University Medical Center
Durham, North Carolina

 Wolters Kluwer | Lippincott Williams & Wilkins
Health

Philadelphia · Baltimore · New York · London
Buenos Aires · Hong Kong · Sydney · Tokyo

Senior Executive Editor: Jonathan Pine
Product Manager: Ryan Shaw
Vendor Manager: Bridgett Dougherty
Senior Manufacturing Manager: Benjamin Rivera
Senior Marketing Manager: Caroline Foote
Design Coordinator: Holly McLaughlin
Production Service: Aptara, Inc.

Library of Congress Cataloging-in-Publication Data

Fundamentals of diagnostic radiology / editors, William E. Brant, Clyde A. Helms. — 4th ed.
   p. ; cm.
   Includes bibliographical references and index.
   ISBN 978-1-60831-912-1 (alk. paper)
   I. Brant, William E.   II. Helms, Clyde A.
[DNLM: 1. Diagnostic Imaging.   WN 180]

616.07′57—dc23

2011050542

Care has been taken to confirm the accuracy of the information presented and to describe generally accepted practices. However, the authors, editors, and publisher are not responsible for errors or omissions or for any consequences from application of the information in this book and make no warranty, expressed or implied, with respect to the currency, completeness, or accuracy of the contents of the publication. Application of the information in a particular situation remains the professional responsibility of the practitioner.

The authors, editors, and publisher have exerted every effort to ensure that drug selection and dosage set forth in this text are in accordance with current recommendations and practice at the time of publication. However, in view of ongoing research, changes in government regulations, and the constant flow of information relating to drug therapy and drug reactions, the reader is urged to check the package insert for each drug for any change in indications and dosage and for added warnings and precautions. This is particularly important when the recommended agent is a new or infrequently employed drug.

Some drugs and medical devices presented in the publication have Food and Drug Administration (FDA) clearance for limited use in restricted research settings. It is the responsibility of the health care provider to ascertain the FDA status of each drug or device planned for use in their clinical practice.

To purchase additional copies of this book, call our customer service department at (800) 638-3030 or fax orders to (301) 223-2320. International customers should call (301) 223-2300.

Visit Lippincott Williams & Wilkins on the Internet: at LWW.com. Lippincott Williams & Wilkins customer service representatives are available from 8:30 am to 6 pm, EST.

10 9 8 7 6 5 4 3 2 1

RRS1112

SECTION III

■ PULMONARY

SECTION EDITOR: Jeffrey S. Klein

CHAPTER 12 ■ METHODS OF EXAMINATION, NORMAL ANATOMY, AND RADIOGRAPHIC FINDINGS OF CHEST DISEASE

JULIO LEMOS AND JEFFREY S. KLEIN

Imaging Modalities

Normal Chest Anatomy
  Posteroanterior Chest Radiograph
  Lateral Chest Radiograph
  Anatomy of the Normal Mediastinum and
    Thoracic Inlet
  Normal Hilar Anatomy
  Pleural Anatomy
  Chest Wall Anatomy
  Anatomy of the Diaphragm

Radiographic Findings in Chest Disease
  Pulmonary Opacity

Pulmonary Lucency
Mediastinal Masses
Mediastinal Widening
Pneumomediastinum and Pneumopericardium
Hilar Disease
Pleural Effusion
Pneumothorax
Localized Pleural Thickening
Diffuse Pleural Thickening
Pleural and Extrapleural Lesions
Chest Wall Lesions
Diaphragm

There are many imaging techniques available to the radiologist for the evaluation of thoracic disease (1). The decision about which imaging procedures to perform depends upon many factors, with the most important one being the availability of various modalities and the type of information sought. Although conventional radiographs of the chest still constitute 25% to 35% of the volume of any general radiology department, there has been a steady decline in favor of CT despite the considerable increase in radiation to the patient. The recent years have seen near disappearance of diagnostic thoracic vascular interventions, thanks to multidetector CT and MR. The recent advent of multichannel, parallel MR imaging might allow for gradual replacement of CT for thoracic vascular diagnostics. Although the imaging algorithm for specific problems may seem relatively straightforward, medical judgment should be preferred. For example, a thin-section CT showing a suspicious solitary pulmonary nodule might be followed directly by a thoracotomy, or rather, in selected patients, by transthoracic needle biopsy. This type of flexible approach will often streamline the diagnostic workup and ultimately lead to better patient care.

IMAGING MODALITIES

Conventional Chest Radiography. Posteroanterior (PA) and lateral chest radiographs are the mainstays of thoracic imaging. Conventional radiographs should be performed as the initial imaging study in all patients with thoracic disease. These radiographs are obtained in most radiology departments on a dedicated chest unit capable of obtaining radiographs with a focus-to-film distance of 6 ft, a high kilovoltage potential (140 kVp) technique, a grid to reduce scatter, and a phototimer to control the length of exposure (2).

The recognition of proper radiographic technique on frontal radiographs involves assessment of four basic features: *penetration*, *rotation*, *inspiration*, and *motion*. Proper penetration is present when there is faint visualization of the intervertebral disk spaces of the thoracic spine and discrete branching vessels can be identified through the cardiac shadow and the diaphragms. Rotation is assessed by noting the relationship between a vertical line drawn midway between the medial cortical margins of the clavicular heads and one drawn vertically through the spinous processes of the thoracic vertebrae. Superimposition of these lines (the former in the midline anteriorly and the latter in the midline posteriorly) indicates a properly positioned, nonrotated patient. An appropriate deep inspiration in a normal individual is present when the apex of the right hemidiaphragm is visible below the tenth posterior rib. Finally, the cardiac margin, diaphragm, and pulmonary vessels should be sharply marginated in a completely still patient who has suspended respiration during the radiographic exposure (Fig. 12.1).

Portable Radiography. Portable anteroposterior (AP) radiographs are obtained when patients cannot be safely mobilized (3). Portable radiographs help monitor a patient's cardiopulmonary status; assess the position of various monitoring and life support tubes, lines, and catheters; and detect complications related to the use of these devices.

There are technical and patient-related compromises as well as inherent physiologic changes with portable bedside radiography. The limited maximal kilovoltage potential of portable units requires longer exposures to penetrate cardiomediastinal

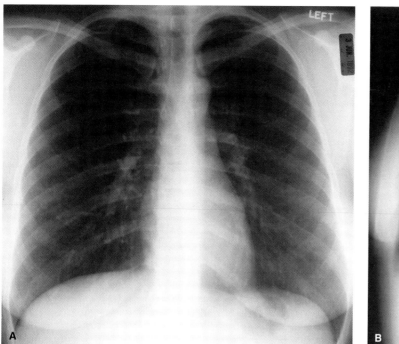
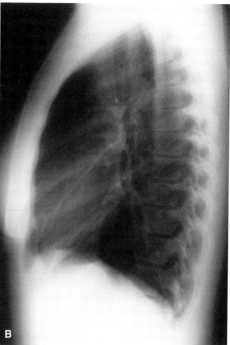

FIGURE 12.1. Normal PA (**A**) and lateral (**B**) radiographs of the chest.

structures, which results in greater motion artifact. Because critically ill patients are difficult to position for portable radiographs, the images are often rotated. Inaccuracies in directing the x-ray beam perpendicular to the patient lead to kyphotic or lordotic radiographs. The short focus-to-film distance (typically 40 in) and AP technique result in magnification of intrathoracic structures. For instance, the apparent cardiac diameter increases by 15% to 20%, bringing the upper limit of normal for the cardiothoracic ratio from 50% on a PA radiograph to 57% on an AP. Physiologically, the supine position of critically ill patients elevates the diaphragm, thus compressing lower lobes and decreasing lung volumes. The normal gravitational effect evens out the blood flow between upper and lower zones in supine patients, which makes assessment of pulmonary venous hypertension difficult. The increase in systemic venous return to the heart produces a widening of the upper mediastinum or "vascular pedicle." The gravitational layering of free-flowing fluid may hide small effusions. Similarly, a pneumothorax may be difficult to detect because free intrapleural air rises to a nondependent position, producing a subtle anteromedial or inferior radiolucency. A device called the *inclinometer* has been developed to accurately record the position of the bedridden patient from supine to completely upright. This device, which clips onto the portable radiograph cassette, gives an accurate estimate of the patient's position at the time of the radiograph, which helps assess the distribution of pulmonary blood flow, pleural effusions, and pneumothorax.

Digital (Computed) Radiography. The main advantages of computed chest radiography are superior contrast resolution and the availability of the image on any computer monitor through a PACS (picture archiving and communication system). Contrast levels and windows can be adjusted to enhance visualization of various regions in the chest or compensate partly for faulty exposure. Although digital images have poorer spatial resolution than their analog counterparts, these benefits render the system appealing.

Dual energy subtraction, a form of computed radiography that utilizes low-energy (60 keV) and high-energy (120 keV) photons to produce selective bone and soft tissue images, respectively, allows improved visualization of lung nodules, calcification, chest wall and pleural lesions, hilar masses, and localization of indwelling tubes, lines and catheters (4).

Special Techniques. A *lateral decubitus* radiograph is obtained with a horizontal x-ray beam while the patient lies in the decubitus position. It is used to detect small effusions, to characterize free-flowing effusions on the decubitus side (Fig. 12.2), or to detect a small pneumothorax on the contralateral side. As little as 5 mL of fluid or 15 mL of air can be demonstrated by this view. Normally, the downside diaphragm assumes a higher position than the upside one. Air trapping can be demonstrated in the dependent lung in patients with a check valve bronchial obstruction who are unable to cooperate for inspiratory/expiratory radiographs or chest fluoroscopy.

An *expiratory radiograph* obtained at residual volume (end of maximal forced expiration) can detect focal or diffuse air trapping and eases detection of a small pneumothorax. In the absence of a direct communication between the pleura and the bronchi, the volume of air in the pleural space remains stable, whereas the volume of air in the lung parenchyma decreases. Because the lung is also displaced away from the chest wall, the visceral pleural line becomes more visible.

An *apical lordotic view* improves visualization of the lung apices, which are obscured on routine PA radiographs by the clavicles and first costochondral junctions. Caudocephalad angulation of the tube projects these anterior bony structures superiorly, providing an unimpeded view of the apices. This view enhances the visualization of middle lobe atelectasis by placing the inferiorly displaced minor fissure in tangent with the x-ray beam and by increasing the AP thickness of the atelectatic middle lobe.

Chest fluoroscopy is used mainly to assess chest dynamics on patients with suspected diaphragmatic paralysis. Although it has been widely abandoned to the benefit of CT, fluoroscopy can still often bring the same answers as CT at a fraction of the radiation exposure: evaluation of a nodular opacity seen on only one view, evaluation of apparent pseudotumor images

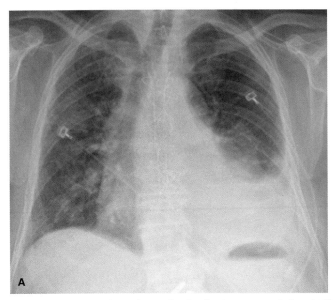 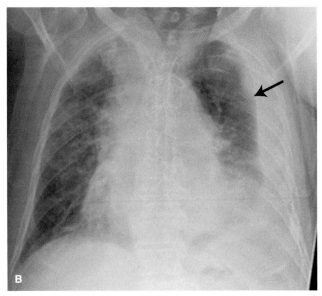

FIGURE 12.2. Lateral Decubitus Film for the Assessment of Pleural Effusion. An upright radiograph (A) in a patient recovering from coronary bypass graft surgery shows a left-sided meniscus indicative of a pleural effusion. A left lateral decubitus film (B) demonstrates free-flowing effusion laterally on the dependent side (*solid arrows*).

caused by vertebral lamina, osteophytes, vertebral transverse processes, healed rib fractures, skin lesions, nipples, or other external objects.

CT and HRCT (Thin-Section CT). Thoracic chest CTs can be acquired in an incremental "stop, acquire, and go" mode, such as for high-resolution CT, in a helical mode, whereby acquisition occurs while the patient translates through the gantry on the CT scan table, or in a step-and-shoot mode, in which data is acquired in contiguous 12 to 16 cm long stacks of images triggered to one phase of the ECG tracing. The latter technique markedly reduces radiation dose and maximizes longitudinal coverage and is therefore most useful for coronary and aortic CTA. Multidetector scanners with 256 to 320 detectors now allow for full chest coverage with collimation as narrow as 1.0 mm in approximately 3 to 5 seconds. Scans without contrast are usually performed for evaluation or follow-up of parenchymal disease. Iodinated contrast material is administered for mediastinal mass or cancer staging evaluation, systemic or pulmonary arterial evaluation, or for cardiac studies.

The field of view for image reconstruction is determined by measuring the widest transverse diameter, as seen on the CT scout view. An edge-enhancing computer reconstruction algorithm ("bone" or "sharp" algorithm) improves the spatial resolution of parenchymal structures and is used for all types of thoracic CT scans. Most frequently, the image is reconstructed in a 512 × 512 matrix size. Matrix sizes up to 1,024 × 1,024 are now available, but studies would be needed to assess whether there is any diagnostic benefit to this fourfold increase in image size. Although images can still be filmed using a laser camera, PACS workstation viewing offers the possibility to modify window width (WW) and window level (WL) as needed. Routine settings for CT display of mediastinal structures are WW = 400 and WL = 40 and for the lungs are WW = 1,500 and WL = −700.

HRCT, thin-section CT, technique involves incremental thinly collimated scans (1.0 to 1.5 mm) obtained at evenly spaced intervals through the thorax for the evaluation of diffuse bronchial or parenchymal lung disease. Image acquisition time is limited to minimize the effects of respiratory and cardiac motion. Expiratory HRCT scans are useful for the detection of air trapping in patients with small airways disease. Normal and abnormal HRCT findings are reviewed in Chapter 17.

The volume of data of a helical CT is acquired with a thickness (collimation) of 0.5 to 10 mm, and the user can then determine the reconstruction interval, which is chosen according to the amount of desired overlap. For example, a helical scan covering 25 cm with a 2.0-mm collimation can be reconstructed with a 2.0-mm interval, yielding 125 contiguous images with no overlap, but could also be reconstructed at a 1.25-mm interval, yielding 200 images, each of which overlaps the following image by 0.75 mm (5).

The major advantages of CT are its superior contrast resolution and cross-sectional display format. Superior contrast resolution allows for the differentiation of calcium, soft tissue, and fat within lung nodules or mediastinal structures. Intravenous enhancement improves contrast within structures or masses as well as within blood vessels (e.g., pulmonary emboli, aortic dissection). The cross-sectional display eliminates the superimposition of structures and allows visualization of parenchymal nodules as small as 2 mm.

The clinical indications for thoracic CT will vary among institutions. The indications for thoracic CT and HRCT are shown in Tables 12.1 and 12.2.

MR. As MR usage expands, studies must be tailored to the individual patient. Morphologic studies usually require only spin echo T1W and T2W sequences in the axial plane. Coronal and sagittal planes are used in selected cases. Mass evaluation might benefit from fat-suppressed sequences, such as STIR, or from gadolinium-enhanced sequences. Angiographic acquisitions are most often performed with GRE volumetric acquisitions. Cardiac sequences benefit from cardiac-gated balanced steady-state free precession (SSFP) techniques. Respiratory motion is minimized by performing rapid single breath-hold acquisitions or by using respiratory compensation techniques. The latest generation of multichannel scanners with parallel imaging and faster gradients show promise in evaluation of embolic disease, without the radiation cost of multidetector CTs (5).

The major advantages of MR are the superior contrast resolution between tumor and fat, the ability to characterize tissues on the basis of T1 and T2 relaxation times, the ability to scan in direct sagittal and coronal planes, and the lack of need for intravenous iodinated contrast (6). In addition, the ability to obtain images along the long axis of the aorta and the advent of cine-MR techniques have made MR the primary

TABLE 12.1

INDICATIONS FOR THORACIC CT

■ INDICATION	■ EXAMPLE
Evaluation of an abnormality identified on conventional radiographs	Densitometry of a solitary pulmonary nodule Localization and characterization of a hilar or mediastinal mass
Staging of lung cancer	Assessment of extent of the primary tumor and the relationship of the tumor to the pleura, chest wall, airways, and mediastinum Detection of hilar and mediastinal lymph node enlargement
Detection of occult pulmonary metastases	Extrathoracic malignancies with a propensity to metastasize to the lung (osteogenic sarcoma and breast and renal cell carcinoma)
Detection of mediastinal nodes	Lymphoma, metastases Infections
Distinction of empyema from lung abscess	Contrast-enhanced CT can usually distinguish a peripheral lung abscess from loculated empyema
Detection of central pulmonary embolism	Angio-CT with high injection rate, thin collimation, and precise contrast bolus timing
Detection and evaluation of aortic disease: aneurysm, dissection, intramural hematoma, aortitis, trauma	Detection and localization of extent, including aortic branch involvement

TABLE 12.2

INDICATIONS FOR THORACIC HRCT

■ INDICATION	■ EXAMPLE
Solitary pulmonary nodule	Breath-hold volumetric examination with thin collimation for accurate density determination without respiratory misregistration
Detection of lung disease in a patient with pulmonary symptoms or abnormal pulmonary function studies and a normal or equivocal chest film	Emphysema Extrinsic allergic alveolitis Small airways disease Immunocompromised patient
Evaluation of diffusely abnormal chest film	
A baseline for evaluation of patients with chronic diffuse infiltrative lung disease for follow-up changes with therapy	Cystic fibrosis Sarcoidosis Interstitial lung disease Histiocytosis X Adult respiratory distress syndrome
To determine approach (type and location) of biopsy	Bronchoscopy versus VATS or needle biopsy

VATS, video-assisted thoracic surgery.

modality for the imaging of most congenital and acquired thoracic vascular disorders. Direct coronal scans are of benefit in imaging regions that lie within the axial plane and are therefore difficult to depict on CT. For this reason, superior sulcus tumors, subcarinal and aortopulmonary window lesions, and certain hilar masses are better depicted by MR than CT. MR is superior to CT in the diagnosis of chest wall or mediastinal invasion because of the high contrast between tumor and chest wall fat and musculature and tumor and mediastinal fat, respectively. The characterization of tissues by their T1 and T2 relaxation times allows for the diagnosis of fluid-filled cysts, hemorrhage, and hematoma formation. The ability to distinguish tumor from fibrosis, based on their T1 and T2 relaxation times, has proven particularly useful in the follow-up of patients irradiated for Hodgkin disease. MR is currently unable to distinguish benign masses from malignant masses or lymph nodes.

The major disadvantages of thoracic MR scanning are the limited spatial resolution, the inability to detect calcium, and the difficulties in imaging the pulmonary parenchyma. MR is also more time-consuming and expensive than CT. These factors, along with the ability of CT to provide superior or equivalent information in most situations, have limited the use of thoracic MR for most noncardiovascular thoracic disorders. The primary indications for thoracic MR are listed in Table 12.3.

PET. Fluorodeoxyglucose (FDG) PET is an imaging modality based on the metabolic activity of neoplastic and inflammatory tissues and therefore can be considered complementary to the anatomic information provided by chest radiography and CT. The role of PET in oncologic diagnosis and staging has developed gradually over the past decade. There is a grow-

ing published experience of whole-body PET in the evaluation of patients with malignancy, particularly bronchogenic carcinoma, and of thoracic PET for the evaluation of the solitary pulmonary nodule (7).

Sonography. Transthoracic sonography is now commonly used for the detection, characterization, and sampling of pleural, peripheral parenchymal, and mediastinal lesions (see Chapter 39). The aspiration of small pleural effusions visualized on real-time sonography is preferable to blind thoracentesis. Similarly, sampling of visible pleural masses in patients with malignant effusions can diminish the number of negative pleural biopsies. The aspiration of pleural-based masses and abscesses can be safely performed by US-guided needle placement into the lesion through the point of contact between the mass and pleura. Large anterior mediastinal masses that have a broad area of contact with the parasternal chest wall may be biopsied without transgressing the lung.

Real-time sonography can also confirm phrenic nerve paralysis without the use of ionizing radiation. It easily detects

TABLE 12.3

INDICATIONS FOR MR OF THE THORAX

Evaluation of aortic disease in stable patients:
   Dissection, aneurysm, intramural hematoma, aortitis
Assessment of superior sulcus tumors
Evaluation of mediastinal, vascular, and chest wall invasion of lung cancer
Staging of lung cancer patients unable to receive intravenous iodinated contrast
Evaluation of posterior mediastinal masses

subpulmonic and subphrenic fluid collections, which may cause apparent diaphragmatic elevation. In emergency room and critical care settings, thoracic sonography is used to detect pneumothorax and to guide central venous catheterization.

Ventilation/Perfusion Lung Scanning. The nuclear medicine examinations for the evaluation of noncardiac thoracic disease are ventilation/perfusion (V/Q) lung scintigraphy (see Chapter 55) and gallium scintigraphy. V/Q scanning is used almost exclusively for the diagnosis of pulmonary embolism, although quantitative V/Q imaging may be useful in the planning of bullectomy, lung volume reduction surgery for emphysema, and lung transplantation. Gallium-67 scanning of the chest is used in the detection of pulmonary infection (e.g., *Pneumocystis carinii* pneumonia in a patient with a normal radiograph) or inflammation (e.g., disease activity in idiopathic pulmonary fibrosis) and in the evaluation of suspected sarcoidosis.

Diagnostic Arteriography has largely been replaced by MDCT angiography. Pulmonary angiograms are only performed in cases where CT pulmonary angiography is suboptimal or equivocal.

Thanks to the newer scanners and to the improvement of three-dimensional rendering tools, thoracic aortography has also been largely replaced by CT, MR, or US. On occasion, an equivocal diagnosis of an aortic laceration following blunt chest trauma can be resolved with this technique. Inflammatory changes of infectious aortitis are also better imaged with MR or CT.

Active bleeding through a bronchial artery is still best addressed by bronchial arteriography, as an active bleeding site is often difficult to pinpoint. When massive or recurrent hemoptysis occurs, most commonly from bronchiectasis, neoplasm, or mycetoma, arteriography and embolization can be performed in the same setting.

Transthoracic Needle Biopsy guided by CT, fluoroscopy, or US is a diagnostic technique used in selected patients with pulmonary, pleural, or mediastinal lesions (7).

Percutaneous Catheter Drainage of intrathoracic air or fluid collections, performed by imaging-guided placement of small-bore multihole catheters, is used for the treatment of empyema, pneumothorax, malignant pleural effusion, and other intrathoracic fluid collections (3).

NORMAL LUNG ANATOMY

Tracheobronchial Tree. The trachea is a hollow cylinder composed of a series of C-shaped cartilaginous rings (Fig. 12.3). The rings are completed posteriorly by a flat band of muscle and connective tissue called the *posterior tracheal membrane.* The tracheal mucosa consists of pseudostratified, ciliated columnar epithelium, which contains scattered neuroendocrine (APUD) cells. The submucosa contains cartilage, smooth muscle, and seromucous glands. The left lateral wall of the distal trachea is indented by the transverse portion of the aortic arch.

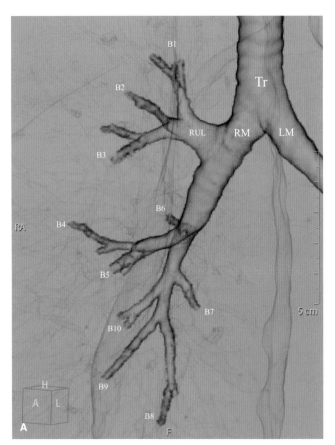
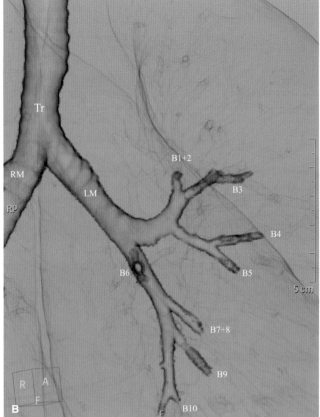

FIGURE 12.3. Prevailing Pattern of Segmental Bronchi. Virtual bronchography three-dimensional rendered images of the usual bronchial anatomy. **A.** Right bronchial tree. **B.** Left bronchial tree. Tr, trachea; RUL, right upper lobe; LUL, left upper lobe; RM, right main bronchus; LM, left main bronchus; BT, left lower lobe basal trunk; RML, right middle lobe; B1, apical (upper lobe); B2, posterior (upper lobe); B3, anterior (upper lobe); B4, lateral (middle lobe) and superior (lingula); B5, medial (middle lobe) and inferior (lingula); B6, superior (lower lobe); B7, medial basilar (lower lobe); B8, anterior (lower lobe); B9, lateral basilar (lower lobe); B10, posterior (lower lobe).

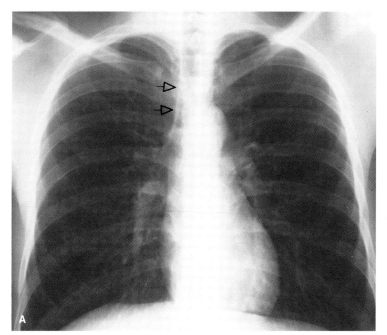
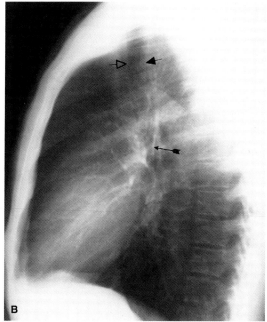

FIGURE 12.4. **Trachea. A.** The right paratracheal stripe (*open arrows*) is composed of the right lateral tracheal wall, a small amount of mediastinal fat, paratracheal lymph nodes, and the visceral and parietal pleural layers of the right upper lobe. **B.** Left lateral chest film shows the anterior (*open arrow*) and posterior (*short solid arrow*) walls of the trachea. The posterior wall of the bronchus intermedius (*long solid arrow*) is readily visible on lateral radiographs as it crosses the end-on view of the left upper lobe bronchus. Because these structures are central, their relationship tends to remain even on rotated films. This is easily seen on CT (see Fig 12.5B, image 3).

The trachea is approximately 12 cm long in adults, with an upper limit of normal coronal tracheal diameter of 25 mm in men and 21 mm in women. In cross section, the trachea is oval or horseshoe-shaped, with a coronal-to-sagittal diameter ratio of 0.6:1.0. A narrowing of the coronal diameter producing a coronal-to-sagittal ratio of <0.6 is termed a *saber sheath trachea* and is seen in patients with chronic obstructive pulmonary disease.

On chest radiographs, the trachea is seen as a vertically oriented cylindric lucency extending from the cricoid cartilage superiorly to the main bronchi inferiorly. A slight tracheal deviation to the right after entering the thorax can be a normal radiographic finding. The interface of the right upper lobe (RUL) with the right lateral tracheal wall is called the *right paratracheal stripe* (Fig. 12.4A). This stripe should be uniformly smooth and should not exceed 4 mm in width; thickening or nodularity reflects disease in any of the component tissues, including medial tracking pleural effusion. The left lateral wall is surrounded by mediastinal vessels and fat and is not normally visible radiographically. The posterior trachea can be visualized on the lateral chest (Fig. 12.4B). The presence of air in the esophagus produces the tracheoesophageal stripe, which represents the combined thickness of the tracheal and esophageal walls and intervening fat. This stripe should measure less than 5 mm; thickening is most commonly seen with esophageal carcinoma.

The bronchial system exhibits a branching pattern of asymmetric dichotomy, with the daughter bronchi of a parent bronchus varying in diameter, length, and the number of divisions. The bronchial generation "n" indicates the number of divisions since the trachea, which bears generation number 1 (8). The main bronchi arise from the trachea at the carina, with the right bronchus forming a more obtuse angle with the long axis of the trachea. The right main bronchus is considerably shorter than the left main bronchus (mean lengths of 2.2 and 5 cm, respectively). The tracheal and main, lobar, and segmental bronchial anatomy are easily seen on CT (Fig. 12.5). Bronchi

on end can be seen as a ring shadow on chest radiographs. Bronchi gradually lose their cartilaginous support between generations 1 and 12 to 15. Once this happens, these 1- to 3-mm airways are called *bronchioles* (9). Bronchioles bearing alveoli on their walls are termed *respiratory bronchioles*. The latter divide into alveolar ducts and alveolar sacs. The airway just before the first respiratory bronchiole is the *terminal bronchiole*. It is the smallest bronchiole without respiratory exchange structures. In average, a total of 21 to 25 generations are found between the trachea and the alveoli.

Lobar and Segmental Anatomy (Fig. 12.6). The lungs are divided by the *interlobar fissures*, which are invaginations of the visceral pleura. On the right, the minor fissure separates the middle from the upper lobe. The major fissure separates the lower lobe from the upper lobe superiorly and from the middle lobe inferiorly. The upper lobe bronchus and its artery, arising from the truncus anterior, branch into three segmental branches: anterior, apical, and posterior. The middle lobe bronchus arises from the intermediate bronchus and divides into medial and lateral segmental branches, with its blood supplied by a branch of the right interlobar pulmonary artery. The right lower lobe (RLL) is supplied by the RLL bronchus and pulmonary artery. It is subdivided into a superior segment and four basal segments: anterior, lateral, posterior, and medial.

The left lung is divided into upper and lower lobes by the left major fissure. The left upper lobe (LUL) is analogous to the combined right upper and middle lobes. The LUL is subdivided into four segments: anterior, apicoposterior, and the superior and inferior lingular segments. Arterial supply to the anterior and apicoposterior segments parallels the bronchi and is via branches of the upper division of the left main pulmonary artery. The superior and inferior lingular arteries are proximal branches of the left interlobar pulmonary artery, analogous to the middle lobe's blood supply. The left lower lobe (LLL) has a superior segment and three basal segments: anteromedial, lateral, and posterior.

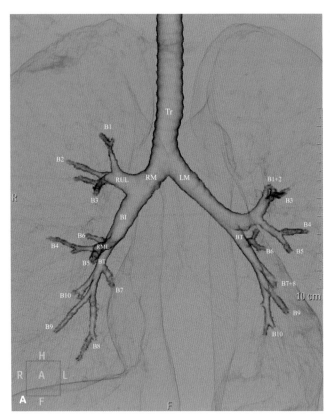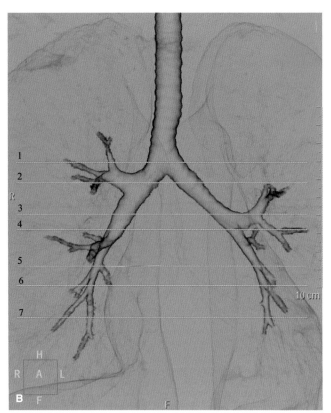

FIGURE 12.5. **Tracheobronchial and Hilar Anatomy. A.** Three-dimensional volume-rendered virtual bronchographic view of the bronchial tree. Tr, trachea; RM, right main bronchus; LM, left main bronchus; RUL, right upper lobe; RML, right middle lobe; LUL, left upper lobe; BI, bronchus intermedius; BT, basal trunk. **B.** Levels of the CT images depicting the bronchial and hilar anatomy. **1. Level of tracheal carina.** Right apical bronchus (1); right superior posterior pulmonary vein (rv); left apicoposterior bronchus (1 and 2 on the left). **2. Level of right upper lobe bronchus.** Right main bronchus (RM); right upper lobe bronchus (ru); right upper lobe anterior (3) and posterior (2) segmental bronchi; right superior pulmonary vein (rv); left main bronchus (LM); left apicoposterior segmental bronchus (1 + 2); left superior pulmonary vein (lv). **3. Level of left upper lobe bronchus, superior division.** Bronchus intermedius (BI), with its posterior border at the level of the left main (LM); right superior pulmonary vein (rv); superior division of left upper lobe bronchus (small arrows); left upper lobe anterior (3) and apicoposterior (1 + 2) segmental bronchi; left descending pulmonary artery (Ld). **4. Level of left upper lobe bronchus, inferior (lingular) division.** Bronchus intermedius (BI); right descending pulmonary artery (Rd); lingular bronchus (4 + 5); left lower lobe bronchus (LL); left lower lobe superior segmental bronchus (6); left descending pulmonary artery (Ld). **5. Level of middle lobe bronchus.** Middle lobe bronchus (4 + 5); right lower lobe bronchus (RL); right descending pulmonary artery (Rd); lingular superior segmental bronchus (4); left lower lobe basal trunk (BT); left lower lobe segmental arteries (a). **6. Level of lower lobe basal trunks.** Lateral (4) and medial (5) segmental bronchi of the middle lobe; right lower lobe basal trunk (BT); right lower lobe basal segmental arteries (a, on right); lingular segmental bronchus (5); left lower lobe anteromedial segmental bronchus (7 + 8); left lower lobe lateral and posterior basal segmental bronchi (9 + 10); left lower lobe basal segmental arteries (a, on left). **7. Level of basal segmental bronchi.** Right lower lobe medial (7, on right), anterior (8, on right), lateral (9, on right), and posterior (10, on right) basal segmental bronchi; right inferior pulmonary vein (v, on right); left lower lobe medial (7, on left), anterior (8, on left), lateral (9, on left), and posterior (10, on left) basal segmental bronchi; left inferior pulmonary vein (v, on left).

Respiratory Portion of Lung. The respiratory bronchioles contain a few alveoli along their walls and give rise to the gas-exchanging units of the lung: the *alveolar ducts* and the *alveolar sacs*. The pulmonary alveolus is lined by two types of epithelial cells (pneumocytes). Type 1 pneumocytes are flattened squamous cells covering 95% of the alveolar surface area and are invisible by light microscopy. These cells are incapable of mitosis or repair. The rarer type 2 pneumocytes are cuboidal cells, which are visible under light microscopy and are capable of mitosis. Type 2 pneumocytes are the source of new type 1 pneumocytes and provide a mechanism for repair following alveolar damage. These cells are also thought to be the source of alveolar surfactant, a phospholipid that lowers the surface tension of alveolar walls and prevents alveolar collapse at low lung volumes.

Pulmonary Subsegmental Anatomy is discussed in Chapter 17, along with the HRCT description of these anatomic structures.

Fissures. The interlobar pulmonary fissures represent invaginations of the visceral pleura deep into the substance of the lung (Fig. 12.6) (10). These fissures may completely or incompletely separate the lobes from one another. An incomplete fissure has important consequences regarding interlobar spread of parenchymal consolidation, collateral air drift in patients with lobar bronchial obstruction, and the appearance of pleural effusion in the supine patient. The fissures are well delineated on CT or HRCT (Fig. 12.7).

In most individuals, there are two interlobar fissures on the right and one on the left. The fissures are complete laterally and incomplete medially, fusing with the adjacent lobe. The *minor fissure* is complete in about 25% of individuals but fuses with the RUL in about 50%. The inferior fissure of the right middle lobe (RML) is well developed and there is very little fusion between the RML and the RLL. This oblique fissure is complete in less than 35% of individuals, with fusion between the lobes most common along the posteromedial portion of the fissure. The *left major fissure* is similar to the *right major fissure*, with fusion along the posterior aspect in approximately 35% of individuals.

The major and minor fissures are best visualized on lateral radiographs. Variable portions of the major fissures are seen

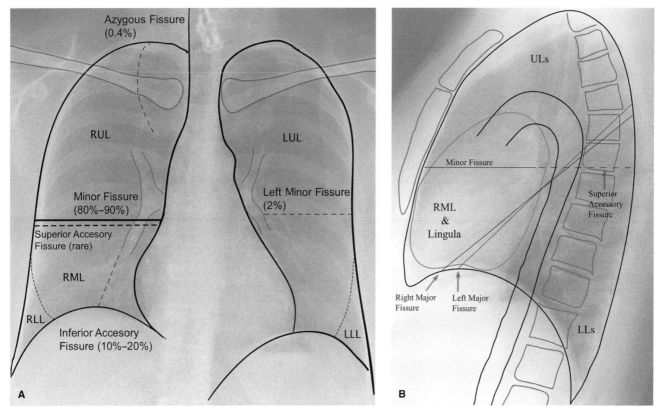

FIGURE 12.6. Normal Lobar and Fissural Anatomy. A. Frontal view. **B.** Lateral view. RUL, right upper lobe; LUL, left upper lobe; RML, right middle lobe; RLL, right lower lobe; LLL, left lower lobe; ULs, upper lobes; LLs, lower lobes.

as obliquely oriented, thin white lines coursing anteroinferiorly from posterior to anterior. The left major fissure usually begins more superiorly and has a slightly more vertical course than the right major fissure. At their points of contact with the diaphragm or chest wall, the fissures often have a triangular configuration, with the apex of the triangle pointing toward the fissure. This appearance is the result of the presence of a small amount of fat within the distal aspect of the fissure. Although the major fissures are not usually visualized on frontal radiographs because of their oblique course relative to the x-ray beam, occasional extrapleural fat infiltration along their superolateral aspect can give rise to a curvilinear edge in the upper thorax. The minor fissure projects at the level of the right fourth rib and is seen as a thin undulating line on frontal radiographs in approximately 50% of individuals. On a lateral radiograph, the minor fissure is often seen as a thin curvilinear line with a convex superior margin. Not uncommonly, the posterior aspect of the minor fissure extends posterior to the margin of the right major fissure. This is because the minor fissure abuts the entire convexity of the anterior lower lobe, but the major fissure interface is caused by the crest of the convexity.

The *inferior accessory fissure* is the most common accessory fissure and is found in approximately 10% to 20% of individuals. This fissure, which separates the medial basal from the remaining basal segments of the lower lobe, is often incomplete (Fig. 12.6). It may be seen on frontal radiographs as a thin curvilinear line extending superiorly from the medial third of the hemidiaphragm toward the lower hilum. The inferior accessory fissure has been misidentified as the inferior pulmonary ligament (invisible on normal chest radiographs) and is responsible for the juxtaphrenic peak described in upper lobe volume loss. A small triangle of extrapleural fat, seen at its point of insertion on the diaphragm, helps identify the inferior accessory fissure. An inferior accessory fissure can be seen

on CT scans through the lower thorax, where it is identified as a curvilinear line extending anterolaterally from just in front of the inferior pulmonary ligament toward the major fissure.

The *azygos fissure* is seen in 0.5% of individuals (Fig. 12.6). It is composed of four layers of pleura (two visceral and two parietal) and represents an invagination of the right apical pleura by the azygos vein, which has incompletely migrated to its normal position at the right tracheobronchial angle. The azygos fissure appears as a vertical curvilinear line, convex laterally, which extends inferiorly from the lung apex and ends in a teardrop, which is the azygos vein. The significance of this fissure lies in its ability to limit the spread of apical segmental consolidation to the azygos lobe (that portion of the apical segment delineated by the azygos fissure) and in excluding pneumothorax from the apical portion of the pleural space.

The *superior accessory fissure* separates the superior segment from the basal segments of the lower lobe. On the right side it may be distinguished from the minor fissure on lateral radiographs because it extends posteriorly from the major fissure to the chest wall.

The *left minor fissure* is a rarely seen normal variant that separates the lingula from the remaining portions of the upper lobe.

Ligaments. The *inferior pulmonary ligament* is a sheet of connective tissue that extends from the hilum superiorly to a level at or just above the hemidiaphragm. Thus, it comprises fused visceral and parietal pleura and binds the lower lobe to the mediastinum and runs alongside the esophagus. The ligament contains the inferior pulmonary vein superiorly and a variable number of lymph nodes. The inferior pulmonary ligament is sometimes seen on CT scans through the lower thorax as a small laterally directed beak of mediastinal pleura adjacent to the esophagus (Fig. 12.8). The tethering effect of this ligament on the lower lobe accounts for the medial location

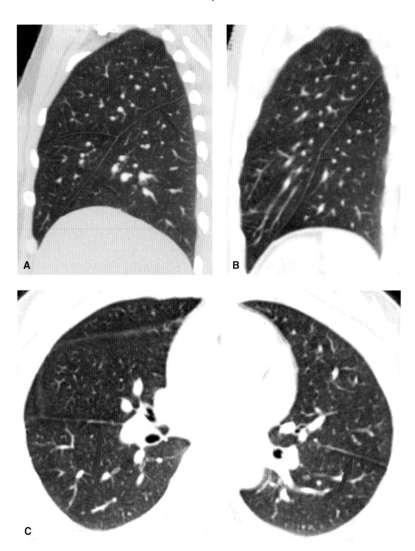

A

B

C

FIGURE 12.7. **Fissural Anatomy on Multidetector CT. A.** CT with sagittal reconstruction through the right lung shows major (*arrows*) and minor (*arrowhead*) fissures. **B.** CT with sagittal reconstruction through the left lung shows major fissure (*arrows*). **C.** Axial CT shows the oblique fissures as thin lines (*arrows*). The minor fissure (*arrowhead*) is indistinct owing to its domed shape and oblique orientation.

and triangular appearance of lower lobe collapse. The ligament may also act as a barrier to the spread of pleural and mediastinal fluid and may marginate medial pleural or mediastinal air collections to produce a characteristic appearance on radiographs.

The *sublobar septum* (Fig. 12.8) has been mistaken for the inferior pulmonary ligament. It is a linear structure seen on CT near the inferior pulmonary ligament extending into the lung from the mediastinal pleura.

The *pericardiophrenic ligament* is a triangular density extending toward the lung that is seen along the posterior aspect of the right heart border on lung windows on chest CT (Fig. 12.8). It represents a reflection of pleura over the inferior portion of the phrenic nerve and pericardiophrenic vessels. It is distinguished from the sublobar septum by its more anterior location and by its characteristic ramifications as branches of the nerve and vessel reflect over the hemidiaphragm.

Pulmonary Arteries (Fig. 12.9A–C) (11). The pulmonary artery is an elastic artery that arises from the right ventricle at approximately 1-o'clock position relative to the ascending aorta. These two structures then rotate from right to left as they ascend in the mediastinum until the pulmonary artery lies at the 5-o'clock position. The left pulmonary artery is a direct continuation of the main pulmonary artery. The right artery branches just below the carina, with an angle close to 90°. Within the left hilum, the artery envelopes the upper margin of the left main bronchus, at which point it divides into the upper and lower lobe arteries. The arch formed by

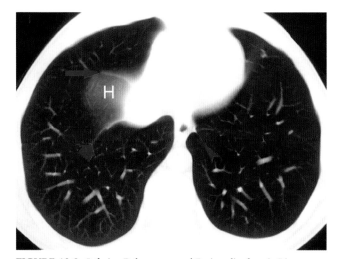

H

FIGURE 12.8. **Inferior Pulmonary and Pericardiophrenic Ligaments.** A CT scan just above the diaphragm demonstrates a thin line (*arrowhead*) extending posterolaterally at the level of the esophagus that represents the sublobar septum extending to the inferior pulmonary ligament. On the right, a curvilinear line (*fat arrow*) extending from just lateral to the inferior vena cava represents the right pericardiophrenic ligament containing branches of the phrenic nerve and pericardiophrenic vessels. More anteriorly, a thin line (*arrow*) is seen just above the apex of the right hemidiaphragm (*H*), which represents fat within the inferior aspect of the major fissure.

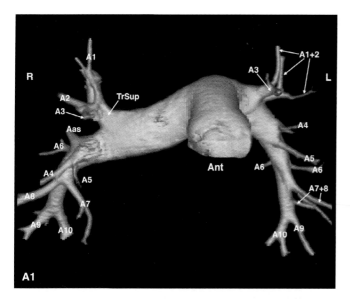
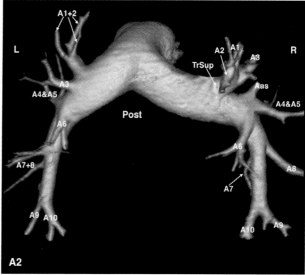
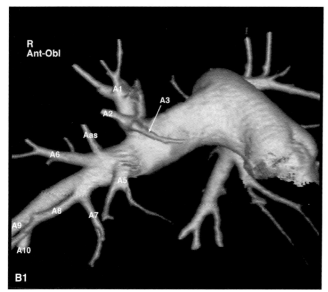
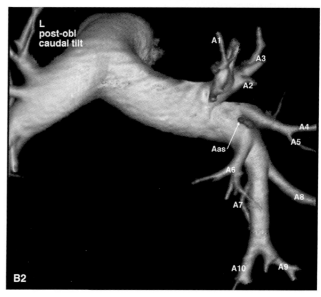

FIGURE 12.9. Prevailing Pattern of Segmental Arteries and Venous Returns. Three-dimensional volume-rendered images of the pulmonary arterial system in different views depict the most usual arterial anatomy. The branches of the right and left pulmonary arteries accompany and divide in parallel with the corresponding bronchi. **A.** Left and right pulmonary arteries; (1) anterior view and (2) posterior view. **B.** Right pulmonary artery; (1) anterior view and (2) posterior view. (*continued*)

the LLL artery over the left hilar bronchi (i.e., the bronchus is hypoarterial) is easily seen on the lateral view. On the other hand, the right pulmonary artery courses laterally and anterior to the main bronchus. The right artery divides within the pericardium into the truncus anterior and interlobar arteries. In contradistinction to the left side, the right interlobar artery courses anterolateral to the bronchus (i.e., the bronchus is epiarterial). The different spatial relationships are essential when determining bronchial and pulmonary situs. At the same level that the bronchi lose their cartilage and become bronchioles, the elastic arteries lose their elastic lamina and become muscular arteries. Thickening of the alveolocapillary membrane from edema fluid or fibrosis impedes gas exchange and results in dyspnea and hypoxemia.

Bronchial Arteries are the primary nutrient vessels of the lung. They supply blood to the bronchial walls to the level of the terminal bronchioles. In addition, several mediastinal structures receive a variable amount of blood supply from the bronchial circulation. These include the tracheal wall, middle

third of the esophagus, visceral pleura, mediastinal lymph nodes, vagus nerve, pericardium, and thymus.

The bronchial arteries usually arise from the proximal descending thoracic aorta at the level of the carina but may show significant variability. Most commonly there are one right-sided and two left-sided arteries. The right bronchial artery usually arises from the posterolateral wall of the aorta in common with an intercostal artery as an intercostobronchial trunk. The left bronchial arteries arise individually from the anterolateral aorta or, rarely, from an intercostal artery. Approximately two-thirds of the blood from the bronchial arterial system returns to the pulmonary venous system via the bronchial veins (a small right-to-left shunt). The remaining blood, which includes veins draining the large bronchi, tracheal bifurcation, and mediastinum, drains into the azygos or hemiazygos systems.

Pulmonary Veins (Fig. 12.9D) arise within the interlobular septa from the alveolar and visceral pleural capillaries. The veins travel in connective tissue envelopes that are separate

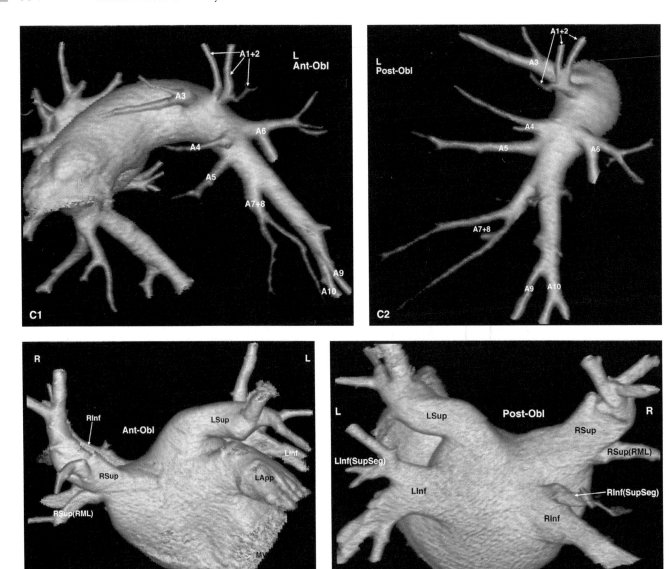

FIGURE 12.9. (*Continued*) **C.** Left pulmonary artery; (1) anterior view and (2) posterior view. TrSup, truncus superior; A1, apical (upper lobe); A2, posterior (upper lobe); A3, anterior (upper lobe); A4, lateral (middle lobe) and superior (lingula); A5, medial (middle lobe) and inferior (lingula); A6, superior (lower lobe); A7, medial basal (lower lobe); A8, anterior basal (lower lobe); A9, lateral basal (lower lobe); A10, posterior basal (lower lobe). Note that the right upper lobe receives an accessory branch from the proximal right interlobar pulmonary artery (Aas). **D.** Left atrium and venous returns; (1) anterior view and (2) posterior view. Three-dimensional volume-rendered images of the left atrium and venous returns depict the most usual venous return anatomy. Significantly more variation exists than in the bronchial/arterial systems. Although only the main returns are depicted here, the reader will find an extensive discussion in Yamashita (11). RSup, Right superior venous return; LSup, left superior venous return; RInf, right inferior venous return; LInf, left inferior venous return. Several branches can join the left atrium separate from their lobar venous return. The most common ones are RSup (RML), right middle lobe branch of the RSup; LInf(SupSeg) and RInf(SupSeg), branches from the superior segments of the lower lobes. Lapp, Left atrial appendage; MV, mitral valve plane.

from the bronchoarterial trunks. The pulmonary veins, which may number from three to eight, drain into the left atrium.

Pulmonary Lymphatics help clear fluid and particulate matter from the pulmonary interstitium. There are two major lymphatic pathways in the lung and pleura. The visceral pleural lymphatics, which reside in the vascular (innermost) layer of the visceral pleura, form a network over the surface of the lung that roughly parallels the margins of the secondary pulmonary lobules. These peripheral lymphatics penetrate the lung to course centrally within interlobular septa, along with the pulmonary veins, toward the hilum. The parenchymal lymphatics originate in proximity to the alveolar septa ("juxta-alveolar lymphatics") and course centrally with the bronchoarterial bundle. The perivenous and bronchoarterial lymphatics com-

municate via obliquely oriented lymphatics located within the central regions of the lung. These perivenous lymphatics and their surrounding connective tissue, when distended by fluid, account for the radiographic appearance of Kerley A lines.

Pulmonary Interstitium is the scaffolding of the lung and as such provides support for the airways and pulmonary vessels (Fig. 12.10) (10). It begins within the hilum and extends peripherally to the visceral pleura. The interstitial compartment that extends from the mediastinum and envelopes the bronchovascular bundles is termed the *axial interstitium*. The axial fiber system continues distally as the *centrilobular interstitium* along with the arterioles, capillaries, and bronchioles to provide support for the air-exchanging portions of the lung. The *subpleural interstitium* and interlobular septa are parts of

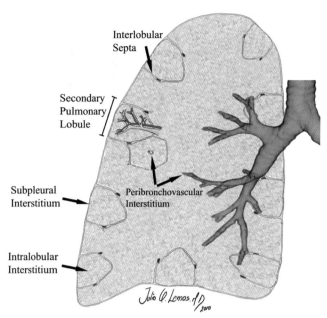

FIGURE 12.10. Diagram of the Pulmonary Interstitium.

the *peripheral interstitium*, which divides secondary pulmonary lobules. The pulmonary veins and lymphatics lie within the peripheral interstitium. The *intralobular interstitium* is a thin network of fibers that bridges the gap between the centrilobular and peripheral compartments.

Edema involving the axial interstitium is recognized radiographically as peribronchial cuffing. Pathologic involvement of the intralobular interstitium is difficult to discern radiographically, but may account for some cases of so-called "ground-glass" opacity on chest radiographs and HRCT scans. Thickening of portions of this interstitium are occasionally seen as intralobular lines on HRCT. Radiographically, edema of the peripheral and subpleural interstitium accounts for Kerley B lines (or interlobular lines on HRCT) and "thickened" fissures on chest radiographs.

Posteroanterior Chest Radiograph

A firm knowledge of the normal anatomy displayed on the frontal (usually PA) chest radiograph is key to detecting and localizing pathologic conditions and to avoid mistaking normal structures for pathologic findings (Fig. 1A).

Soft Tissues of the chest wall consist of the skin, subcutaneous fat, and muscles. The lateral edges of the sternocleidomastoid muscles are readily visible in most patients. The visualization of normal fat in the supraclavicular fossae and the companion shadows of skin and subcutaneous fat paralleling the clavicles helps exclude mass, adenopathy, or edema in this region. The inferolateral edge of the pectoralis major muscle is normally seen curving toward the axilla. Both breast shadows should be evaluated routinely to detect evidence of prior mastectomy or distorting mass. The soft tissues lateral to the bony thorax should be smooth, symmetric, homogeneous densities.

Bones. The thoracic spine, ribs and costal cartilages, clavicles, and scapulae are routinely visible on frontal chest radiographs. The bodies of the thoracic vertebrae should be vertically aligned, with endplates, pedicles, and spinous processes visualized. Twelve pairs of symmetric ribs should be seen; the upper ribs have smooth superior and inferior cortical margins, while the middle and lower ribs have flanged inferior

cortices where the intercostal neurovascular bundles run. Cervical ribs are identified in approximately 2% of individuals and may be associated with symptoms of thoracic outlet syndrome. Companion shadows paralleling the inferior margins of the first and second ribs represent extrapleural fat, which may be abundant in obese individuals. Costal cartilage calcification is seen in a majority of adults, increases in prevalence with advancing age, and can add multiple shadows to the PA view. Men typically show calcification at the upper and lower margins, while the majority of women develop central cartilaginous calcification.

Lung–Lung Interfaces. A familiarity with the normal mediastinal interfaces is key to the interpretation of frontal chest radiographs (2). The lung–mediastinal interfaces are seen as sharp edges where the lung and adjacent pleura reflect off of various mediastinal structures. The lung–lung interfaces as seen on frontal radiographs relate directly to the space available in three regions viewed on the lateral film: the retrosternal space, the retrotracheal triangle, and the retrocardiac space (Fig. 12.11).

The retrosternal airspace reflects contact of the anterosuperior aspect of the upper lobes (Fig. 12.11). On frontal radiographs, the *anterior junction line* is seen as a thin vertical line that overlies the thoracic spine (Fig. 12.12). The anterior junction anatomy is an inferior extension of the upper lobe reflections off the innominate veins, with the latter producing an inverted V-shaped retromanubrial opacity. The anterior junction line often disappears after sternotomy, or when abundant anterior mediastinal fat precludes retrosternal contact of the upper lobes.

A second potential lung–lung interface is seen on the lateral chest radiograph as the *retrotracheal triangle,* a radiolucent region representing contact of the posterosuperior portions of the upper lobes (Fig. 12.11). If the retrotracheal

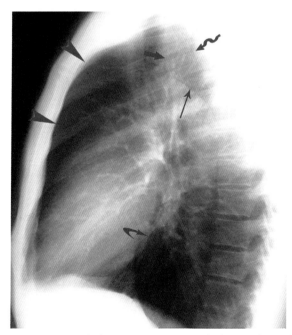

FIGURE 12.11. Radiolucent Spaces on Lateral Chest Radiographs. The retrosternal space is demarcated anteriorly by the posterior margin of the sternum (*arrowheads*) and the heart and ascending aorta posteriorly and accounts for the anterior junction line seen on frontal radiographs. The retrotracheal triangle is marginated by the posterior wall of the trachea anteriorly (*fat arrow*), the spine posteriorly (*squiggly arrow*), and the aortic arch inferiorly (*solid triangle*). The retrocardiac space is demarcated anteriorly by the posterior cardiac margin (*curved arrow*) and the inferior vena cava (*small arrow*).

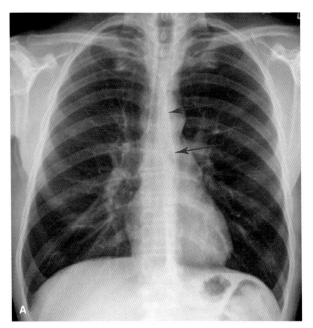
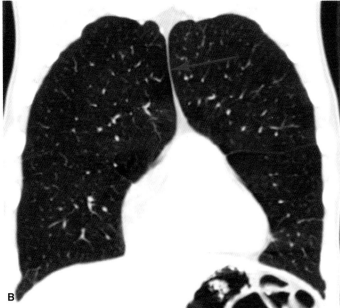

FIGURE 12.12. Anterior Junction Line. A. A PA chest film shows the anterior junction line (*arrows*). **B.** Coronal-reformatted CT at lung windows through the anterior thorax shows the anterior junction line (*arrow*).

space available is small, only a right paraesophageal interface is visualized on the PA view (Fig. 12.13). If the space is large, a posterior junction line is seen (Fig. 12.12) (Table 12.4).

The third potential lung–lung interface occurs in the *retrocardiac space* (Fig. 12.11). If that space is large, the azygoesophageal recess of the RLL can abut the preaortic recess of the LLL to produce an inferior *posterior junction line*.

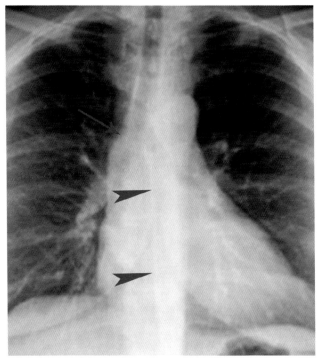

FIGURE 12.13. Lung–Lung Interfaces on Frontal Radiograph. Coned down view of a PA film shows the azygos arch (*arrow*) that separates the supra-azygos lung from the infra-azygos lung, which creates the azygoesophageal recess interface (*arrowheads*).

Lung–Mediastinal Interfaces (Table 12.5). The right lateral margin of the superior vena cava is commonly seen as a straight or slightly concave interface with the RUL extending from the level of the clavicle to the superior margin of the right atrium. Prominence or convexity of the caval interface may represent caval dilatation or lateral displacement by a dilated or tortuous aortic arch or other mediastinal mass.

Along the right upper mediastinum, the RUL contacts the right lateral tracheal wall in a majority of individuals. This produces the right paratracheal stripe (Fig. 12.4A). The thickness of this line, measured above the level of the azygos vein, should not exceed 4 mm. Thickening or nodularity of the paratracheal stripe is seen in abnormalities of the tissues comprising the strip, including tracheal tumors, paratracheal lymph node enlargement, and right pleural effusion (Fig. 12.2).

The arch of the azygos vein separates the right paraesophageal from the upper azygos esophageal space (Fig. 12.13). The measurement should be made through the midpoint of the azygos arch perpendicular to the right main bronchus. Supine positioning or performance of the Müller maneuver (forced inspiration against a closed glottis) will increase azygos venous diameter. In general, a diameter of >10 mm on a PA radiograph should raise the possibility of mass, adenopathy, or dilatation of the azygos vein; the latter may be seen with right

TABLE 12.4

ANTERIOR AND POSTERIOR JUNCTION LINES

■ LINE	■ FEATURES
Anterior junction line	Obliquely oriented from right superior to left inferior
	Extends from upper sternum to base of heart
Posterior junction line	Vertically oriented in the midline
	Extends from upper thoracic spine to level of azygos and aortic arches

TABLE 12.5

NORMAL LUNG–MEDIASTINAL INTERFACES

Right sided	Right paraesophageal interface
	Superior vena cava/right paratracheal stripe
	Anterior arch of the azygos vein
	Right paraspinal interface
	Azygoesophageal recess
	Lateral margin of right atrium
	Confluence of right pulmonary veins (right border of left atrium)
	Lateral margin of inferior vena cava
Left sided	Lateral margin of left subclavian artery
	Transverse aortic arch
	Left superior intercostal vein ("aortic nipple")
	Aortopulmonary window interface
	Aortopulmonary interface
	Lateral margin of main pulmonary artery
	Preaortic recess
	Left paraspinal interface
	Left atrial appendage
	Left ventricle
	Epipericardial fat pad

heart failure, obstruction of venous return to the heart, or a congenital venous anomaly such as azygos continuation of the inferior vena cava. An increase in the diameter of the azygos vein from prior comparable radiographs is more important than the actual measurement.

The *azygoesophageal recess* interface is a vertically oriented interface overlying the thoracic spine (Fig. 12.13). While normally straight or concave in contour, the middle third of the interface may have a slight rightward convexity at the level of the right inferior pulmonary veins. Convexity of the superior third of the interface should suggest subcarinal lymph node enlargement or a mass. Convexity of the middle third of this recess is usually a result of the confluence of right pulmonary veins or the right border of the left atrium. Left atrial dilatation will enlarge and laterally displace this interface, producing a double-density interface composed of the right lateral borders of both the right and the left atria. Convexity of the inferior third is most commonly due to a sliding hiatal hernia. Occasionally, a tortuous descending aorta or enlarged paraesophageal lymph nodes can cause this recess to be convex to the right in its lower third. When air is present in the distal portion of the esophagus and the azygoesophageal recess interfaces with the right lateral wall of the esophagus, a line (the right inferior esophagopleural stripe) rather than an edge is seen.

The *paraspinal interface* is a straight, vertical interface extending the length of the right hemithorax and represents contact of the right lung with a small amount of tissue lateral to the thoracic spine. It is inconsistently visualized on the right side. A focal convexity of this interface suggests spinal or paraspinal disease.

The right heart projects just to the right of the lateral margin of the thoracic spine on a normal PA radiograph (Fig. 12.11). This portion of the heart is the lateral margin of the right atrium, which creates a smooth convex interface with the medial segment of the middle lobe. Individuals with pectus excavatum have leftward cardiac displacement and may not demonstrate this interface. In patients with right atrial dilatation, this interface may extend well into the right lung.

The right lateral border of the inferior vena cava may be seen at the level of the right hemidiaphragm as a concave lateral interface. The inferior vena caval interface is best visualized on

lateral radiographs (Fig. 12.11). This interface may be absent in patients with azygos continuation of the inferior vena cava.

In the uppermost portion of the left mediastinum, one or more interfaces may be recognized cephalad to the aortic arch. The interface most often visualized is the subclavian artery (Fig. 12.14). It is unusual for the LUL to interface with the left lateral wall of the trachea to form the left paratracheal stripe because the subclavian artery and adjacent fat usually intervene.

The transverse portion of the aortic arch ("aortic knob") creates a small convex indentation on the left lung in normal individuals (Fig. 12.14). As the aorta elongates and dilates with age, this interface projects more laterally, and lung may be seen to encircle a greater circumference of the knob.

In approximately 5% of individuals, the left superior intercostal vein may be seen on frontal radiographs as a rounded or triangular opacity that focally indents the lung immediately superolateral to the aortic arch. This density, termed the "aortic nipple" (Fig 12.15), represents the superior intercostal vein as it arches anteriorly from its paraspinal position around the aortic arch to drain into the posterior aspect of the left innominate vein. This structure, which normally measures <5 mm, may enlarge with elevation of right atrial pressure or with congenital or acquired obstruction of venous return to the right heart.

Immediately inferior to the aortic arch, the LUL contacts the mediastinum to produce the *aortopulmonary window* interface (Fig. 12.14). This interface is usually straight or concave toward the lung; the latter appearance is seen with a tortuous aorta, emphysema, or congenital absence of the left pericardium. A convex lateral interface should suggest mass or lymph node enlargement in the aortopulmonary window.

Immediately inferior to the aortopulmonary window is the left lateral border of the main pulmonary artery (Fig. 12.14). The interface of this structure may be convex, straight, or concave toward the lung. Enlargement of the main pulmonary artery is seen as an idiopathic condition in young women, as a result of poststenotic dilatation in valvular pulmonic stenosis,

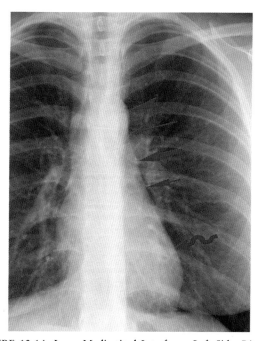

FIGURE 12.14. Lung–Mediastinal Interfaces, Left Side. PA chest radiograph shows the normal contours along the left mediastinum (from superior to inferior): aortic knob (*arrowhead*), aortopulmonary window (*skinny arrow*), main pulmonary artery (*fat arrow*), left atrial appendage (*small arrow*), and left ventricle (*squiggly arrow*).

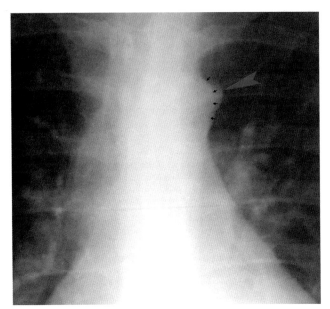

FIGURE 12.15. Aortic Nipple. The contour of the "aortic nipple" is formed by the left superior intercostal vein (*arrowhead*). The small black arrows denote the contour of the aortic knob.

or in conditions where there is increased flow or pressure in the pulmonary arterial system, such as left-to-right intracardiac shunts.

The preaortic recess interface is seen in a small percentage of normal individuals as a reflection of the LLL with the esophagus anterior to the descending aorta, extending vertically from the undersurface of the aortic knob a variable distance toward the diaphragm. It is usually etched in black (negative Mach effect).

The left paraspinal interface represents the reflection of the left lung off the paraspinal soft tissues, which largely consist of fat but also contain the sympathetic chain, proximal intercostal vessels, intercostal lymph nodes, and hemiazygos and accessory hemiazygos veins. The left paraspinal interface, which is etched in white (positive Mach effect), is seen in a majority of individuals, in contrast to the right paraspinal interface. Neurogenic tumors, hematoma, paraspinal abscess, lipomatosis, and medial pleural effusion can cause lateral displacement of this interface.

The left atrial appendage forms a concave interface immediately below the main pulmonary artery (Fig. 12.14). Straight ening or convexity of this interface used to be seen commonly in rheumatic mitral valve disease but may be seen in patients with left atrial enlargement of any cause.

The left ventricle comprises most of the left heart border. A gentle convex margin with the lingula is normal (Fig. 12.14). Abnormalities of the left ventricular contour will be discussed in detail in the section on cardiovascular disease.

Fat adjacent to the cardiac apex may create a focal bulge in the left cardiac contour that obscures the heart border at the left cardiophrenic angle. This epipericardial fat pad is usually unilateral or more prominent on the left and is most often seen in obese patients and those on corticosteroids. A typical appearance on the lateral radiograph is usually diagnostic; CT is helpful in equivocal cases.

The Lungs (Fig. 12.14). The opacity of the lungs as visualized radiographically is attributable solely to the presence of the pulmonary vasculature and enveloping interstitial structures. The arteries are solid cylinders branching along the airways. Both gradually diminish in caliber as they divide.

Bronchi smaller than subsegmental are not visible radiographically. The pulmonary veins can often be traced horizontally to the left atrium, whereas the arteries can be followed to their hilar origin, which lies more cephalad than the left atrium. The effects of gravity explain the predominance of vasculature in an upright patient as well as the isodistribution of vessels in the supine patient. The normal dark gray opacity of the upper lungs increases inferiorly in women as a result of summation of overlying breast tissue or in men with prominent pectoralis muscles. The opacity of the lung may be increased by processes that render the interstitium or airspaces opaque or decreased by any process associated with diminished blood flow to the lung or destruction of parenchymal structures.

Diaphragm. The diaphragm is the major inspiratory muscle comprising muscular origins along the costal margins and insertions into the membranous dome. The right hemidiaphragm overlies the liver, and the left hemidiaphragm overlies the stomach and spleen. On frontal radiographs exposed in deep inspiration, the apex of the right hemidiaphragm typically lies at the level of the sixth anterior rib, approximately one-half interspace above the apex of the left hemidiaphragm (Fig. 12.14). A scalloped appearance to the hemidiaphragm is not uncommon. Focal bulges in the diaphragmatic contour are usually a result of acquired diaphragmatic eventration (thinning).

Upper Abdomen. Portions of the liver, spleen, and gastric fundus are routinely visualized on most frontal chest radiographs. Abnormalities of abdominal situs may be identified by noting the location and appearance of the liver, stomach, and spleen. Enlargement of the liver may cause right diaphragmatic elevation and right lateral compression of the stomach. Intrahepatic air may be seen within the biliary tree, portal vein, or a hepatic abscess. Calcified hepatic lesions or calcified gallstones overlying the lower portion of the liver may be visible. A mass arising within the gastric fundus can occasionally be seen as a soft tissue opacity protruding into a gas-filled gastric lumen. Splenomegaly may be identified by noting a soft tissue mass in the left upper quadrant that displaces the stomach bubble anteromedially and the splenic flexure of the colon inferiorly.

Lateral Chest Radiograph

The normal lateral chest film is a challenge because of summation of the right hemithorax over the left (Fig 12.1B). However, knowledge of normal lateral radiographic anatomy can greatly aid in detection and localization of parenchymal and cardiomediastinal processes (12, 13).

Soft Tissues. Air outlining the anterior axillary folds may render the anterior edges of these skin folds visible overlying the superior aspect of the thorax. The edges are seen as bilateral opacities that are concave anteriorly and can be followed through the level of the thoracic inlet to merge with the soft tissues of the arms.

Bones. The anterior margins of the scapulae project as oblique straight edges overlying the superior and posterior aspects of the thorax, often over the retrotracheal triangle. The anterior and posterior cortical margins of the thoracic vertebral bodies should be aligned, forming a gradual kyphosis.

Lung Interfaces. The retrotracheal (or Raider) triangle is bordered by the posterior border of the trachea/esophagus, the anterior border of the spine, and the top of the aortic arch (Fig. 12.11). Masses and air-space disease near the apices, retrotracheal masses (e.g., aberrant subclavian artery or posterior thyroid goiter), or esophageal masses may produce an abnormal opacity in this region.

If the descending aorta is tortuous, its posterior margin and occasionally its anterior margin may be followed for varying distances, depending upon where the aorta returns to a prespinal position to traverse the aortic hiatus and enter the abdomen. Rarely, the superior margin of the arch of the azygos vein is visible projecting over the lower aspect of the aortic arch. In certain individuals, the posterior edges of the innominate or left subclavian arteries may be visible in relation to the tracheal air column.

The appearance of the retrosternal space depends upon the shape of the sternum and the amount of anterior mediastinal fat. On well-penetrated lateral radiographs, the body of the sternum is readily visible (Fig. 12.11). A thin retrosternal stripe from a small amount of fat immediately behind the body of the sternum is usually seen. Sternal fracture, infection, tumor, or prior sternotomy can distort or thicken this stripe. Enlargement of internal mammary arteries (e.g., coarctation of the aorta) or lymph nodes (typically with lymphoma or metastatic breast carcinoma) produces masses seen projecting through the concavities between the costal cartilages. Inferiorly, the left lung may be excluded from contacting the anteromedial chest wall by a round or triangular opacity, which represents the cardiac apex and adjacent extrapleural fat. This impression on the anterior surface of the lingula has been termed the *cardiac incisura* and should not be mistaken for a mass. CT will prove helpful in equivocal cases. A mass arising within the anterior mediastinum may not be visible on a PA view but will usually encroach on this retrosternal clear space.

The anterior pericardium can be identified separately from the myocardium in 20% of subjects. This thin line represents the pericardial layers between the epicardial and pericardial fat. Nodularity or thickness >2.0 mm suggests disease or effusion.

The posterior aspect of the inferior vena cava is visible in a majority of individuals as a concave posterior or straight edge that is visible at the posteroinferior cardiac margin, just above the diaphragm (Fig. 12.11). In the pediatric population, its absence often concurs with cardiac abnormalities.

The hemidiaphragms appear as parallel domed structures on lateral radiographs (Fig. 12.1). The posterior portion lies at a more inferior level than the anterior portion, creating a deep posterior costophrenic sulcus and a shallow anterior sulcus. There are several methods of distinguishing the right from the left hemidiaphragm on the lateral view. The anterior left hemidiaphragm is obliterated (silhouetted) by the cardiac contact, whereas the right hemidiaphragm is seen in its entire anteroposterior course. On a well-positioned left lateral chest radiograph, with the right side of the thorax farther from the x-ray cassette than the left, the right anterior and posterior costophrenic sulci should project beyond the corresponding left-sided sulci as a result of x-ray beam divergence. Identification of the right and left costophrenic sulci allows identification of the corresponding hemidiaphragms. The presence of air in the stomach or splenic flexure projecting above one hemidiaphragm and below another identifies the more cephalad structure as the left hemidiaphragm. Occasionally, when the right and left major fissures are distinguishable (the left is more vertically oriented than the right), following a major fissure to its point of contact with the diaphragm will allow identification of that hemidiaphragm.

Anatomy of the Normal Mediastinum and Thoracic Inlet

The mediastinum is a narrow, vertically oriented structure that resides between the medial parietal pleural layers of the lungs. It contains central cardiovascular, tracheobronchial structures and the esophagus enveloped in fat with intermixed lymph nodes (Fig. 12.16) (Table 12.6) (14). The thoracic inlet structures are best depicted by CT and MR (Fig 12.17A). Several

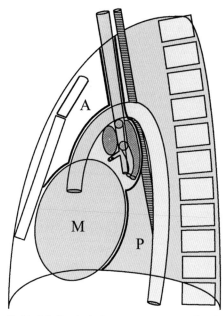

FIGURE 12.16. Mediastinal Compartments as Defined on Lateral View. *A*, Anterior mediastinum; *M*, middle mediastinum; *P*, posterior mediastinum.

TABLE 12.6

CONTENTS OF THE THORACIC INLET AND MEDIASTINUM

■ COMPARTMENT	■ CONTENTS
Thoracic inlet	Thymus Confluence of right and left internal jugular and subclavian veins Right and left carotid arteries Right and left subclavian arteries Trachea Esophagus Prevertebral fascia Phrenic, vagus, recurrent laryngeal nerves Muscles
Anterior mediastinum	Internal mammary vessels Internal mammary and prevascular lymph nodes Thymus
Middle mediastinum	Heart and pericardium Ascending and transverse aorta Main and proximal right and left pulmonary arteries Confluence of pulmonary veins Superior and inferior vena cava Trachea and main bronchi Lymph nodes and fat within mediastinal spaces
Posterior mediastinum	Descending aorta Esophagus Azygos and hemiazygos veins Thoracic duct Sympathetic ganglia and intercostal nerves Lymph nodes

schemes have been described to divide the mediastinum into separate compartments. We will use an anatomic method, in which a line drawn through the sternal angle anteriorly and fourth thoracic intervertebral space posteriorly divides the mediastinum into superior and inferior compartments. The inferior mediastinum is further subdivided into anterior, middle, and posterior compartments. This division of the mediastinum is purely arbitrary, as there are no true anatomic boundaries between the three compartments. However, by using the most easily recognizable mediastinal structure—the heart—as the focal point, the relationship of mediastinal masses to the heart allows for simple and consistent compartmentalization. Furthermore, this division of the mediastinum corresponds to easily recognizable regions seen on the lateral chest radiograph. A minor variation of the anatomic method, in which there is no superior and inferior division and the anterior, middle, and posterior compartments extend vertically from the thoracic inlet superiorly to the diaphragm inferiorly, is most practical to radiologists and is used here (Fig. 12.16). Within each compartment are readily identifiable structures and a number of spaces, in free communication with one another, which contain fat and lymph nodes. The structures and spaces native to each compartment and their normal appearance are reviewed here.

Anterior Mediastinum. The anterior (prevascular) mediastinal compartment includes all structures behind the sternum and anterior to the heart and great vessels as well as the internal mammary vessels and lymph nodes, thymus, and the brachiocephalic veins (Table 12.6). The internal mammary vessels reside within the parasternal fat and lie on either side of the sternum. Normal lymph nodes accompany the vessels but are not routinely visualized on CT. The interface of the retrosternal space with the anterior portion of the right and left lungs may be visualized on lateral chest radiographs (see the section "Lateral Chest Radiograph"). The thymus is a triangular or bilobed structure that is maximal in size at puberty and then undergoes gradual fatty involution. In most individuals older than 35 years, the thymus is predominantly fatty, with little or no intermixed glandular (soft tissue) component (Fig. 12.17A). The margins of the gland in an adult should be flat or concave toward the lung. The left lobe is commonly larger than the right. Anatomically, the thymus lies in the prevascular space, which is continuous with the retrosternal space anteriorly. It lies immediately anterior to the superior vena cava, aortic arch and great vessels, the main pulmonary artery, and, more inferiorly, the heart. The prevascular space generally retains the triangular configuration of the involuted thymus. Normal lymph nodes may be visible on CT within the fat of the prevascular space. Beginning at the level of the aortic arch in most individuals, the anterior portion of the prevascular space tapers to form a thin, vertically oriented linear density that represents the anterior junction line. The right and left brachiocephalic veins occupy the posterior aspect of the prevascular space at the level of the root of the great vessels. The right brachiocephalic vein is seen on CT as a round density owing to its vertical orientation, while the crossing left brachiocephalic vein appears oval or tubular in configuration.

Middle Mediastinum. The middle (vascular) mediastinal compartment comprises the pericardium and its contents, the aortic arch and proximal great arteries, the central pulmonary arteries and veins, the trachea and main bronchi, and lymph nodes (Table 12.6). The hila may be considered as extensions of the middle mediastinal compartment. The phrenic and vagus nerves are not visible on CT scans, but run together in the space between the subclavian arteries and brachiocephalic veins. The recurrent laryngeal nerves lie on each side within the tracheoesophageal groove. Four middle mediastinal spaces surrounding the trachea and carina can be distinguished (Fig. 12.17C). The

right paratracheal space, containing lymph nodes and a small amount of fat, appears as the right paratracheal stripe on PA views. This space extends from the thoracic inlet superiorly to the azygos vein inferiorly. The *pretracheal space* is seen between the trachea posteriorly and the posterior margin of the ascending aorta anteriorly and is contiguous with the precarinal space inferiorly. It contains fat, lymph nodes, and the retroaortic portion of the superior pericardial recess and is the anatomic route used during routine transcervical mediastinoscopy. The *retrotracheal space* varies in AP dimension, depending upon the degree of invagination of the RUL behind the upper trachea. To the left of the trachea lies the *aortopulmonary window*. The borders of the aortopulmonary window are the aortic arch superiorly; the left pulmonary artery inferiorly; the distal trachea, left main bronchus, and esophagus medially; the mediastinal pleural surface of the LUL laterally; the posterior surface of the ascending aorta anteriorly; and the anterior surface of the proximal descending aorta posteriorly. This space contains fat, lymph nodes, the ligamentum arteriosum, and the left recurrent laryngeal nerve.

Continuing inferiorly, the main and left pulmonary arteries occupy the left anterolateral portion of the middle mediastinum (Fig. 12.17D). The tracheal carina forms the posterior margin of the middle mediastinum. The RUL bronchus is seen just below the tracheal carina. More inferiorly, the right pulmonary artery is seen coursing toward the right and slightly posteriorly, just behind the ascending aorta and anterior to the bronchus intermedius (Fig. 12.17E). The subcarinal space is outlined posteriorly by air in the azygoesophageal recess and anteriorly by the posterior aspect of the transverse right pulmonary artery. The left superior pulmonary vein lies immediately anterior to the left main and upper lobe bronchi.

The main pulmonary artery can be followed inferiorly to the level of the outflow tract of the right ventricle. At this level, the right and left atrial appendages and the top of the left atrium proper may be seen (Fig. 12.17F). Also at this level, the right superior pulmonary vein lies anterior to the middle lobe bronchus, which in turn lies immediately anterior to the RLL bronchus. Inferiorly, the right atrium proper, right ventricle, and left ventricle are identified (Fig. 12.17G).

ATS Nodal Stations. To provide greater uniformity in the evaluation of nodal disease and thereby help guide diagnostic nodal sampling, the American Thoracic Society (ATS) has devised a standard classification scheme for mediastinal lymph nodes (see Fig. 13.11). A simplified version of this classification to aid in accurate nodal staging of lung cancer has recently been proposed (see Fig. 15.20).

Posterior Mediastinum. The posterior (postvascular) mediastinal compartment lies behind the pericardium and includes the esophagus, the descending aorta, the azygos and hemiazygos veins, the thoracic duct, and the intercostal and autonomic nerves (Table 12.5). The esophagus lies posterior or posterolateral to the trachea, from the level of the thoracic inlet superiorly to the tracheal carina inferiorly. From the thoracic inlet to the level of the aortic arch, the RUL and LUL of the lungs meet behind the esophagus and anterior to the spine to form the narrow posterior junction line seen on CT scans through the upper thorax and appearing as a vertical line through the tracheal air column on frontal radiographs. The esophagus then maintains a constant relationship with the descending thoracic aorta, usually lying anteromedial to the aorta (Figs. 12.17 and 12.18) down to the level of the aortic hiatus, where the aorta is in a direct prevertebral position while the esophagus crosses the aorta anteriorly to exit the thorax via the esophageal hiatus. There are lymph nodes about the descending aorta that are not normally visible. The descending aorta lies anterolateral to the thoracic spine at the level of the aortopulmonary window. In young adults, the aorta maintains this position

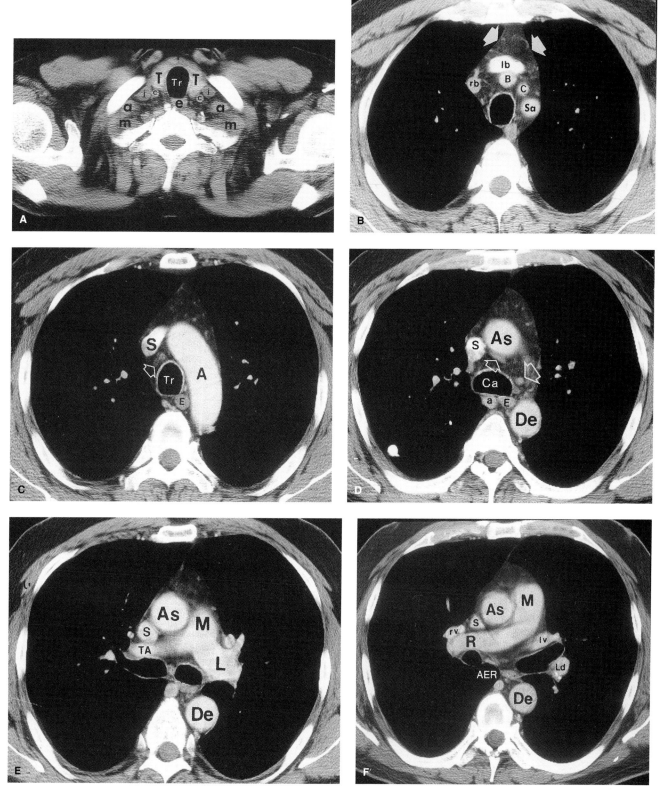

FIGURE 12.17. Normal Mediastinal Anatomy on CT. A. Thoracic inlet. Tr, trachea; t, thyroid; e, esophagus; j, internal jugular vein; c, common carotid artery; a, anterior scalene muscle; m, middle scalene muscle. **B.** Supra-aortic level. CT scan demonstrates the triangular appearance of the fatty thymus (*arrows*) occupying the anterior mediastinum. lb, left brachiocephalic vein; rb, right brachiocephalic vein; B, brachiocephalic artery; C, common carotid artery; Sa, left subclavian artery. **C.** Aortic arch level. Four main structures are identified at this level: A, aortic arch; S, superior vena cava; Tr, trachea; E, esophagus. Normal-sized lymph nodes are seen in the retrocaval, pretracheal space (*open arrow*). **D.** Aortopulmonary window level. The aortopulmonary window contains fat and small lymph nodes (*large open arrow*). The retroaortic portion of the superior pericardial recess is seen as a crescent-shaped fluid-filled structure (*small open arrow*). As, ascending aorta; De, descending aorta; S, superior vena cava; Ca, tracheal carina; a, azygos vein; E, esophagus. **E.** Main and left pulmonary artery level. As, ascending aorta; S, superior vena cava; De, descending aorta, M, main pulmonary artery; L, left pulmonary artery; TA, truncus anterior branch of right pulmonary artery. **F.** Right pulmonary artery and azygoesophageal recess level. M, main pulmonary artery; R, right pulmonary artery; As, ascending aorta; De, descending aorta; S, superior vena cava; rv, right superior pulmonary veins; lv, left superior pulmonary veins; Ld, left descending pulmonary artery; AER, azygoesophageal recess. (*continued*)

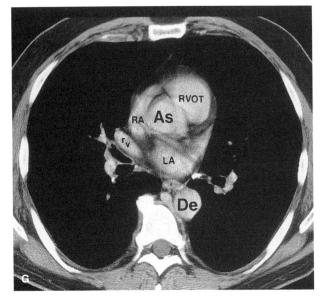
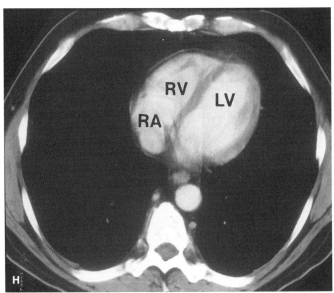

FIGURE 12.17. *(Continued)* **G.** Right ventricular outflow tract/atrial appendages. RVOT, Right ventricular outflow tract; RA, right atrium; LA, left atrium; rv, right superior pulmonary vein; As, ascending aorta; De, descending aorta. **H.** Ventricles and intraventricular septum. RA, right atrium; RV, right ventricle; LV, left ventricle.

to the level of the aortic hiatus of the diaphragm, where it lies directly in the midline. In older patients and those with a tortuous or dilated aorta, the vessel lies more laterally and protrudes into the LLL as it descends, carrying the esophagus with it before returning to a midline position at the level of the aortic hiatus. The azygos and hemiazygos veins lie on the right and left sides, respectively, posterolateral to the descending aorta within a fat-containing space that contains the thoracic duct and the sympathetic chains (normally not visible) and small lymph nodes (Fig. 12.18). Inferiorly, this space is continuous with the retrocrural space and laterally with the

paraspinal space, which contains the intercostal arteries, veins, and lymph nodes.

Normal Hilar Anatomy

Frontal View. The hilum represents the junction of the lung with the mediastinum and is composed of upper lobe pulmonary veins and branches of the pulmonary artery and corresponding bronchi (Fig. 12.19). These are all enveloped by small amounts of fat, with intermixed lymph nodes.

The shape of the right hilum on frontal radiographs has been likened to a sideways V, with the opening pointing rightward (Fig. 12.19A and B). The upper portion of the V is composed primarily of the truncus anterior and the posterior division of the right superior pulmonary vein. The right interlobar artery forms the lower half of the V, as it descends lateral to the bronchus intermedius. The right inferior pulmonary vein crosses the lower right hilar shadow but does not contribute to its opacity (Fig. 12.19A).

On CT, the upper portion of the right hilum is composed of the right superior pulmonary vein, truncus anterior division of the right pulmonary artery, and the RUL bronchus. The RUL pulmonary vein courses vertically, anterolateral to the truncus anterior (Figs. 12.5B and 12.17D–F). Here again, the epiarterial position of the bronchus can be recognized. The lower portion of the right hilum is composed of the right descending (or interlobar) pulmonary artery laterally and the bronchus intermedius and proximal RLL bronchus medially (Fig. 12.17E and F).

The upper left hilar shadow is composed centrally of the distal left main pulmonary artery and, more peripherally, of one or more branches of its LUL division and the posterior division of the left superior pulmonary vein (Fig. 12.19). The left pulmonary artery and left descending artery arch over the left mainstem bronchus and are thus named *hypoarterial*. The descending artery then forms the lower portion of the left hilar shadow as it descends behind the left heart.

On CT of the upper left hilum, the left superior pulmonary vein courses anterior to the left pulmonary artery and, more inferiorly, anterior to the LUL bronchus to empty into the

FIGURE 12.18. Posterior Mediastinal Anatomy. A CT scan shows a contrast-filled esophagus (*fat arrow*) anteromedial to the proximal descending aorta (*Ao*). Also visible within the posterior mediastinum are the azygos vein (*a*), hemiazygos vein (*skinny arrow*), and thoracic duct (*arrowhead*).

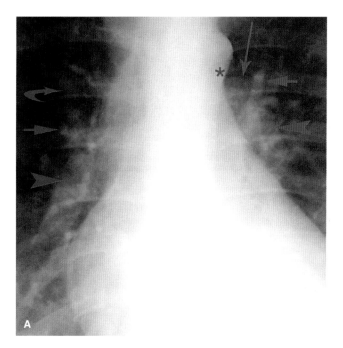

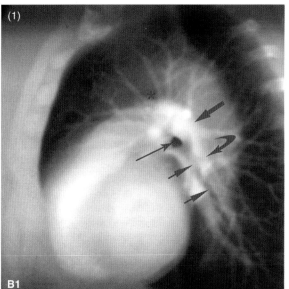

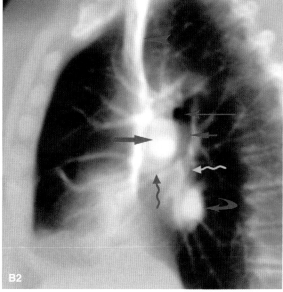

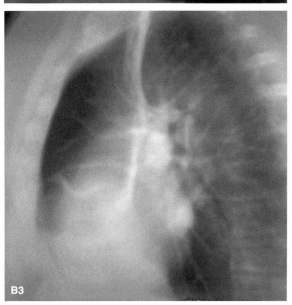

FIGURE 12.19. Normal Frontal and Lateral Hilar Anatomy. A. Cone-down frontal view. Right hilum: *red arrowhead*, right interlobar artery; *short red arrow*, right superior pulmonary vein; *curved red arrow*, truncus anterior. Left hilum: *skinny blue arrow*, left pulmonary artery; *blue arrowhead*, left descending pulmonary artery; *blue short arrow*, left superior pulmonary vein; The *blue asterisk* is in the AP window. **B.** Using two-dimensional imaging techniques, one can gain adequate insight of the complex lateral hilar anatomy. This view shows a 50-mm average sagittal projection over the hila of a contrast CT with 3-mm collimation reconstructed at 2-mm. (1) Left hilum: *Skinny blue arrow* outlines the left upper lobe bronchus; *short blue arrows* show the left lower lobe bronchus; *curved blue arrow* indicates the left descending artery; AP window (*asterisk*) lies between the inferior border of the aorta and the left pulmonary artery (*fat blue arrow*). (2) Right hilum: Note the relationship between the right upper lobe bronchus (*skinny red arrow*) and the right pulmonary artery (*fat red arrow*). *Short red arrow* indicates the posterior border of the bronchus intermedius; *squiggly red arrow* shows the middle lobe bronchus; *squiggly green arrows* indicates the right lower lobe bronchus; *curved red arrow* indicates the right lower venous return; *red arrowhead* delineates the superior vena cava. The differential density is the result of the heavier contrast layering along the posterior aspect of the vessel in a supine acquisition. (3) Two-dimensional average merge of (1) and (2). Using the data from (1) and (2), note the relationship between the different structures described above.

superolateral aspect of the left atrium (Fig. 12.17D–F). The left pulmonary artery arches posteriorly, superiorly, and to the left, over the left main and upper lobe bronchi (thus being hypoarterial), to bifurcate into upper and lower lobe arteries (Fig. 12.17D and E). The lower portion of the left hilum is composed of the left descending artery, which lies posterolateral to the LLL bronchus (Fig. 12.17E). The left inferior pulmonary vein courses horizontally at a level slightly behind that of the right inferior vein to empty into the left atrium, just medial to the left basal trunk bronchus.

As seen on frontal radiographs, the right and left pulmonary arteries comprise the predominant portion of the hilar opacity, with the superior pulmonary veins, lobar bronchi, bronchopulmonary lymph nodes, and a small amount of fat contributing little to the overall hilar density (Fig. 12.19A). In more than 90% of normal individuals, the left hilar shadow is higher than the right. This is because the left pulmonary artery, which comprises the predominant portion of the left hilar shadow, ascends over the left main and upper lobe bronchus, whereas the right pulmonary artery lies inferior to the RUL bronchus. In the remainder of individuals, the right and left hila lie at the same level; a right hilum that lies above the left suggests volume loss in the RUL or LLL.

Left Lateral View. On a true lateral radiograph, the right and left hilar shadows are not completely superimposed and comprise a combination of the right and left pulmonary arteries and the superior pulmonary veins (Fig. 12.19C and D). The anterior aspect of the hilar shadow is composed of the transverse portion of the right pulmonary artery, which produces a vertically oriented oval opacity projecting immediately anterior to the bronchus intermedius. The confluence of right superior pulmonary veins overlaps the lower portion of the right pulmonary artery and contributes to its opacity. Superiorly and posteriorly, the comma-shaped left pulmonary artery passes above and behind the round or oval lucency representing the horizontally oriented LUL bronchus summating on a portion of the left mainstem bronchus and then descends behind the LLL bronchus. The confluence of left superior pulmonary veins, which lies behind the level of the right superior pulmonary vein, creates an opacity that occupies the posteroinferior aspect of the composite hilar shadow. The avascular aspect of the composite hilar shadow, inferior to the shadow of the right pulmonary artery and veins and anterior to the descending left pulmonary artery and left superior vein, is called the *inferior hilar window.* This region is roughly triangular in shape, with its apex at the junction of the LUL and LLL bronchi and its base directed anteriorly and inferiorly. The RML and lingular veins cross the inferior hilar window, but because of their small size, they do not contribute significant opacity to this area.

The vascular structures of the composite hilar shadow are suspended around the central bronchi (Fig. 12.19). Beginning superiorly, the RUL bronchus is seen in approximately 50% of individuals as an end-on, round lucency at the upper margin of the composite hilar shadow. Recognition of this bronchus, when not visible on prior radiographs, should suggest a mass or lymph node enlargement about the bronchus. The posterior wall of the bronchus intermedius is a thin vertical line, 2 mm or thinner, extending inferiorly from the posterior aspect of the RUL bronchus. The line is seen in 95% of patients and extends inferiorly to bisect the end-on lucency of the LUL bronchus on a lateral film. This structure is rendered visible because air within the intermediate bronchus anteriorly and lung within the azygoesophageal recess posteriorly outlines its posterior wall. Thickening or nodularity of this line is seen in bronchogenic carcinoma, pulmonary edema, or enlargement of azygoesophageal recess lymph nodes. The LUL bronchus, which is seen in 75% of individuals, lies no more than 4 cm directly inferior to the RUL bronchus. This

bronchus is visualized with greater frequency than the RUL bronchus because it is outlined by the left pulmonary artery and by other mediastinal structures, while the RUL bronchus is contacted only by the right main pulmonary artery anteroinferiorly and the azygos arch superiorly. The projection of the posterior wall of the bronchus intermedius over the LUL bronchus also helps identify the LUL bronchus. Below the oval lucency of the latter, the basal trunk of the LLL bronchus can sometimes be identified, with its anterior wall visible as a white line, outlined by air in the bronchial lumen and air in the lung. The LLL bronchus is seen immediately below and continuous with the horizontal LUL bronchus.

The appearance of the hila changes with a slight degree of rotation. If on a left lateral radiograph, the patient is rotated slightly right side back and left side forward, the more posteriorly positioned left pulmonary artery will be summated on the more anterior right main pulmonary artery, and the hila are termed "closed." If on the other hand, the rotation is slightly left side back and right side forward, the left pulmonary artery is further separated from the right and the hila are termed "open." If the patient is in a true lateral position, the beam divergence will magnify the right-sided structures and simulate minimal "closing" of the hila. The relationship of the right-sided bronchus intermedius to the round hole of the end-on LUL bronchus can be helpful in evaluating differences in rotation between serial lateral views on the same patient. Analyzing this normal hilar relationship is helpful in determining the side of the posterior costophrenic sulcus if the ribs are not completely superimposed.

Pleural Anatomy

The pleura is a serosal membrane that envelops the lung and lines the costal surface, diaphragm, and mediastinum (15). It is composed of two layers, the visceral and the parietal pleura, that join at the hilum. Blood supply to the parietal pleura is via the systemic circulation, while the visceral pleura is supplied by the pulmonary circulation. The parietal pleura is contiguous with the chest wall and diaphragm and therefore extends deep posteriorly into the costophrenic sulci, while the visceral pleura is adherent to the surface of the lung. The pleural space is a potential space between the two pleural layers and normally contains a small amount of fluid (<5 mL) that reduces friction during breathing.

The normal costal, diaphragmatic, and mediastinal pleura is not visible on plain radiographs or CT. On HRCT, a 1- to 2-mm stripe may be seen lining the intercostal spaces between adjacent ribs (Fig. 12.20). This "intercostal stripe" represents the combination of the two pleural layers, the endothoracic fascia, and the innermost intercostal muscle (Fig. 12.21). Internal to the ribs, the normal pleura is not seen and the inner cortex of rib appears to contact the lung. The presence of soft tissue density between the inner rib and the lung, best appreciated on HRCT studies, indicates pleural thickening. The innermost intercostal muscle is anatomically absent in the paravertebral area, and if a thin line is visible between the lung and paravertebral fat or rib, it represents a combination of the two pleural surfaces and the endothoracic fascia.

Chest Wall Anatomy

The radiographic anatomy of the soft tissues and bony structures of the chest wall have been discussed in the section on the normal frontal radiograph. CT provides detailed anatomic information about the normal chest wall and axillae. A detailed knowledge of normal cross-sectional chest wall and axillary anatomy is key to accurate localization and characterization

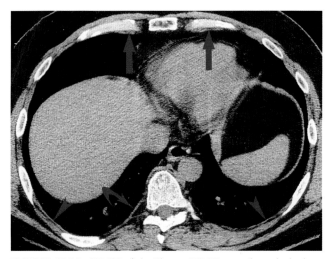

FIGURE 12.20. HRCT of the Pleura. HRCT scan through the lung bases demonstrates normal intercostal stripes (*arrowheads*) that are separated from the intercostal muscles by a layer of fat. An intercostal vein (*curved arrow*) is seen in the paravertebral region. Anteriorly, the transverse thoracic muscles (*arrows*) line the parasternal pleural surface.

of disease processes. Chest wall anatomy as seen on CT at six representative levels is shown in Fig. 12.22.

Anatomy of the Diaphragm

The diaphragm is composed of striated muscle and a large central tendon separating the thoracic and abdominal cavities. The diaphragmatic muscle arises anteriorly from the posterior aspect of the xiphoid process and anterolaterally, laterally, and posterolaterally from the sixth to the twelfth costal cartilages and ribs. The diaphragmatic crura originate from the upper lumbar vertebrae and course to the posterior aspect of the central tendon. They have no direct action on the rib cage (Fig. 12.23). The diaphragm has three normal openings and two potential gaps. The *aortic hiatus* lies in the midline, immediately behind the diaphragmatic crura and anterior to the twelfth thoracic vertebral body. The aorta, thoracic duct, and azygos and hemiazygos veins traverse this opening. The *esophageal hiatus* usually lies slightly to the left of midline, cephalad to the aortic hiatus, and transmits the esophagus and vagus nerves. The inferior vena cava pierces the central tendon of the diaphragm at the level of the eighth thoracic intervertebral disk space. The foramina of Morgagni are triangular gaps in the muscles of the anteromedial diaphragm. This cleft is normally

occupied by fat and the internal mammary vessels; it is a site of potential intrathoracic herniation of abdominal contents. The foramina of Bochdalek are defects in the closure of the posterolateral diaphragm at the junction of the pleuroperitoneal membrane with the transverse septum. Hernias through the foramina of Morgagni and Bochdalek are discussed in Chapter 19.

On CT scans, the domes of the diaphragms appear as rounded opacities on either side of the chest at the level of the base of the heart. In some patients scanned on deep inspiration, the diaphragm has an undulating or nodular appearance from contraction of slips of diaphragmatic muscle. This appearance is seen with increasing frequency in older patients, and is more common on the left than the right. Posteriorly, the superior aspects of the diaphragmatic crura are seen. The crura are curvilinear opacities that arise from the upper two to three lumbar vertebrae. Their associated esophageal and aortic openings within the bundles of the crura are well visualized on CT (Fig. 12.23). Continuing inferiorly into the upper abdomen, the inferior aspects of the diaphragmatic crura may have a rounded appearance in cross section and should not be mistaken for enlarged retrocrural lymph nodes. Review of contiguous CT images will allow for proper identification of these structures.

RADIOGRAPHIC FINDINGS IN CHEST DISEASE

Parenchymal lung disease can be divided into those processes that produce an abnormal increase in the density of all or a portion of the lung on chest radiographs (pulmonary opacity) and those that produce an abnormal decrease in lung density (pulmonary lucency). The normal density of the lungs is a result of the relative proportion of air to soft tissue (blood or parenchyma) in a ratio of 11:1. Therefore, it stands to reason that processes that increase the relative amount of soft tissue will create a significant decrease in this ratio and be more easily discernible than diffuse processes, which destroy blood vessels and parenchyma and cause little change in this ratio, thereby producing only small decreases in overall lung density. CT, by virtue of its superior contrast resolution, is more sensitive than plain radiography to subtle decreases in overall radiographic density.

Abnormal pulmonary opacities may be classified into airspace-filling opacities, opacity resulting from atelectasis, interstitial opacities, nodular or masslike opacities, and branching opacities (Table 12.7). These patterns have been shown to accurately represent pulmonary pathologic processes in correlative radiographic–pathologic studies and are a practical means of generating a differential diagnosis based on the known patterns of parenchymal involvement in a wide variety of pulmonary diseases.

FIGURE 12.21. Normal Pleural and Chest Wall Anatomy. The visceral pleura is 0.1 to 0.2 mm thick and is composed of a single layer of mesothelial cells and its associated fibroelastic fascia, called the subpleural interstitium, that is part of the peripheral interstitial network. The parietal pleura is 0.1 mm thick and is composed of a single layer of mesothelial cells lining a loose connective tissue layer containing systemic capillaries, lymphatic vessels, and sensory nerves. Outside the parietal pleura is the fibroelastic endothoracic fascia, which is separated from the pleura by a thin layer of extrapleural fat. The endothoracic fascia lines the ribs and intercostal muscles.

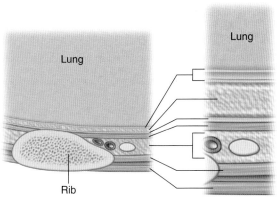

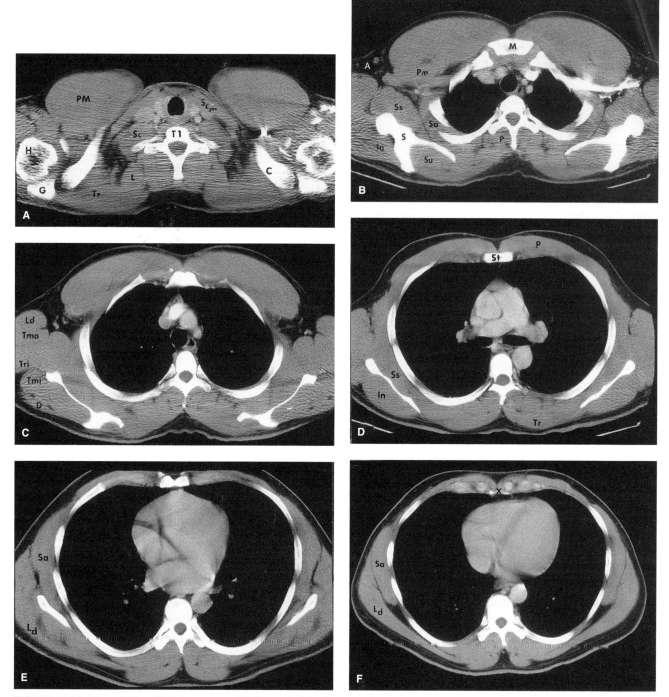

FIGURE 12.22. Normal Chest Wall Anatomy on CT. A. Level of the thoracic inlet. PM, pectoralis major muscle; Tr, trapezius muscle; L, levator scapulae muscle; Sc, scalene muscle; Scm, sternocleidomastoid muscle; H, humeral head; G, glenoid; C, distal clavicle; T1, first thoracic vertebral body. **B.** Level of the axillary vessels. Pm, pectoralis minor muscle; Sa, serratus anterior muscle; Su, supraspinatus muscle; In, infraspinatus muscle; Ss, subscapularis muscle; P, paraspinal muscles; M, manubrium of the sternum; S, body of the scapula; A, axilla with normal lymph nodes. **C.** Level of the sternomanubrial joint. Ld, latissimus dorsi muscle; Tma, teres major muscle; Tri, long head of the triceps muscle; Tmi, teres minor muscle; D, deltoid muscle. **D.** Level of the body of the sternum. P, pectoralis muscles; Ss, subscapularis muscle; In, intraspinatus muscle; Tr, trapezius muscle; St, body of the sternum. **E.** Level of tip of scapula. Ld, Latissimus dorsi muscle; Sa, serratus anterior muscle. **F.** Level of the xiphoid process. Ld, latissimus dorsi muscle; Sa, serratus anterior muscle; X, xiphoid process of the sternum.

Pulmonary Opacity

Airspace Disease. Radiographic findings of airspace disease are listed in Table 12.8. Airspace patterns of opacity develop when the air normally present within the terminal airspaces of the lung is replaced by material of soft tissue density, such as blood, transudate, exudate, or neoplastic cells. A segmental distribution of disease may be seen in a process such as pneumococcal pneumonia, which begins in the terminal airspaces and spreads from involved to uninvolved airspaces

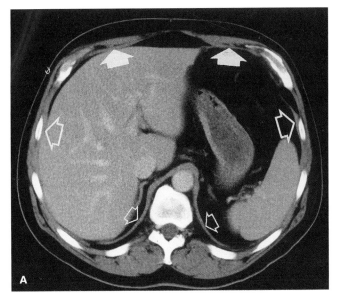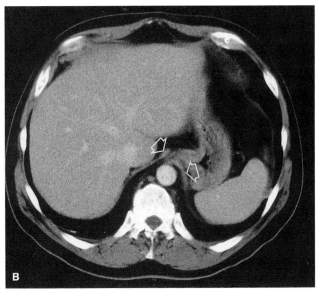

FIGURE 12.23. Normal Anatomy of the Diaphragm on CT. A. A scan through the upper abdomen demonstrates the crura of the diaphragm posteriorly (*small open arrows*), the costal origins of the diaphragm laterally (*large open arrows*), and the costal cartilaginous origins anterolaterally (*solid arrows*). **B.** More inferiorly, the esophageal hiatus is seen between the crura (*open arrows*).

via interalveolar channels (pores of Kohn) and channels bridging preterminal bronchioles with alveoli (canals of Lambert). Initially, the opacity is poorly margined because the airspace-filling process extends in an irregular fashion to involve adjacent airspaces, creating an irregular interface with the x-ray beam. Not uncommonly, airspace nodules, which are poorly margined, rounded opacities 6 to 8 mm in diameter, may be seen at the leading edge of an airspace-filling process. These nodules represent filling of acini or other sublobular structures and are most often seen in diffuse alveolar pulmonary edema and transbronchial spread of cavitary tuberculosis.

A characteristic of airspace-filling processes is the tendency of airspace shadows to coalesce as they extend through the lung (16). When the airspaces are rendered opaque by the presence of intra-alveolar cellular material and fluid, the normally aerated bronchi become visible as tubular lucencies called *air bronchograms* (Fig. 12.24). Occasionally, small intra-acinous bronchi or groups of uninvolved alveoli may be visible within an airspace nodule as air bronchiolograms or air alveologram, respectively. Rarely, severe interstitial disease encroaching upon the airspaces may produce an air bronchogram; this is most typically seen in "alveolar" sarcoid. When the airspace-filling process extends to the interlobar fissure, it is seen as a sharply marginated lobar opacity.

A pattern of parenchymal opacity that reliably represents an airspace-filling process is the "bat's wing" or "butterfly" pattern of disease. In this pattern, dense opacities occupy the central regions of lung and extend laterally to abruptly marginate before reaching the peripheral portions of the lung; hence the term "bat's wing" (see Fig. 14.2). To date, there is no explanation for this distribution of disease, which appears almost exclusively in patients with pulmonary edema or hemorrhage. Another feature of airspace-filling processes is the tendency to rapidly change in appearance over short intervals of time. The development or resolution of parenchymal opacities within hours usually indicates an airspace-filling process; prominent exceptions include atelectasis and interstitial pulmonary edema. The differential diagnosis of diffuse confluent airspace opacities is reviewed in Table 12.9.

The CT and HRCT findings of airspace disease are similar to those described on plain chest radiographs. These are (1) lobar, segmental, and/or lobular distribution of disease; (2) poorly marginated opacities that tend to coalesce; (3) airspace nodules; and (4) air bronchograms. A lobar or segmental

TABLE 12.7

PATTERNS OF PARENCHYMAL OPACITY

■ TYPE	■ EXAMPLE
Airspace (alveolar) filling	Pneumococcal pneumonia
Interstitial opacities	
Reticular/linear	Idiopathic pulmonary fibrosis
Reticulonodular	Sarcoidosis
Branching	Allergic bronchopulmonary aspergillosis
Nodular	
Miliary (<2 mm)	Miliary tuberculosis
Micronodule (2–7 mm)	Acute hypersensitivity pneumonitis
Nodule (7–30 mm)	Metastatic disease, granuloma
Mass (>30 mm)	Bronchogenic carcinoma
Atelectasis	Endobronchial neoplasm

TABLE 12.8

RADIOGRAPHIC CHARACTERISTICS OF AIRSPACE DISEASE

Lobar or segmental distribution
Poorly marginated
Airspace nodules
Tendency to coalesce
Air bronchograms
Bat's wing (butterfly) distribution
Rapidly changing over time

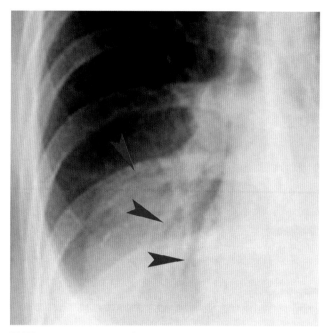

FIGURE 12.24. Air Bronchograms in Airspace Disease. Cone-down view of the right lower lobe in a patient with pneumococcal pneumonia shows homogeneous lobar airspace disease with air bronchograms (*arrows*) within the opacified lobe.

distribution of disease is easily appreciated on cross-sectional imaging. CT and HRCT are further capable of showing individually opacified lobules, termed a "patchwork quilt" appearance, which is seen in many airspace processes, most classically bronchopneumonia (see Fig. 17.3). Coalescence of opacities, commonly seen in pulmonary edema and pneumonia, is best assessed on serial CT studies. With isolated airspace disease, the interlobular septa are normal or obscured. As with plain films, the presence of airspace nodules provides

TABLE 12.9

DIFFUSE CONFLUENT AIRSPACE OPACITIES: DIFFERENTIAL DIAGNOSIS

■ TYPE	■ EXAMPLE
Pulmonary edema	Cardiogenic Fluid overload/renal failure Noncardiogenic (ARDS) (see Table 14.2)

Pneumonia	*Pneumocystis carinii*
	Gram-negative bacteria
	Influenza
	Fungi
	   Histoplasmosis
	   Aspergillosis

Hemorrhage	See Table 14.3
Neoplasm	Bronchoalveolar cell carcinoma Lymphoma
Alveolar proteinosis	Acute silica inhalation Lymphoma Leukemia AIDS

TABLE 12.10

TYPES OF PULMONARY ATELECTASIS

■ TYPE	■ EXAMPLE
Obstructive (resorptive)	Bronchogenic carcinoma (endo- bronchial)
Passive (relaxation)	Pleural effusion Pneumothorax
Compressive	Bulla
Cicatricial	Post-primary tuberculosis Radiation fibrosis
Adhesive	Respiratory distress syndrome of the newborn

further evidence of an airspace process. On HRCT studies, these nodules are usually seen within the peribronchiolar (centrilobular) region of the pulmonary lobule. Air bronchograms or bronchiolograms are usually better appreciated on CT and HRCT than on plain radiographs owing to superior contrast resolution and the cross-sectional nature of CT. This is particularly true in those regions of the lung where bronchi course in the transverse plane (anterior segments of upper lobes, middle lobe and lingula, and superior segments of the lower lobes).

Atelectasis literally means "incomplete expansion." It is used to describe any condition in which there is loss of lung volume, and it is usually but not invariably associated with an increase in radiographic density. There are four basic mechanisms of atelectasis: resorptive, relaxation, cicatricial, and adhesive (Table 12.10) (17).

The most common form of atelectasis is *obstructive* or *resorptive atelectasis* and is secondary to complete endobronchial obstruction of a lobar bronchus with resorption of gas distally. Incomplete bronchial obstruction more often produces air trapping from a check-valve effect rather than atelectasis, because air enters but cannot exit the lung. Complete obstruction of a central bronchus may not produce atelectasis if collateral airflow to the obstructed lung (via pores of Kohn, canals of Lambert, or incomplete interlobar fissures) allows the lung to remain inflated. An obstructed lobe or lung containing 100% oxygen, as may be seen in some mechanically ventilated patients, will collapse more rapidly (sometimes within minutes) than lung containing ambient air. This is the result of the rapid absorption of oxygen from the alveolar spaces into the alveolar capillaries. Bronchogenic carcinoma, foreign bodies, mucous plugs, and malpositioned endotracheal tubes are the most common causes of endobronchial obstruction and secondary resorptive atelectasis.

Passive or *relaxation atelectasis* results from the mass effect of an air or fluid collection within the pleural space on the subjacent lung. Since the natural tendency of the lung is to collapse when dissociated from the chest wall, pleural collections will produce atelectasis. The degree of atelectasis depends upon the size of the pleural collection and upon the compliance of the lung and visceral pleura. A large pleural or chest wall mass or an elevated diaphragm can also produce passive atelectasis. *Compressive atelectasis* is a form of passive atelectasis in which an intrapulmonary mass compresses adjacent lung parenchyma; common causes include bullae, abscesses, and tumors.

Processes resulting in parenchymal fibrosis reduce alveolar volume and produce *cicatricial atelectasis*. Localized cicatricial atelectasis is most often seen in association with chronic upper lobe fibronodular tuberculosis. The radiographic appearance is

TABLE 12.11

RADIOGRAPHIC SIGNS IN LOBAR ATELECTASIS

■ DIRECT SIGNS	■ INDIRECT SIGNS
Displacement of interlobar fissure	Increased density of atelectatic lung
	Bronchovascular crowding
	Ipsilateral diaphragm elevation
	Ipsilateral tracheal/cardiac/mediastinal shift
	Hilar elevation (upper lobe atelectasis) or depression (lower lobe atelectasis)
	Compensatory hyperinflation of other lobe(s)
	Shifting granuloma
	Ipsilateral small hemithorax
	Ipsilateral rib space narrowing

that of severe lobar volume loss with scarring, bronchiectasis, and compensatory hyperinflation of the adjacent lung. Diffuse cicatricial atelectasis is seen in interstitial fibrosis of any etiology. An overall increase in lung density, with reticular opacities and diminished lung volumes, is characteristic of this condition.

Adhesive atelectasis occurs in association with surfactant deficiency. Type 2 pneumocytes, the cells responsible for surfactant production, may be injured as a result of general anesthesia, ischemia, or radiation. Surfactant deficiency causes increased alveolar surface tension and results in diffuse alveolar collapse and volume loss. Radiographs show a diminution in lung volume, which may be associated with an increase in density.

Lobar atelectasis. The only direct radiographic finding of lobar atelectasis is the displacement of an interlobar fissure (Table 12.11) (18). There are several indirect findings of atelectasis, most of which reflect attempts to compensate for the volume loss (Fig. 12.25). Diminished aeration results in increased density

in the affected portion of lung and bronchovascular crowding. Ipsilateral shift of the trachea, heart, or mediastinum and hilar structures is a common finding in lobar atelectasis. Shift of the entire mediastinum is typical of collapse of an entire lung. Compensatory hyperinflation represents an attempt by the remaining normal lung to partially fill the space lost by the affected lung. This mechanism usually develops with chronic volume loss and is not seen in acute collapse. It is seen as increased lucency with attenuation of pulmonary vascular markings. In complete lung or upper lobe atelectasis, the contralateral upper lobe may herniate across the midline, bowing the anterior junction line toward the affected side. A characteristic but seldom seen plain radiographic finding of compensatory hyperinflation is the "shifting granuloma," in which a preexisting granuloma in an adjacent aerated lung changes position as it moves toward the collapsed lobe. In chronic atelectasis of a lung, a decrease in size of the hemithorax with approximation of the ribs may be seen. The absence of an air bronchogram helps distinguish resorptive lobar atelectasis from lobar pneumonia, particularly if the atelectatic lobe is only slightly diminished in volume. A triangular configuration with the apex at the pulmonary hilum is common to all types of lobar atelectasis. The fissure bordering the collapse typically assumes a concave configuration. Complete lobar atelectasis can easily be missed on PA and lateral radiographs but is easily appreciated on CT.

Segmental atelectasis. Atelectasis of one or several segments of a lobe is difficult to determine on plain radiographs. The appearance ranges from a thin linear opacity to a wedge-shaped opacity that does not abut an interlobar fissure. Segmental atelectasis is better appreciated on CT.

Subsegmental (platelike) atelectasis. Bandlike linear opacities representing linear atelectasis are commonly associated with hypoventilation. This is seen in patients with pleuritic chest pain, postoperative patients, or patients with massive hepatosplenomegaly or ascites. Subsegmental atelectasis tends to occur at the lung bases. The linear shadows are 2 to 10 cm in length and are typically oriented perpendicular to the costal pleura (Fig. 12.26). Pathologically, these areas of linear collapse are deep to invaginations of visceral pleura formed by incomplete fissures or scars.

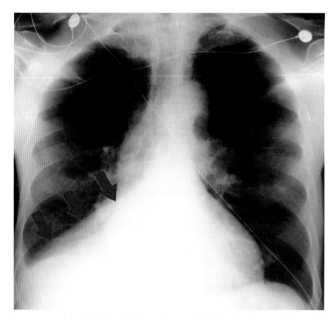

FIGURE 12.25. Lobar Atelectasis. Upright frontal chest radiograph in a postoperative patient with right lower lobe atelectasis shows a homogeneous triangular opacity in the right lower lung that partially obscures the right hemidiaphragm. The upper margin of the collapsed lobe is marginated by the inferiorly displaced major fissure (*arrows*). Bronchoscopy retrieved a mucous plug from the right lower lobe bronchus, and the lobe subsequently re-expanded.

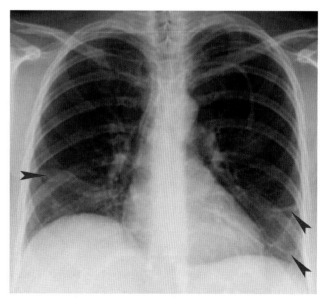

FIGURE 12.26. Subsegmental (Platelike) Atelectasis. Frontal chest radiograph in a woman with abdominal pain shows diminished lung volumes and bilateral lower zone linear opacities (*arrowheads*) coursing perpendicular to the costal pleura, representing areas of subsegmental atelectasis.

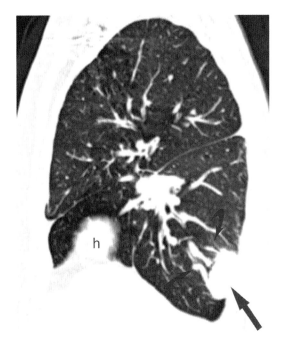

FIGURE 12.27. Round Atelectasis. CT with sagittal reformation at lung windows through the right lung in a patient with rounded atelectasis shows a pleural-based mass (*straight arrow*) in the posterior right lower lobe associated with pleural thickening. Note the vessels coursing into the mass (*curved arrows*). *h*, portion of the right atrium.

Rounded atelectasis is an uncommon form of atelectasis in which the collapsed lung forms a round mass in the lower lobe. This condition is most closely associated with asbestos-related pleural disease but may be seen in any condition associated with an exudative (proteinaceous) pleural effusion. The process develops when pleural adhesions form in the resolving phase of a pleural effusion and cause the adjacent lung to roll up into a ball as it re-expands. The round opacity is most often found along the inferior and posterior costal pleural surfaces adjacent to an area of pleural fibrosis or plaque formation. Plain radiographs reveal a well-defined, pleural-based mass between 2 and 7 cm adjacent to an area of pleural thickening in the lower lung. The identification of a curvilinear bronchovascular bundle or "comet tail" entering the anterior inferior margin of the mass, as seen on lateral radiographs or tomograms, is characteristic. The CT appearance of round atelectasis is characteristic (Fig. 12.27). The round or wedge-shaped mass forms an acute angle with the pleura and is seen adjacent to an area of pleural thickening, usually in the inferior and posterior thorax. The "comet tail" of vessels and bronchi is seen curving between the hilum and the apex of the mass. The atelectatic lung enhances following intravenous contrast administration. When the characteristic CT findings are seen in a patient with a known history of pleural disease, the appearance is diagnostic and no further evaluation is necessary. However, if any of the above criteria are not satisfied, the lesion should be biopsied to exclude malignancy.

Right upper lobe atelectasis (Fig. 12.28A) (19). In RUL atelectasis, the lung collapses superiorly and medially, with superomedial displacement of the minor fissure and anteromedial displacement of the upper half of the major fissure, producing a right upper paramediastinal density on frontal radiographs, which can obliterate the normal right paratracheal stripe and azygos vein. A central convex mass will prevent part of the usual fissure concavity. This appearance produces the S sign of Golden. The trachea is deviated toward the right,

and the right hilum and hemidiaphragm are elevated. "Tenting" or "peaking" of the diaphragm is occasionally seen and represents fat within the inferior aspect of a stretched inferior accessory fissure. Compensatory hyperinflation of the middle and lower lobes may be seen in chronic atelectasis, and the LUL may herniate across the midline anteriorly toward the right. Scarring from tuberculosis, endobronchial tumor, and mucous plugging are common causes of RUL atelectasis.

LUL/lingular atelectasis (Fig. 12.28B) has a different appearance from RUL atelectasis because of the absence of a minor fissure. The LUL collapses anteriorly, maintaining a broad area of contact with the anterior costal pleural surface. The major fissure shifts anteriorly and is seen marginating a long, narrow band of increased opacity paralleling the anterior chest wall on lateral radiographs. Diagnosis on frontal radiographs may be difficult. There is a veil of increased opacity over the left upper thorax, which can obliterate the aortic knob, AP window, and left upper cardiac margin. The apex of the left hemithorax remains lucent as a result of hyperinflation of the superior segment of the LLL. Leftward tracheal displacement, hilar and diaphragmatic elevation, and leftward bulging of the anterior junction line from an overinflated RUL are additional clues to the diagnosis. An uncommon finding on the frontal radiograph in LUL atelectasis is a crescent of air ("Luftsichel") along the left upper mediastinum, which represents a portion of the overinflated superior segment of the LLL interposed between the aortic arch medially and the collapsed upper lobe laterally (see Fig. 15.9). Postinflammatory cicatrization and endobronchial tumor are the most common causes of LUL atelectasis.

Middle lobe atelectasis (Fig. 12.28C) displaces the minor fissure inferiorly and the major fissure superiorly. Because of the minimal thickness of the collapsed middle lobe and the oblique orientation of the inferiorly displaced minor fissure, the detection of middle lobe atelectasis on frontal radiographs is difficult. The only finding on frontal radiographs may be a vague density over the right lower lung, with obscuration of the right heart margin. The lateral radiograph shows a typical triangular density, with its apex at the hilum. A lordotic frontal radiograph, which projects the minor fissure tangent to the frontal x-ray beam, will depict the atelectatic middle lobe as a triangular opacity, which is sharply marginated superiorly by the minor fissure, with its apex directed laterally. Middle lobe atelectasis is most often cicatricial and follows middle lobe infection with secondary fibrosis and bronchiectasis.

RLL Atelectasis (Fig. 12.28D). The RLL collapses toward the lower mediastinum owing to the tethering effect of the inferior pulmonary ligament. This results in inferior displacement of the upper half of the major fissure and posterior displacement of the lower half, producing a triangular opacity in the right lower paravertebral space that obscures the medial right hemidiaphragm on frontal radiographs (Fig. 12.25). The lateral margin of this triangular opacity is formed by the displaced major fissure. The right hemidiaphragm may be elevated. The right interlobar pulmonary artery is obscured within the opaque collapsed lower lobe, a finding that helps distinguish the triangular opacity of RLL atelectasis from a medial pleural effusion, which tends to displace the interlobar artery laterally rather than obscure it. On lateral radiographs, a vague triangular opacity with its apex at the hilum and its base over the posterior portion of the right hemidiaphragm and posterior costophrenic sulcus may be seen. Mucous plugs, foreign bodies, and endobronchial tumors are the most common etiologic agents.

LLL atelectasis (Fig. 12.28D) is similar in appearance to atelectasis of the RLL. A triangular opacity in the left lower paramediastinal region, with loss of the medial retrocardiac diaphragmatic outline, is seen on frontal radiographs. In addition, the left hilum is displaced inferiorly and the interlobar

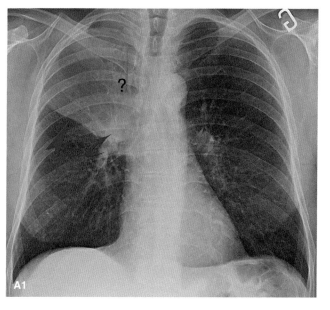

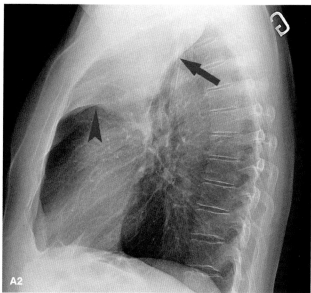

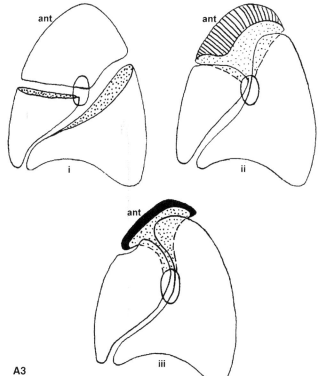

FIGURE 12.28. Lobar Atelectasis, PA, Lateral, and Schematic Representations. A. Right upper lobe. *Arrowheads* show the elevated and bowed minor fissure; *arrow* shows the right major fissure, as in diagram ii. Note the elevated right hilum, with the *curved arrow* showing the interlobar artery, and the silhouetting of the normal contours of the SVC and upper hilum (*question mark*). The significant density is caused by mucus retention within the atelectatic lobe (courtesy of Dr. Louise Samson). (*continued*)

artery is obscured. The diaphragm may be elevated and the heart shifted toward the left. Compensatory hyperinflation of the LUL may be seen. The LLL commonly is atelectatic in patients with large hearts and in postoperative patients, particularly those who have had coronary bypass surgery.

Combined middle and RLL atelectases may be seen with obstruction of the bronchus intermedius by a mucous plug or tumor. The radiographic appearance on the frontal radiograph is characteristic, with a homogeneous triangular opacity sharply marginated superiorly by the depressed minor fissure and obscuration both of the right heart border and the right hemidiaphragm. Cardiac and mediastinal shift toward the right is common.

Collapse of an entire lung is most often seen with obstructing masses in the main bronchus. The lung is opacified, with an absence of air bronchograms. The trachea and heart are shifted toward the side of collapse, with herniation of the contralateral anteromedial lung across the midline to widen the retrosternal space on lateral radiographs and bulge the anterior junction line on frontal radiographs. The chest wall may show approximation of the ribs in chronic collapse. Compensatory diaphragmatic elevation in left lung atelectasis may be recognized by noting superior displacement of the gastric air bubble or splenic flexure of the colon.

Interstitial Disease. Interstitial opacities are produced by processes that thicken the interstitial compartments of the lung. Water, blood, tumor, cells, fibrous tissue, or any combination of these may render the interstitial space visible on radiographs. Interstitial opacities are usually divided into reticular, reticulonodular, nodular, and linear patterns on plain radiographs

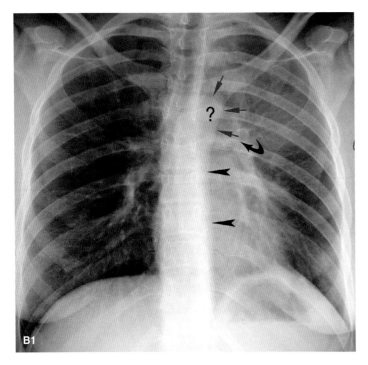

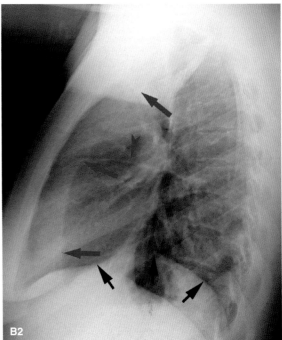

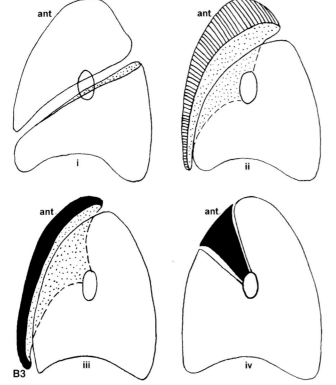

FIGURE 12.28. (*Continued*) **B.** Left upper lobe (LUL). On the lateral view *red arrows* outline the anteriorly displaced major fissure, as in diagram iii, reaching down to the slightly elevated left hemidiaphragm (*small black arrows*). The nondisplaced right minor fissure (*red arrowhead*) indicates that this is a left-sided process. On the PA view, we note the diffuse opacity of the LUL. Note that the contours of the aortic knob and AP window are silhouetted (*black question mark*). The *small red arrows* outline the manubrium, not to be mistaken for the aortic knob. The LUL bronchus is retracted superiorly (*curved black arrow*). The *black arrowheads* outline the descending aorta, which remains visible in LUL atelectasis. Narrowing of the rib cage with closer spacing of the ribs is seen on the left resulting from the volume loss in the left lung.

(Fig. 12.29) (Table 12.12) (20,21). The predominant pattern of opacity produced by an interstitial process depends upon the nature of the underlying disease and the portion of the interstitium affected.

Reticular pattern refers to a network of curvilinear opacities that usually involves the lungs diffusely. The subdivision of reticular opacities into fine, medium, and coarse opacities refers to the size of the lucent spaces created by these intersecting curvilinear opacities (Fig. 12.29). A fine reticular pattern, also known as a "ground-glass pattern," is seen in processes that thicken or line the parenchymal interstitium of

the lung to produce a fine network of lines with intervening lucent spaces on the order of 1 to 2 mm in diameter. Diseases that most commonly produce this appearance include interstitial pulmonary edema and usual interstitial pneumonitis. Medium reticulation, also termed "honeycombing," refers to reticular interstitial opacities where the intervening spaces are 3 to 10 mm in diameter. This pattern is most commonly seen in pulmonary fibrosis involving the parenchymal and peripheral interstitial spaces. Coarse reticular opacities with spaces greater than 1 cm in diameter are seen most commonly in diseases that produce cystic spaces as a result of

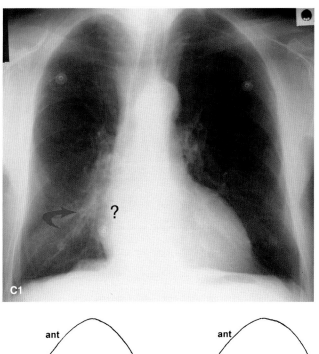

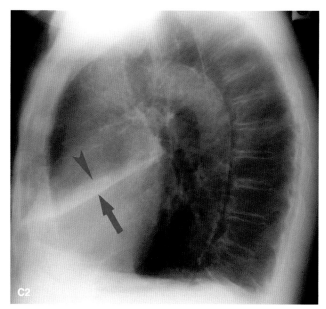

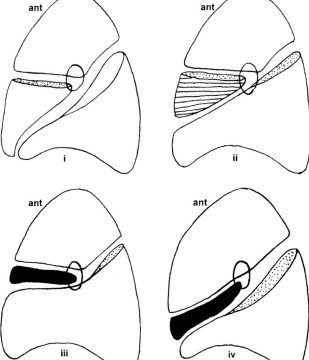

FIGURE 12.28. (*Continued*) **C. Right middle lobe.** On the lateral view, the *arrowhead* points out the downward displaced minor fissure and the *arrow* points out the minimally upward displaced major fissure, as in diagram **iv**. On the PA view, we note that the midcardiac portion of the right mediastinal contour (*curved arrow*) is silhouetted and indistinct (*question mark*). (*continued*)

parenchymal destruction. The most common interstitial diseases associated with coarse reticulation are idiopathic pulmonary fibrosis, sarcoidosis, and Langerhans cell histiocytosis of the lung.

Nodular opacities represent small rounded lesions within the pulmonary interstitium. In contrast to airspace nodules, interstitial nodules are homogeneous (they lack air bronchiolograms or air alveolograms) and well defined, as their margins are sharp and they are surrounded by normally aerated lung. In addition, unlike airspace nodules, which tend to be uniform in diameter (approximately 8 mm), these opacities can be divided into miliary opacities (<2 mm), micronodules (2 to 7 mm), nodules (7 to 30 mm), or masses (>30 mm). A micronodular or miliary pattern is seen predominantly in granulomatous pro-

cesses (e.g., miliary tuberculosis or histoplasmosis) (see Fig. 16.9), hematogenous pulmonary metastases (most commonly thyroid and renal cell carcinoma), and pneumoconioses (silicosis) (see Fig. 17.10). Nodules and masses are most often seen in metastatic disease to the lung.

Reticulonodular opacities may be produced by the overlap of numerous reticular shadows or by the presence of both nodular and reticular opacities. Although this appearance seems to be frequent on radiographs, only a few diseases actually show reticulonodular involvement on pathology specimens. Silicosis, sarcoidosis, and lymphangitic carcinomatosis are diseases that may give rise to true reticulonodular opacities.

Linear patterns of interstitial opacities are seen in processes that thicken the axial (bronchovascular) or peripheral

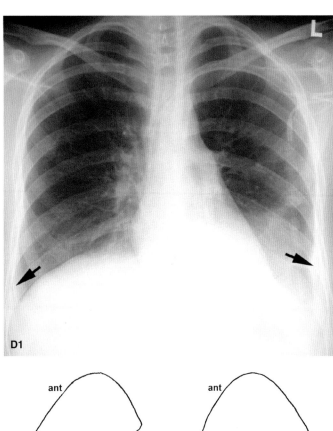

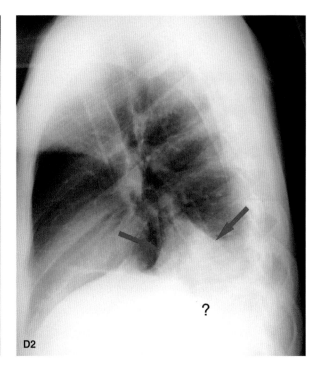

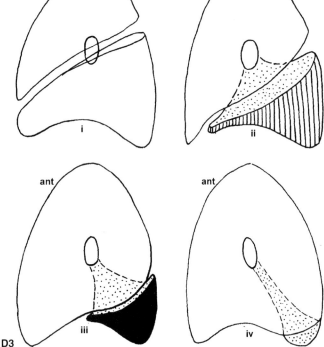

FIGURE 12.28. (*Continued*) **D.** Right and left lower lobes. Both lower lobes collapse in a similar fashion. In this example of left lower lobe atelectasis in a patient with bilateral pleural effusions (*small black arrows*), note on the lateral view how the major fissure (*large red arrows*) outlines the opacity of the atelectatic lobe, as depicted on diagram iii. The contour of the left hemidiaphragm is lost (*question mark*). On the frontal view inferior and medial displacement of the hilum (*curved red arrow*) and increase opacity behind the heart indicates volume loss. Note the vertical migration of the left mainstem bronchus, and the contour of the left descending pulmonary artery. (Diagrams from Reed (19); used with permission from RSNA.)

interstitium of the lung. Because the axial interstitium surrounds the bronchovascular structures, thickening of this compartment produces parallel linear opacities radiating from the hila when visualized in length or peribronchial "cuffs" when viewed end-on. A central distribution of linear interstitial disease is most often seen with interstitial pulmonary edema or "increased markings" emphysema. This pattern of interstitial disease may be impossible to distinguish from airways diseases, such as bronchiectasis and asthma, which primarily thicken the walls of airways. Thickening of the peripheral interstitium of the lung produces linear opacities that are either 2 to 6 cm long, <1-mm-thick lines that are obliquely oriented and course through the substance of the lung toward the hila (Kerley A lines) or shorter (1 to 2 cm) thin lines that are peripheral and course perpendicular to and contact the pleural surface (Kerley B lines). Kerley A lines correspond to thickening of connective tissue sheets within the lung, which contain lymphatic communications between the perivenous and bronchoarterial lymphatics, while Kerley B lines represent thickened peripheral subpleural interlobular septa (see Fig. 14.1) (22). A linear pattern of disease is seen in pulmonary edema, lymphangitic carcinomatosis, and acute viral or atypical bacterial pneumonia.

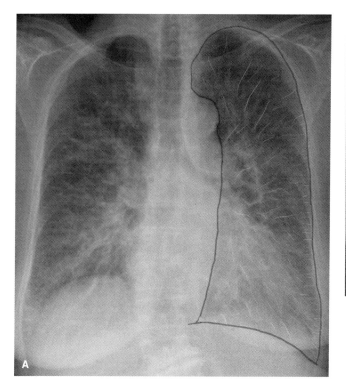

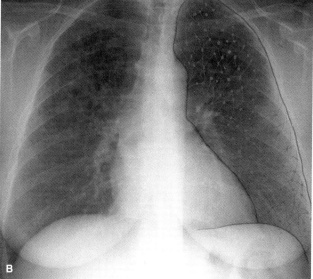

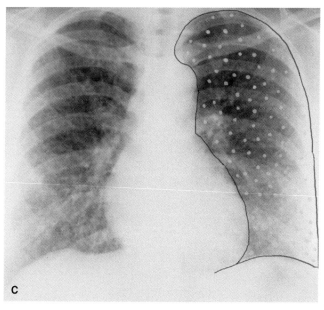

FIGURE 12.29. **Patterns of Interstitial Opacity on Chest Radiographs.** **A.** Linear interstitial disease in pulmonary edema. **B.** Reticulonodular disease of sarcoidosis. **C.** Nodular disease in military tuberculosis.

The HRCT findings of interstitial lung disease are reviewed in Chapter 17.

Pulmonary Nodule refers to a discrete rounded opacity within the lung, measuring less than 3 cm in diameter. A round opacity greater than 3 cm in diameter is termed a *pulmonary mass*. A solitary pulmonary nodule presents a common diagnostic dilemma (discussed in a subsequent section).

Mucoid Impaction. Branching tubular opacities that are distinguished from normal vascular shadows invariably represent mucus-filled, dilated bronchi and are termed *bronchoceles* or *mucoid impactions*. Their appearance has been likened to that of a gloved finger or the shape of the letters V or Y, depending upon the length of airway and number of branches involved. When in a central perihilar location, these bronchoceles are a result of nonobstructive bronchiectasis, as in cystic fibro-

sis or allergic bronchopulmonary aspergillosis, or of postobstructive bronchiectasis distal to an endobronchial tumor or a congenitally atretic bronchus. In the latter condition, a typical location—immediately distal to the expected location of the apical segmental bronchus and a hyperlucent segment or lobe distal to the bronchocele owing to collateral air drift—should suggest the diagnosis. Peripheral bronchoceles are most often seen in cystic fibrosis and posttuberculous bronchiectasis.

Pulmonary Lucency

Abnormal lucency of the lung may be localized or diffuse (Table 12.13) (21). Focal radiolucent lesions of the lung include cavities, cysts, bullae, blebs, and pneumatoceles (Fig. 12.30).

TABLE 12.12

PATTERNS OF PULMONARY INTERSTITIAL OPACITIES

Predominantly linear		
Chronic interstitial edema		
Lymphangitic carcinomatosis		
Interstitial fibrosis of any etiology		
Predominantly reticular: acute		
Edema	Heart failure	
	Fluid overload	
	Nephropathy	
Infection	Viral	
	Mycoplasma	
	Pneumocystis carinii	
	Malaria	
Drug reactions		
Predominantly reticular: chronic		
Postinfectious scarring	Tuberculosis (postprimary)	
	Histoplasmosis (chronic)	
	Coccidioidomycosis (chronic)	
	Pneumocystis carinii	
Chronic interstitial edema	Mitral valve disease	
Collagen vascular disease	Rheumatoid lung	
	Scleroderma	
	Dermatomyositis/polymyositis	
	Ankylosing spondylitis	
	Mixed connective tissue disease	
	Idiopathic pulmonary hemorrhage	
Granulomatous disease	Sarcoidosis	
	Eosinophilic granuloma	
Neoplasm	Lymphangitic carcinomatosis	
	Lymphoma and lymphocytic disorders	
	Lymphocytic interstitial pneumonitis	
Inhalational	Asbestosis	
	Silicosis and coal worker's pneumoconiosis	
	Hypersensitivity pneumonitis (chronic phase)	
	Chronic aspiration	
Drug reaction	Nitrofurantoin	
	Chemotherapeutic agents	
	Amiodarone	
	Radiation pneumonitis (chronic)	
Idiopathic	Idiopathic pulmonary fibrosis	
	Lymphangioleiomyomatosis	
	Tuberous sclerosis	
	Neurofibromatosis	
	Amyloidosis (alveolar septal form)	

Predominantly nodular		
Infection	Mycobacteria	
	Tuberculosis	
	Nontuberculous mycobacteria	
	Fungi	
	Histoplasmosis	
	Blastomycosis	
	Coccidioidomycosis	
	Cryptococcosis	
	Virus	
	Varicella (healed)	
	Bacterial	
	Septic emboli	
	Parasites	
Inhalation diseases	Inorganic (pneumoconiosis)	
	Silicosis[a] and coal worker's pneumoconiosis[a]	
	Berylliosis[a]	
	Siderosis	
	Heavy metal dust	
	Talcosis	
	Organic	
	Hypersensitivity pneumonitis	
	Toxic inhalants	
	Isocyanates	
Granulomatous disease	Sarcoidosis[a]	
	Langerhans cell histiocytosis (early)	
Vascular	Arteriovenous malformation	
	Vasculitis	
	Wegener	
	Lymphomatoid granulomatosis	
	Systemic lupus erythematosus	
Neoplasm		
Primary	Synchronous bronchogenic carcinoma	
Metastatic	Lymphoma[a]	
	Hodgkin	
	Non-Hodgkin	
	Bronchogenic carcinoma[a]	
	Thyroid carcinoma	
	Renal cell carcinoma[a]	
	Breast carcinoma[a]	
	Melanoma	
	Choriocarcinoma	
	Osteogenic carcinoma	
Idiopathic	Alveolar microlithiasis	
	Amyloidosis (nodular form)	

[a]These entities can also present as reticulonodular disease.
Adapted from Reed (21); information used with permission.

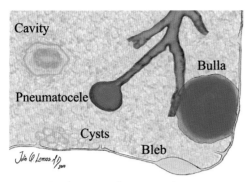

FIGURE 12.30. Focal Lucent Pulmonary Lesions.

These lesions are usually recognized by identification of the wall that marginates the lucent lesion.

Cavities form when a pulmonary mass undergoes necrosis and communicates with an airway, leading to gas within its center. The wall of a cavity is usually irregular or lobulated and, by definition, is greater than 1 mm thick. Lung abscess and necrotic neoplasm are the most common cavitary pulmonary lesions. A *bulla* is a gas collection within the pulmonary parenchyma, with >1 cm diameter and a thin wall <1 mm thick. It represents a focal area of parenchymal destruction (emphysema) and may contain fibrous strands, residual blood vessels, or alveolar septa. An *air cyst* is any well-circumscribed intrapulmonary gas collection with a smooth thin wall >1 mm thick. While some of these lesions will have a true epithelial lining (bronchogenic cyst that communicates with a bronchus), most do not and likely represent postinflammatory or posttraumatic lesions (23). A *bleb* is a collection of gas <1 cm in size within the layers of the visceral pleura. It is usually found in the apical portion of the lung. These small gas collections are not seen on plain radiographs but may be visualized on chest CT, where they are indistinguishable from paraseptal emphysema. Rupture of an apical bleb can lead to spontaneous pneumothorax. *Pneumatoceles* are thin-walled, gas-containing structures that represent distended airspaces distal to a check-valve obstruction of a bronchus or bronchiole, most commonly secondary to staphylococcal pneumonia. A *traumatic air cyst* results from pulmonary laceration following blunt trauma. These lesions generally resolve within 4 to 6 months. *Bronchiectatic cysts* are usually multiple, rounded, thin-walled lucencies found in clusters in the lower lobes, and represent saccular dilatations of airways in varicose or cystic bronchiectasis.

Unilateral pulmonary hyperlucency must be distinguished from differences in lung density resulting from technical factors or overlying soft tissue abnormalities. Grid cutoff from a combination of lateral and near or far focus-grid decentering may lead to a graduated increase in density across the width of the chest film, simulating unilateral hyperlucency. Rotation of the patient will produce an increase in density over the lung rotated away from the film cassette. Congenital absence of the pectoralis muscle (Poland syndrome) or mastectomy can produce apparent hyperlucency.

True unilateral hyperlucent lung is a result of decreased blood flow to the lung. Diminished blood flow may result from a primary vascular abnormality, shunting of blood away from a lung that traps air, or a combination of the two. Hypoplasia of the right or left pulmonary artery produces a lung that is hyperlucent and diminished in size. A similar appearance may be produced by lobar resection or atelectasis, where the remaining lobe or lung hyperinflates to accommodate the hemithorax, thereby attenuating pulmonary vessels and producing hyperlucency. Pulmonary arterial obstruction may be

secondary to extrinsic compression or invasion by a hilar mass or to pulmonary embolism. A check-valve effect from an endobronchial tumor or foreign body can produce air trapping, resulting in shunting of blood and unilateral hyperlucency. The Swyer-James syndrome or unilateral hyperlucent lung is a condition that follows adenoviral infection during infancy (see Fig. 18.13). An asymmetric obliterative bronchiolitis with severe air trapping on expiration and secondary unilateral pulmonary artery hypoplasia produces the hyperlucency in this condition. Finally, asymmetric involvement of lung by emphysema can produce a hyperlucent lung; this is most common with severe bullous disease.

Bilateral hyperlucent lungs may be simulated by an overpenetrated film or by a thin patient. As with unilateral hyperlucency, true bilateral hyperlucent lungs are the result of diminished pulmonary blood flow. This may be the result of congenital pulmonary stenosis, most commonly associated with the tetralogy of Fallot, or secondary to an acquired obstruction of the pulmonary circulation, as in pulmonary arterial hypertension or

TABLE 12.13

CAUSES OF PULMONARY LUCENCY

Localized	Cavity
	Cyst
	Bulla
	Bleb
	Pneumatocele
Diffuse Unilateral	Technical factors
	Grid cutoff
	Patient rotation
	Extrapulmonary disorder
	Soft tissue abnormalities
	Absent pectoralis muscle
	Mastectomy
	Contralateral pleural effusion/thickening
	Pneumothorax
	Pulmonary disease
	Diminished pulmonary blood flow
	Hypoplastic lung/pulmonary artery
	Obstruction of pulmonary artery
	Pulmonary embolism
	Mediastinal/hilar tumor
	Fibrosing mediastinitis
	Diminished pulmonary blood flow and hyperinflation
	Lobar atelectasis/resection
	Swyer-James syndrome
	Endobronchial tumor/foreign body producing a check-valve effect
Bilateral	Technical factors
	Overpenetrated radiograph
	Diminished pulmonary blood flow
	Congenital pulmonary outflow obstruction
	Mediastinal tumor
	Pulmonary arterial hypertension
	Chronic thromboembolic disease
	Fibrosing mediastinitis
	Diminished pulmonary blood flow and hyperinflation
	Emphysema
	Asthma

Adapted from Reed (21); information used with permission.

chronic thromboembolic disease. Pulmonary emphysema results in hyperinflation with air trapping on expiration, destruction of the pulmonary microvasculature, and attenuation of lobar and segmental vessels, thereby producing bilateral hyperlucency (24). Asthma produces transient air trapping and diffuse bilateral vascular attenuation, resulting in both hyperinflation and hyperlucency.

Mediastinal Masses

Mediastinal masses are recognized on frontal radiographs by the presence of a soft tissue density that causes obliteration or displacement of the mediastinal contours or interfaces. The lung–mass interface typically is well defined laterally, where it is convex with the adjacent lung, and it creates obtuse angles with the lung at its superior and inferior margins. This latter characteristic is diagnostic of an extrapulmonary lesion, whether intramediastinal or pleural. Lateral displacement of the trachea or heart may be seen with large mediastinal masses, sometimes first recognized by displacement of an indwelling endotracheal tube, nasogastric tube, or intravascular catheter. The presence of calcification, fat, or, rarely, a fat–fluid level (as in a cystic teratoma) can limit the differential diagnosis of a mediastinal mass.

Virtually every patient with a mediastinal mass will have thoracic CT or MR performed, with US usually limited to evaluation of vascular masses and for real-time imaging guidance during transthoracic needle biopsy.

The vascular origin of a mediastinal mass is readily apparent on contrast-enhanced CT, MR, and, occasionally, transthoracic or transesophageal US. The recognition of fat within a mediastinal mass on CT or MR limits the differential diagnosis to a small number of entities, including diaphragmatic hernia, lipoma, teratoma, epicardial fat pad, and thymolipoma. A fat–fluid level is virtually diagnostic of a mature teratoma. Although calcification is occasionally detected radiographically within mediastinal masses, CT is considerably more sensitive and provides more specific characterization of the calcification. The presence of coarse calcification within an anterior mediastinal mass should suggest the diagnosis of a teratoma (especially if a tooth is seen) or thymoma (coarse calcification). Curvilinear rimlike calcification should suggest a cyst or aneurysm. Conversely, the presence of calcification within an untreated mediastinal mass virtually excludes the diagnosis of lymphoma.

Frontal and lateral chest radiographs usually localize a mediastinal mass to a structure within the anterior, middle, or posterior mediastinal compartments (see Chapter 13). For instance, if the contours of a lesion are outlined by air and seen above the clavicles, then the lesion must be in the posterior mediastinum. Conversely, if the contours of a lesion are lost at the thoracic inlet level, it must be anterior. Obviously, CT and MR provide more precise information regarding structures involved by the mass. This not only helps narrow the differential diagnosis but is key in guiding further diagnostic procedures (Fig. 12.31). For example, a posterior mediastinal mass intimately related to the esophagus may best be evaluated by esophagoscopy and transesophageal biopsy, while a subcarinal mass is best approached by bronchoscopy and transcranial needle aspiration biopsy.

Mediastinal Widening

Mediastinal widening is described as a smooth, uniform increase in the transverse diameter of the mediastinum on frontal chest radiographs. True mediastinal disease is often difficult to distinguish from technical factors, including AP technique, supine positioning, and rotation. Clues to the presence of disease include change in mediastinal width from prior frontal radiographs, mass effect on adjacent mediastinal structures (tracheal deviation or displacement of an indwelling nasogastric tube or central venous catheter), increased density

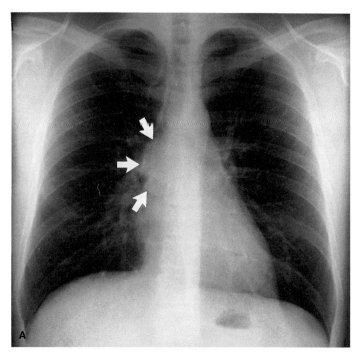
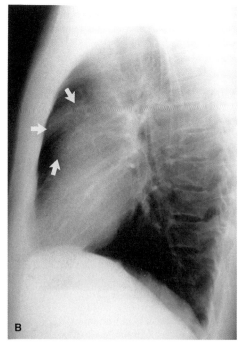

FIGURE 12.31. Anterior Mediastinal Mass Resulting From Seminoma. Frontal (**A**) and lateral (**B**) chest radiographs in a 35-year-old man with a history of cough and fatigue demonstrate a lobulated mass (*arrows*) in the right anterior mediastinum. A CT-guided biopsy showed seminoma.

of the mediastinum, and obscuration of the normal mediastinal contours, most specifically the aortic knob and paratracheal stripe. While normal measurements have been developed for mediastinal width, there is such great individual variability that absolute measurements are somewhat useless.

Pneumomediastinum and Pneumopericardium

The diagnosis of *pneumomediastinum* is usually made by findings on conventional radiographs. Small amounts of extraluminal air appear as linear or curvilinear lucencies lining anatomic structures within the mediastinal contours (see Fig. 13.20). Larger collections may be seen outlining the cardiac silhouette, mediastinal vessels, tracheobronchial tree, or esophagus. The most common finding is air outlining the left heart border, where a curvilinear lucency representing pneumomediastinum is paralleled by a thin curvilinear opacity representing the combined thickness of the visceral and parietal pleura of the lingula. Another sign of pneumomediastinum is the "continuous diaphragm" sign, in which air dissects between the pericardium above and central diaphragm below to allow visualization of the central portion of the diaphragm in contiguity with the right and left hemidiaphragms, each of which is outlined by air in the lower lobes, respectively. While this sign is fairly specific for pneumomediastinum, pneumopericardium may produce a similar finding. Small amounts of mediastinal air are often more easily appreciated on the lateral film, with air outlining the aortic root or main or central pulmonary arteries.

Pneumomediastinum should be distinguished from three entities that may mimic some of the radiographic findings and have significantly different etiologies and therapeutic implications: pneumopericardium, medial pneumothorax, and Mach bands. Air in the pericardial sac is limited by the normal pericardial reflections and extends superiorly to the proximal ascending aorta and main pulmonary artery. Additionally, pneumopericardium is often secondary to an infectious process with associated pericardial fluid and thickening, which will produce an air–fluid level on horizontal beam radiographs. Air within the pericardial sac will rise to a nondependent position on decubitus positioning, unlike mediastinal air, which is not mobile. The differentiation of pneumomediastinum from a medial pneumothorax is also aided by decubitus views because pleural air will rise nondependently along the lateral pleural space. In contrast to pneumothorax, pneumomediastinum may be seen to outline intramediastinal structures (pulmonary artery, trachea) and is often bilateral. However, the distinction between pneumomediastinum and pneumothorax may be impossible, and the two conditions often coexist, particularly in the neonatal period. Paramediastinal lucent bands created by Mach effect are easily distinguished from pneumomediastinum. The lateral margin of lucent Mach bands consists of lung parenchyma, as opposed to the thin pleural line seen with mediastinal air. These bands represent an optical illusion (caused by a retinal reinforcement response [25]) that disappears when the interface between mediastinal soft tissues and lung is covered.

Hilar Disease

Signs of enlarged bronchopulmonary lymph nodes or hilar mass on frontal chest radiographs include hilar enlargement, increased hilar density, lobulation of the hilar contour, and distortion of central bronchi (26). An abnormal hilum is most easily appreciated by comparison with the contralateral hilum and by review of prior chest radiographs (Fig. 12.32). CT will often show a left hilar mass that is not evident on routine radiographs. On the right, the normally sharp right hilar angle, formed by the intersection of the lower lateral aspect of the right superior pulmonary vein with the upper lateral aspect of the right interlobar pulmonary artery, is often distorted or obscured by a right hilar mass. An increase in density of the hilar shadow is seen with a hilar mass that lies primarily

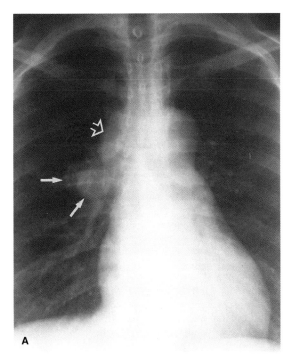
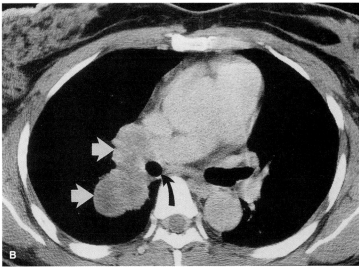

FIGURE 12.32. Hilar Lymph Node Enlargement. A. A PA radiograph in a 49-year-old woman with metastatic renal cell carcinoma demonstrates a lobulated enlargement and increased density of the right hilum (*solid arrows*) with concomitant paratracheal lymph node enlargement (*open arrow*). **B.** A CT scan through the hila shows the lobulated soft tissue mass (*short arrows*) within the right hilum surrounding the bronchus intermedius (*curved arrow*).

anterior or posterior to the normal hilar vascular shadows. In such patients, the enlarged hilar nodes will produce an increase in density on frontal views and a lobulated appearance when viewed in profile on a lateral radiograph.

When an abnormally dense hilum is noted, the relationship between the vessels and the density must be assessed. A density through which the normal hilar vessels (interlobar artery, upper lobe arteries, left descending artery) can be seen constitutes a "hilum overlay" sign, which indicates a mass superimposed on the hilum. Conversely, vascular structures that converge only as far as the lateral margin of the increased hilar density indicate enlargement of intrahilar vascular structures (the "hilum convergence" sign). The lateral radiograph or a CT will clarify the abnormality. In patients with small lung volumes or exaggerated kyphosis, a mass in the lower right hilum on frontal radiographs may be simulated by the end-on projection of a horizontally oriented right interlobar artery. Comparison with prior radiographs will usually resolve the matter, with CT reserved for equivocal cases.

Tumors involving the lobar bronchi or bronchus intermedius may produce luminal narrowing of the bronchi with enlargement of the hilar shadow. Occasionally, an endobronchial mass produces an abrupt cutoff of the bronchial air column, which is associated with lobar atelectasis or obstructive pneumonitis. In a small percentage of normal individuals, the right or left anterior segment, upper lobe bronchi are visualized as end-on ring shadows at the superolateral margin of the hila. The presence of a soft tissue density greater than 5 mm in thickness lateral to an anterior segmental bronchus is suspicious for mass or adenopathy in this region; the posterior division of the superior vein that lies immediately lateral to the anterior segmental bronchus should not exceed this thickness. Abnormal thickening of the walls of the main or lobar bronchi is a prominent feature of hilar abnormality on lateral chest films.

Enlargement of the right or left hilar shadow from pulmonary artery dilatation is produced by increased flow or increased pressure in the pulmonary arterial circulation. Pulmonary artery dilatation is usually assessed by measurement of the right interlobar pulmonary artery on PA radiographs. The margins of this vessel are readily visible, with the lateral margin outlined by air in the lower lobe and the medial margin outlined by air in the bronchus intermedius. The upper limit of normal for the transverse diameter of the proximal right interlobar artery, as measured on a PA radiograph at a level immediately lateral to the proximal portion of the bronchus intermedius, is 17 mm in men and 15 mm in women (see Fig. 14.14).

The lateral radiograph can confirm the impression of hilar abnormality seen on frontal radiographs and may demonstrate a mass when the frontal radiograph is normal. Hilar masses that lie predominantly anterior or posterior to the hilar vessels are best visualized on the lateral view. Because the lateral radiograph is a composite of both hilar shadows, the cumulative density of bilateral hilar masses may produce a significant increase in the normal density of the composite shadow, which is more easily appreciated on a lateral than on a frontal view.

The radiographic findings of a hilar mass on lateral radiographs are an abnormal size of or a lobulated contour to the normal vascular shadows, the presence of soft tissue in a region that is normally radiolucent, an increase in density of the composite hilar shadow, and abnormalities of the central bronchi. An increase in the size and density of the composite hilar shadow is best appreciated by comparison with prior radiographs, as is usually seen with bilateral hilar lymph node enlargement from sarcoidosis. Hilar lymph node enlargement produces lobulation of the normally smooth outlines of the right and left main pulmonary arteries. There are additional findings unique to the lateral radiograph that suggest the presence of a hilar mass and may allow lateralization of the hilar abnormality. Because the RUL bronchus is visualized on the

lateral radiograph in only a minority of individuals, visualization of the RUL bronchial lumen, particularly if it was invisible on a prior lateral radiograph, is a strong evidence of mass or adenopathy in the upper right hilum. A lobulated posterior wall of the bronchus intermedius, or a thickness >3 mm, indicates an abnormality of the bronchus (bronchitis or bronchogenic carcinoma), edema of the axial interstitium (pulmonary edema or lymphangitic carcinomatosis), or enlargement of lymph nodes in the posterior aspect of the lower right hilum.

The normal anatomy of the inferior hilar window was reviewed earlier in this chapter. The identification of a soft tissue mass >1 cm in diameter within this radiolucent region is an accurate indicator of unilateral or bilateral hilar mass. Occasionally, the silhouetting of the anterior wall of the LLL bronchus, recognized as a concave anterior curvilinear structure contiguous with the anterior aspect of the LUL bronchus, allows lateralization of a mass to the left lower hilum (Fig. 12.33). The added opacity of a mass within the normally radiolucent inferior hilar window produces an oval opacity to the composite hilar shadow on lateral radiographs.

On a lateral radiograph, enlargement of pulmonary arteries is assessed by measuring the left descending pulmonary artery as it arches over the left mainstem/LUL bronchus at a 2:00 position (Fig 12.19B).

Helical CT is the most sensitive method of detecting and localizing enlarged hilar (bronchopulmonary) lymph nodes and masses. Although contrast enhancement is almost never necessary to assess mediastinal nodes, it simplifies identification of enlarged vascular structures or nonenhancing hilar nodes (defined as nodes that exceed 10 mm in short-axis diameter) or masses. Hilar masses are seen on axial or coronal spin echo MR as round masses of low or intermediate signal intensity, in distinction to the signal void of flowing blood within the hilar vessels or of air in the bronchi. Coronal MR may be superior to CT in the detection of enlarged hilar lymph nodes because it displays the hilar vessels, which are oriented in the cephalocaudad direction, in length rather than in cross section. Displacement or distortion of the hilar vessels provides indirect evidence of hilar disease. Tumor invasion of a branch of the pulmonary artery or vein within the hilum produces a filling defect within the vessel on contrast-enhanced CT or intraluminal signal on MR. The density characteristics of hilar masses on CT can help provide important information for differential diagnosis; for example, a round, cystic hilar mass with imperceptible walls in an asymptomatic young person is typical of a bronchogenic cyst.

Enlarged hilar lymph nodes can be detected by CT without the use of intravenous contrast. A detailed knowledge of the normal hilar vascular and bronchial anatomy, as seen on CT, is necessary for the identification of subtle hilar contour abnormalities. In those portions of the hilum where lung directly contacts a wall of a bronchus, thickening or lobulation of the normal thin linear shadow of the bronchial wall indicates hilar abnormality. This is particularly well seen where the RLL and LLL contact the posterior walls of the bronchus intermedius and the LUL bronchus, respectively (Fig. 12.34). Lymph node enlargement in these regions is obscured on frontal radiographs by the overlying cardiac and hilar vascular shadows. CT is more sensitive than plain radiographs or MR for the detection of soft tissue masses within lobar or proximal segmental bronchi. In most patients with an endobronchial mass, a large extraluminal component produces a radiographically visible hilar soft tissue mass and obstructive atelectasis.

Enlarged hilar lymph nodes may have different appearances on CT. Enlargement of discrete lymph nodes, most commonly seen in sarcoidosis, appears as multiple distinct round masses (Fig. 12.34). When tumor or an inflammatory process extends through the nodal capsule to involve contiguous nodes, a single

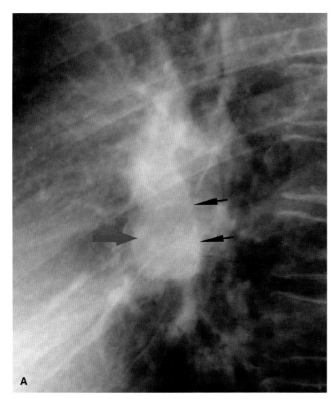

FIGURE 12.33. **Hilar Mass Within the Inferior Hilar Window. A.** A cone-down view of a lateral radiograph in a patient subsequently found to have a plasmacytoma of the left hilum shows a mass (*red arrow*) within the inferior hilar window obliterating the anterior wall of the left lower lobe bronchus (*small black arrows*). **B.** A CT scan through the lower hila confirms the presence of a left hilar mass (*asterisk*).

large mass of confluent lymph nodes is produced and that may be difficult to distinguish from a primary hilar bronchogenic carcinoma. This latter appearance is most often seen in hilar nodal metastases from small cell carcinoma of the lung or lymphoma (see Fig. 15.10). As in enlargement of mediastinal lymph nodes, the CT density of enlarged hilar nodes can provide clues to the diagnosis (see Table 13.5).

An abnormally small hilum indicates a diminution in the size of the right or left pulmonary artery.

Pleural Effusion

The radiographic appearance of pleural effusions depends upon the amount of fluid present, the patient's position during the radiographic examination, and the presence or absence of adhesions between the visceral and parietal pleura. Small amounts of pleural fluid initially collect between the lower lobe and diaphragm in a subpulmonic location. As more fluid accumulates, it spills into the posterior and lateral costophrenic sulci. A moderate amount of pleural fluid (>175 mL) in the erect patient will have a characteristic appearance on the frontal radiograph, with a homogeneous lower zone opacity seen in the lateral costophrenic sulcus with a concave interface toward the lung. This concave margin, known as a *pleural meniscus*, appears higher laterally than medially on frontal radiographs because the lateral aspect of the effusion, which surrounds the costal surface of the lung, is tangent to the frontal x-ray beam. Similarly, the meniscus of pleural fluid as seen on lateral radiographs peaks anteriorly and posteriorly (Fig. 12.35) (27).

In patients with suspected pleural effusion, a lateral decubitus film with the affected side down is the most sensitive technique to detect small amounts of fluid. With this technique, pleural fluid collections as small as 5 mL may be seen layering between the lung and lateral chest wall. While a moderate-size, free-flowing collection should be obvious on upright radiographs, a large pleural effusion can cause passive atelectasis of the entire lung, producing an opaque hemithorax. It may be difficult to distinguish the latter condition from collapse of an entire lung. While a massive effusion should produce contralateral mediastinal shift,

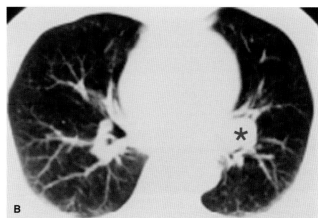

FIGURE 12.34. **Enlarged Hilar Nodes on CT.** Contrast-enhanced CT with coronal reformation through the level of the hila in a patient with biopsy-proven sarcoidosis demonstrates bilateral hilar lymph node enlargement (*arrows*).

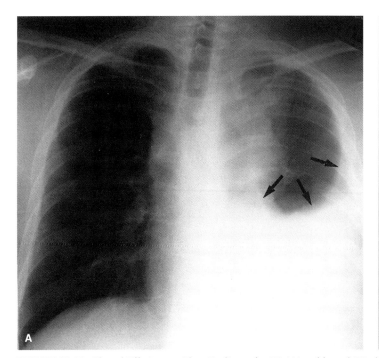
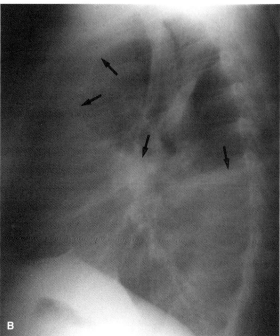

FIGURE 12.35. Pleural Effusion on Chest Radiographs. PA (**A**) and lateral (**B**) chest radiographs demonstrate the typical meniscoid appearance (*arrows*) in a patient with a left pleural effusion resulting from mediastinal Hodgkin lymphoma.

a collapsed lung without pleural effusion will show shift toward the opaque side. In some patients, CT or US may be necessary to distinguish pleural fluid from collapsed lung.

CT is quite sensitive in the detection of free pleural fluid. On axial scans, pleural fluid layers posteriorly with a characteristic meniscoid appearance and has a CT attenuation value of 0 to 20 H. Small effusions may be difficult to differentiate from pleural thickening, fibrosis, or dependent atelectasis, and decubitus scans are useful in making this distinction. The pleural and peritoneal spaces are oriented in the axial plane at the level of the diaphragm. This may cause some difficulty in localizing the fluid to one or both spaces. Fluid in either the pleural or peritoneal space can displace the liver and spleen medially, away from the chest wall. A key to distinguishing ascites from pleural fluid on axial CT scans is to observe the relationship of the fluid to the diaphragmatic crus. Pleural fluid in the posterior costophrenic sulcus will lie posteromedial to the diaphragm and displace the crus laterally. In contrast, peritoneal fluid lies within the confines of the diaphragm and therefore will displace the crus medially. Another useful distinguishing feature is the quality of the interface of the fluid with the liver or spleen. Intraperitoneal fluid will show a distinct, sharp interface with the liver and spleen as it directly contacts these organs, whereas pleural effusions will have a hazy, indistinct interface with these viscera because of the interposed hemidiaphragms. Because the peritoneal space does not extend posterior to the bare area of the liver, right-sided fluid extending posteromedially must be pleural. A large effusion will allow the inferior edge of the adjacent atelectatic lower lobe to float in the fluid, creating a curvilinear opacity that can be misinterpreted as the diaphragm separating pleural fluid from ascites. This "pseudodiaphragm" is recognized as a broad band that does not extend far laterally or anteriorly and is contiguous superiorly with an atelectatic lung containing air bronchograms (Fig. 12.36). US is particularly useful in detecting free flowing pleural effusions, which are usually seen as anechoic collections at the base of the pleural space surrounding atelectatic lung (see Chapter 39).

Pleural fluid may become loculated between the pleural layers to produce an appearance indistinguishable from that of a pleural mass. Fluid loculated within the costal pleural layers appears as a vertically oriented elliptical opacity with a broad area of contact with the chest wall, producing a sharp, convex interface with the lung when viewed in tangent. CT is commonly utilized to detect and localize loculated pleural fluid collections. The characteristic finding is a sharply marginated lenticular mass of fluid attenuation conforming to the concavity of the chest wall that forms obtuse angles at its edges and compresses and displaces the subjacent lung. Multiple fluid locules can mimic pleural metastases or malignant mesothelioma radiographically; CT or US can confirm the fluid characteristics of these pleural "masses."

Pleural fluid may extend into the interlobar fissures, producing characteristic findings. Free fluid within the minor fissure is usually seen as smooth, symmetric thickening on a frontal radiograph. Fluid within the major fissure is normally not visible on frontal radiographs, as the fissures are viewed en face. An exception is fluid extending into the lateral aspect of an incomplete major fissure, which produces a curvilinear density extending from the inferolateral to the superomedial aspect of the lung. Fluid loculated between the leaves of visceral pleura within an interlobar fissure results in an elliptic opacity oriented along the length of the fissure. These loculated collections of pleural fluid are termed "pseudotumors" and are most often seen within the minor fissure on frontal radiographs in patients with congestive heart failure. The tendency for these opacities to disappear rapidly with diuresis has led to the term "vanishing lung tumor." Although a characteristic appearance on plain radiographs is usually sufficient for diagnosis, the CT demonstration of a localized fluid collection in the expected location of the major or minor fissure is confirmatory.

An uncommon appearance of pleural effusion is seen when fluid accumulates between the lower lobe and diaphragm and is termed a *subpulmonic* effusion. While small amounts of pleural fluid normally accumulate in this location, it is uncommon for larger effusions to remain subpulmonic without spilling into the posterior and lateral costophrenic sulci. A subpulmonic effusion may be difficult to appreciate on upright chest radiographs because the fluid collection mimics an elevated

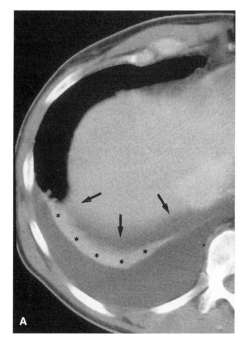 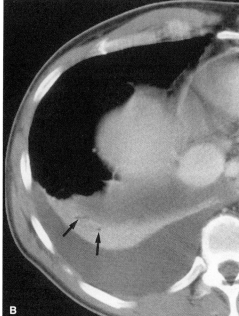

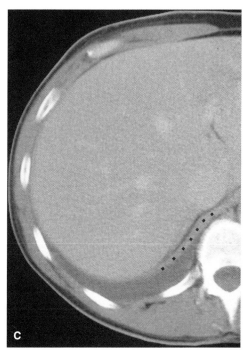

FIGURE 12.36. Subpulmonic Pleural Effusion on CT. A. A CT scan through the lower chest shows fluid surrounding an enhancing broad curvilinear structure (*asterisks*). The fluid creates an ill-defined interface with the liver (*arrows*). B. A scan 1 cm more cephalad shows that the curvilinear density represents the tip of an atelectatic right lower lobe containing air bronchograms (*arrows*). C. More inferiorly, the crus of the diaphragm (*dotted structure*) is displaced laterally by posteromedial pleural fluid.

hemidiaphragm. Clues to its presence on frontal radiographs include apparent and new elevation of the diaphragm, lateral peaking of the hemidiaphragm that is accentuated on expiration, a minor fissure that is close to the diaphragm (right-sided effusions), and an increased separation of the gastric air bubble from the base of the lung (left-sided effusions). Despite the atypical subpulmonic accumulation of fluid with the patient upright, the effusion will layer dependently on lateral decubitus radiographs (Fig. 12.37).

The radiographic detection of pleural effusion in the supine patient can be difficult because fluid accumulates in a dependent location posteriorly. The most common finding is a hazy opacification of the affected hemithorax with obscuration of the hemidiaphragm and blunting of the lateral costophrenic angle. Fluid extending over the apex of the lung may produce a

soft tissue cap with a concave interface inferiorly, while medial fluid may cause an apparent mediastinal widening.

Pneumothorax

The classic radiographic finding of pneumothorax on upright chest films is visualization of the visceral pleura as a curvilinear line that parallels the chest wall, separating the partially collapsed lung centrally from pleural air peripherally (Fig. 12.38). An expiratory radiograph aids in the detection of a small pneumothorax by increasing the volume of intrapleural air relative to lung, thereby displacing the visceral pleural reflection away from the chest wall and by exaggerating the differences in density of pneumothorax (black) to lung (gray) at the end of expiration. In

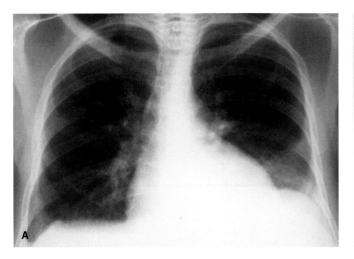

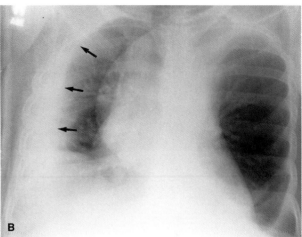

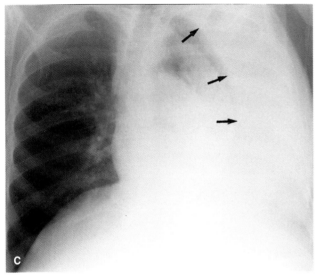

FIGURE 12.37. Bilateral Subpulmonic Pleural Effusions. A. An upright PA radiograph in a 41-year-old woman with ascites demonstrates apparent elevation of both hemidiaphragms. Right (**B**) and left (**C**) decubitus films demonstrate dependent layering of the subpulmonic pleural fluid (*arrows*).

a small percentage of patients, a pneumothorax will be visible only on a lateral or decubitus film or a frontal radiograph obtained in full inspiration. This suggests that when there is a strong clinical suspicion of pneumothorax and the frontal expiratory radiograph is normal, a lateral or inspiratory film may be beneficial for proper diagnosis.

The detection of a pneumothorax is difficult when chest films are obtained in the supine position. Approximately 30% of pneumothoraces imaged on supine radiographs go undetected. Because many portable radiographs are obtained with the patient supine, the recognition of a pneumothorax on a supine film is particularly important in the critically ill patient, who is at high risk from iatrogenic trauma or barotrauma. In a supine patient, the most nondependent portion of the pleural space is anterior or anteromedial. Small pneumothoraces will initially collect in these regions and will fail to produce a visible pleural line. The affected hemithorax may appear hyperlucent. Anteromedial air may sharpen the borders of mediastinal soft tissue structures, resulting in improved visualization of the cardiac margin and the aortic knob. The lateral costophrenic sulcus may appear abnormally deep and hyperlucent—a finding known as the "deep sulcus" sign. Visualization of the anterior costophrenic sulcus owing to air anteriorly and inferiorly produces the "double diaphragm" sign, as the dome and anterior portions of the diaphragm are outlined by lung and pleural air, respectively. When an anterior pneumothorax is suspected on a supine radiograph, an upright film, lateral decubitus film with the affected side up, or CT scan should be obtained (Fig. 12.39).

Subpulmonic pneumothoraces are rare. Radiographically, a localized area of hyperlucency is seen inferiorly, with the visceral pleural line paralleling the hemidiaphragm. Loculated pneumothoraces develop as the result of adhesions between visceral and parietal pleura and may be found anywhere in the pleural space.

CT is often necessary for diagnosis.

Several entities produce a curvilinear line or interface or hyperlucency on chest radiographs and must be distinguished from a pneumothorax. Skin folds resulting from the compression of redundant skin by the radiographic cassette can produce a curvilinear interface that simulates the visceral pleural line. A skin fold produces an edge or interface with atmospheric air, in distinction to the visceral pleural line seen in a pneumothorax. The interface produced by a skin fold rarely continues over the lung apex and is often seen to extend beyond the chest wall. Pulmonary vascular opacities may be followed peripheral to the skin fold interface. Bullae may simulate pneumothorax by producing localized or unilateral hyperlucency. They are marginated by thin curvilinear walls that are concave rather than convex to the chest wall. The distinction of pneumothorax from bullous disease may be difficult but is usually evident by the clinical presentation. However, since this distinction has important therapeutic implications, certain patients may require CT.

CT is more sensitive than conventional radiographs in the detection of pneumothorax because of its cross-sectional nature and superior contrast resolution. The CT demonstration of linear parenchymal bands of tissue traversing large

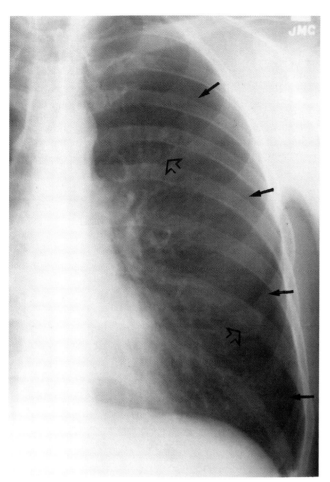

FIGURE 12.38. The Visceral Pleural Line in Pneumothorax. PA radiograph in a patient with a cystic fibrosis and a spontaneous pneumothorax demonstrates a curvilinear visceral pleural line (*arrows*) separating the left lung medially from the chest wall laterally. Note the presence of extensive coarse reticular opacities reflecting the underlying bronchiectasis seen in this disease.

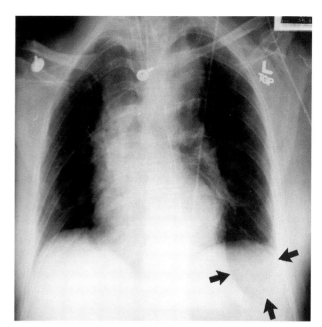

FIGURE 12.39. Deep Sulcus Sign in Supine Patient with Pneumothorax. A supine chest film obtained in a ventilated patient following placement of a left subclavian central venous catheter shows a deep sulcus sign at the left base (*arrows*), representing a pneumothorax. Note hyperlucent region over the left upper quadrant (arrows) reflecting pleural air in the costophrenic sulcus anterior to the spleen.

avascular areas helps distinguish bullae from loculated pneumothoraces. CT may be used to detect and drain loculated pneumothoraces in critically ill patients.

Localized Pleural Thickening

Localized pleural thickening is seen as a flat, smooth, slightly raised soft tissue opacity extending over one or two intercostal spaces that displaces the lung from the innermost cortical margin of the ribs when viewed in tangent. Localized pleural thickening viewed en face is usually undetectable radiographically because the lesion does not significantly attenuate the x-ray beam and does not present a raised edge to be recognized as a distinct opacity. An exception is the presence of pleural calcification, which can usually be recognized as discrete thin linear or curvilinear calcific opacities paralleling the inner surface of the ribs when viewed end-on or as geographic areas of increased density with round or lobulated borders when viewed en face. Focal areas of pleural fibrosis are best appreciated on conventional and high-resolution CT scans, where they are easily distinguished from deposits of subpleural fat by their density.

There are two additional radiographic findings that mimic the appearance of focal pleural thickening. The apical cap is a curvilinear subpleural opacity <5 mm thick with a sharp or slightly irregular inferior margin that represents nonspecific fibrosis of the apical lung and adjacent visceral pleura. While it is usually bilateral and symmetric, slight asymmetry in thickness is common. Any growth of the opacity, significant asymmetry, inferior convexity of the opacity, rib destruction, or symptoms should prompt a CT or MR examination followed by biopsy to exclude an apical neoplasm (Pancoast or superior sulcus tumor). The companion shadows of the inferior aspects of the first and second ribs are smooth apical linear opacities that parallel the lower cortical margins of the first two ribs and represent the pleural layers and subpleural fat viewed in tangent. These are most prominent in obese individuals and should not be mistaken for pleural fibrosis.

Diffuse Pleural Thickening

Fibrothorax appears as a thin, smooth band of soft tissue with a sharp internal margin seen immediately beneath and parallel to the inner margin of the ribs and intercostal spaces. It is usually unilateral and extends over large areas of the dependent (posterior and inferior) portions of the pleural space. Anterior or posterior costal pleural thickening creates a veil-like opacity without sharp margins when viewed en face on frontal radiographs. Blunting of the lateral costophrenic sulcus may be seen on frontal radiographs, while sparing of the posterior costophrenic sulcus and an absence of layering fluid on decubitus positioning help distinguish pleural fibrosis from a small effusion. Fibrothorax tends to spare the interlobar fissures and mediastinal pleura. CT and HRCT are more sensitive than conventional radiographs in the detection of pleural thickening. The diminished volume of the affected hemithorax seen with extensive fibrothorax is more easily appreciated on axial CT images than on frontal radiographs (see Fig. 19.9). CT and HRCT provide an unimpeded view of the underlying lung in patients with diffuse pleural thickening, allowing detection of associated interstitial pulmonary fibrosis. This is important in evaluating patients with suspected asbestosis and in assessing the extent of pulmonary disease in patients being considered for pleurectomy.

Pleural and Extrapleural Lesions

The shape and margins of a peripheral opacity as seen on conventional radiographs help define the opacity as parenchymal, pleural, or extrapleural. Pleural masses form obtuse angles with the adjacent normal pleura, in distinction to peripheral lung lesions, which usually contact the normal pleura at acute angles. Pleural and extrapleural masses are usually vertically oriented elliptic opacities. Pleural lesions tend to have smooth, well-defined margins as they compress normal lung. These smooth margins are best appreciated on radiographic projections with the x-ray beam tangent to the interface between the mass and the lung. Another feature of pleural lesions is the clarity of the margin of the lesion on frontal and lateral radiographs; a mass sharply outlined by lung on one view but poorly marginated on the orthogonal view should suggest a pleural or extrapleural process. In contrast, intraparenchymal lesions are surrounded by air and will have similar margins on both views. Pleural lesions, unlike parenchymal lesions, do not change position with respiratory motion. Lung disease is often confined to a lobe, while pleural disease may extend across fissures. Pedunculated pleural lesions such as fibromas are rare but can present with radiographic features of both pleural and parenchymal lesions.

Despite the aforementioned features, the distinction of pleural from peripheral parenchymal lesions may be difficult. This distinction has important diagnostic implications; while parenchymal processes are best evaluated by examination of expectorated sputum or by bronchoscopy, pleural lesions will require thoracentesis or pleural biopsy. CT is often used to help distinguish between pleural and parenchymal disease (see Chapter 19). A peripheral lesion that is completely surrounded by lung on CT is intraparenchymal, with the exception being the rare pleural lesion arising within an interlobar fissure. Peripheral lung masses generally have irregular margins and may contain air bronchograms. Those parenchymal lesions that contact the pleura will form acute angles with the chest wall as on plain films. The CT appearance of pleural and extrapleural or chest wall lesions are similar. Both pleural and extrapleural lesions are sharply defined and form obtuse angles with the chest wall (see Fig. 19.10); rib destruction or subcutaneous mass are the only findings that localize an extrapulmonary lesion to the chest wall. When a peripheral parenchymal lesion invades the pleura, determining the origin of the mass may be impossible. CT can further characterize peripheral lesions by their density; a smooth fatty mass is almost certainly a pleural lipoma (see Fig. 19.10), whereas a homogeneous pleural or extrapleural soft tissue mass is most likely a fibroma or neurogenic tumor (see Fig. 19.11). The signal intensity on T1W and T2W spin echo MR images may be useful in the characterization of focal pleural masses. On T1WIs and T2WIs, loculated fluid collections will show homogeneous low and high signal, respectively. Lipomas will show homogeneous high signal intensity on T1WI and intermediate signal intensity on T2WI, while fibromas are typically of intermediate and high signal intensity, respectively, as a result of the high cellularity of these tumors.

Chest Wall Lesions

Chest wall lesions become evident radiographically when (1) they extend into the thorax and become outlined by displaced lung, (2) there is bone displacement or destruction by the mass, or (3) they protrude externally from the skin surface to be outlined by air in the atmosphere. CT, MR, and US are all useful in assessing the characteristics of chest wall lesions. While CT and MR are most useful in determining the extent of intrathoracic involvement by chest wall lesions, US is the least expensive and simplest method of characterizing the nature of palpable chest wall lesions, particularly if they are thought to be vascular or cystic in nature. The radiographic findings of chest wall lesions related to specific bony or soft tissue components of the chest wall are detailed in the section on chest wall disease in Chapter 19.

Diaphragm

Radiographic findings of diaphragmatic disorders include elevation and depression of the diaphragm and abnormalities of diaphragmatic contour. The diagnostic considerations of diaphragmatic disease are reviewed in Chapter 19.

References

1. Wilkinson GA, Fraser RG. Roentgenography of the chest. Appl Radiol 1975;4:41–53.
2. Ravin CE, Chotas HG. Chest radiography. Radiology 1997;204:593–600.
3. Wandtke JC. Bedside chest radiography. Radiology 1994;192:282–284.
4. Kuhlman JE, Collins J, Brooks GN, Yandow D, Broderick LS. Dual-energy subtraction chest radiography: what to look for beyond calcified nodules. Radiographics 2006;26:79–92.
5. Cody DD, Mahesh M. Technologic advances in multi-detector CT with a focus on cardiac imaging. Radiographics 2007;27:1829–1837.
6. Duerden RM, Pointon KS, Habib S. Review of clinical cardiac MRI. Imaging 2006;18:178–186.
7. Kostakoglu L, Agress H, Goldsmith SJ. Clinical role of FDG PET in evaluation of cancer patients. Radiographics 2003;23:315–340.
8. Horsfield K, Cumming G. Morphology of the bronchial tree in man. J Appl Physiol 1968;24:373–383.
9. Vanpeperstraete F. The cartilaginous skeleton of the bronchial tree. Adv Anat Embryol Cell Biol 1974;48:1–15.
10. Raasch BN, Carsky EW, Lane EJ, et al. Radiographic anatomy of the interlobar fissures: a study of 100 specimens. AJR Am J Roentgenol 1982;138:1043–1049.
11. Yamashita H. Roentgenologic Anatomy of the Lung. 1st ed. Tokyo: Igaku-Shoin, 1978.
12. Proto AV, Speckman JM. The left lateral radiograph of the chest 1. Med Radiogr Photogr 1979;55:30–74.
13. Proto AV, Speckman JM. The left lateral radiograph of the chest 2. Med Radiogr Photogr 1980;56:38–64.
14. Heitzman R. The Mediastinum: Radiologic Correlations with Anatomy and Pathology. Berlin: Springer-Verlag, 1988:311–349.
15. Im JG, Webb WR, Rosen A, Gamsu G. Costal pleura: appearances at high-resolution CT. Radiology 1989;171:125–131.
16. Felson B. The roentgen diagnosis of disseminated pulmonary alveolar diseases. Semin Radiol 1967;2:3.
17. Fraser RS, Colman N, Müller NL, Paré PD. Diseases of the Chest. 4th ed. Philadelphia, PA: Saunders, 1999:534–560.
18. Proto AV, Tocino I. Radiographic manifestations of lobar collapse. Semin Roentgenol 1980;15:117–173.
19. Lubert M, Krause GR. Patterns of lobar collapse as observed radiographically. Radiology 1951;56:165–172.
20. Felson B. Disseminated interstitial diseases of the lung. Ann Radiol 1966;9:325.
21. Reed JC. Plain Film Patterns and Differential Diagnosis. 5th ed. St Louis, MO: Mosby, 2003.
22. Kerley P. Radiology in heart disease. Br Med J 1933;2:594–597.
23. Godwin JD, Webb WR, Savoca CJ, et al. Multiple thin-walled cystic lesions of the lung. AJR Am J Roentgenol 1980;135:593–604.
24. Simon G. Radiology and emphysema. Clin Radiol 1964;15:293–306.
25. Lane EJ, Proto AV, Philips TW. Mach bands and density perception. Radiology 1976;121:9–13.
26. Müller NL, Webb WR. Imaging of the pulmonary hila. Invest Radiol 1985;20:661–671.
27. Raasch BN, Carsky EW, Lane EJ, et al. Pleural effusion: explanation of some typical appearances. AJR Am J Roentgenol 1982;139:899–904.

CHAPTER 13 ■ MEDIASTINUM AND HILA

JEFFREY S. KLEIN

This chapter reviews the radiologic approach to mediastinal masses, diffuse mediastinal disease, and hilar abnormalities.

MEDIASTINAL MASSES

Localized mediastinal abnormalities are common diagnostic challenges for the radiologist. Patients with mediastinal masses tend to present in one of two fashions: with symptoms related to local mass effect or invasion of adjacent mediastinal structures (stridor in a patient with thyroid goiter) or incidentally with an abnormality on a routine chest radiograph. Occasionally, a mediastinal mass is discovered in the course of an evaluation for known malignancy (e.g., a patient with non-Hodgkin lymphoma [NHL]) or for a condition such as myasthenia gravis, in which there is an association with thymoma. Multidetector-row CT (MDCT) is the primary cross-sectional modalities used to evaluate mediastinal masses, with PET useful to assess the response of mediastinal tumors to therapy, particularly lymphoma, and to distinguish residual or recurrent tumor from fibrosis.

For the purposes of the following discussion, the mediastinum is divided into superior (thoracic inlet) and inferior components, with the inferior mediastinum subdivided into anterior, middle, and posterior compartments, as described in Chapter 12 (1).

Thoracic Inlet Masses

The thoracic inlet is the region of the upper thorax marginated by the first rib and represents the junction between the neck and thorax. Masses in this region commonly present as neck masses or with symptoms of upper airway obstruction resulting from tracheal compression. Tortuous/dilated vascular structures, thyroid masses, lymphomatous nodes, and lymphangiomas are the most common thoracic inlet masses (Table 13.1).

Vascular Structures. Perhaps the most common thoracic inlet mass is seen in older patients as the tortuous arterial structures (Fig. 13.1), in particular the confluence of the right brachiocephalic and right subclavian arteries as they bulge laterally into the right upper lobe to produce a right thoracic inlet mass. Since the "mass" is situated anteriorly in the thoracic inlet, its lateral border above the clavicle is indistinct. This is in distinction to thoracic inlet masses that are posterior or

paravertebral in location, which are sharply outlined by apical lung which extends higher posteriorly than anteriorly. This finding is termed the "thoracic inlet" or "cervicothoracic" sign and helps localize thoracic inlet masses, thereby suggesting the etiology of such lesions. Tortuous arterial structures may be identified by the presence of atherosclerotic calcification within their walls and can often be seen on a lateral chest radiograph as a "mass" projecting posterior to the tracheal air column which is sharply outlined posteriorly. In contrast to other masses in the thoracic inlet, a tortuous vessel is usually associated with tracheal deviation toward the side of the mass, whereas most goiters and other inlet masses displace the trachea contralaterally.

Thyroid Masses. In a small percentage of patients with a cervical thyroid goiter, a thyroid carcinoma, or an enlarged gland from thyroiditis, extension of the thyroid through the thoracic inlet into the superior mediastinum may occur. These lesions are usually discovered as incidental findings on chest radiographs; a minority of patients will present with complaints of dyspnea or dysphagia as a result of tracheal or esophageal compression by the mass. Thyroid goiters arising from the lower pole of the thyroid or the thyroid isthmus can enter the superior mediastinum anterior to the trachea (80% of cases) or to the right and posterolateral to the trachea (20% of cases).

On chest radiographs, an anterosuperior mediastinal mass typically deviates the trachea laterally and either posteriorly (anterior masses) or anteriorly (posterior masses). Coarse, clumped calcifications are common in thyroid goiters. Radio-iodine studies should be performed as the initial imaging procedure, although false-negative results do occur. CT usually shows characteristic findings: (1) well-defined margins, (2) continuity of the mass with the cervical thyroid, (3) coarse calcifications, (4) cystic or necrotic areas, (5) baseline high CT attenuation (because of intrinsic iodine content), and (6) intense enhancement (>25 H) as a result of the hypervascularity of most thyroid masses and prolonged enhancement (resulting from active uptake of iodine from contrast media) following IV contrast administration (Fig. 13.2). MR is useful in depicting the longitudinal extension of thyroid goiters without the use of IV contrast.

Parathyroid Masses. In approximately 2% of patients, the parathyroid glands fail to separate from the thymus in the neck and descend with the gland into the anterosuperior mediastinum. These glands can be found near the thoracic inlet in or about the thymus. This becomes important in the small

TABLE 13.1

THORACIC INLET MASSES

Vascular	Tortuous brachiocephalic/subclavian artery
Thyroid mass	Goiter Malignancy Thyromegaly resulting from thyroiditis
Parathyroid mass	Hyperplasia Adenoma Carcinoma

Lymph node mass	Lymphoma
	  Hodgkin
	  Non-Hodgkin
	Metastases
	Inflammatory
	  Tuberculosis

Lymphangioma	

percentage of patients with persistent clinical and biochemical evidence of hyperparathyroidism following routine neck exploration and parathyroidectomy. Most of these ectopic parathyroid lesions are small (<3 cm) adenomas; rarely, they represent hyperplastic glands or parathyroid carcinoma. When

US and nuclear medicine studies have failed to localize a lesion in the neck, CT, MR, or technetium[99] sestamibi scanning may be useful in detecting mediastinal lesions.

Lymphangiomas. These uncommon masses are tumors comprised of dilated lymphatic channels. The cystic or cavernous form (cystic hygroma) is most commonly discovered in infancy and is often associated with chromosomal abnormalities, including Turner syndrome and trisomies 13, 18, and 21. In infants, these lesions tend to extend from the neck into the anterior mediastinum; less commonly they may arise primarily within the anterior mediastinum in older patients. Histologically, these tumors are composed of cystic spaces lined by epithelium and contain clear, straw-colored fluid. Although these lesions are benign histologically, they tend to insinuate themselves between vascular structures and the trachea. This makes complete surgical resection of lymphangiomas difficult, and they frequently recur. CT demonstrates a well-defined cystic mass within the thoracic inlet or superior mediastinum. MR typically shows a mass of high-signal intensity on T2WIs because of the fluid content.

Anterior Mediastinal Masses

A number of neoplasms and nonneoplastic conditions arise in the anterior mediastinum and produce anterior mediastinal masses. These include thymic neoplasms, lymphoma, germ cell neoplasms, and primary mesenchymal tumors (Table 13.2).

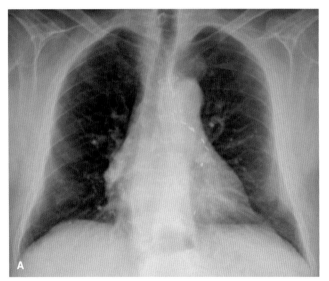

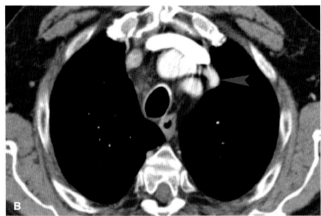

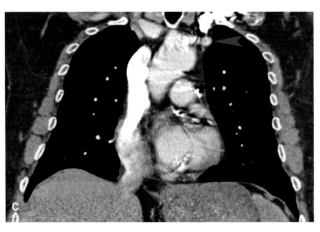

FIGURE 13.1. **Tortuous Left Common Carotid Artery Producing a Superior Mediastinal Mass. A.** Chest radiograph demonstrates a left superior mediastinal mass (*arrowhead*). Axial (**B**) and coronal (**C**) reformatted contrast-enhanced scans show a tortuous left common carotid artery (*arrowheads*) arising from the aortic arch as producing the "mass."

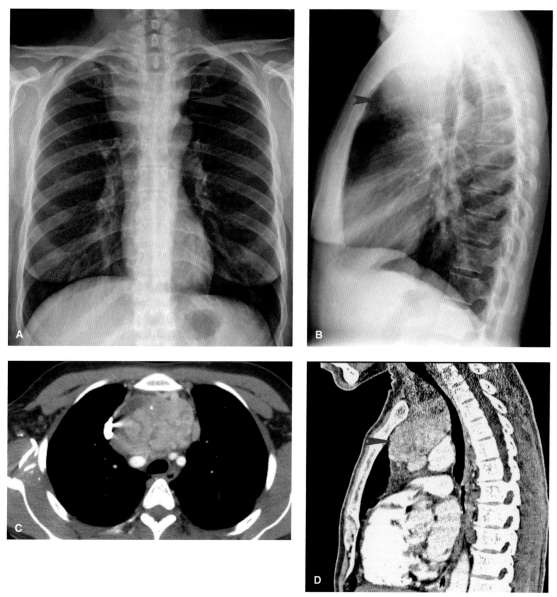

FIGURE 13.2. Thyroid Goiter. Posteroanterior (**A**) and lateral (**B**) radiographs show a lobulated anterior and superior mediastinal mass (*arrowheads*). **C.** Axial contrast-enhanced CT at the level of the manubrium shows a mixed attenuation mass with foci of calcification and regions of low attenuation anterior to the trachea and great vessels. **D.** Sagittal-reformatted midline scan shows the mass (*arrowhead*) extending from the thoracic inlet into the anterior mediastinum.

Thymomas or ***thymic epithelial neoplasms*** are the second most common primary mediastinal neoplasms in adults after lymphoma. These lesions are neoplasms that arise from the thymic epithelium and contain varying numbers of intermixed lymphocytes. The traditional classification of these tumors is into *thymomas,* which are histologically benign but may be either encapsulated (noninvasive) or invasive, and *thymic carcinomas,* in which the epithelial component shows signs of frank malignancy. The World Health Organization has recently reclassified these neoplasms based upon the morphology of the epithelial component and the ratio of epithelial cells to lymphocytes. The classification system divides these neoplasms into types A, AB, B1, B2, B3, and C, with a spectrum of histologic changes ranging from the classic encapsulated thymoma (A), which has a favorable prognosis, to thymic carcinoma (C), which generally carries a poor prognosis (2).

The average age at diagnosis of thymoma is 45 to 50; these lesions are rare in patients under the age of 20. While most often associated with myasthenia gravis, thymoma has been associated with other autoimmune diseases, such as pure red cell aplasia, Graves disease, Sjögren syndrome, and hypogammaglobulinemia. Of patients with myasthenia gravis, 10% to 28% have a thymoma, while a larger percentage of patients with thymoma (30% to 54%) have or will develop myasthenia.

On chest radiographs, thymomas are seen as round or oval, smooth or lobulated soft tissue masses arising near the origin of the great vessels at the base of the heart (2). CT is best for characterizing thymomas and detecting local invasion preoperatively (Fig. 13.3). As a result of their firm consistency, thymomas characteristically maintain their shape where they contact the sternum anteriorly and heart and great vessels posteriorly. Compared to type A tumors, higher-grade thymomas, particularly types B3 and C, tend to show larger size, more irregular margins, heterogeneous enhancement, regions of necrosis, mediastinal nodal metastases, and calcification. Invasion of

TABLE 13.2

ANTERIOR MEDIASTINAL MASSES

Thymic masses	Thymoma
	Thymic cyst
	Thymolipoma
	Thymic hyperplasia
	Thymic neuroendocrine tumors
	Thymic carcinoma
	Thymic lymphoma
Lymphoma	Hodgkin
	Non-Hodgkin
Germ cell neoplasms	Teratoma (benign or malignant)
	Seminoma
	Embryonal cell carcinoma
	Endodermal sinus tumor
	Choriocarcinoma
Thyroid mass	Goiter
	Tumor
	Adenoma
	Carcinoma
	Thyroiditis
Ectopic parathyroid mass	Hyperplasia
	Adenoma
	Carcinoma
Mesenchymal tumor	Lipoma
	Hemangioma
	Leiomyoma
	Liposarcoma
	Angiosarcoma

tumor through the thymic capsule is present in 33% to 50% of patients (Fig. 13.4; invasive tumor). In the majority of these patients, this determination cannot be made by CT or MR and may even be difficult to determine on examination of the resected specimen. Local invasion of pleura, lung, pericardium, chest wall, diaphragm, and great vessels occurs in decreasing order of frequency in 10% to 15% of patients. Contiguity of a thymoma with the adjacent chest wall or mediastinal structures cannot be used as reliable evidence of invasion of these structures. Drop metastases to dependent portions of the pleural space are a recognized route of spread of thymoma that has invaded the pleura. Extrathoracic metastases are rare, although transdiaphragmatic spread of a pleural tumor into the retroperitoneum has been described. For these reasons, it is important to image the entire thorax and upper abdomen in any patient with suspected invasive disease.

In patients with myasthenia gravis who are being evaluated for thymoma, CT can demonstrate tumors that are invisible on conventional radiographs. However, very small thymic tumors may not be distinguishable from a normal or hyperplastic gland with CT, particularly in younger patients with a large amount of residual thymic tissue.

Thymic cysts may be congenital or acquired. Congenital unilocular thymic cysts are rare lesions that represent remnants of the thymopharyngeal duct and contain thin or gelatinous fluid. They are characterized histologically by an epithelial lining, with thymic tissue in the cyst wall, which distinguishes thymic cysts histologically from other congenital cystic lesions within the anterior mediastinum. Acquired multilocular thymic cysts are postinflammatory in nature and have been associated with AIDS, prior radiation or surgery, and autoimmune conditions such as Sjögren syndrome, myasthenia gravis, and aplastic anemia. In these latter conditions,

clinical and radiologic distinction of multilocular thymic cyst from thymoma may be difficult; in fact, the two conditions can coexist. Large cysts will be evident as soft tissue masses on conventional radiographs, and CT or MR will demonstrate the cystic nature of the lesion (3). If the distinction between a true thymic cyst, cystic degeneration of a thymoma or lymphoma, a germ cell neoplasm, or lymphangioma is impossible on clinical and radiologic grounds, the lesion should be biopsied or resected.

Thymolipoma is a rare, benign thymic neoplasm that consists primarily of fat with intermixed rests of normal thymic tissue. These masses are asymptomatic and therefore are typically large when first detected. Chest radiographs show a large anterior mediastinal mass that, because of its pliable nature, tends to envelope the heart and diaphragm. CT demonstrates a fatty mass with interspersed soft tissue densities. Resection is curative.

Thymic Carcinoid. Neuroendocrine tumors of the thymus are rare malignant neoplasms believed to arise from thymic cells of neural crest origin (amine precursor uptake and decarboxylation—APUD or Kulchitsky cells). The most common histologic type is carcinoid tumor, which, as with similar lesions arising within the bronchi, ranges in differentiation and behavior from typical carcinoid to atypical carcinoid to small cell carcinoma. Approximately 40% of patients have Cushing syndrome as a result of adrenocorticotropic hormone secretion by the tumor; these patients tend to have smaller lesions at the time of diagnosis since they present early with signs of corticosteroid excess. The carcinoid syndrome is uncommon. This lesion is indistinguishable from thymoma on plain radiographs and CT scans.

Thymic hyperplasia is defined as enlargement of a thymus that is normal on gross and histologic examination. This rare entity occurs primarily in children as a rebound effect in response to an antecedent stress, discontinuation of chemotherapy, or treatment of hypercortisolism. An association with Graves disease has also been noted. The term *thymic hyperplasia* has been used incorrectly to describe the histologic findings of lymphoid follicular hyperplasia of the thymus, found in 60% of patients with myasthenia gravis. In contrast to most cases of true thymic hyperplasia, lymphoid hyperplasia does not produce thymic enlargement. Most patients with thymic hyperplasia have normal or diffusely enlarged glands on CT (Fig. 13.5); occasionally thymic hyperplasia will present as a mass that is radiographically indistinguishable from thymoma. Most cases can be resolved by noting a decrease in size on follow-up studies, thereby obviating the need for biopsy.

Thymic Lymphoma. The thymus is involved in 40% to 50% of patients with the nodular sclerosing subtype of Hodgkin disease. Its radiographic appearance is indistinguishable from that of other solid neoplasms arising within the thymus. The presence of lymph node enlargement in other portions of the mediastinum or anterior chest wall involvement should suggest the diagnosis.

Lymphoma—either Hodgkin disease or non-Hodgkin lymphoma (NHL)—is the most common primary mediastinal neoplasm in adults. Hodgkin disease involves the thorax in 85% of patients at the time of presentation. The majority (90%) of patients with intrathoracic involvement have mediastinal lymph node enlargement; this most commonly involves the anterior mediastinal and hilar nodal groups. The anterior mediastinum is the most frequent site of a localized nodal mass in patients with Hodgkin disease, particularly those with the nodular sclerosing type (Fig. 13.6). Isolated enlargement of mediastinal or hilar nodes outside the anterior mediastinum should suggest an alternative diagnosis. Only 25% of patients with Hodgkin lymphoma have disease limited to the mediastinum at the time of diagnosis. NHL involves the thorax in approximately 40% of patients at presentation. In contrast to

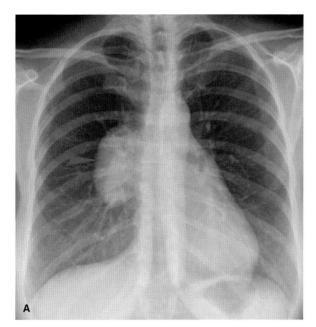

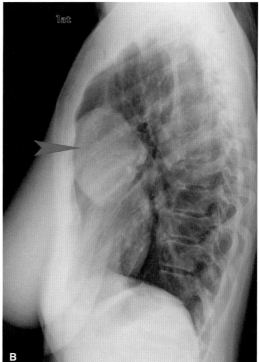

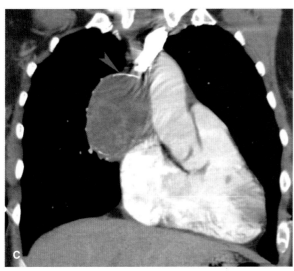

FIGURE 13.3. **Thymoma. A.** Chest radiograph shows a right mediastinal mass (*arrowhead*). Note the right hilum visible through the mass, producing the hilum overlay sign indicating the mass is anterior in location. **B.** Lateral radiograph confirms the anterior location of the mass (*arrowhead*). **C.** Coronal-reformatted contrast-enhanced scan shows a mixed attenuation mass with peripheral calcification (*arrowhead*). Surgical resection revealed a noninvasive thymoma.

Hodgkin disease, only 50% of patients with NHL and intrathoracic disease have mediastinal nodal involvement, and only 10% of NHL patients have disease that is limited to the mediastinum. Of the various subtypes of NHL that present with mediastinal masses, lymphoblastic lymphoma and diffuse large B-cell lymphoma are the most common (Fig. 13.7). Lymphoma involving a single mediastinal or hilar nodal group is much more common in NHL than in Hodgkin disease. NHL most commonly involves middle mediastinal and hilar lymph nodes; juxtaphrenic and posterior mediastinal nodal involvement is uncommon but is seen almost exclusively in NHL. Patterns of pulmonary parenchymal involvement in lymphoma are discussed in Chapter 15.

While Hodgkin disease spreads in a fairly predictable pattern from one nodal group to an adjacent group, NHL is felt to be a multifocal disorder in which patterns of involvement are unpredictable. Localized intrathoracic Hodgkin disease is usually treated with radiation therapy, with 90% response

rates. More widespread Hodgkin disease and NHL are treated with chemotherapy, with better response rates for Hodgkin disease than for NHL.

On conventional radiographs, lymphoma involving the anterior mediastinum is indistinguishable from thymoma or germ cell neoplasm and presents as a lobulated mass projecting to one or both sides (Figs. 13.6, 13.7). Calcification in untreated lymphoma is extremely uncommon, and its presence within an anterior mediastinal mass should suggest another diagnosis. Involvement of other lymph nodes in the mediastinum or hila makes lymphoma more likely. An enlarged spleen displacing the gastric air bubble medially, seen in the upper abdominal portion of the frontal chest film, provides an additional clue to the diagnosis.

CT is performed in virtually all patients with lymphoma. The advantages of chest CT include the ability to better characterize and localize masses seen on chest radiographs; detection of subradiographic sites of involvement that can alter disease

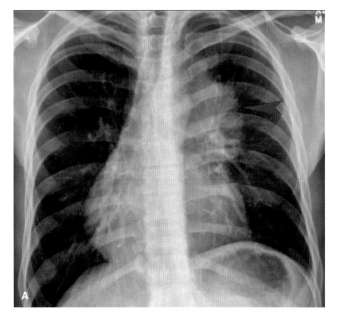

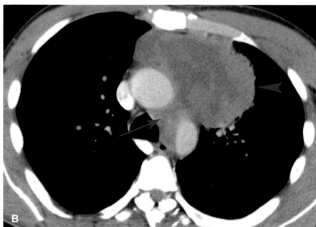

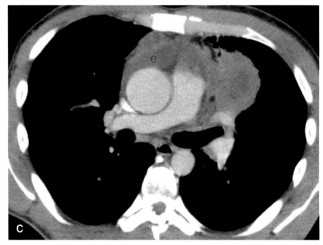

FIGURE 13.4. Invasive Thymoma. A. Posteroanterior chest radiograph reveals a left mediastinal mass (*arrowhead*) with an irregular lateral border. **B.** CT confirms a solid left anterior mediastinal mass (*arrowhead*) with foci of necrosis. Note soft tissue infiltration of the aortopulmonary window (*arrow*) indicating mediastinal invasion. **C.** Axial scan more inferiorly shows broad mediastinal contact by the tumor with associated pericardial effusion (*e*). Mediastinal and pericardial invasion were confirmed at sternotomy.

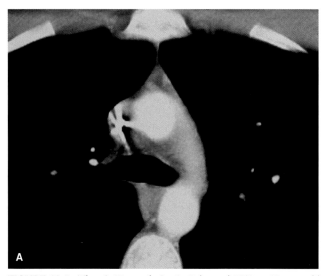

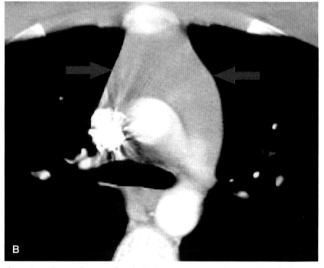

FIGURE 13.5. Thymic Hyperplasia. A. Enhanced CT in a 12-year-old undergoing chemotherapy for rhabdomyosarcoma shows virtual absence of thymic tissue. **B.** Scan 3 months following the completion of chemotherapy shows uniform enlargement of thymus (*arrows*), reflecting rebound hyperplasia.

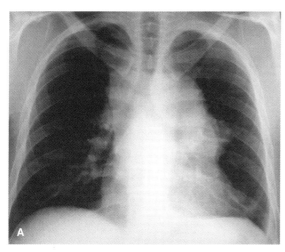
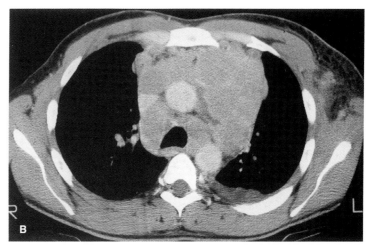

FIGURE 13.6. Hodgkin Lymphoma. A. Posteroanterior chest radiograph in a 35-year-old man shows a large, lobulated mediastinal mass. B. Contrast-enhanced CT at the level of the aortic arch shows bulky anterior and middle mediastinal lymphadenopathy.

staging, prognosis, and therapy; guidance for transthoracic or open biopsy; the ability to monitor response to therapy; and detection of relapse. The appearance of nodal involvement in lymphoma varies; most commonly, discrete enlarged solid lymph nodes or conglomerate masses of nodes are seen (Fig. 13.6B). Central necrosis, seen in 20% of patients, has no prognostic significance. Nodal calcification is rare in the absence of previous mediastinal radiation or systemic chemotherapy. Parenchymal involvement is usually the result of direct extranodal extension of a tumor from hilar nodes along the bronchovascular lymphatics; this is better appreciated on axial CT images than on chest radiographs (4,5). Likewise, a tumor extending from the mediastinum to the pericardium, subpleural space, and chest wall is best appreciated on CT or MR. On MR, untreated lymphoma appears as a mass of uniform low-signal intensity on T1WIs and uniform high-signal intensity or intermixed areas of low- and high-signal intensity on T2WIs. The areas of low-signal intensity on T2WIs of untreated patients may be a result of foci of fibrotic tissue in nodular sclerosing Hodgkin disease.

CT and fluorodeoxyglucose (FDG) PET are used to monitor the response of lymphoma to therapy. While CT can accurately assess tumor regression and detect relapse within nodal groups outside the treated region, the ability to distinguish residual tumor from sterilized fibrotic masses is limited. Residual soft tissue masses have been reported in up to 50% of patients, most commonly with nodular sclerosing Hodgkin disease, and are more common when the pretreatment mass is large. Some patients with residual masses on CT or MR will have tumor recurrence within 6 to 12 months after the completion of therapy. In general, the appearance of high-signal intensity regions on T2WIs more than 6 months after treatment should suggest recurrence. Radionuclide scintigraphy with gallium-67, particularly SPECT, has been largely replaced by FDG-PET in the initial diagnosis and staging of thoracic lymphoma. PET is clearly superior to CT or MR in distinguishing recurrent tumor from fibrosis in both Hodgkin disease and NHL.

Germ cell neoplasms, which include teratoma, seminoma, choriocarcinoma, endodermal sinus tumor, and embryonal cell carcinoma, arise from collections of primitive germ cells

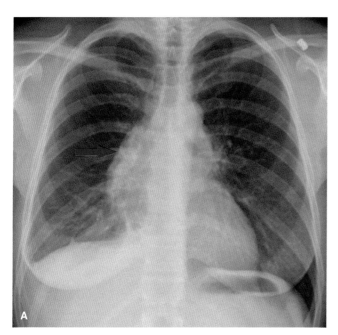
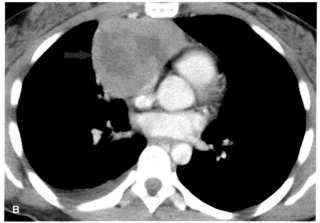

FIGURE 13.7. Non-Hodgkin Lymphoma, Diffuse Large B-cell Type. A. Chest radiograph shows a right anterior mediastinal mass (*arrow*). There is a small right pleural effusion. B. Contrast-enhanced CT scan shows a large anterior mediastinal mass with mixed attenuation (*arrow*) with associated small right pleural effusion. Core needle biopsy showed diffuse large B-cell lymphoma.

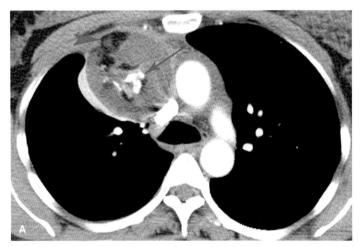 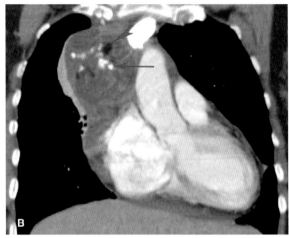

FIGURE 13.8. Mature Teratoma. Axial (**A**) and coronal-reformatted (**B**) contrast-enhanced CT in a 46-year-old female reveals an anterior mediastinal mass with foci of calcification (*arrow*) and fat (*arrowhead*). Surgical resection confirmed a mature teratoma.

that arrest in the anterior mediastinum on their journey to the gonads during embryologic development. Since they are histologically indistinguishable from germ cell tumors arising in the testes and ovaries, the diagnosis of a primary malignant mediastinal germ cell neoplasm requires exclusion of a primary gonadal tumor as a source of mediastinal metastases. A key in distinguishing primary from metastatic mediastinal germ cell neoplasm is the presence of retroperitoneal lymph node involvement in metastatic gonadal tumors.

The most common benign mediastinal germ cell neoplasm is teratoma, comprising 60% to 70% of mediastinal germ cell neoplasms. Teratomas may be cystic or solid. Cystic or mature teratoma is the most common type of teratoma seen in the mediastinum. In contrast to a dermoid cyst, which is an ovarian neoplasm containing only elements derived from the ectodermal germinal layer, a cystic teratoma of the mediastinum commonly contains tissues of ectodermal, mesodermal, and endodermal origins. For this reason, it is inaccurate to use the term "dermoid cyst" to describe cystic mediastinal germ cell neoplasms. Solid teratomas are usually malignant, with seminoma comprising 25% to 50% of such lesions (6). Most germ cell neoplasms are detected in patients in the third or fourth decade of life. While benign tumors have a slight female preponderance (female/male, 60%/40%), malignant tumors are seen almost exclusively in men.

Radiographically, these tumors have a distribution similar to that of thymomas. While the majority are located in the anterior mediastinum, up to 10% are found in the posterior mediastinum. Benign lesions are often round or oval and smooth in contour; an irregular, lobulated, or ill-defined margin suggests malignancy. Calcification is present in 33% to 50% of tumors but is nonspecific unless in the form of a tooth. On CT, benign teratomas are usually cystic and may contain soft tissue, bone, teeth, fat, or, rarely, fat–fluid levels (Fig. 13.8). Seminoma, choriocarcinoma, and endodermal sinus (yolk sac) tumors are malignant lesions seen primarily in young men. Seminoma is the most common malignant germ cell neoplasm, accounting for 30% of these tumors. The radiographic findings are nonspecific. CT typically shows a large, lobulated soft tissue mass that may contain areas of hemorrhage, calcification, or necrosis (Fig. 13.9). Elevated serum levels of α-fetoprotein or human chorionic gonadotropin are helpful in the diagnosis of suspected malignant mediastinal germ cell neoplasm, while clinical and CT evidence of gynecomastia is an additional clue.

Thyroid Masses. While masses arising from the thyroid can present as anterior and superior mediastinal masses, these lesions are best considered as thoracic inlet masses, as discussed earlier.

Mesenchymal Tumors. Benign and malignant tumors arising from the fibrous, fatty, muscular, or vascular tissues of the mediastinum may present as mediastinal masses, most commonly in the anterior mediastinum. Lipomas can occur in any location in the mediastinum but are most often anterior. The diagnosis is made by the recognition of a well-defined mass of uniform fatty attenuation (under –50 H). The presence of soft tissue elements should raise the possibility of a thymolipoma or liposarcoma; the latter may show evidence of invasion of adjacent structures at the time of diagnosis. Fat within a mature teratoma or transdiaphragmatic herniation of omental fat is usually easily distinguished from a lipoma.

Hemangiomas are benign tumors composed of vascular channels and may be associated with the syndrome of hereditary hemorrhagic telangiectasia. A pathognomonic sign on chest radiographs is the recognition of phleboliths within a smooth or lobulated soft tissue mass. Angiosarcomas are rare malignant vascular neoplasms that are indistinguishable from other invasive neoplasms arising within the anterior mediastinum.

Leiomyomas are rare benign neoplasms that arise from smooth muscle within the mediastinum. Similarly, fibromas and mesenchymomas (tumors that contain more than one mesenchymal element) can appear as anterior mediastinal masses.

Middle Mediastinal Masses

Lymph Node Enlargement and Masses (Table 13.3). Most middle mediastinal lymph node masses are malignant, representing metastases from bronchogenic carcinoma (Fig. 13.10), extrathoracic malignancy, or lymphoma (7). Benign causes of middle mediastinal lymph node enlargement include sarcoidosis, mycobacterial and fungal infection, angiofollicular lymph node hyperplasia (Castleman disease), and angioimmunoblastic lymphadenopathy.

On plain radiographs, several findings suggest that a middle mediastinal mass represents lymph node enlargement. The presence of multiple bilateral mediastinal masses that distort the lung/mediastinal interface is relatively specific for lymph node enlargement. Solitary masses resulting from lymph node enlargement tend to be elongated and lobulated rather than spherical, since usually more than a single node in a vertical chain of nodes is involved. Occasionally, calcification can be detected within enlarged lymph nodes on plain radiographs;

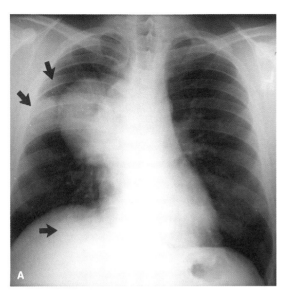
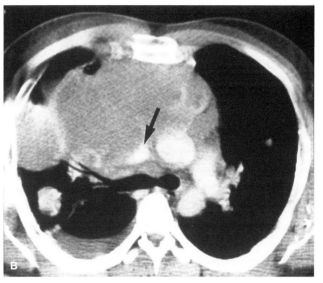

FIGURE 13.9. Malignant Germ Cell Tumor. A. Posteroanterior chest radiograph in a 38-year-old man reveals a right mediastinal mass with discrete right lung nodules (*arrows*). **B.** Contrast-enhanced CT demonstrates a large anterior mediastinal mass invading the superior vena cava (*arrow*) with right lung nodules and a small pleural effusion. CT-guided biopsy showed choriocarcinoma.

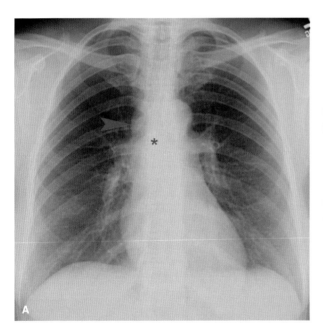
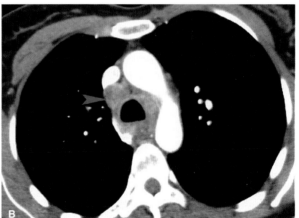
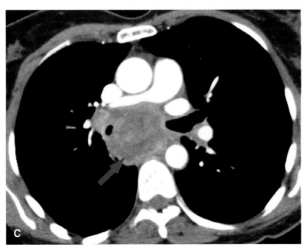

FIGURE 13.10. Adenocarcinoma With Enlarged Middle Mediastinal and Hilar Nodes. A. Chest radiograph shows enlarged right paratracheal (*arrowhead*) and subcarinal (*asterisk*) nodes. **B** and **C.** Axial contrast-enhanced scans shows enlarged, necrotic right paratracheal (*arrowhead*) and subcarinal (*arrow*) nodes. Bronchoscopic biopsy revealed adenocarcinoma.

TABLE 13.3

MIDDLE MEDIASTINAL MASSES

Lymph node masses	Malignancy
	Bronchogenic carcinoma
	Lymphoma
	Leukemia
	Kaposi sarcoma
	Extrathoracic malignancy
	Head and neck tumors (squamous cell carcinoma of skin, larynx; thyroid carcinoma)
	Genitourinary tumors (renal cell carcinoma, seminoma)
	Breast carcinoma
	Melanoma
	Infection
	Bacteria
	Anaerobic lung abscess
	Anthrax
	Plague
	Tularemia
	Tuberculosis
	Fungi
	Histoplasmosis
	Coccidioidomycosis
	Cryptococcosis
	Viral infection
	Measles
	Mononucleosis
	Idiopathic
	Sarcoidosis
	Castleman disease
	Angioimmunoblastic lymphadenopathy
Foregut and mesothelial cysts	Bronchogenic cyst
	Pericardial cyst
Tracheal and central bronchial neoplasms	Malignant
	Carcinoid tumor (bronchi)
	Adenoid cystic carcinoma (trachea)
	Squamous cell carcinoma
Diaphragmatic hernias	Foramen of Morgagni hernia
	Traumatic hernia
Vascular lesions	Arterial
	Double arch/right arch
	Tortuous innominate/subclavian artery
	Aneurysm of the aortic arch
	Venous
	Dilated azygos vein
	Dilated hemiazygos vein
	Dilated SVC
	Left-sided SVC
	Dilated left superior intercostal vein
	Dilatation of the main pulmonary artery

SVC, superior vena cava.

CT is more sensitive in detecting nodal calcification and its distribution within lymph nodes.

One of the prime indications for performing thoracic CT is to detect the presence of enlarged mediastinal lymph nodes. CT is most often obtained to confirm an abnormal chest radiographic

TABLE 13.4

DENSITY OF MEDIASTINAL/HILAR NODES ON CT

Calcification		
Central	Mycobacteria	
	Fungus	
Peripheral (eggshell)	Silicosis	
	Sarcoidosis	
Hypervascular	Carcinoid tumor/small cell carcinoma	
	Kaposi sarcoma	
	Metastases	
	Renal cell carcinoma	
	Thyroid carcinoma	
	Castleman disease	
Necrosis	Mycobacteria	
	Fungus	
	Metastases	
	Squamous cell carcinoma	
	Seminoma	
	Lymphoma	

finding or to evaluate a patient with suspected mediastinal disease despite normal radiographs (a patient with a suspicious solitary pulmonary nodule or with cervical Hodgkin disease). The ability of CT to image in the axial plane and its inherent high-contrast resolution allow for the recognition of abnormally enlarged lymph nodes that would not be evident on chest radiographs. In general, abnormal lymph nodes are seen as round or oval soft tissue masses that measure larger than 1.0 cm in their short-axis diameter. Although CT is unable to distinguish between benign inflammatory nodes and those involved by malignancy based upon size criteria alone, CT can provide useful information about the internal density of the nodes (Table 13.4).

A standardized classification system for hilar and mediastinal lymph nodes is the American Thoracic Society (ATS) map (Fig. 13.11). This scheme correlates with easily identifiable CT and anatomic landmarks and is most important when reporting lymph node enlargement in patients with bronchogenic carcinoma. A recently recommended new lymph node map has been proposed by the International Association for the Staging of Lung Cancer (8). A diagram of this simplified seven-station nodal map is illustrated in Chapter 15, Figure 15.20.

MR is as sensitive as CT in detecting enlarged mediastinal lymph nodes. Advantages of MR include the absence of iodinated contrast, easy distinction between vascular and soft tissue structures, exquisite contrast resolution between mediastinal nodes and fat on T1W sequences, and the ability to image in the direct coronal or sagittal plane. The latter feature is an advantage in those mediastinal regions that parallel the axial plane (subcarinal space, aortopulmonary window) and therefore tend to suffer from partial volume-averaging effects on CT. The major disadvantages of MR at present are the inability to detect nodal calcification and limited spatial resolution; the latter can result in an inability to distinguish between a group of normal size nodes and a single enlarged node, thereby leading to false-positive results.

In addition to the detection and characterization of enlarged mediastinal nodes, CT can help guide diagnostic nodal tissue sampling. This is usually most helpful in the setting of suspected bronchogenic carcinoma, where accurate staging of mediastinal nodal disease is important for prognostic purposes and treatment planning. The recognition of enlarged subcarinal or pretracheal nodes on CT may suggest biopsy via transcarinal Wang needle or mediastinoscopy, respectively.

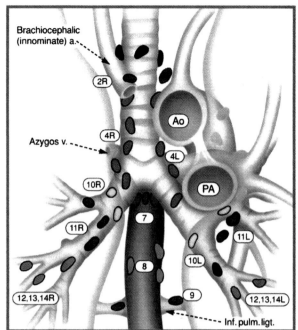

Superior Mediastinal Nodes

- **1** Highest Mediastinal
- **2** Upper Paratracheal
- **3** Pre-vascular and Retrotracheal
- **4** Lower Paratracheal (including Azygos Nodes)

N_2 = single digit, ipsilateral
N_3 = single digit, contralateral or supraclavicular

Aortic Nodes

- **5** Subaortic (A-P window)
- **6** Para-aortic (ascending aorta or phrenic)

Inferior Mediastinal Nodes

- **7** Subcarinal
- **8** Paraesophageal (below carina)
- **9** Pulmonary Ligament

N_1 Nodes

- **10** Hilar
- **11** Interlobar
- **12** Lobar
- **13** Segmental
- **14** Subsegmental

(Mountain/Dresler modifications from Naruke/ATS-LCSG Map)

© 1997 Reprints are permissible for educational use only.

FIGURE 13.11. **American Thoracic Society Nodal Stations.** Ao, aorta; PA, pulmonary artery. (From Mountain CF, Dresler CM. Regional lymph node classification for lung cancer staging. Chest 1997;111:1718–1723; reprinted with permission.)

As mentioned above, mediastinal lymph node enlargement is common in Hodgkin disease and NHL. Lymphoma accounts for 20% of all mediastinal neoplasms in adults, and most patients with intrathoracic lymphoma have concomitant extrathoracic disease. In most patients, the nodal enlargement is bilateral but asymmetric (Fig. 13.12). Nodular sclerosing Hodgkin disease commonly results in lymph node enlargement, predominantly within the anterior mediastinum and thymus. Isolated posterior nodal enlargement is usually seen only in patients with NHL.

Leukemia, particularly the T-lymphocytic varieties, can cause intrathoracic lymph node enlargement. The lymph node enlargement is usually confined to the middle mediastinal and hilar nodes.

The most common source of metastases to middle mediastinal nodes is bronchogenic carcinoma. In the majority of patients, symptoms or plain radiographic findings suggest the presence of a primary tumor in the lung. In a small percentage of patients, particularly those with small cell carcinoma,

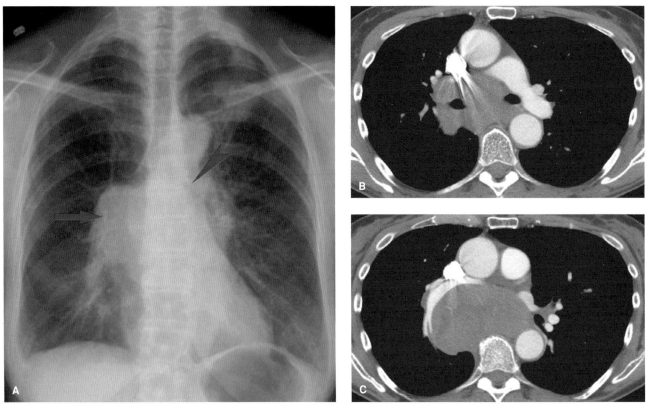

FIGURE 13.12. Right Hilar/Middle Mediastinal Mass Due to Non-Hodgkin Lymphoma. A. Chest radiograph shows a right hilar and subcarinal mass (*arrow*). Note splaying of the carina and narrowing of the left main bronchus (*arrowhead*). The density overlying the left upper lobe is an artifact. **B** and **C.** Axial contrast-enhanced CT scans show a right hilar and subcarinal soft tissue mass. CT-guided core biopsy revealed non-Hodgkin lymphoma.

the primary carcinoma may be inconspicuous or invisible on plain radiographs, with nodal metastases being the only visible abnormality. Lymph node enlargement is often unilateral on the side of the visible pulmonary or hilar abnormality (Fig. 13.13). Paratracheal and aorticopulmonary nodes are most commonly involved. Since the accuracy of CT in predicting the presence or absence of mediastinal lymph node metasta-

ses is approximately 60% to 70%, PET—and in particular integrated CT/PET—should be performed in most patients with bronchogenic carcinoma. A more thorough discussion of mediastinal nodal involvement in bronchogenic carcinoma may be found in Chapter 15.

Lymph node metastases from extrathoracic malignancies can result in mediastinal node enlargement, either with or

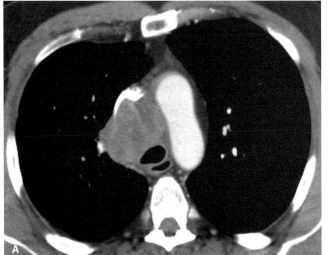
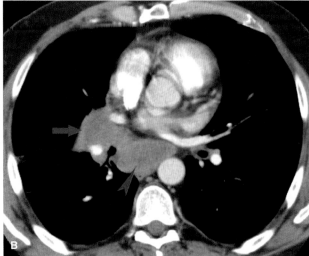

FIGURE 13.13. Middle Mediastinal Lymph Node Enlargement From Small Cell Carcinoma of Lung. Axial contrast-enhanced CT scans at the level of the aortic arch (**A**) and top of left atrium (**B**) show enlarged right lower paratracheal, right hilar-interlobar (*arrow*), and subcarinal (*arrowhead*) lymph nodes.

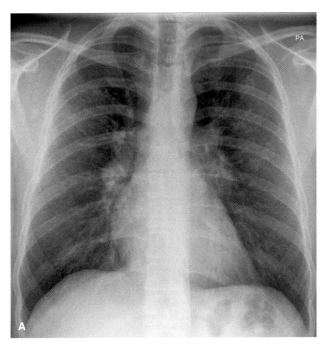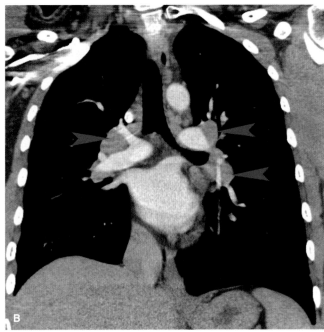

FIGURE 13.14. **Lymphadenopathy in Sarcoidosis. A.** Posteroanterior radiograph in a 46-year-old man with sarcoidosis reveals bilateral hilar lymph node enlargement with upper and mid lung reticulonodular opacities. **B.** Coronal reformatted contrast-enhanced CT at the level of the carina shows bilateral hilar lymph node enlargement (*arrowheads*).

without concomitant pulmonary metastases. These mediastinal nodal metastases may result from inferior extension of neck masses (thyroid carcinoma, head and neck tumors); extension along the lymphatic channels from below the diaphragm (testicular or renal cell carcinoma, and GI malignancies); or hematogenous extension (breast carcinoma, melanoma, and Kaposi sarcoma) (9).

Mediastinal lymph node enlargement is very common in patients with sarcoidosis, occurring in 60% to 90% of patients at some stage of their disease. Nodal enlargement is typically bilateral and symmetric and involves the hila as well as the mediastinum (Fig. 13.14); this usually allows for differentiation of sarcoidosis from lymphoma and metastatic disease. In sarcoidosis, the enlarged nodes produce a lobulated appearance on chest radiographs and CT, because the enlarged nodes do not coalesce. This is in contrast to lymphoma and nodal metastases, in which the intranodal tumor extends through the nodal capsule to form conglomerate enlarged nodal masses. Right and left paratracheal lymph nodes are typically involved; anterior or posterior mediastinal nodal enlargement has been described with greater frequency recently, probably as a result of the improved sensitivity of CT for detecting nodal involvement in these regions.

A variety of infections, most commonly histoplasmosis, coccidioidomycosis, cryptococcosis, and tuberculosis, can cause mediastinal nodal enlargement (Fig. 13.15). Typically these patients have parenchymal opacities on chest radiographs, but isolated lymph node enlargement may be seen, particularly in children and young adults. Bacterial infections such as anthrax, bubonic plague, and tularemia are uncommon causes of lymph node enlargement. Typically, there will be symptoms and signs of acute infection, and chest radiographs will show evidence of pneumonia. Bacterial lung abscesses also may be associated with reactive lymph node enlargement. Hilar and mediastinal lymph nodes may be enlarged in patients with measles pneumonia and infectious mononucleosis.

Angiofollicular lymph node hyperplasia (Castleman disease) is characterized by enlargement of hilar and mediastinal lymph

nodes, predominantly in the middle and posterior mediastinal compartments. In the more common hyaline vascular type, the disease is localized to one lymph node region and presents as an asymptomatic mediastinal soft tissue mass. Histologically, there is replacement of normal nodal architecture with multiple germinal centers and multiple small vessels with hyalinized walls that course perpendicularly toward the germinal centers to give

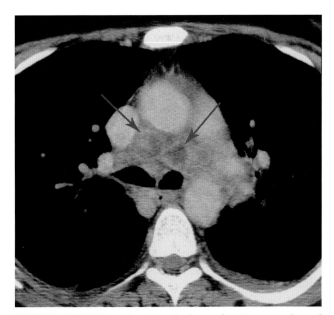

FIGURE 13.15. **Tuberculous Lymphadenopathy.** Contrast-enhanced CT at the level of the tracheal carina demonstrates enlarged precarinal and left peribronchial lymph nodes (*arrows*) with central necrosis and peripheral enhancement. Material obtained by mediastinoscopy revealed *Mycobacterium tuberculosis*.

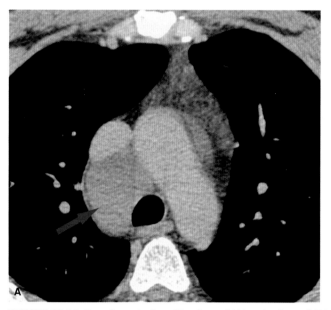 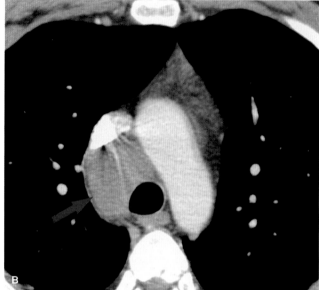

FIGURE 13.16. Bronchogenic Cyst. Unenhanced (**A**) and enhanced (**B**) CT scans in a 38-year-old man demonstrate a smooth, low-attenuation paratracheal mass (*arrows*) that fails to enhance, consistent with a bronchogenic cyst.

a characteristic "lollipop" appearance on light microscopy. The vascular nature of these masses accounts for the intense enhancement seen on contrast-enhanced CT or angiography. Calcification within these masses has been described. These lesions are cured by resection.

Angioimmunoblastic lymphadenopathy is a rare disorder seen in older adults; it is characterized by constitutional symptoms, lymphadenopathy, hepatosplenomegaly, and skin rash. Hemolytic anemia and hypergammaglobulinemia may be seen. Histologically, the enlarged nodes contain a chronic inflammatory infiltrate and are hypervascular. Chest radiographs and CT show hilar and mediastinal lymph node enlargement that are indistinguishable from other etiologies. As with Castleman disease, the vascular nature of the involved lymph nodes accounts for the contrast enhancement seen on CT. These patients manifest signs of immunodeficiency similar to those associated with AIDS, with one-third developing high-grade lymphoma and many succumbing to opportunistic infections such as *Pneumocystis carinii* pneumonia and cytomegalovirus inclusion disease.

Foregut and mesothelial cysts are common mediastinal lesions that typically present as asymptomatic masses on routine chest radiographs in young adults. CT and MR show findings characteristic of the cystic nature of these lesions.

Congenital bronchogenic cysts result from anomalous budding of the tracheobronchial tree during development. To be characterized as bronchogenic in origin, the wall of the cyst must be lined by a respiratory epithelium with pseudostratified columnar cells and contain seromucous glands; some may contain cartilage and smooth muscle within their walls. It is often difficult to distinguish between bronchogenic and enteric cysts based on their location and pathologic appearance; the term *foregut cyst* has been used to describe those lesions that cannot be specifically characterized. The majority of bronchogenic cysts (80% to 90%) arise within the mediastinum in the vicinity of the tracheal carina. Most mediastinal lesions are asymptomatic; occasionally, compression of the tracheobronchial tree or esophagus may produce dyspnea, wheezing, or dysphagia. Rarely, mediastinal cysts become secondarily infected after communication with the airway or esophagus, or they cause symptomatic compression after rapid enlargement following

hemorrhage. Bronchogenic cysts are seen as soft tissue masses in the subcarinal or right paratracheal space on frontal chest radiographs; less common sites of involvement include the hilum, posterior mediastinum, and periesophageal region. They appear as a single smooth, round, or elliptic mass; a minority are lobulated in contour. CT is the method of choice for the diagnosis of a mediastinal cyst. If a well-defined, thin-walled mass of fluid density (0 to 10 H) is seen that fails to enhance following IV contrast administration, it can be assumed to represent a benign cyst (Fig. 13.16) (10). High CT numbers (>40 H) suggesting a solid mass can be seen when the cyst is filled with mucoid material, milk of calcium, or blood. Calcification of the cyst wall has been described but is uncommon. MR shows characteristic low-signal intensity on T1WIs and high-signal intensity on T2WIs. The presence of proteinaceous material within the cyst will shorten T1 relaxation times, yielding high-signal intensity on T1WIs. In many patients, resection is required for definitive diagnosis. Both transbronchoscopic and percutaneous needle aspiration and drainage have been used successfully for the diagnosis and treatment of these lesions.

Pericardial cysts arise from the parietal pericardium and contain clear serous fluid surrounded by a layer of mesothelial cells. Most often, they arise in the anterior cardiophrenic angles, with right-sided lesions being twice as common as left-sided lesions; approximately 20% arise more superiorly within the mediastinum. These lesions usually present as incidental asymptomatic round or oval masses in the cardiophrenic angle (Fig. 13.17). Their pliable nature can be demonstrated with a change in patient position. CT typically shows a unilocular cystic mass adjacent to the heart; MR or US via a subxiphoid approach shows findings characteristic of a simple cyst. As with bronchogenic cysts, there have been reports of cysts with high attenuation on CT that on resection are found to be filled with proteinaceous or mucoid material.

Tracheal and central bronchial masses commonly produce upper airway symptoms with obstructive pneumonitis and atelectasis and rarely present as asymptomatic mediastinal masses. Occasionally, central airway masses present as radiographic abnormalities when they distort the tracheal air column or mediastinal contour. These masses are discussed in Chapter 18.

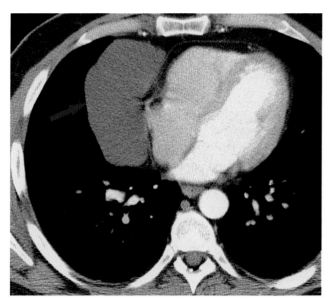

FIGURE 13.17. Pericardial Cyst. Enhanced CT scan through heart shows a smooth, sharply marginated, low-attenuation mass (*arrow*) in the right cardiophrenic angle, consistent with a pericardial cyst.

Diaphragmatic hernias, which may present as pericardiac masses, are discussed in Chapter 19.

Vascular Lesions. Congenital or acquired anomalies of the heart and great vessels are common middle mediastinal masses and are discussed in Chapter 14.

Neurogenic Lesions. Rarely, a neurofibroma arising from the phrenic nerve may present as a middle mediastinal juxtacardiac mass.

Posterior Mediastinal Masses

Neurogenic Tumors (Table 13.5). Posterior mediastinal masses arising from neural elements are classified by their tissue of origin. Three groups have been recognized: (*1*) tumors arising from intercostal nerves (neurofibroma, schwannoma); (*2*) sympathetic ganglia (ganglioneuroma, ganglioneuroblastoma, and neuroblastoma); and (*3*) paraganglionic cells (chemodectoma, pheochromocytoma). Tumors in each of these three groups may be benign or malignant neoplasms (6). Although neurogenic tumors can occur at any age, they are most common in young patients. Neuroblastoma and ganglioneuroma are most common in children, whereas neurofibroma and schwannoma affect adults more frequently.

Histologically, both neurofibroma and schwannoma are comprised of spindle cells that arise from the Schwann cell. While neurofibroma is an encapsulated tumor that contains interspersed neurons, schwannoma is not encapsulated and contains no neuronal elements. Both tumors are more common in patients with neurofibromatosis. Multiple lesions in the mediastinum, particularly bilateral apicoposterior masses, are virtually diagnostic of neurofibromatosis. A small percentage of schwannomas (10%) are locally invasive (malignant schwannoma).

Radiographically, intercostal nerve tumors appear as round or oval paravertebral soft tissue masses. CT shows a smooth or lobulated paraspinal soft tissue mass, which may erode the adjacent vertebral body or rib. CT demonstration of tumor extension from the paravertebral space into the spinal canal via an enlarged intervertebral foramen is characteristic of a "dumbbell" neurofibroma. MR is the modality of choice for

TABLE 13.5	
POSTERIOR MEDIASTINAL MASSES	
Neurogenic tumors	Peripheral (intercostal) nerves
	Neurofibroma
	Schwannoma
	Sympathetic ganglia
	Ganglioneuroma
	Ganglioneuroblastoma
	Neuroblastoma
	Paraganglion cells
	Chemodectoma
	Pheochromocytoma
Esophageal lesions	Duplication (enteric) cyst
	Diverticulum
	Neoplasm
	Leiomyoma
	Squamous cell carcinoma
	Esophageal dilatation
	Achalasia
	Scleroderma
	Peptic stricture
	Carcinoma
	Paraesophageal varices
	Hiatal hernia
	Sliding
	Paraesophageal
Foregut cysts	Enteric
	Neurenteric
Vertebral lesion	Trauma
	Paraspinal hematoma
	Infection
	Paraspinal abscess
	Tuberculosis
	Staphylococcus
	Tumor
	Metastases (bronchogenic, breast, renal cell carcinoma)
	Multiple myeloma
	Lymphoma
	Degenerative disease (osteophytosis)
	Extramedullary hematopoiesis
Lateral thoracic meningocele	
Pancreatic pseudocyst	

imaging a suspected neurofibroma. In addition to the occasional demonstration of both intra- and extra-spinal canal components, MR of neurofibromas shows typical high-signal intensity on T2WIs.

Tumors that arise from the sympathetic ganglia represent a continuum from the histologically benign ganglioneuroma found in adolescents and young adults to the highly malignant neuroblastoma seen almost exclusively in children under the age of 5 years. These tumors generally present as elongated, vertically oriented paravertebral soft tissue masses with a broad area of contact with the posterior mediastinum (Figs. 13.18, 13.19). These findings may help distinguish these lesions from neurofibromas, which usually maintain an acute angle with the vertebral column and posterior mediastinum and therefore tend to show sharp superior and inferior margins on lateral chest radiographs. Large masses may erode vertebral bodies

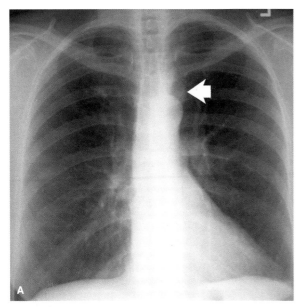
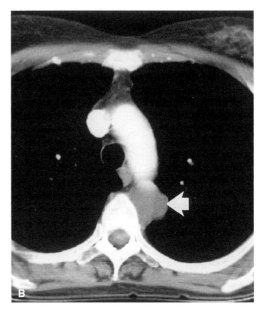

FIGURE 13.18. Neurofibroma. A. Frontal chest radiograph shows a left upper mediastinal mass (*arrow*). **B.** Contrast-enhanced CT confirms the presence of a left paravertebral soft tissue mass (*arrow*). Surgical resection confirmed a neurofibroma.

or ribs. Calcification, seen in up to 25% of cases, is a helpful diagnostic feature of these tumors but does not help distinguish benign from malignant neoplasms. Because these tumors often produce catecholamines, urinary levels of vanillylmandelic acid or metanephrines, which are byproducts of catecholamine metabolism, may be elevated. Prognosis depends upon the histologic features of the tumor and the patient's age and extent of disease at the time of diagnosis.

Paragangliomas are tumors that arise in the aorticopulmonary paraganglia of the middle mediastinum or the aortico-sympathetic ganglia of the posterior mediastinum. They are divided into nonfunctioning neoplasms (chemo-dectomas), which occur almost exclusively in or about the aortopulmonary window, and functioning neoplasms (pheochromocytomas), which are found in the posterior sympathetic chain or in or about the heart or pericardium. Approximately 2% of

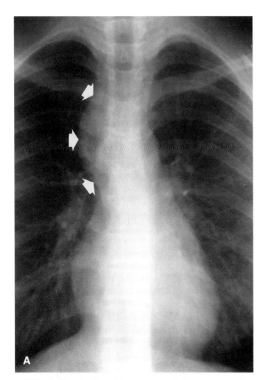
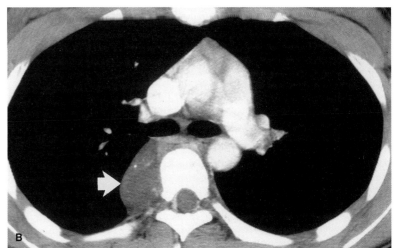

FIGURE 13.19. Ganglioneuroma. A. Posteroanterior radiograph in a 15-year-old woman reveals an oval, vertically oriented, right-sided mediastinal mass (*arrows*). **B.** Contrast-enhanced CT shows a low-attenuation posterior mediastinal mass (*arrow*) with calcification. This was surgically proven to be ganglioneuroma.

all pheochromocytomas arise in the mediastinum. The posterior mediastinum is the site of fewer than 25% of mediastinal paragangliomas, with the majority arising in the anterior or middle mediastinum. Radiographically, these tumors are indistinguishable from other neurogenic tumors. However, most patients have hypertension and biochemical evidence of excess catecholamine production. CT and angiography demonstrate hypervascular masses; radionuclide iodine-131-meta-iodobenzylguanidine scanning is diagnostic in functioning tumors.

Esophageal Lesions. Because most of the intrathoracic esophagus is intimately associated with the thoracic spine and descending thoracic aorta, lesions in the middle or distal third of the esophagus may present as posterior mediastinal masses. Common presenting symptoms include dysphagia and aspiration pneumonia, although many patients are asymptomatic.

The majority of esophageal neoplasms, excluding lesions that arise at the esophagogastric junction, are squamous cell carcinomas. Unlike benign neoplasms of the posterior mediastinum, these lesions, when seen on chest radiographs, are rarely asymptomatic. Typically, these patients have a history of dysphagia and significant weight loss. Difficulty in detecting asymptomatic lesions and the absence of a serosa account for the advanced stage of most esophageal carcinoma at presentation and a 5-year survival rate of less than 20%. Most patients with esophageal carcinoma have abnormal plain radiographic findings, including an abnormal azygoesophageal interface,

widening of the mediastinum (resulting from the tumor itself or a dilated esophagus proximal to the obstructing lesion), abnormal thickening of the tracheoesophageal stripe, and tracheal deviation and compression. The diagnosis is usually made on barium esophagram and confirmed by endoscopic biopsy. CT scanning has proved accurate for staging esophageal carcinoma: findings include an intraluminal mass; thickening of the esophageal wall; loss of fat planes between the esophagus and adjacent mediastinal structures (usually the trachea, with upper esophageal lesions, and the descending aorta, with lower esophageal lesions); and evidence of nodal and distant metastases.

Several benign esophageal neoplasms, including leiomyoma, fibroma, and lipoma, can present as smooth, solitary mediastinal masses projecting laterally from the posterior mediastinum on frontal chest radiographs. They generally involve the lower third of the esophagus from the level of the subcarinal space to the esophageal hiatus. Initial evaluation is with barium studies, which show a smooth, broad-based mass forming obtuse margins with the esophageal wall. CT demonstrates a smooth, well-defined soft tissue mass adjacent to the esophagus without obstruction. The absence of esophageal dilatation above the mass helps distinguish benign tumors from carcinoma.

Pulsion diverticula arising at the cervicothoracic esophageal junction or distal esophagus (Fig. 13.20) are false diverticula representing mucosal outpouchings through defects in

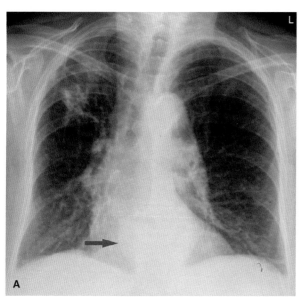

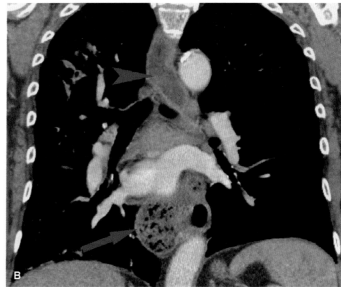

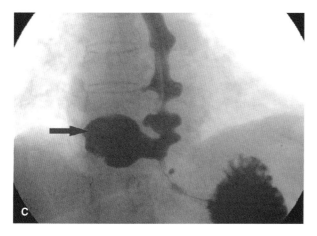

FIGURE 13.20. **Esophageal Pulsion Diverticulum in Achalasia. A.** Frontal radiograph demonstrates a mass in the azygoesophageal recess (*arrow*) containing an air–fluid level. Patchy right upper lobe consolidation reflects aspiration pneumonia. **B.** Coronal reformatted contrast-enhanced CT through the esophagus shows a focal outpouching (*arrow*) extending right lateral from a distended esophagus. Note the fluid-filled dilated proximal esophagus (*arrowhead*). **C.** Contrast esophagram shows a diverticulum (*arrow*) above a narrowed esophagogastric junction.

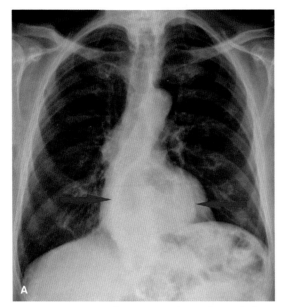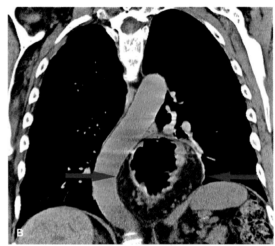

FIGURE 13.21. Hiatal Hernia. A. Chest radiograph shows a retrocardiac mass containing air (*arrows*). **B.** Coronal reformatted CT scan at the level of the descending aorta shows a hiatal hernia (*arrows*).

the muscular layer of the esophagus. A large proximal pulsion diverticulum (Zenker) may extend through the thoracic inlet and appear as a retroesophageal superior mediastinal mass containing an air–fluid level on upright chest radiographs. A distal pulsion diverticulum appears as a juxtadiaphragmatic mass with an air–fluid level projecting to the right of midline. Barium swallow is diagnostic.

A dilated esophagus resulting from functional (achalasia, scleroderma) or anatomic (stricture, carcinoma) obstruction may produce a mass that courses vertically over the length of the mediastinum, projecting toward the right side on frontal chest radiographs. An air–fluid level on upright films is usually present. A completely air-filled, dilated esophagus appears as a thin curvilinear line along the medial right thorax, because the right lateral wall of the esophagus is outlined by intraluminal air medially and the right lung laterally. Barium study or CT will confirm the diagnosis of a dilated esophagus; determination of the cause of obstruction often requires endoscopy or esophageal manometry.

Esophageal varices may produce a round or lobulated retrocardiac mass in patients with portal hypertension. The diagnosis is usually made by endoscopic recognition of submucosal varices involving the distal esophagus. The varices are readily recognized on contrast CT, MR, or portal venography.

A common cause of a mass in the posteroinferior mediastinum is a hiatal hernia. This results from a separation of the superior margins of the diaphragmatic crura and stretching of the phrenicoesophageal ligament. The stomach is by far the most common structure in the hernia sac (Fig. 13.21); the gastric cardia (sliding hernia) or fundus (paraesophageal hernia) may be involved. Rarely, omental fat, ascitic fluid, or a pancreatic pseudocyst herniates through the esophageal hiatus into the mediastinum. The characteristic location at the esophageal hiatus and the presence of a rounded density containing an air or air–fluid level on upright films are diagnostic. Barium swallow or a CT scan will confirm the diagnosis (see Fig. 19.25).

Enteric/Neurenteric Cysts. Enteric cysts are fluid-filled masses lined by enteric epithelium. Esophageal cysts usually arise intramurally or immediately adjacent to the esophagus. When an enteric cyst has a persistent communication with

the spinal canal (canal of Kovalevski) and is associated with congenital defects of the thoracic spine (anterior spina bifida, hemivertebrae, or butterfly vertebrae), it is termed a *neurenteric cyst*. CT or MR can confirm the cystic nature of these masses (Fig. 13.22). If the cyst communicates with the GI tract, it may contain air or an air–fluid level or opacify with contrast during an upper GI series.

Vertebral Abnormalities. A variety of conditions that affect the thoracic spine may manifest as posterior mediastinal masses. These lesions typically produce lateral deviation of the paraspinal reflection on frontal radiographs. Often, the bony

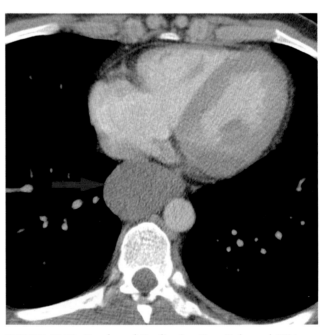

FIGURE 13.22. Esophageal Duplication Cyst. Enhanced CT in an 18-year-old man with a posterior mediastinal mass on chest radiography (not shown) demonstrates a low-attenuation right paraesophageal mass (*arrow*), consistent with an esophageal duplication cyst.

origin of these lesions is not obvious on initial examination, making distinction from neurogenic tumors and other posterior mediastinal masses difficult.

Neoplastic, infectious, metabolic, traumatic, or degenerative processes of the thoracic spine may produce a paraspinal mass by one of four mechanisms: (*1*) expansion of vertebral body or posterior elements (multiple myeloma, aneurysmal bone cyst); (*2*) extraosseous extension of infection, tumor, or marrow elements (infectious spondylitis, metastatic carcinoma, extramedullary hematopoiesis, respectively); (*3*) pathologic fracture and paraspinal hematoma formation (any destructive neoplastic or inflammatory process, trauma); or (*4*) protrusion of degenerative osteophytes. Neoplastic processes are usually easily identified by expansion and destruction of vertebral bodies, with sparing of intervertebral disks. Bronchogenic, breast, or renal cell carcinoma are the most common primary sites of thoracic spinal metastases. Infectious spondylitis is distinguished from neoplastic processes by the presence of a paravertebral mass centered at the point of maximal bone destruction. In patients with a paravertebral abscess secondary to tuberculosis or bacterial infection, narrowing of the adjacent disk space and destruction of vertebral endplates are important clues to the diagnosis. Extramedullary hematopoiesis is seen almost exclusively in conditions associated with ineffective production or excessive destruction of erythrocytes, such as thalassemia major, congenital spherocytosis, and sickle cell anemia. It is recognized by noting expansion of the medullary space and cyst formation within long bones, ribs, and vertebral bodies, with associated lobulated paraspinal soft tissue masses. These masses, which represent hyperplastic bone marrow that has extruded from the vertebral bodies and posterior ribs, are typically seen in the lower thoracic and upper lumbar region. Traumatic injuries to the thoracic spine are usually obvious from the patient's history and recognition of spine fracture on conventional and CT studies of the spine. Degenerative disk disease may produce a localized paraspinal mass on frontal radiographs. Well-penetrated films will show the characteristic interolaterally projecting osteophytes at the level of the mass, which are most commonly right-sided because of the inhibitory effect of the pulsating descending aorta on left-sided osteophyte formation.

Lateral thoracic meningoceles represent an anomalous herniation of the spinal meninges through an intervertebral foramen, resulting in a paravertebral soft tissue mass. Most meningoceles are discovered in middle-aged patients as asymptomatic masses. They are slightly more common on the right and are multiple in 10% of cases. There is a high association between lateral thoracic meningoceles and neurofibromatosis. A meningocele is the most common posterior mediastinal mass in patients with neurofibromatosis; conversely, approximately two-thirds of patients with meningoceles have neurofibromatosis. Chest radiographs typically reveal a round, well-defined paraspinal mass that is indistinguishable from a neurofibroma. Additional clues to the diagnosis include rib erosion, enlargement of the adjacent neural foramen, vertebral anomalies, or kyphoscoliosis. When a lateral meningocele is associated with kyphoscoliosis, it is usually found at the apex of the scoliotic curve on the convex side. MR demonstration of a herniated subarachnoid space is the diagnostic technique of choice (Fig. 13.23); conventional or CT myelography, which demonstrates filling of the meningocele with contrast, is reserved for equivocal cases.

Miscellaneous Conditions. A pancreatic pseudocyst rarely produces a posterior mediastinal mass by extending cephalad from the retroperitoneum through the esophageal or aortic hiatus of the diaphragm. The diagnosis relies on CT demonstration of continuity of a predominantly cystic mass with its retroperitoneal portion (Fig. 13.24). The presence of a left

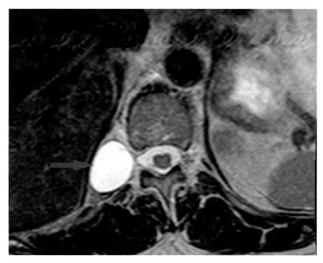

FIGURE 13.23. Lateral Thoracic Meningocele in Neurofibromatosis. Axial T2-weighted MR through the lower thoracic spine shows a high-signal mass in the right paravertebral region (*arrow*) in a patient with neurofibromatosis type 1.

pleural effusion is a further clue to the diagnosis. Hernias through the foramen of Bochdalek, which produce a posterior mediastinal mass, are discussed in Chapter 19.

Rarely, malignant lymph node enlargement may produce a recognizable paraspinal mass. This is most often seen in NHL, metastatic lung cancer, and seminoma (Fig. 13.25); other mediastinal or extrathoracic sites of involvement are invariably present.

Despite the advances in detection and characterization of mediastinal masses with cross-sectional imaging, most patients will require tissue sampling for definitive diagnosis. However, the radiologist can use the information provided by CT or MR to help limit the differential diagnosis and thereby guide the appropriate evaluation and treatment. In a large percentage of cases, when tissue sampling is required, it can be accomplished by CT- or US-guided transthoracic biopsy.

DIFFUSE MEDIASTINAL DISEASE

The differential diagnosis of diffuse widening of the mediastinum is reviewed in Table 13.6.

Mediastinal infection is an uncommon condition that may be divided into acute and chronic forms based upon etiology, clinical features, and radiologic findings. The distinction between acute and chronic infection is important because there are considerable differences in treatment and prognosis.

Acute mediastinitis is caused by bacterial infection that most often develops following esophageal perforation or is a complication of cardiothoracic or esophageal surgery (Fig. 13.26). Esophageal perforation may complicate esophageal instrumentation (e.g., endoscopy, biopsy, dilatation, or stent placement), penetrating chest trauma, esophageal carcinoma, foreign body or corrosive ingestion, or vomiting. Spontaneous esophageal perforation following prolonged vomiting is termed *Boerhaave syndrome*. In this condition, a vertical tear occurs along the left posterolateral wall of the distal esophagus, just above the esophagogastric junction, leading to signs and symptoms of acute mediastinitis. Less commonly, acute mediastinitis may develop from intramediastinal extension of infection in the neck, retropharyngeal space, lungs, pleural space, pericardium, or spine.

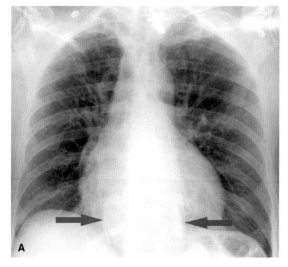

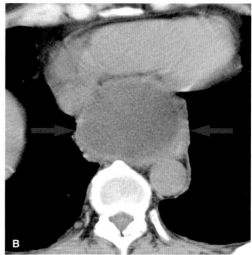

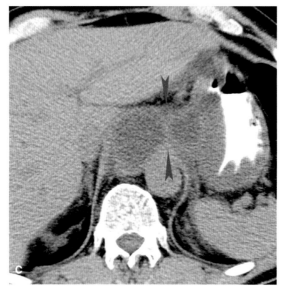

FIGURE 13.24. Pancreatic Pseudocyst as Posterior Mediastinal Mass. A. Portable chest radiograph in a 62-year-old man with an episode of severe pancreatitis 7 months earlier shows a posteroinferior mediastinal mass (*arrows*). **B.** Unenhanced CT through the lower chest shows a thick-walled cystic posterior mediastinal mass (*arrows*). **C.** Scan through the upper abdomen shows communication of the abdominal and thoracic components of the pseudocyst (*arrowheads*) via the esophageal hiatus.

The clinical presentation of acute mediastinitis is usually dramatic and is characterized by severe retrosternal chest pain, fever, chills, and dysphagia, often accompanied by evidence of septic shock. Physical examination may reveal findings associated with pneumomediastinum, with subcutaneous emphysema in the neck and an apical, systolic crunching sound on chest auscultation (Hamman sign).

The most common chest radiographic findings are widening of the superior mediastinum in 66% of patients and pleural effusion in 50% of patients. Specific findings such as mediastinal air or air–fluid levels are less common. When mediastinitis occurs in association with Boerhaave syndrome, pneumoperitoneum and left hydropneumothorax may be seen.

When esophageal perforation is suspected, an esophagram should be performed to detect leakage of contrast into the mediastinum and to localize the exact site of perforation. In a patient not at risk for aspiration, a water-soluble contrast agent is administered initially. Once gross contrast extravasation has been excluded, barium is then given for superior radiographic detail. The sensitivity of the esophagram for detecting contrast leakage is highest when the study is obtained within 24 hours of the perforation.

MDCT is the radiologic study of choice for the diagnosis of acute mediastinitis (11). CT findings include extra luminal gas, bulging of the mediastinal contours, and focal or diffuse soft tissue infiltration of mediastinal fat. Localized fluid collections suggest focal abscess formation. Associated findings include mediastinal venous thrombosis, pneumothorax, pleural effusion or empyema, subphrenic abscess, and vertebral osteomyelitis.

While the clinical and radiographic diagnosis of mediastinitis is often straightforward, it may be difficult in postoperative patients who have undergone recent median sternotomy. In these patients, infiltration of mediastinal fat and focal air or fluid collections may be normal findings on postoperative CT scans performed days to weeks following the removal of intraoperatively placed mediastinal drains. In such patients, the progression of findings on follow-up CT scans will correctly identify the majority of those with postoperative mediastinal infection.

The prognosis for patients with acute mediastinitis varies with the underlying etiology and the extent of mediastinal involvement at the time of diagnosis. Esophageal perforation is associated with the poorest outcome, with a mortality approaching 50%. A delay in diagnosis and treatment of the mediastinal infection of greater than 24 hours is associated with a significant increase in overall morbidity and mortality.

In addition to its sensitivity in the diagnosis of mediastinitis, CT can be used to guide treatment and predict outcome. Those patients with evidence of extensive mediastinal infection, seen

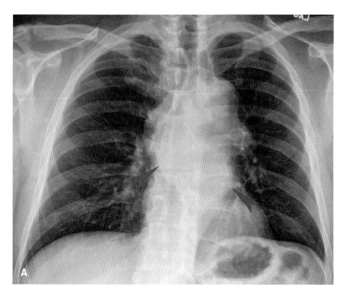

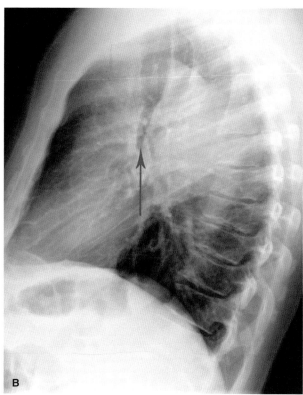

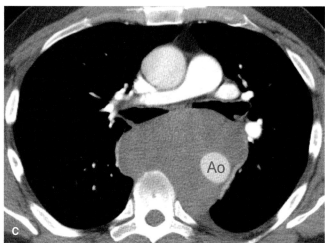

FIGURE 13.25. Posterior Mediastinal Nodal Metastases From Seminoma. Frontal (**A**) and lateral (**B**) chest radiographs in a 48-year-old male with metastatic seminoma shows a posterior mediastinal mass distorting the azygoesophageal recess (*arrowheads*) and displacing the distal trachea and carina anteriorly (*arrow*). **C.** Axial contrast-enhanced CT through the mid chest shows a large posterior mediastinal soft tissue mass encasing and displacing the descending aorta (*Ao*) and extending into the pre- and left paravertebral region.

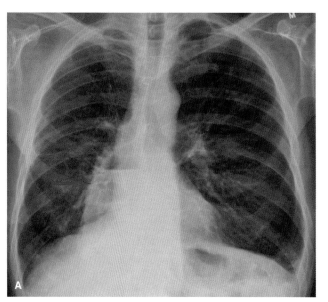

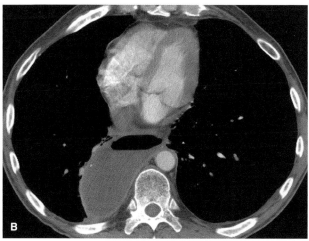

FIGURE 13.26. Posterior Mediastinal Abscess Complicating Esophagectomy. A. Frontal chest radiograph in a patient status post esophagectomy without gastric pull-through shows a large extrapulmonary air–fluid collection in the posteromedial right hemithorax (*arrow*). **B.** Axial contrast-enhanced CT through the lower chest shows a peripherally enhancing air–fluid collection in the right paravertebral region. Percutaneous aspiration revealed purulent material.

TABLE 13.6

DIFFUSE MEDIASTINAL WIDENING

Smooth	Mediastinal lipomatosis
	Malignant infiltration
	Lymphoma
	Small cell carcinoma
	Adenocarcinoma
	Mediastinal hemorrhage
	Arterial bleeding
	Traumatic aortic arch/great vessel laceration
	Aneurysmal rupture
	Venous bleeding
	SVC/right atrial laceration
	Mediastinitis
	Acute (suppurative)
	Chronic (sclerosing)
	Histoplasmosis
	Tuberculosis
	Idiopathic
Lobulated	Lymph node enlargement (see Table 14.4)
	Thymic mass (see Table 13.3)
	Germ cell neoplasm (see Table 13.3)
	Vascular lesions
	Tortuosity of great vessels
	SVC occlusion (dilated venous collaterals)
	Malignancy
	Sclerosing mediastinitis
	Catheter-induced thrombosis
	Neurofibromatosis

SVC, superior vena cava.

on CT as diffuse infiltration of the mediastinal fat without evidence of abscess formation, have a mortality approaching 50%. In contrast, patients with discrete mediastinal abscesses that are amenable to surgical or percutaneous drainage, or with small localized abscesses that are amenable to antibiotic therapy alone, have a more favorable prognosis. In addition, patients with mediastinal abscesses and contiguous empyema or subphrenic abscess may respond favorably to drainage of these extramediastinal collections.

Chronic Sclerosing (Fibrosing) Mediastinitis. The hall marks of chronic sclerosing mediastinitis are chronic inflammatory changes and mediastinal fibrosis. The most common cause of this rare condition is granulomatous infection, usually secondary to *Histoplasma capsulatum*. Tuberculous infection, radiation therapy, and drugs (methysergide) are less common causes. Idiopathic mediastinal fibrosis, which is probably an autoimmune process, is related to fibrosis in other regions, including the retroperitoneum, intraorbital fat, and thyroid gland.

Several theories have been advanced to explain the pathogenesis of sclerosing mediastinitis owing to histoplasmosis. The most widely accepted theory suggests that affected patients develop an idiosyncratic hypersensitivity response to a fungal antigen that "leaks" from infected mediastinal lymph nodes.

Clinically, this condition occurs in adults and presents with a variety of symptoms, depending upon the extent of fibrosis and the mediastinal structures compromised by the fibrotic process. The superior vena cava (SVC) is the most commonly affected structure, with involvement in over 75% of symptomatic patients. The SVC syndrome manifests with headache, epistaxis, cyanosis, jugular venous distention, and edema of the face, neck, and upper extremities. The most serious and potentially fatal manifestation of sclerosing mediastinitis is obstruction of the central pulmonary veins, which produces pulmonary edema that may mimic severe mitral stenosis. Patients with involvement of the tracheobronchial tree may have cough, dyspnea, wheezing, hemoptysis, and obstructive pneumonitis. Dysphagia or hematemesis can be seen with esophageal involvement. Less commonly, pulmonary arterial hypertension and cor pulmonale can develop from narrowing of the pulmonary arteries.

The most common finding noted on chest radiographs is asymmetric lobulated widening of the upper mediastinum, most often on the right. When the process is secondary to granulomatous infection, enlarged calcified lymph nodes may be seen. Narrowing of the tracheobronchial tree may be evident. The sequelae of vascular involvement may be seen, including oligemia from pulmonary arterial compression or venous hypertension and pulmonary edema from involvement of the central pulmonary veins. Postobstructive atelectasis or consolidation may also be seen.

CT is the modality of choice for the diagnosis and assessment of chronic sclerosing mediastinitis. Enlarged lymph nodes with calcification are the most common finding (Fig. 13.27). The fibrotic infiltration of the mediastinal fat that is characteristic of this condition is seen as abnormal soft tissue density replacing the normal mediastinal fat with obliteration of the normal mediastinal interfaces. CT delineates the degree of involvement of the mediastinal vessels, trachea, and central bronchi. In patients with significant SVC involvement, collateral venous channels within the mediastinum and chest wall are well demonstrated (12).

MR is superior to CT for the assessment of vascular involvement. The ability to examine the mediastinal vessels in both the axial and coronal planes without the need for IV contrast helps detect vascular compromise. A significant disadvantage of MR is its inability to detect nodal calcification, a finding that is key to the diagnosis. For this reason, MR is most often utilized as an adjunct to CT when findings of vascular involvement are equivocal.

A definitive diagnosis of chronic sclerosing mediastinitis and the establishment of the underlying etiology are difficult. Skin tests for histoplasmosis and tuberculosis may add additional information but are usually not helpful. The precise diagnosis, and more important the distinction from infiltrating malignancy, usually requires biopsy.

Mediastinal Hemorrhage. Injury to mediastinal vessels resulting from blunt or penetrating thoracic trauma is the most common cause of mediastinal hemorrhage. Blunt chest trauma most often occurs in the setting of a motor vehicle accident, when rapid deceleration and thoracic cage compression produce shearing effects at the aortic isthmus. Iatrogenic trauma, usually from attempts at central line placement, can also cause mediastinal hemorrhage. Spontaneous hemorrhage may develop in patients with a coagulopathy, or with aortic rupture from aneurysm or dissection. Chronic hemodialysis, radiation vasculitis, and bleeding into a mediastinal mass are rare causes of mediastinal hemorrhage.

In the nontraumatic setting, the symptoms and signs of mediastinal hemorrhage are often mild or absent. The patient may complain of retrosternal chest pain radiating toward the back. Rarely, SVC compression may result in the SVC syndrome. Extension of blood from the mediastinum superiorly into the retropharyngeal space may result in neck stiffness, odynophagia, or stridor.

The main radiographic finding in mediastinal hemorrhage of any cause is a focal or diffuse widening of the mediastinum that obscures the normal mediastinal contours (13). In mediastinal hemorrhage, the mediastinum develops a flat or slightly convex outward contour, unlike the round, lobulated,

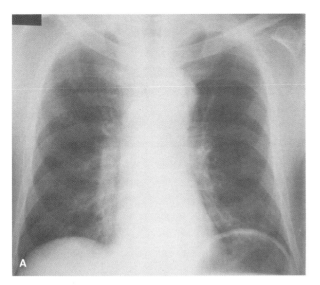

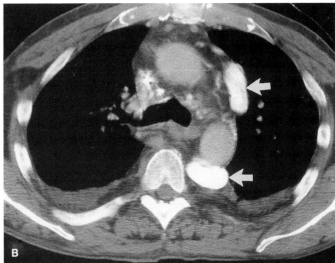

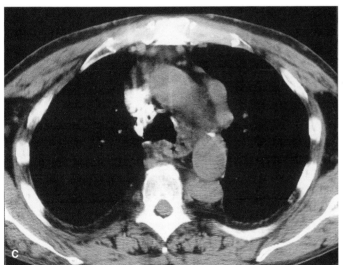

FIGURE 13.27. Sclerosing Mediastinitis From Histoplasmosis. **A.** Posteroanterior chest film in an asymptomatic 68-year-old man shows lobulated widening of the upper mediastinum. **B.** Contrast-enhanced CT reveals marked dilatation of the left superior intercostal vein (*arrows*), high-attenuation material in and around the superior vena cava, and numerous collaterals within the mediastinal fat. **C.** A noncontrast scan at approximately the same level reveals mediastinal calcification obliterating the superior vena cava. The patient was a former resident of Ohio where histoplasmosis is endemic.

or irregular contour seen with enlarged lymph nodes or a localized mediastinal mass. Blood extending from the mediastinum into the pleural or extrapleural space produces a free-flowing effusion or a loculated extrapleural collection, respectively. Rarely, extension of blood into the lungs via the bronchovascular interstitium produces interstitial opacities that mimic pulmonary edema. Serial radiographs may show rapid changes in mediastinal or pleural fluid collections in patients with persistent hemorrhage. CT demonstrates abnormal soft tissue within the mediastinum that obliterates the normal interfaces between the mediastinal fat, the vessels, and the airways (Fig. 13.28). Freshly clotted blood is high in attenuation and is usually easily appreciated on helical CT. CT is also superior to plain radiography in demonstrating the extramediastinal extent of hemorrhage and is useful in demonstrating associated thoracic injuries in patients following blunt chest trauma.

Mediastinal lipomatosis is a benign, asymptomatic condition characterized by excessive deposition of fat in the mediastinum. Predisposing conditions include obesity, Cushing disease, and corticosteroid therapy. However, this entity is unassociated with identifiable conditions in approximately 50% of patients.

On conventional radiographs, the most common finding is smooth, symmetric widening of the superior mediastinum. If the amount of fat deposition is marked, the mediastinum may

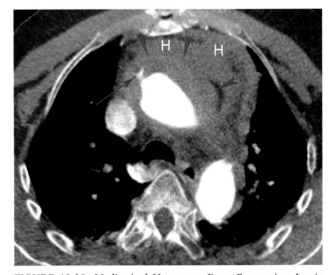

FIGURE 13.28. Mediastinal Hematoma From Penetrating Aortic Ulcer and Intramural Hematoma. Axial scan from CT aortogram demonstrates a focal outpouching (*arrow*) extending right anterolateral from the ascending aorta with an aortic intramural hematoma (outlined by *arrowheads*) and an associated mediastinal hematoma (*H*).

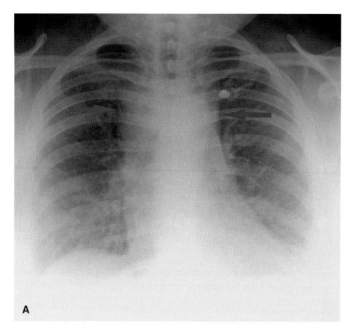
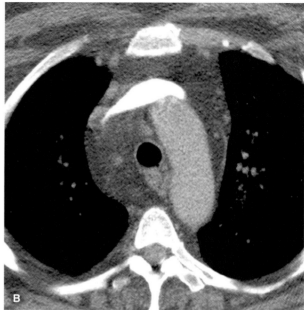

FIGURE 13.29. Mediastinal Lipomatosis. A. Frontal chest radiograph shows a widened superior mediastinum (*arrows*), particularly on the right. **B.** Unenhanced CT at the level of the aortic arch shows abundant mediastinal fat responsible for the mediastinal widening.

show lobulated margins. Unlike mediastinal tumor infiltration or hemorrhage, which usually cause tracheal deviation or narrowing, the trachea remains at midline in mediastinal lipomatosis. Fat may also accumulate in the paraspinal regions, chest wall, and cardiophrenic angles; the latter produces enlargement of the epipericardial fat pads that is a clue to the proper diagnosis.

CT provides a definitive diagnosis by demonstrating abundant, homogeneous, unencapsulated fat that bulges the mediastinal contours (Fig. 13.29). Displacement or compression of mediastinal structures, particularly the trachea, is notable by its absence. Heterogeneity within the fat suggests other primary or superimposed conditions, such as neoplastic infiltration, infection, hemorrhage, or fibrosis.

Multiple symmetric lipomatosis is a rare entity that resembles simple mediastinal lipomatosis radiographically. The distinction between these two conditions is made by the distribution of abnormal fat and mass effect on mediastinal structures. In multiple symmetric lipomatosis, the cardiophrenic angles, paraspinal areas, and the anterior mediastinum are spared; periscapular lipomas may also be seen. The trachea is often compressed or displaced by fat in patients with this condition, whereas this is not seen in simple lipomatosis.

Malignancy. Malignant involvement of the mediastinum is typically seen as discrete masses or lymph node enlargement. Rarely, diffuse soft tissue infiltration of the mediastinal fat may occur, either alone or in association with focal lesions. Plain radiographs are nonspecific, usually demonstrating mediastinal widening. CT shows soft tissue infiltration of the normal mediastinal fat and obliteration of the normal tissue planes. This pattern is most common with extracapsular spread of lymphoma or small cell carcinoma of the lung. The latter disease has a high propensity to invade mediastinal structures and therefore may present with symptoms of airway obstruction or SVC syndrome.

Pneumomediastinum is the presence of extraluminal gas within the mediastinum. Possible sources of such gas include the lungs, trachea, central bronchi, esophagus, and extension of gas from the neck or abdomen (Table 13.7) (see Fig. 18.10) (14).

Air from the lungs is the most common source of pneumomediastinum. The mechanism of pneumomediastinum formation involves a sudden rise in intrathoracic and intra-alveolar pressure that leads to alveolar rupture. The extra-alveolar air first collects within the bronchovascular interstitium and then dissects centrally to the hilum and mediastinum (the Macklin effect). Less commonly, the air may dissect peripherally toward the subpleural interstitium and rupture through the visceral pleura to produce a pneumothorax.

Pneumomediastinum most commonly complicates mechanical ventilation in patients with ARDS, because the combination of positive pressure ventilation and abnormally stiff lungs

TABLE 13.7

PNEUMOMEDIASTINUM

Intrathoracic source	Alveoli
	Valsalva maneuver
	Positive pressure ventilation
	Esophagus
	Boerhaave syndrome
	Endoscopic interventions (biopsy, dilatation, sclerotherapy)
	Carcinoma
	Tracheobronchial tree
	Bronchial stump dehiscence
	Tracheobronchial laceration
	Fistula formation
	Tracheal/esophageal malignancy
	Infection (tuberculosis, histoplasmosis)
Extrathoracic source	Recent sternotomy/thoracotomy
	Pneumoperitoneum/pneumoretroperitoneum
	Subcutaneous emphysema in neck
	Stab wound
	Laryngeal fracture

predisposes to alveolar rupture. Spontaneous pneumomediastinum can occur with deep inspiratory or Valsalva maneuvers during strenuous exercise, childbirth, weightlifting, and inhalation of drugs such as marijuana, nitrous oxide, and crack cocaine. Patients with asthma are prone to pneumomediastinum; this is related to the airway obstruction that characterizes this disease. Prolonged vomiting from any cause may lead to intrathoracic pressures that are sufficiently high to produce pneumomediastinum. In patients with diabetic ketoacidosis, the increased respiratory effort that accompanies attempts at correcting the underlying metabolic acidosis can lead to pneumomediastinum. Blunt chest trauma can result in pneumomediastinum as a result of an abrupt increase in intra-alveolar pressure and shearing forces affecting the alveolar walls.

Pneumomediastinum arising from the tracheobronchial tree or esophagus usually is a result of traumatic disruption of these structures. The marked shearing forces that develop with blunt trauma may lead to fracture of the trachea or mainstem bronchi. Penetrating trauma to the tracheobronchial tree is usually iatrogenic and may follow endotracheal intubation, bronchoscopy, or tracheostomy. Rarely, neoplasms or inflammatory lesions (e.g., tuberculosis) may erode through the tracheal wall and into the peritracheal fat. Esophageal rupture is most often spontaneous, usually in the setting of severe, prolonged vomiting (Boerhaave syndrome). In addition to pneumomediastinum, a left hydropneumothorax and pneumoperitoneum may be present in this condition. Spontaneous esophageal rupture may occur during childbirth, during a severe asthmatic episode, or with blunt chest trauma. Endoscopic procedures, stent placement, esophageal dilatation, corrosive ingestion, and carcinoma may lead to esophageal perforation. Mediastinal gas may be produced by bacterial organisms in acute mediastinitis.

Air within the soft tissues of the neck from penetrating trauma or laryngeal fracture may lead to pneumomediastinum by extending inferiorly through the retropharyngeal and prevertebral spaces, or along the sheaths of the great vessels. Deep space infections in the neck can spread along the same fascial planes and lead to mediastinitis. The term *Ludwig angina* describes the substernal chest pain caused by the intramediastinal extension of such infections. Rarely, pneumomediastinum develops as air dissects superiorly from the retroperitoneum through the aortic hiatus or from the peritoneal cavity along the internal mammary vascular sheaths.

The symptoms associated with pneumomediastinum vary with the underlying etiology, extent of mediastinal air, and presence of mediastinitis. Mediastinal air without infection is generally asymptomatic and does not require treatment. In some patients with spontaneous pneumomediastinum, there may be substernal, pleuritic type chest pain of sudden onset that can be related to a specific inciting incident, such as vomiting or the Valsalva maneuver. Dyspnea may be present. In adults, mediastinal air under pressure usually escapes into the neck, producing crepitus over the neck, supraclavicular regions, and chest wall. Rarely, mediastinal air under pressure may produce a tension pneumomediastinum in which the clinical findings are those of cardiac tamponade. Patients with mediastinitis and pneumomediastinum are usually seriously ill with chest pain, high fevers, dyspnea, and signs of sepsis. The radiographic findings of pneumomediastinum are reviewed in Chapter 12.

THE HILA

Hilar abnormalities are first appreciated on conventional posteroanterior and lateral chest radiographs. CT and MR are used to confirm and characterize hilar masses or to detect subradiographic involvement of the hila, the latter most often in patients with bronchogenic carcinoma.

Unilateral Hilar Enlargement

Malignancy (Table 13.8). A hilar mass usually represents bronchogenic carcinoma or confluent lymph node metastases (Fig. 13.30). Unilateral hilar enlargement may be the presenting radiographic feature of squamous cell carcinoma, where the hilar mass represents the central extension of an endobronchial tumor from its origin within a segmental bronchus. Concomitant hilar lymph node involvement may contribute to hilar enlargement in some of these patients. Approximately 20% of patients with squamous cell carcinoma have a hilar mass on chest radiograph. In contrast, patients with adenocarcinoma and large cell carcinoma more commonly present with a peripheral pulmonary nodule or mass. In many patients, the hilar mass may be obscured by adjacent lung collapse or obstructive pneumonitis.

Unilateral hilar enlargement resulting from metastatic lymph node involvement is most often seen in small cell carcinoma. The propensity of this tumor for early invasion of the bronchial submucosa and peribronchial lymphatics accounts

TABLE 13.8

UNILATERAL HILAR ENLARGEMENT

Lymph node enlargement	
Malignancy	Bronchogenic carcinoma
	Lymph node metastases
	Bronchogenic carcinoma
	Head and neck malignancy
	Squamous cell carcinoma of skin, larynx
	Thyroid carcinoma
	Breast carcinoma
	Melanoma
	Genitourinary malignancy
	Renal cell carcinoma
	Testicular neoplasm
	Lymphoma
Infection	Tuberculosis
	Histoplasmosis
	Coccidioidomycosis
	Pneumonic plague
	Tularemia
	Anaerobic lung abscess
	Measles
	Mononucleosis
Pulmonary artery enlargement	Valvular pulmonic stenosis
	Pulmonary artery aneurysm
	Infection
	Tuberculosis (Rasmussen aneurysm)
	Left-to-right shunts
	Patent ductus arteriosis
	Atrial and ventricular septal defects
	Arteritis (see below)
	Tetralogy of Fallot
	Central pulmonary embolus
	Chronic thromboembolic disease
	Pulmonary arteritis
	Behçet disease
	Hughes–Stovin syndrome
	Takayasu arteritis
Cyst	Bronchogenic cyst

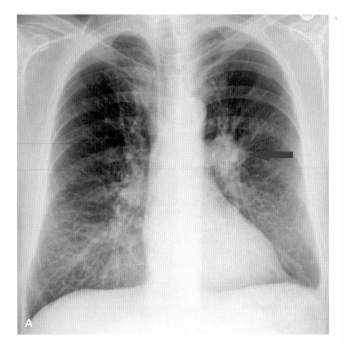

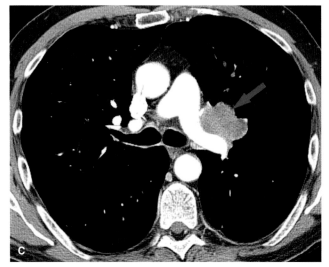

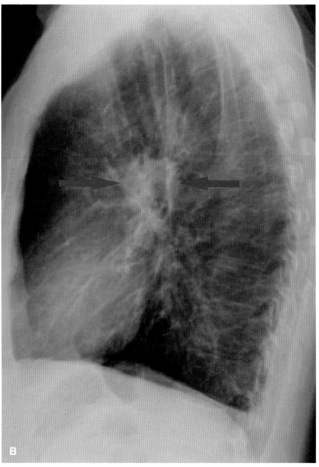

FIGURE 13.30. Bronchogenic Carcinoma as Left Hilar Mass. Frontal (**A**) and lateral (**B**) chest radiographs show an enlarged and abnormally dense left hilum (*arrows*). **C.** Axial contrast-enhanced CT through the right upper lobe bronchus shows a lobulated left hilar mass (*arrow*). Biopsy revealed adenocarcinoma.

for the high incidence of widespread hematogenous and hilar and mediastinal lymph node metastases at the time of diagnosis. Plain film evidence of enlarged hilar lymph nodes resulting from metastases from adenocarcinoma of lung or large cell carcinoma are seen in only 10% to 15% of patients. Contrast-enhanced CT or MR is more sensitive for detecting enlarged hilar nodes and should be performed in all patients to guide further staging procedures and for proper preoperative or treatment planning.

Metastases to hilar and mediastinal lymph nodes from extrathoracic malignancies are uncommon, occurring in approximately 2% of patients. The malignancies that are most often associated with intrathoracic nodal metastases are genitourinary (renal and testicular), head and neck (skin, larynx, and thyroid), breast, and melanoma (7). In renal cell carcinoma and seminoma, lymphatic spread of tumor to retroperitoneal nodes and up the thoracic duct to the posterior mediastinum is the mode of spread to thoracic nodes. Although there is no direct communication between the thoracic duct and anterior mediastinal lymph nodes, reflux of tumor emboli through incompetent valves may allow tumor spread to hilar, para-

tracheal, and intraparenchymal lymphatics. Head and neck tumors reach the mediastinum via lymphatic spread from cervical lymph nodes. Intrathoracic nodal metastases from breast carcinoma are often seen late in the course of disease, often years after the initial diagnosis. Malignant melanoma is the extrathoracic neoplasm with the highest incidence of intrathoracic nodal metastases (Fig. 13.31); patients with nodal disease will almost invariably have radiographic evidence of parenchymal metastases.

Although 75% of patients presenting with Hodgkin lymphoma have evidence of intrathoracic lymph node enlargement, isolated unilateral hilar lymph node enlargement is uncommon. The thoracic manifestations in NHL differ in primary pulmonary lymphoma versus lymphoma that primarily involves extrathoracic sites with secondary pulmonary involvement. Thoracic involvement in primary pulmonary lymphoma is largely limited to parenchymal and pleural disease, whereas secondary pulmonary lymphoma generally manifests as intrathoracic lymph node enlargement, with 35% showing hilar or middle mediastinal lymph node enlargement and some presenting as an isolated finding.

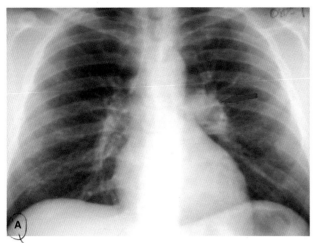
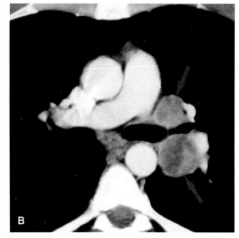

FIGURE 13.31. Hilar Nodal Metastases From Melanoma. A. Posteroanterior radiograph in a patient with melanoma shows left hilar enlargement (*arrow*). B. Enhanced CT scan shows enlarged left hilar lymph nodes (*arrows*) from metastatic disease.

Infection. Unilateral hilar or mediastinal lymph node enlargement is a characteristic feature in primary pulmonary tuberculosis (see Fig. 16.8) in distinction to postprimary tuberculosis; an exception is the severely immunocompromised patient with AIDS. Isolated lymph node enlargement as a manifestation of primary tuberculosis is more common in children than in adults. There is almost always concomitant parenchymal disease in immunocompetent patients with lymph node enlargement. Fungal infections such as histoplasmosis and coccidioidomycosis may present with hilar lymph node enlargement, typically associated with patchy or lobar airspace consolidation in the ipsilateral lung (see Fig. 16.16). A variety of bacterial infections have been associated with unilateral hilar lymph node enlargement, including plague, tularemia, and anaerobic lung abscess. A characteristic finding in patients with pneumonic plague is the detection on unenhanced CT of increased attenuation within hilar and mediastinal nodes that drain regions of

parenchymal involvement owing to intranodal hemorrhage. Tularemia (*Francisella tularensis*) causes parenchymal consolidation in association with hilar lymph node enlargement and pleural effusion.

The viral infections most commonly associated with hilar lymph node enlargement are infectious mononucleosis and measles pneumonia. The thorax is infrequently involved in mononucleosis, but hilar lymph node enlargement is the most common manifestation of intrathoracic disease. Lymph node enlargement may accompany the reticular interstitial opacities of typical measles pneumonia, or it may be associated with nodular, segmental, or lobar opacities and pleural effusion in atypical measles pneumonia.

Pulmonary Artery Enlargement. Although unilateral hilar enlargement is most often the result of a mass or enlarged lymph nodes, abnormal enlargement of the right or left PA may cause hilar prominence (Fig. 13.32). Vascular disorders that produce unilateral PA enlargement include poststenotic

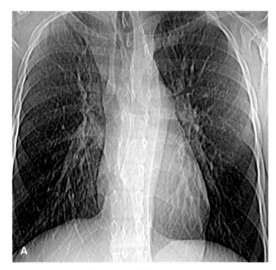
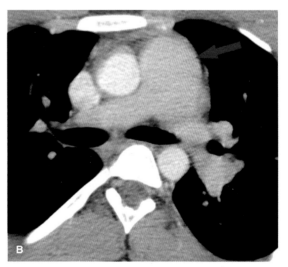

FIGURE 13.32. Unilateral Hilar Enlargement From Idiopathic Dilatation of the Pulmonary Artery. A. Scout view from chest CT shows abnormal convexity in the region of the main PA (*arrow*). Note thoracic scoliosis. B. Enhanced CT scan shows dilated main PA (*arrow*) with normal right and left PAs. Physical examination and echocardiogram showed no evidence of pulmonic valve disease.

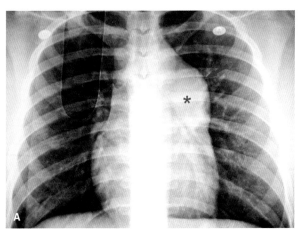
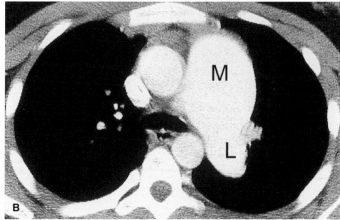

FIGURE 13.33. Left Hilar Enlargement in Valvular Pulmonic Stenosis. A. Chest radiograph shows a middle mediastinal mass (*arrow*) with left hilar enlargement (*asterisk*). **B.** Axial contrast-enhanced CT shows marked main (*M*) and left (*L*) pulmonary arterial dilatation as a result of valvular pulmonic stenosis.

dilatation from valvular or postvalvular pulmonic stenosis (Fig. 13.33), PA aneurysms, and distension of the PA by thrombus or tumor. Patients with congenital valvular pulmonic stenosis may develop poststenotic dilatation or aneurysms of the main and left PAs from the jet effect of blood upon these vessels. Rarely, stenoses resulting from PA vasculitis, congenital rubella, or Williams syndrome may lead to poststenotic dilatation of a PA. Aneurysms of the central PAs are usually associated with congenital heart disease, such as pulmonic stenosis and left-to-right shunts from ventricular septal defect and patent ductus arteriosus. Rare vasculitides such as Behçet disease and Hughes–Stovins syndrome may present with PA aneurysms. A large pulmonary embolus lodging in the proximal portion of a PA may cause proximal dilatation. Obviously, these patients are symptomatic and will show characteristic findings on perfusion lung scan, helical CT, and pulmonary arteriography.

Bronchogenic cyst is an uncommon cause of a hilar mass. CT and MR will show a round, smooth, thin-walled cyst, usually found in an asymptomatic young adult. Because the hilum is an unusual location for a bronchogenic cyst, and distinction from a necrotic tumor or lymph node mass cannot be made radiographically, these lesions should be biopsied or removed.

Bilateral Hilar Enlargement

Bilateral hilar enlargement is the result of enlargement of either the hilar lymph nodes or the central PAs (Table 13.9).

Malignancy. The malignancies producing bilateral hilar lymph node enlargement are similar to those producing unilateral enlargement. In distinction to unilateral nodal enlargement, metastases are uncommon causes of bilateral hilar nodal enlargement. The most frequent solid tumors producing bilateral hilar disease are small cell carcinoma of the lung and malignant melanoma.

Bilateral hilar lymph node involvement by lymphoma is more common in Hodgkin disease than NHL. Hilar involvement is virtually never seen without concomitant anterior mediastinal nodal enlargement in Hodgkin disease, whereas NHL may produce isolated hilar disease.

The most common chest radiographic manifestation of leukemic involvement of the thorax is hilar and mediastinal lymph node enlargement; it is seen in up to 25% of patients. Lymph node enlargement is much more common in the lymphocytic than the myelogenous form, particularly in chronic lymphocytic leukemia.

Infection. Mediastinal and hilar lymph node enlargement from infection is most often seen in tuberculous and fungal infection with histoplasmosis and coccidioidomycosis. In these diseases, the lymph node enlargement may be unilateral or bilateral. With bilateral disease, the enlargement is asymmetric in distinction to sarcoidosis, which is typically symmetric. Bacterial infection from *Bacillus anthracis* (anthrax) and *Yersinia pestis* (plague) may produce bilateral hilar enlargement. In anthrax infection, the lymph node enlargement is often associated with patchy airspace opacities in the lower lobes. The bubonic form of plague may produce marked hilar and mediastinal adenopathy without pneumonia. Recurrent bacterial infection complicating cystic fibrosis is often associated with bilateral hilar lymph node enlargement, and distinction from PA enlargement owing to pulmonary hypertension may be difficult.

TABLE 13.9

BILATERAL HILAR ENLARGEMENT

Lymph node enlargement	Malignancy (see Table 13.2)
	Infection (see Table 13.2)
	Inflammatory disease
	Sarcoidosis
	Berylliosis
	Angioimmunoblastic lymphadenopathy
	Inhalational disease
	Silicosis
Pulmonary artery enlargement	Pulmonary arterial hypertension
	Left-to-right intracardiac shunt
	High output state
	Anemia
	Thyrotoxicosis
	Cystic fibrosis

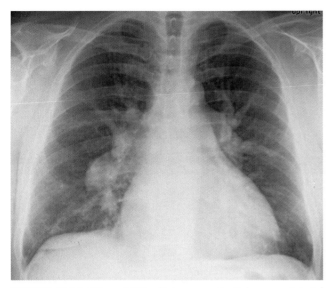

FIGURE 13.34. Bilateral Hilar Enlargement in Pulmonary Arterial Hypertension. Frontal chest radiograph shows marked central pulmonary arterial dilatation with attenuation of peripheral vasculature ("pruning") in a patient with severe pulmonary arterial hypertension due to chronic obstructive pulmonary disease.

Sarcoidosis is associated with bilateral hilar lymph node enlargement in 80% of patients. Most of these patients have concomitant paratracheal lymph node enlargement, and nearly half have concomitant radiographic parenchymal disease. The pattern of lymph node involvement in sarcoidosis has been termed the 1-2-3 sign, with 1 = right paratracheal, 2 = right hilar, and 3 = left hilar lymph node enlargement (Fig. 13.14; see Fig. 17.25). The enlarged nodes produce symmetric, lobulated hilar masses on plain film, since the enlarged nodes remain separate. In 20% of patients, the involved lymph nodes will calcify; usually the calcifications are punctate in appearance, but occasionally peripheral "eggshell" calcification is seen. In some patients, the involved nodes can be seen to enhance after contrast administration on CT. In the majority of patients, the enlarged nodes resolve within 2 years of discovery. In a small percentage, the nodes remain enlarged for many years.

Berylliosis and Silicosis. The hilar and mediastinal lymph node enlargement of chronic berylliosis is radiographically indistinguishable from that of sarcoidosis. Similarly, silicosis can produce hilar and mediastinal lymph node enlargement; eggshell calcification of hilar nodes is highly suggestive of this entity, although peripheral nodal calcification may also be seen with sarcoidosis, histoplasmosis, or amyloidosis.

Bilateral pulmonary artery enlargement is seen with increased flow or increased resistance in the pulmonary circulation (Fig. 13.34). The conditions associated with bilateral pulmonary arterial enlargement are reviewed in Chapter 14.

Small Hila

Bilaterally small hila (Table 13.10) can be seen in some adults with severe pulmonary overinflation from emphysema or in those with diminished pulmonary blood flow due to congenital pulmonary outflow obstruction (tetralogy of Fallot, Ebstein anomaly).

The most common causes of a small hilum are atelectasis and resection of a portion of lung, which leave a small residual hilar artery supplying the remaining lobe or lobes. Hypoplasia

TABLE 13.10

SMALL HILUM (HILA)

Unilateral	Absence or hypoplasia of the pulmonary artery
	Hypoplastic or hypogenetic lung
	Swyer–James syndrome
	Lobar atelectasis
	Lobar resection
	Compression/invasion of the pulmonary artery
	Cyst
	Neoplasm
	Fibrosing mediastinitis
Bilateral	Emphysema
	Obstruction to pulmonary flow
	Fibrosing mediastinitis
	Tetralogy of Fallot
	Valvular pulmonic stenosis
	Ebstein anomaly

of the PA, often with associated abnormalities of the ipsilateral lung (hypogenetic lung syndrome, Swyer–James syndrome) (see Fig. 18.13), is another cause of a small hilum. Less commonly, invasion of the proximal PA by mediastinal tumor, or obstruction of the PA on account of fibrosing mediastinitis, can produce a diminutive hilar shadow. In any patient in whom a small hilum is a new radiographic finding, a CT scan should be performed to assess the mediastinum for central obstructing lesions. The left hilum can appear small in patients in whom the hilar shadow is obscured by the upper left heart margin or by fat in the region of the aortopulmonic interface. In these cases, the lateral radiograph will usually show a left PA of normal size.

References

1. Whitten CR, Khan S, Munneke GJ, Grubnic S. A diagnostic approach to mediastinal abnormalities. Radiographics 2007;27:657–671.
2. Tomiyama N, Johkoh T, Mihara N, et al. Using the World Health Organization classification of thymic epithelial neoplasms to describe CT findings. AJR Am J Roentgenol 2002;179:881–886.
3. Strollo DC, Rosado-de-Christenson ML. Tumors of the thymus. J Thorac Imaging 1999;14:152–171.
4. Uffmann M, Schaefer-Prokop C. Radiological diagnostics of Hodgkin and non-Hodgkin lymphomas of the thorax. Radiologe 2004;44:444–456.
5. Strollo DC, Rosado-de-Christenson ML, Jett JR. Primary mediastinal tumors. Part 1: tumors of the anterior mediastinum. Chest 1997;112:511–522.
6. Duwe BV, Sterman DH, Musani AI. Tumors of the mediastinum. Chest 2005;128:2893–2909.
7. Strollo DC, Rosado-de-Christenson ML, Jett JR. Primary mediastinal tumors. Part 2: tumors of the middle and posterior mediastinum. Chest 1997;112:1344–1357.
8. Rusch VW, Asamura H, Watanabe H, et al. The IASLC lung cancer staging project: a proposal for a new international lymph node map in the forthcoming seventh edition of the TNM classification for lung cancer. J Thorac Oncol 2009;4:568–577.
9. McLoud TC, Kalisher L, Stark P, Greene R. Intrathoracic lymph node metastases from extrathoracic neoplasm. AJR Am J Roentgenol 1978;131:403–407.
10. McAdams HP, Kirejczyk WM, Rosado-de-Christenson ML, Matsumoto S. Bronchogenic cyst: imaging features with clinical and histopathologic correlation. Radiology 2000;217:441–446.
11. Carrol CL, Jeffrey RB, Federle MP, Vernacchia FS. CT evaluation of mediastinal infections. J Comput Assist Tomogr 1987;11:449–454.
12. Rossi SE, McAdams HP, Rosado-de-Christensen ML, et al. Fibrosing mediastinitis. Radiographics 2001;21:737–757.
13. Woodring JH, Loh FK, Kryscio RJ. Mediastinal hemorrhage: an evaluation of radiographic manifestations. Radiology 1984;151:15–21.
14. Zylak CM, Standen JR, Barnes GR, Zylak CJ. Pneumomediastinum revisited. Radiographics 2000;20:1043–1057.

CHAPTER 14 ■ PULMONARY VASCULAR DISEASE

CURTIS E. GREEN AND JEFFREY S. KLEIN

Pulmonary Edema

Pulmonary Hemorrhage and Vasculitis

Pulmonary Embolism

Pulmonary Arterial Hypertension

PULMONARY EDEMA

Basic Principles. Under normal conditions, the interstitial space of the lung is kept dry by pulmonary lymphatics located within the axial and peripheral interstitium of the lung. The lymphatics drain the small amounts of transudated fluid that enters the interstitial spaces as an ultrafiltrate of plasma. Because there are no lymphatic structures immediately within the alveolar walls (parenchymal interstitium), filtered interstitial fluid is drawn to the lymphatics by a pressure gradient from the alveolar interstitium to the axial and peripheral interstitium. When the rate of fluid accumulation in the interstitium exceeds the lymphatic drainage capabilities of the lung, fluid accumulates first within the interstitial space. As the amount of extravascular fluid increases, fluid accumulates in the corners of the alveolar spaces. Progressive fluid accumulation eventually produces flooding of the alveolar spaces, resulting in airspace pulmonary edema. While interstitial edema may leave the gas-exchanging properties of the lung unaffected, flooding of the alveolar spaces leads to impaired oxygen and carbon dioxide exchange.

Excess fluid accumulation in the lung is caused by one of three basic mechanisms. The most common mechanism involves a change in the normal Starling forces that govern fluid movement in the lung. Because normal fluid movement is determined by the differences in hydrostatic and oncotic pressure between the pulmonary capillaries and surrounding alveolar interstitium, an imbalance in these forces may lead to pulmonary edema. This imbalance of forces is most commonly the result of increased capillary hydrostatic pressure (hydrostatic pulmonary edema) and less commonly diminished plasma oncotic or interstitial hydrostatic pressure. A second mechanism is obstruction or absence of the normal pulmonary lymphatics, which leads to the excess accumulation of interstitial fluid. Thirdly, a wide variety of disorders can injure the epithelium of the capillaries and alveoli, causing an increase in capillary permeability that allows protein-rich fluid to escape from the capillaries into the pulmonary interstitium.

Imaging findings in pulmonary edema result from both the interstitial and the airspace components and depend to some extent on the cause of the edema, as will be discussed later. The radiographic appearance of interstitial pulmonary edema results from thickening of the components of the interstitial spaces by fluid (1). Thickening of the axial interstitium results in the loss of definition of the intrapulmonary vascular shadows and thickening of the peribronchovascular interstitium causing peribronchial cuffing and tram tracking. Edema within alveolar septa is not discernible as discrete opacities but produces ground-glass opacity initially in only the dependent lung zones and then throughout the lungs, but still worse in the dependent zones. Involvement of peripheral and subpleural interstitial structures produces Kerley lines and subpleural edema. Kerley A and B lines represent thickening of central connective tissue septa and peripheral interlobular septa, respectively, whereas Kerley C lines represent a network of thickened interlobular septa (Fig. 14.1). Subpleural edema is the accumulation of fluid within the innermost (interstitial) layer of the visceral pleura and is best seen on the lateral radiograph as smooth thickening of the interlobar fissures. The radiographic changes of interstitial pulmonary edema may progress to those of airspace edema or, if successfully treated, resolve within 12 to 24 hours.

Airspace pulmonary edema develops when fluid in the interstitial spaces spills into the alveoli. The upright chest radiograph typically shows bilaterally symmetric airspace opacities predominantly in the mid and lower lung zones. Airspace nodules and the findings of interstitial edema (Kerley B lines and subpleural edema) are usually present peripherally. As with interstitial edema, the airspace opacities of alveolar edema may change rapidly, often within hours. The differential diagnosis of diffuse airspace opacities has been reviewed (see Table 12.9).

Thin-section CT can on occasion be quite useful for identification and assessment of pulmonary edema as the findings are fairly specific (2). Thickening of subpleural, septal, and bronchovascular structures is well depicted. Mild parenchymal edema produces a ground-glass pattern around the hila (Fig. 14.2). Early alveolar edema is seen as centrilobular airspace nodules surrounding the arteries within the lobular core, whereas severe alveolar edema produces dense perihilar airspace opacification.

Hydrostatic pulmonary edema (normal capillary permeability) is the most common form of pulmonary edema. It is usually caused by an elevation in the pulmonary venous pressure (pulmonary venous hypertension [PVH]). The classic cause of PVH is left ventricular systolic failure, but renal failure and a variety of cardiac and noncardiac abnormalities have the same physiology. Decreased capillary oncotic pressure, such as present in patients with hypoalbuminemia secondary to the nephrotic syndrome or liver failure, can cause findings identical to those in patients with elevated hydrostatic pressure.

The *causes of PVH* may be divided into four major categories: obstruction to left ventricular inflow, left ventricular systolic dysfunction (LV failure), mitral valve regurgitation, and systemic or pulmonary volume overload. The classic cause of obstruction to left ventricular inflow is mitral stenosis, but

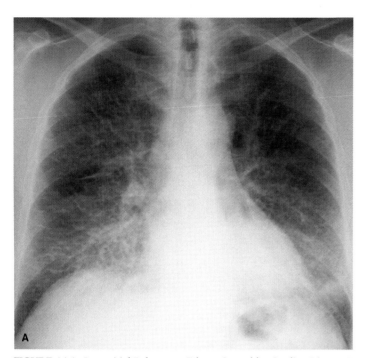

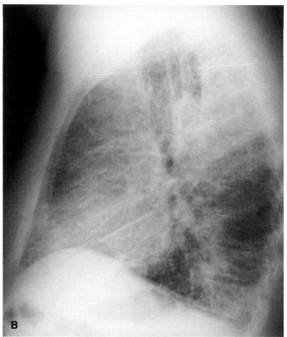

FIGURE 14.1. Interstitial Pulmonary Edema Caused by Cardiac Disease. Posteroanterior (**A**) and lateral (**B**) chest films in a 65-year-old man with an anterior wall myocardial infarction show hydrostatic interstitial edema as evidenced by prominent upper lobe vessels (redistribution of pulmonary blood flow), indistinct lower lung zone pulmonary vessels, peripheral linear opacities (thickened interlobular septa or Kerley B lines), and thickened fissures (subpleural edema) resulting from acute left ventricular failure. Note the absence of cardiomegaly.

poor left ventricular compliance (diastolic dysfunction), such as caused by hypertrophy or chronic ischemic subendocardial fibrosis, is more common. Mimickers of mitral stenosis such as left atrial myxomas are rare. Obstruction of the central pulmonary veins from tumor, fibrosing mediastinitis, or pulmonary vein thrombosis may also be associated with the radiographic findings of PVH. Common causes of LV failure include ischemic heart disease, aortic valve stenosis and

regurgitation, and nonischemic cardiomyopathy (Table 14.1). Severe mitral valve regurgitation can cause PVH directly by elevating left atrial pressure or secondarily by causing LV failure. Acute pulmonary volume overload is relatively common and most frequently due to iatrogenic overhydration. Acute postinfarction ventricular septal defect is a rare cause. Patients with acute or chronic renal failure may develop pulmonary edema because of increased pulmonary capillary hydrostatic

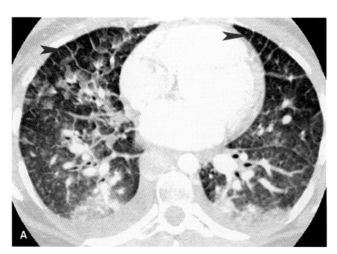

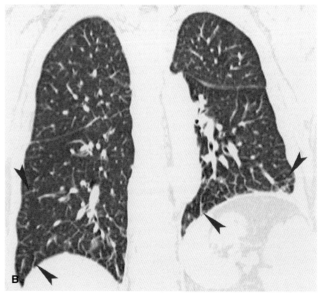

FIGURE 14.2. Thin-Section CT of Hydrostatic Interstitial Pulmonary Edema. A. Axial scan in a 28-year-old woman with postpartum cardiomyopathy shows thickening of the interlobular septal (*arrowheads*) and bronchovascular bundles with dependent patchy ground-glass and airspace opacities and bilateral pleural effusions. **B.** Coronal reconstruction in a different patient with hydrostatic interstitial edema. Thickened septal lines (*arrowheads*) and bronchovascular bundles and scattered ground-glass opacities are present, but there is no airspace consolidation.

TABLE 14.1

CAUSES OF PULMONARY VENOUS HYPERTENSION AND PULMONARY EDEMA

Left ventricular systolic dysfunction	Ischemic heart disease Left ventricular outflow obstruction (aortic stenosis, hypertension, coarctation, hypertrophic obstructive cardiomyopathy) Aortic stenosis Hypoplastic left heart syndrome
Obstruction to left ventricular inflow	Mitral valve stenosis Decreased left ventricular compliance (hypertrophy, pericardial constriction or tamponade, restrictive cardiomyopathy) Left atrial myxoma Cor triatriatum and supravalvular mitral ring
Mitral regurgitation	Endocarditis Papillary muscle rupture or dysfunction Ruptured chordae Mitral prolapse
Systemic or pulmonary volume overload	Overhydration Renal failure Ventricular septal rupture
Pulmonary venous obstruction Central pulmonary veins	Fibrosing mediastinitis Pulmonary vein stenosis (tumor invasion, post-cardiac ablation or surgery) Pulmonary venous thrombosis
Intrapulmonary veins	Pulmonary veno-occlusive disease

pressure caused by a combination of hypervolemia and LV dysfunction.

The classic radiographic findings of PVH are enlargement of pulmonary veins and redistribution of pulmonary blood flow to the nondependent lung zones (1). Pulmonary venous enlargement is seen as progressive dilatation of horizontally oriented pulmonary veins on serial chest radiographs. The redistribution of pulmonary blood flow results from lower zone pulmonary venous constriction causing increased resistance to lower zone blood flow, with resultant preferential flow into upper lobe vessels. Therefore, with PVH in the upright patient with normal lung parenchyma, the upper zone vessels are frequently as large as or larger in diameter than the lower zone vessels. This is the opposite of the normal appearance, in which the lower zone vessels are larger than the upper zone vessels as a result of the normal gravitational effects on pulmonary blood flow. It should be noted that in patients with basilar lung disease, pulmonary blood flow may appear to be redistributed in the absence of PVH and with upper lobe lung disease (e.g., centrilobular emphysema) distribution may not change.

The sequence of events following the development of PVH has been studied in patients with acute cardiac decompensation following myocardial infarction. Several studies have correlated the radiographic findings of PVH in the erect patient with measurements of pulmonary capillary wedge pressure (PCWP) using flow-directed balloon occlusion (e.g., Swan-Ganz) catheters. When PCWP is normal (8 to 12 mm Hg), the chest radiograph is normal. Mild elevation of PCWP (12 to 18 mm Hg) produces constriction of lower lobe vessels and

enlargement of upper lobe vessels. Progressive elevation of PCWP (19 to 25 mm Hg) leads to the findings of interstitial pulmonary edema: loss of vascular definition, peribronchial cuffing, and Kerley lines (Fig. 14.1). PCWP above 25 mm Hg produces alveolar filling with radiographic findings of bilateral airspace opacities in the perihilar and lower lung zones.

Atypical Radiographic Appearances of PVH. Several conditions may give rise to atypical radiographic appearances of PVH. Because the distribution of edema is affected by gravity, it is not surprising that edema fluid accumulates posteriorly or unilaterally in patients maintaining a prolonged supine or decubitus position, respectively. The diagnosis of unilateral edema is suggested by typical radiographic and clinical findings of pulmonary edema in one lung that resolve rapidly or redistribute with changes in patient positioning. Another cause of asymmetric or unilateral pulmonary edema is an interruption in the blood supply to one lung. This may be seen in pulmonary artery hypoplasia or in an acquired obstruction to pulmonary arterial blood flow, such as central pulmonary embolus or extrinsic compression of the pulmonary artery from tumor or fibrosis. In these conditions, the lung with diminished pulmonary blood flow is "protected" from the transudation of fluid and the development of pulmonary edema. Bronchogenic carcinoma, lymphoma, or other causes of unilateral lymph node enlargement can impede normal lymphatic drainage and predispose to unilateral pulmonary edema. Similarly, unilateral pulmonary venous obstruction from tumor or fibrosing mediastinitis will predispose to edema on the affected side. Unilateral pulmonary edema may develop in the lung that is reexpanded by the rapid evacuation of a large pleural fluid collection or pneumothorax. This is known as *reexpansion pulmonary edema* and is discussed in a subsequent section.

Alveolar pulmonary edema localized to the right upper lung may be seen in patients with severe mitral regurgitation. Edema formation is likely the result of preferential regurgitant flow of blood into the right upper lobe pulmonary vein across the superiorly and posteriorly oriented mitral valve. These patients will usually have typical radiographic findings of interstitial edema elsewhere in the lungs.

Patients with pulmonary emphysema frequently have unusual appearances of alveolar edema. Areas of bullae, most commonly in the apical portions of the lungs, are spared from the development of alveolar edema because the pulmonary blood flow to these regions has already been obliterated by the emphysematous process. These emphysematous regions within adjacent areas of airspace opacification can simulate cavity formation and may be difficult to distinguish radiographically from necrotizing pneumonia or pneumatocele formation. Comparison with previous radiographs and correlation with the clinical course will aid in the proper diagnosis.

Increased Capillary Permeability Edema. Rapidly progressive respiratory compromise caused by leakage of protein-rich edema fluid into the lung, resulting from damage to the pulmonary microcirculation, may develop as a complication of a variety of systemic conditions. When respiratory failure develops as a result of this condition and is associated with increased lung stiffness (noncompliance) it is termed *acute respiratory distress syndrome* (ARDS) (3). The edema associated with this syndrome is called *lung injury* or *increased capillary permeability edema*, as compared to the normal alveolocapillary permeability of hydrostatic edema. Many pulmonary and nonpulmonary disorders have been associated with increased-permeability edema (Table 14.2); the most common are shock, severe trauma, burns, sepsis, narcotic overdose, and pancreatitis. Although the precise pathogenesis of capillary permeability edema has yet to be completely elucidated, current evidence suggests that recruitment and activation of neutrophils in the lung with release of enzymes and oxygen radicals are key factors in the development of capillary endothelial damage.

TABLE 14.2

ETIOLOGIES OF INCREASED PERMEABILITY PULMONARY EDEMA

Septicemia	Gram-negative bacteria
Shock	
Major surgery	
Burns	
Acute pancreatitis	
Disseminated intravascular coagulation	
Drugs	Narcotics
	Heroin
	Crack cocaine
	Aspirin
Inhalation of noxious fumes	Nitrogen dioxide (silo filler's disease)
	Hydrocarbons
	Smoke
	Chlorine
	Phosgene
Aspiration of fluid	Fresh or salt water near drowning
	Gastric fluid aspiration (Mendelson syndrome)
Fat embolism	
Amniotic fluid embolism	

The pathologic changes associated with ARDS are those of diffuse alveolar damage and are common to all patients regardless of the underlying etiology. Within 12 to 24 hours following the initial insult (stage 1 ARDS), damage to capillary endothelium produces engorged capillaries and proteinaceous interstitial edema. Within the first week (stage 2), the injury to type 1 pneumocytes leads to the flooding of alveoli with edema fluid and proteinaceous and cellular debris, which form hyaline membranes lining the distal airways and alveoli. In stage 3 ARDS, type 2 pneumocytes proliferate in an attempt to reline the denuded alveolar surfaces, and fibroblastic tissue proliferates within the airspaces. This fibroblastic tissue may resolve and leave minimal scarring or, particularly in those with severe disease and long-standing oxygen requirements, result in extensive interstitial fibrosis.

Radiographically, ARDS follows a predictable pattern. Chest radiographs become abnormal by 12 to 24 hours following the onset of dyspnea and demonstrate patchy peripheral airspace opacities (Fig. 14.3) (2). CT scans show diffuse ground-glass and airspace opacities which may have a striking nondependent distribution. Interlobular septal thickening is usually absent (Fig. 14.4). These opacities coalesce over the next several days to produce confluent bilateral airspace opacities with air bronchograms. Radiographic improvement in the opacities may be seen within the first week, but this is often caused by the effects of increasing positive pressure ventilation rather than true histologic improvement. After 1 week, the airspace opacities gradually give way to a coarse reticulonodular pattern that may resolve over the course of several months or remain unchanged, in which case the pattern represents irreversible pulmonary fibrosis (i.e., honeycombing). Pneumonia complicating ARDS is difficult to diagnose radiographically, but it should be suspected when a focal area of airspace opacification or a significant pleural effusion develops during the

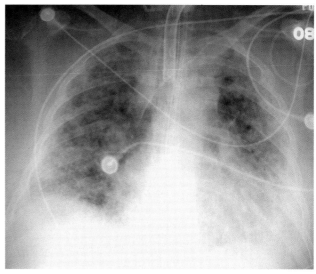

FIGURE 14.3. Increased Permeability (Lung Injury) Edema in Acute Respiratory Distress Syndrome. Portable chest radiograph in a 46-year-old woman with severe pancreatitis and respiratory failure reveals bilateral airspace opacification with a somewhat peripheral distribution, representing diffuse alveolar damage and permeability edema.

course of the disease. Likewise, the superimposition of LV failure may be impossible to recognize but is suggested by rapid clinical and radiographic deterioration associated with changes in measured PCWP and edema fluid protein content. Pneumomediastinum and pneumothorax may result as a complication of positive pressure ventilation to stiff lungs and should be sought on portable chest radiographs.

Radiographic Distinction of Hydrostatic From Increased Capillary Permeability Edema. Beyond identifying the presence of pulmonary edema, the ability to distinguish between types of pulmonary edema has significant diagnostic and therapeutic importance. Measurements of PCWP and transbronchial sampling of pulmonary edema fluid are techniques that accurately distinguish hydrostatic from increased capillary permeability edema. In hydrostatic edema, PCWP measurements are elevated and a protein-poor transudative edema

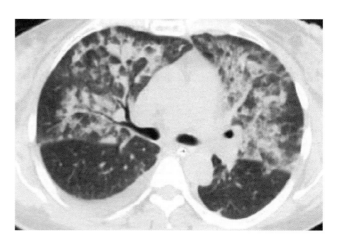

FIGURE 14.4. Thin-Section CT of Lung Injury Edema. Geographic, nondependent ground-glass and airspace opacities are present, but interlobular septal thickening is absent.

fluid is present, whereas in increased-permeability edema, there is a normal PCWP and proteinaceous edema fluid is seen. Milne and colleagues have described the chest radiographic findings that can be used to distinguish cardiac and overhydration edema from increased capillary permeability edema (3). In pulmonary edema associated with chronic cardiac failure, the heart is usually enlarged and displays an inverted (redistributed) pulmonary blood flow pattern. The distribution of edema is even from central to peripheral over the lower lung zones. The vascular pedicle, which represents the mediastinal width at the level of the superior vena cava and left subclavian artery, is widened (>53 mm on posteroanterior radiograph), reflecting increased circulating blood volume. Lung volumes are diminished because of decreased pulmonary compliance from edema. Peribronchial cuffing, Kerley lines, and pleural effusions represent interstitial and intrapleural transudation of fluid, respectively. These findings may be difficult to interpret, however. Furthermore, cardiac size per se is not particularly useful in distinguishing cardiac-related edema from other causes of hydrostatic and capillary leak edema for the following reasons: many patients with heart failure will not have radiographically evident cardiac enlargement; many patients with cardiac enlargement are not in failure; and enlargement of the cardiac silhouette may be caused by pericardial fluid, mediastinal fat, and poor lung expansion. Cardiomegaly is best considered evidence of a chronic condition rather than an indicator of a specific problem.

Capillary permeability edema can sometimes be distinguished from hydrostatic edema by the following: a nondependent or peripheral distribution of edema, an absence of other signs of hydrostatic edema such as interlobular septal thickening and subpleural edema, and, most importantly, a lack of short-term change. It should be noted that some factors may render radiographic distinction of types of pulmonary edema difficult. Radiographs of supine patients will make evaluation of pulmonary blood flow distribution and vascular pedicle width difficult. The presence of severe alveolar edema will obscure underlying vascular markings. Many patients with capillary permeability edema will be overhydrated in attempts to maintain circulating blood volume, producing complex radiographic findings. Lastly, most intubated patients will suffer from more than one problem.

Neurogenic pulmonary edema following head trauma, seizure, or increased intracranial pressure is a complex phenomenon that appears to involve both hydrostatic and increased permeability mechanisms. Massive sympathetic discharge from the brain in these conditions produces systemic vasoconstriction and increased venous return, with resultant increase in LV diastolic pressure and hydrostatic pulmonary edema. The presence of protein-rich edema fluid and normal PCWP in some patients suggests that increased permeability may be a contributing factor.

High-altitude pulmonary edema develops in certain individuals after rapid ascent to altitudes above 3500 m. Edema typically develops within 48 to 72 hours of ascent and appears to reflect a varied individual response to hypoxemia, in which scattered areas of pulmonary arterial spasm result in transient pulmonary arterial hypertension (PAH). This produces an increase in high-pressure blood flow to uninvolved areas, resulting in damage to the capillary endothelium and increased permeability edema, typically with a patchy distribution. Resolution usually occurs within 24 to 48 hours after the administration of supplemental oxygen or a return to sea level.

Reexpansion Pulmonary Edema. Rapid reexpansion of a lung following severe pneumothorax or collapse from a large pleural effusion present more than 48 hours may result in the development of unilateral pulmonary edema. Marked increases in negative pleural pressure following pleural tube placement, impaired pulmonary lymphatic drainage follow-

ing prolonged lung collapse, and ischemia-induced surfactant deficiency resulting in the need for high negative pleural pressure to reexpand the collapsed lung are proposed mechanisms. Recent evidence points toward prolonged collapse producing ischemia and hypoxemia within the lung, which promotes anaerobic metabolism and formation of free radicals. Reperfusion of the lung upon reexpansion then leads to lung injury and permeability edema. Gradual reexpansion of the lung by slow removal of pleural air or fluid over a 24- to 48-hour period and administration of supplemental oxygen help limit the incidence and severity of this complication.

Acute Upper Airway Obstruction. Pulmonary edema may be seen during or immediately after treatment of acute upper airway obstruction. The proposed mechanism involves the creation of markedly negative intrathoracic pressure by attempts to inspire against an extrathoracic airway obstruction, producing transudation of fluid into the lung. There are no distinguishing radiographic features.

Amniotic Fluid Embolism. A severe and often fatal form of pulmonary edema may develop in a pregnant woman when amniotic fluid gains access to the systemic circulation during labor. There is an association of this entity with fetal distress and demise, because the mucin within fetal meconium plays a key role in the pathogenesis of this disorder. Embolic obstruction of the pulmonary vasculature by mucin and fetal squames within the amniotic fluid leads to sudden PAH and cor pulmonale with decreased cardiac output and pulmonary edema. An anaphylactoid reaction and disseminated intravascular coagulopathy (DIC) from factors within the amniotic fluid contribute to vascular collapse. Radiographically, there are typically bilateral confluent airspace opacities indistinguishable from pulmonary edema of other etiologies. In severe cases, there may be enlargement of the central pulmonary arteries and right heart as a manifestation of cor pulmonale. The diagnosis can be confirmed by identification of fetal squames and mucin in blood samples obtained from indwelling pulmonary artery catheters.

Fat Embolism. The embolization of marrow fat to the lung is a common complication occurring 24 to 72 hours after the fracture of a long bone such as the femur. Within the lung, the fat is hydrolyzed to its component fatty acids, causing increased pulmonary capillary permeability and hemorrhagic pulmonary edema. Radiographically and on CT, confluent ground-glass and airspace opacities are seen (Fig. 14.5). The diagnosis is made by recognizing findings of systemic fat embolism (petechial rash, CNS depression) and pulmonary changes in the

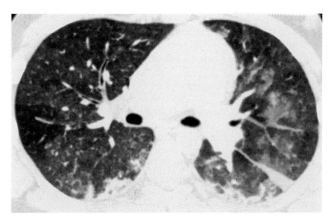

FIGURE 14.5. Fat Embolism Producing Permeability Edema. CT in an 18-year-old man with dyspnea and hypoxemia 48 hours after intramedullary rod placement for a femoral fracture shows asymmetric ground-glass and airspace opacities with small left pleural effusion.

appropriate time period following trauma. Most patients have a mild course with minimal respiratory compromise, whereas a minority will develop progressive respiratory failure leading to death.

PULMONARY HEMORRHAGE AND VASCULITIS

Hemorrhage or hemorrhagic edema of the lung can result from trauma, bleeding diathesis, infections (invasive aspergillosis, mucormycosis, *Pseudomonas*, influenza), drugs (penicillamine), pulmonary embolism, fat embolism, ARDS, and autoimmune diseases (Table 14.3) (4). The autoimmune diseases associated with pulmonary hemorrhage include Goodpasture syndrome, idiopathic pulmonary hemorrhage, Wegener granulomatosis, systemic lupus erythematosus, rheumatoid arthritis, and polyarteritis nodosa.

Goodpasture syndrome is an autoimmune disease characterized by damage to the alveolar and renal glomerular basement membranes by a cytotoxic antibody. The antibody is directed primarily against renal glomerular basement membrane and cross-reacts with alveolar basement membrane to produce the renal injury and pulmonary hemorrhage characteristic of this disorder. Young adult men are most commonly affected and present with cough, hemoptysis, dyspnea, and fatigue. The pulmonary complaints usually precede clinical evidence of renal failure. Chest films show bilateral coalescent airspace opacities that are radiographically indistinguishable from those of pulmonary edema (Fig. 14.6). CT scans demonstrate ground-glass and airspace opacities without interlobular septal thickening acutely (Fig. 14.7). Within several days, the airspace opacities resolve, giving rise to reticular opacities in the same distribution owing to resorption of blood products into the pulmonary interstitium. This results in the so-called crazy paving pattern. Complete radiographic resolution is seen within 2 weeks, except in those with recurrent episodes of hemorrhage, in whom the reticular opacities persist and represent pulmonary fibrosis. The diagnosis is made by immunofluorescent studies of renal or lung tissue, which show a smooth wavy line of fluorescent staining along the basement

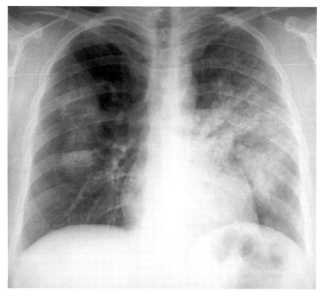

FIGURE 14.6. Pulmonary Hemorrhage in Goodpasture Syndrome. Posteroanterior chest film in a patient with Goodpasture syndrome shows asymmetric bilateral airspace disease presenting intra-alveolar blood.

membrane. The overall prognosis is poor, although the use of immunosuppressive drugs and plasmapheresis has improved survival.

Idiopathic Pulmonary Hemorrhage. The pulmonary manifestations of idiopathic pulmonary hemorrhage are clinically and radiographically indistinguishable from those of Goodpasture syndrome. In distinction to Goodpasture syndrome, this disorder is most common in children, with an equal sex distribution. The diagnosis is one of exclusion and is suggested when pulmonary hemorrhage and anemia are found in a patient with normal renal function and urinalysis and an absence of antiglomerular basement membrane antibodies.

TABLE 14.3

CAUSES OF PULMONARY HEMORRHAGE

Spontaneous	Thrombocytopenia Hemophilia Anticoagulant therapy
Trauma	Pulmonary contusion
Embolic disease	Pulmonary embolism Fat embolism

Vasculitis	Autoimmune
	    Goodpasture syndrome
	    Idiopathic pulmonary hemorrhage
	    Antineutrophil cytoplasmic
	        autoantibody (ANCA) positive
	        vasculitis (see Table 14.5)
	Infectious
	    Gram-negative bacteria
	    Influenza
	    Aspergillosis
	    Mucormycosis

Drugs	Penicillamine

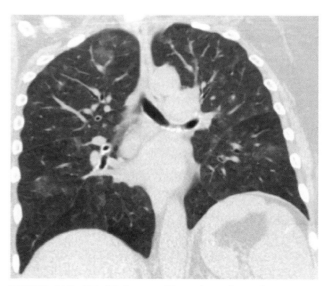

FIGURE 14.7. CT of Pulmonary Hemorrhage. Coronal reconstruction demonstrates diffuse, patchy ground-glass opacities and minimal interlobular septal thickening in the periphery of both lungs, but no pleural fluid or fissural thickening.

Other Vasculitides. Wegener granulomatosis, systemic lupus erythematosus, rheumatoid arthritis, and polyarteritis nodosa are autoimmune disorders associated with a systemic immune complex vasculitis (5). The development of pulmonary hemorrhage in these diseases is secondary to small vessel pulmonary arteritis and capillaritis, which results in spontaneous hemorrhage. The pulmonary manifestations of these diseases are discussed in subsequent sections.

Differentiation of pulmonary hemorrhage from pulmonary edema or pneumonia may be difficult, particularly because many causes of pulmonary edema and pneumonia may have a significant hemorrhagic component. The rapid development of airspace opacities associated with a dropping hematocrit and hemoptysis should suggest the diagnosis. Hemoptysis, however, is not always present. Associated renal disease, hematuria, or findings of a collagen vascular disorder or systemic vasculitis may provide additional clues. The distinction of pulmonary hemorrhage from pneumonia is made by the absence of fever or purulent sputum and the finding of a normal or elevated carbon monoxide–diffusing capacity. This latter determination is directly related to the volume of gas-exchanging intravascular and extravascular intrapulmonary red blood cells and is therefore elevated in pulmonary hemorrhage or hemorrhagic edema but decreased in pneumonia. The presence of hemosiderin-laden macrophages in sputum, bronchoalveolar lavage fluid, or tissue specimens is evidence of chronic or recurrent intrapulmonary hemorrhage. A rapid radiographic improvement of the airspace opacities in pulmonary hemorrhage is common and may aid in diagnosis.

PULMONARY EMBOLISM

Pulmonary embolism (PE) is a common cause of acute chest symptoms. While it is associated with significant morbidity and mortality, treatment with anticoagulation can significantly reduce the likelihood of recurrent emboli that might result in chronic thromboembolic pulmonary hypertension or death. Since anticoagulation has associated morbidity, particularly in elderly and debilitated patients, an accurate determination of the presence or absence of PE is necessary.

The radiologist plays a central role in the diagnostic evaluation of the patient with suspected PE. This section will briefly review the aspects of patient evaluation not related to imaging and then detail the various imaging modalities available to the radiologist. A practical algorithm that serves as a useful guide to the workup of each patient with suspected PE will be provided.

Clinical and Laboratory Findings. The majority of patients with PE have a variety of symptoms, including dyspnea (84%), pleuritic chest pain (74%), anxiety (59%), and cough (53%), and in some patients asymptomatic embolization can occur. Physical examination may reveal tachypnea (respiratory rate >16/min), rales, and a prominent pulmonary component of the second heart sound. Unfortunately, these findings are entirely nonspecific. Only a minority of patients presenting to an emergency department with pleuritic chest pain will be found to have PE.

The main laboratory test obtained in patients with suspected PE is a plasma D-dimer level. D-dimer is a degradation product of fibrin and is a very sensitive indicator of the presence of venous thrombosis. Enzyme-linked immunosorbent assay D-dimer measurements have a sensitivity for deep venous thrombosis (DVT) of 98% to 100%, and therefore a normal value will effectively exclude the possibility of DVT and PE, particularly when the clinical probability for PE is low.

Radiologic Evaluation. A number of imaging techniques are routinely employed in the evaluation of the patient with suspected PE. These include the chest radiograph, ventilation/ perfusion (V/Q) lung scintigraphy, CT angiography, and conventional pulmonary angiography. Noninvasive methods of imaging DVTs include compression and Doppler US of the legs, lower-extremity indirect CT venography, and magnetic resonance venography of the extremities and pelvis. The relatively noninvasive nature and high accuracy of these techniques to diagnose DVT and an increasing familiarity with their performance and interpretation among radiologists have led to their widespread use in the workup of PE.

Chest radiography is the first examination obtained in all patients with suspected PE. Although the majority of patients with PE will have abnormal radiographs, a significant percentage of patients will have normal chest radiographs. The radiographic findings include cardiac, pulmonary arterial, parenchymal, pleural, and diaphragmatic changes (6).

Cardiac enlargement, or more precisely right heart enlargement, is an uncommon finding seen with massive or extensive PE producing cor pulmonale. Enlargement of the central pulmonary arteries from PAH may also be seen but is more commonly a late sequela of chronic thromboembolic disease. The most common radiographic findings in PE without infarction are peripheral airspace opacities and linear atelectasis. Localized peripheral oligemia with or without distended proximal vessels (Westermark sign) is exceedingly rare. The airspace opacification represents localized pulmonary hemorrhage produced by bronchial and pulmonary venous collateral flow to the obstructed region and is seen with peripheral but not central emboli. Volume loss in the lower lung from adhesive atelectasis caused by ischemic injury to type 2 pneumocytes and secondary surfactant deficiency may produce diaphragmatic elevation and the development of linear atelectasis.

Less than 10% of all PEs result in lung infarction. Collateral bronchial arterial and retrograde pulmonary venous flow prevent infarction in most patients. The distinction between embolism without and with infarction is usually impossible radiographically and is of limited importance, as treatment is identical. Infarction from embolism occurs with greater frequency in patients with underlying heart failure because of their limited collateral bronchial arterial flow to the ischemic region. In PEs with infarction, the cardiac, pulmonary arterial, and peripheral vascular changes are indistinguishable from those seen in embolism without infarction.

Radiographic features that suggest infarction include the presence of a pleural effusion and the development of a pleura-based wedge-shaped opacity (Hampton hump). This opacity, typically found in the posterior or lateral costophrenic sulcus of the lung, is wedge-shaped, homogeneous, and lacks an air bronchogram. The blunted apex of the wedge points toward the occluded feeding vessel, whereas the base is against the pleural surface. It is often obscured by surrounding areas of hemorrhage in the early phases following infarction, but becomes more obvious with time as the peripheral areas of hemorrhage resolve. A distinction between PE with and without infarction is usually made by noting changes in the radiographic opacities with time. In embolism without infarction, the airspace opacities should resolve completely within 7 to 10 days, whereas infarcts resolve over the course of several weeks or months and usually leave a residual linear parenchymal scar and/or localized pleural thickening.

None of the aforementioned radiographic findings, either alone or in combination, are useful in making a firm diagnosis of PE. Conversely, a completely normal radiograph may be seen in up to 40% of patients with emboli. The prime utility of the chest radiograph in the evaluation of PE is in the detection of conditions that mimic PE clinically, such as pneumonia or pneumothorax, and as an aid to the interpretation of the ventilation/perfusion lung scan.

Ventilation/Perfusion (V/Q) Lung Scintigraphy. The IV administration of macroaggregates of albumin radiolabeled with technetium (Tc-99m) has given the radiologist a noninvasive method of assessing the patency of the pulmonary circulation. The sensitivity of this technique allows for the confident exclusion of PE when a technically adequate perfusion scan is normal. The addition of ventilation scanning increases the specificity of an abnormal perfusion scan and is always performed in conjunction with the perfusion scan when possible.

Perfusion lung scanning is performed by IV injection of 5 mCi of Tc-99m macroaggregated albumin with the patient supine (see Chapter 56). Images are then obtained in eight projections: anteroposterior, posteroanterior, right and left lateral, and right and left anterior and posterior oblique views. If perfusion abnormalities are present, a ventilation scan using krypton-81m, xenon-133, or aerosolized Tc-99m diethylenetriamine pentaacetic acid (DTPA) is then performed. The use of krypton-81m and Tc-99m DTPA allows for comparable oblique projections identical to the perfusion scan. Perfusion defects can then be characterized as ventilation/perfusion matches (absent ventilation/absent perfusion) or mismatches (normal ventilation/absent perfusion). Ventilation/perfusion mismatch is the hallmark of PE.

Although V/Q scanning is commonly used in the evaluation of the patient with suspected PE, there are limitations to its utility for the diagnosis of PE. First, only a minority of patients (27% in the Prospective Investigation of Pulmonary Embolism Diagnosis [PIOPED] study) undergoing V/Q studies will have either a normal or high-probability study, a result that clinicians can confidently rely upon to guide treatment decisions (5). Second, there is significant interobserver variability in the interpretation of V/Q studies. Finally, there are few well-constructed prospective studies evaluating the accuracy of various patterns of V/Q abnormality in predicting the likelihood of PE.

Several diagnostic schemes have been proposed to assign a probability of PE (as determined by pulmonary angiography) given specific combinations of ventilation, perfusion, and concurrent chest radiographic findings. The V/Q scan interpretation categories published with the results of the PIOPED study have become the standard for radiologists interpreting V/Q studies. A normal V/Q scan effectively excludes PE because of the high sensitivity of the test. A high-probability scan, particularly in a patient with a strong clinical suspicion for embolic disease, allows the patient to be confidently treated for PE. Patients with intermediate or indeterminate (because of extensive obstructive lung disease) probability scans have a 30% to 40% incidence of PE. Likewise, those with a low-probability V/Q scan and a high clinical suspicion for PE should have further noninvasive imaging of the deep venous system or pulmonary arteries. (See Chapter 56 for an expanded discussion of pulmonary scintigraphy.)

Despite its limitations, V/Q scanning can provide useful information and remains a useful noninvasive screening modality for detecting PE. Although uncommon, a normal perfusion study excludes embolism, whereas a high-probability V/Q study, in the appropriate clinical setting, allows for a confident enough diagnosis of PE to initiate anticoagulant therapy. Currently, its role in the evaluation of PE is primarily limited to those patients with a high likelihood of having a diagnostic result (i.e., normal or high probability); such patients are generally young individuals with normal chest radiographs and no history of chronic obstructive pulmonary disease.

CT Pulmonary Angiography. Dynamic CT angiography of the pulmonary arteries (CTPA) using MDCT has proven accurate in the detection of PE (7). Contiguous or overlapping 1- to 2-mm scans through the entire thorax during injection of 80 to 120 mL of 300 to 350 mg I(iodine)/mL nonionic contrast injected through an 18-gauge or larger IV catheter allow routine dense opacification of second- and third-order subsegmental pulmonary arteries. Scans must be interpreted on workstations in a paging or cine mode to allow efficient review and accurate interpretation of the large data sets produced by the current 16- to 64-channel MDCT scanners.

Acute emboli are recognized as intraluminal filling defects (Fig. 14.8) or nonopacified vessels with a convex filling toward the proximal lumen. Secondary findings that can be seen on CT include peripheral oligemia (Westermark sign), pleura-based wedge-shaped consolidation reflecting peripheral hemorrhage or infarct, linear atelectasis, and pleural effusion. The detection of a high-attenuation thrombus in the pulmonary arteries on unenhanced CT in patients with PE has been rarely described. Chronic emboli should be suggested when the filling defect is adherent to the vessel wall rather than in the center of the lumen or a web is present (Fig. 14.9). Common diagnostic pitfalls in the detection of PE on CTPA include motion artifact, streak artifact from dense contrast or catheters, partial volume averaging of obliquely oriented vessels, prominent hilar lymphoid tissue, poorly opacified pulmonary veins, mucus-filled bronchi, and regional areas of increased pulmonary arterial resistance from consolidation or atelectasis, all of which can simulate intraluminal arterial filling defects.

At present MDCT is widely considered the first-line diagnostic modality for the evaluation of suspected PE. Confident detection of a discrete intraluminal filling defect is highly specific for PE. Conversely, multiple studies have shown that the negative predictive value of a good-quality CTPA for PE is greater than 95%. For these reasons, only those patients at high risk for significant morbidity or mortality from recurrent PE (i.e., patients with severe chronic obstructive pulmonary disease or cor pulmonale) should be considered for conventional angiography following a negative or inconclusive CT study; the latter occurs in approximately 5% of patients referred for CTPA, a percentage similar to that of nondiagnostic pulmonary arteriograms.

Although the ability to detect small emboli has improved significantly with MDCT, the main limitation of CTPA remains the reliable detection of small (subsegmental) emboli, although the frequency and clinical significance of such emboli are subjects of significant debate. In addition to the detection of emboli, up to two-thirds of patients with acute chest symptoms who are studied with CTPA to exclude PE have an alternative diagnosis suggested by findings detected on CT, something not possible with techniques that evaluate only the pulmonary vasculature such as perfusion scintigraphy, MR angiography, and conventional angiography.

Pulmonary angiography has traditionally been considered to be the gold standard in the diagnosis of PE (8). Digital subtraction angiography is the technique selectively used when a definitive diagnosis of PE or DVT cannot be achieved by less invasive means. This study, which requires right heart and pulmonary arterial catheterization with selective injection of nonionic contrast, can be performed safely in a majority of patients. The accuracy of pulmonary arteriography in the diagnosis of PE is high. On the basis of clinical follow-up of patients with negative studies, the sensitivity of pulmonary angiography is 98% to 99%, although as with CTPA, the accuracy for the detection of subsegmental PE is closer to 66%.

PE is diagnosed on pulmonary angiography when an intraluminal filling defect or the trailing end of an occluding thrombus is outlined by contrast. Secondary signs, including a prolonged arterial phase, diminished peripheral perfusion, and delay in the venous phase, are nonspecific and are not used to diagnose PE. Once a thrombus is unequivocally identified, the study is terminated. The only exception would be a patient who is considered a candidate for surgical thrombectomy or thrombolytic therapy, where precise knowledge of the laterality, location, and extent of the thrombus is required.

The overall complication rate of pulmonary angiography is 2% to 5% and can be divided into those related to contrast

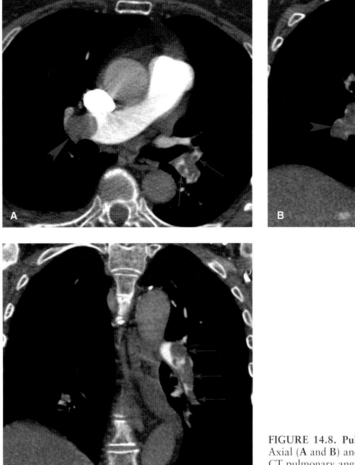

FIGURE 14.8. Pulmonary Embolism on CT Angiography. Axial (**A** and **B**) and coronal (**C**) reconstructed images from a CT pulmonary angiogram show nearly occlusive thrombus in the right main pulmonary artery (*arrowheads*) and the left lower lobe pulmonary artery and its branches (*arrows*).

administration and those secondary to cardiac catheterization and injection of intrapulmonary arterial contrast. Mortality from pulmonary angiography is less than 0.5% and is usually related to sudden RV failure from transient elevation of pul- monary artery pressure secondary to contrast injection. Death from pulmonary angiography is seen almost exclusively in criti- cally ill patients and those with preexisting severe PAH (pulmo- nary artery systolic pressure >70 mm Hg) or RV dysfunction

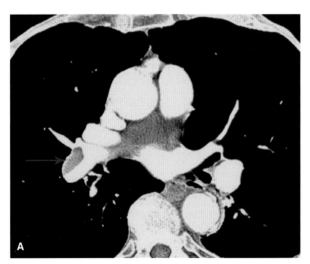

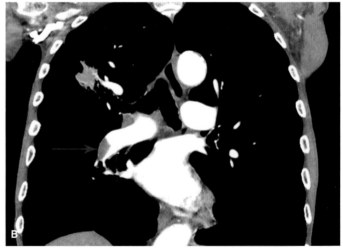

FIGURE 14.9. Chronic Pulmonary Emboli. Axial (**A**) and coronal (**B**) reconstructions demonstrate a large filling defect (*arrows*) adherent to the anterolateral wall of the pulmonary artery to the right lower lobe.

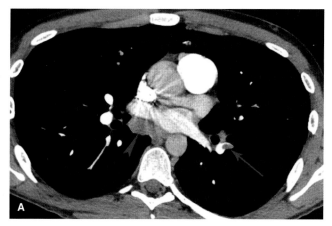
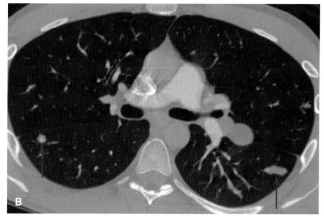

FIGURE 14.10. Pulmonary Tumor Emboli From Metastatic Renal Cell Carcinoma. A. Axial CT image shows a filling defect (*arrow*) representing a tumor embolus in the artery to the anteromedial basal segment artery of the left lower lobe. An enlarged subcarinal lymph node (*arrowhead*) is also present. **B.** Round and ovoid metastases (*arrows*) to the lung are present in the superior segments.

(RV end diastolic pressure >20 mm Hg). There is no significant increase, however, in the incidence of major, nonfatal reactions in patients with PAH. In addition, the majority of patients with severe RV dysfunction have uneventful studies. When one considers the added safety of selective contrast injections using nonionic contrast agents and the high mortality of untreated PE in this population, pulmonary angiography should be performed in these patients when indicated.

Noninvasive Imaging for DVT. The use of noninvasive techniques for the diagnosis of DVT has altered the conventional approach to the evaluation of pulmonary thromboembolic disease (see Chapter 40). Because 90% of PEs arise from the lower extremities, and because the treatment for proximal (i.e., above-the-knee) DVT is identical to that for proven PE, a confident diagnosis of proximal DVT can provide an endpoint in patient evaluation for thromboembolic disease.

When performed by skilled personnel, compression US has a sensitivity of 90% to 95% and a specificity of 95% to 98% for the diagnosis of acute DVT when compared to contrast venography. False-negative studies occur when DVT is limited to the calf or pelvis, or in patients with duplicated deep venous systems. False-positive studies are seen most often in patients with prior DVT. In addition to providing an accurate diagnosis of the presence of DVT, US offers the advantage of imaging the nonvenous structures in the leg, allowing the radiologist to diagnose conditions that may simulate DVT clinically, such as Baker cysts, enlarged lymph nodes, pseudoaneurysms, and pelvic masses compressing the iliac vein.

Although accurate for the diagnosis of proximal DVT, a negative compression US study does not exclude PE. Thus, patients with a negative US study should undergo evaluation of the pulmonary arteries with CT or conventional angiography.

Indirect CT venography (CTV), typically performed after contrast injection has been administered for CTPA, has been used to allow detection of thigh and pelvic DVT. Axial or helical scans performed from the popliteal fossa to the diaphragm obtained approximately 3 minutes after the initiation of contrast injection for CTPA have been shown in preliminary studies to have a high accuracy in the detection of proximal lower-extremity and pelvic DVT. The addition of CTV to CTPA can provide incremental information for the diagnosis of venous thromboembolic disease, particularly when a proximal DVT is detected in a patient with a poor-quality, equivocal, or negative CTPA study.

MR venography and radionuclide scintigraphy can be used to detect DVT, but these are not used routinely in clinical practice for this purpose.

Nonthrombotic pulmonary embolism can occur rarely. The most commonly described conditions are (1) air embolism, usually as a result of air within a venous catheter or air injected during contrast-enhanced CT; (2) macroscopic fat embolism following long bone fracture, with pulmonary embolization of marrow elements; (3) methylmethacrylate embolization complicating vertebroplasty; and (4) radioactive seed implant embolization from prostate brachytherapy.

Pulmonary tumor emboli can develop in a small percentage of patients with malignancies such as bronchoalveolar cell carcinoma, breast cancer, hepatoma, and GI malignancies. These tumor emboli may lead to significant respiratory symptoms because of occlusion of small vessels. Imaging features are uncommon but include central pulmonary arterial dilation and enlarged, nodular peripheral pulmonary artery branches on thin-section CT (Fig. 14.10). In patients suspected of this disorder, aspiration cytology from a wedged pulmonary arterial occlusion (Swan–Ganz) catheter can be useful for diagnosis.

PULMONARY ARTERIAL HYPERTENSION

Pulmonary arterial hypertension (PAH) is defined as a systolic pressure in the pulmonary artery exceeding 30 mm Hg, either measured directly, by catheterization of the pulmonary artery, or estimated by echocardiography. The diagnosis of PAH is usually evident from the clinical history, physical findings, and appearance on chest radiographs. The typical radiographic findings of PAH are enlarged main and hilar pulmonary arteries that taper rapidly toward the lung periphery (Fig. 14.11). Associated enlargement of the RV, seen on lateral radiographs as prominence of the anterosuperior cardiac margin with obliteration of the retrosternal airspace, is an additional clue to the diagnosis. Occasionally, hypertension-induced atherosclerotic lesions in the large elastic arteries can produce mural calcifications on radiographs or CT, a rare finding that is specific for PAH. A useful measurement for enlargement of the central pulmonary arteries, usually indicating PAH in the absence of a left-to-right shunt, is a transverse diameter of the proximal interlobar pulmonary artery on posteroanterior chest radiograph that exceeds 16 mm. CT measurement of the main pulmonary artery is even more useful (9). In patients younger than 50 years, a ratio of the diameter of the main pulmonary artery (measured at the level of the main right pulmonary artery) to the transverse diameter of the ascending aorta at the

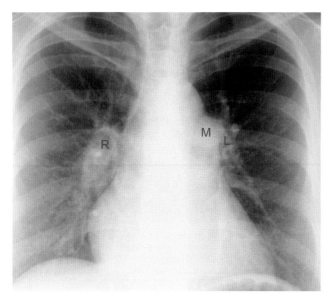

FIGURE 14.11. Pulmonary Arterial Hypertension. Posteroanterior chest radiograph in a 29-year-old woman with idiopathic pulmonary hypertension shows enlarged main (*M*), right (*R*), and left (*L*) pulmonary arteries with diminutive peripheral vessels.

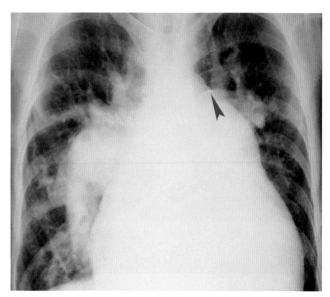

FIGURE 14.13. Acquired Eisenmenger Syndrome. A frontal radiograph of a 56-year-old man with an atrial septal defect shows massive enlargement of the central pulmonary arteries and heart with "pruning" of the peripheral vessels and calcium in the left pulmonary artery (*arrowhead*) consistent with high pulmonary arterial resistance.

same level greater than 1.0 strongly correlates with a mean pulmonary artery pressure greater than 20 mm Hg. Because the aorta normally enlarges with advancing age, in patients older than 50 years, a maximum transverse measurement of the main pulmonary artery greater than 30 mm correlates better (Fig. 14.12). All of this assumes that the patient does not have pulmonary overcirculation, in which case the peripheral vessels will also be enlarged. Flattening or bowing of the interventricular septum toward the LV indicates RV hypertension. A normal measurement of the main or right interlobar pulmonary artery does not exclude PAH, as patients with mild or even moderate elevation of pulmonary artery pressure may have normal-sized arteries. Those patients with long-standing PAH will develop RV hypertrophy, with eventual RV dilatation and failure (cor pulmonale). MR may also demonstrate intraluminal signal during the early diastolic phase of the cardiac cycle, a finding indicative of turbulent flow caused by the increased vascular resistance that is sometimes seen with marked elevation of pulmonary artery pressure.

In addition to PAH, enlargement of the central pulmonary arteries may be seen in conditions associated with increased flow through the pulmonary circulation. This occurs in patients with a high cardiac output, such as anemia, those with thyrotoxicosis, or those with left-to-right shunts. The latter includes atrial and ventricular septal defects, patent ductus arteriosus, and partial anomalous pulmonary venous return. Early in the course of left-to-right shunts, the pulmonary artery pressure is normal or slightly elevated, because pulmonary vascular resistance drops to compensate for the increased flow. In these patients, there is enlargement of both central and peripheral pulmonary arteries, producing "shunt vascularity" on chest radiographs. If uncorrected, some of these individuals will develop muscular hypertrophy of the pulmonary arterioles with medial hyperplasia and intimal fibrosis causing an increase in pulmonary vascular resistance (Eisenmenger syndrome). These patients have typically very large hearts owing to long-standing overcirculation with superimposed pulmonary hypertension (Fig. 14.13). Many patients with Eisenmenger

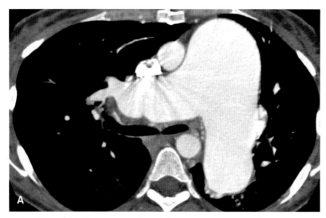
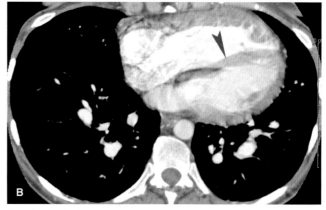

FIGURE 14.12. Pulmonary Arterial Hypertension. Axial CT scans through at the level of the main pulmonary arteries (**A**) and the ventricles (**B**) show marked enlargement of the pulmonary trunk and both main pulmonary arteries. Flattening of the interventricular septum (*arrowhead*) indicates high right ventricular pressure.

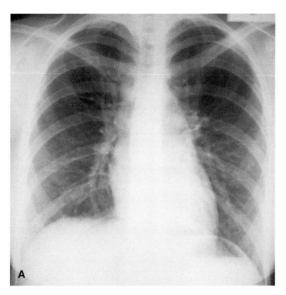 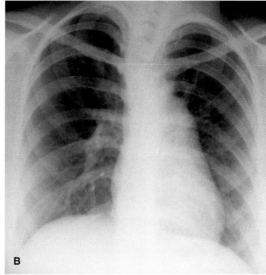

FIGURE 14.14. **Congenital Eisenmenger Syndrome. A.** Frontal chest radiograph in a 19-year-old woman with complete atrioventricular canal. The chest radiograph is normal except for mild prominence of the pulmonary trunk, which could be normal for a patient this age. The history of cyanosis since early childhood strongly suggests congenitally elevated pulmonary arterial resistance. Pulmonary artery pressure was suprasystemic. **B.** Frontal radiograph in a 16-year-old girl with a ventricular septal defect shows an enlarged pulmonary trunk and slightly prominent descending right pulmonary artery. Pulmonary pressures were systemic.

physiology have high pulmonary resistance and are cyanotic since early childhood. They typically present with relatively unimpressive chest radiographs with a normal heart size and slightly enlarged pulmonary trunk (Fig. 14.14).

An increase in resistance to pulmonary blood flow is the most common cause of PAH (Table 14.4). The most common causes are parenchymal lung disease and chronic hypoventilation from obstructive sleep apnea. Other causes include severe chest wall deformity, diffuse pleural fibrosis, recurrent PE, pulmonary vasculitis (e.g., lupus and scleroderma), and idiopathic (primary) pulmonary hypertension. Chronic elevation of pulmonary venous pressure can also result in PAH. This is most commonly the result of mitral stenosis, although any impedance to pulmonary venous return to the left heart can produce venous hypertension. Less common entities in this group include atrial myxoma, cor triatriatum, and pulmonary vein stenosis or occlusion. Chronic LV failure rarely, if ever, results in PAH owing to relatively short chronicity. An important clue to the presence of mitral stenosis is enlargement of the LA and appendage. Unfortunately, the pulmonary trunk may be enlarged in patients with LV failure from ischemic heart disease owing to the presence of concomitant emphysema.

Parenchymal lung diseases, particularly centrilobular emphysema and diffuse interstitial fibrosis, are common causes of PAH. The mechanisms by which these disorders produce increased vascular resistance include chronic hypoxemia and reflex vasoconstriction and the development of irreversible changes in pulmonary arteriolar caliber, with widespread obliteration of the pulmonary vascular bed. The radiographic findings of emphysema and interstitial fibrosis are usually evident on plain radiographs by the time PAH has developed (Fig. 14.15).

Chronic hypoxemia from alveolar hypoventilation is the likely mechanism for PAH that complicates pleural fibrosis, kyphoscoliosis, and the obesity–hypoventilation syndrome. Pleural thickening and kyphoscoliosis are readily evident radiographically. The obesity–hypoventilation (obstructive sleep apnea) syndrome is usually associated with marked truncal obesity and lungs that are diminished in volume (mostly

owing to diaphragmatic elevation) but are normal in appearance.

Disorders of the pulmonary arteries that produce PAH include chronic PEs, vasculitis, and pulmonary arteriopathy resulting from long-standing increased pulmonary blood flow from left-to-right shunt. Occlusion of lobar and segmental vessels producing PAH can result from failure of pulmonary thromboemboli to lyse or completely recanalize (Fig. 14.16).

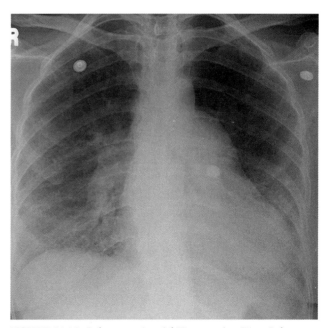

FIGURE 14.15. **Pulmonary Arterial Hypertension From Pulmonary Fibrosis.** Frontal chest radiograph in a 49-year-old woman with scleroderma shows typical findings of pulmonary artery hypertension as well as basilar predominant interstitial lung disease.

TABLE 14.4

CAUSES OF PULMONARY ARTERIAL HYPERTENSION

Chronic pulmonary venous hypertension

Lung disease/chronic hypoxemia
   Emphysema/chronic bronchitis
   Cystic lung disease
      Langerhans cell histiocytosis
      Lymphangioleiomyomatosis
   Cystic fibrosis
   Interstitial fibrosis
      Usual interstitial pneumonitis
      Sarcoidosis
      Radiation fibrosis (rare)
   Small airways disease
      Constrictive bronchiolitis

Chronic hypoventilation
   Obesity and obstructive sleep apnea
   Chest wall deformity (kyphoscoliosis)

Idiopathic (primary) pulmonary hypertension

Eisenmenger syndrome

Pulmonary vasculitis (plexogenic pulmonary arteriopathy)
   Connective tissue diseases (scleroderma, lupus, mixed
     connective tissue disease)
   ANCA-positive vasculitis (see Table 14.5)
   HIV infection

Drugs (fenfluramine, dexfenfluramine, "fen-phen")

Chronic pulmonary thromboembolic disease

ANCA-positive vasculitis
   Wegener vasculitis
   Churg–Strauss vasculitis
   Microscopic polyangiitis
   Drug-induced vasculitis

ANCA, antineutrophil cytoplasmic antibody.

TABLE 14.5

Antineutrophil Cytoplasmic Antibody (ANCA) positive
  vasculitis
Wegener vasculitis
Churg-Strauss vasculitis
Microscopic polyangitis
Drug induced vasculitis

Rarely, pulmonary vasculitis resulting from diseases such as rheumatoid lung disease or Takayasu arteritis produces obliteration of the pulmonary vasculature and leads to PAH.

The diagnosis of large-vessel thromboembolic pulmonary hypertension is usually made by echocardiography, which provides an indirect estimate of pulmonary artery pressure. CT angiographic findings of chronic thromboembolic pulmonary hypertension (CTPH) correlate with conventional angiographic findings and include focal stenoses, bandlike or weblike filling defects, and eccentric wall thickening (Figs. 14.9 and 14.16). Lung windows in patients with CTPH classically demonstrate a pattern of mosaic attenuation, with the hyperlucent regions demonstrating attenuated vascular markings (mosaic oligemia) as compared to areas of increased attenuation that result from hyperemia from intact pulmonary artery branches.

Idiopathic or primary pulmonary hypertension encompasses diseases of the pulmonary arterioles and venules that are not attributable to other etiologies and have characteristic histologic findings. *Plexogenic pulmonary arteriopathy, recurrent microscopic PE,* and *pulmonary veno-occlusive disease* (PVOD) are the three diseases that comprise this category. Plexogenic pulmonary arteriopathy is a disease among young women in whom medial hypertrophy and intimal fibrosis obliterate the muscular arteries. Dilated vascular channels within the periphery of the obliterated vessel produce the plexogenic lesions seen on biopsy in virtually all patients with this disease. Progressive dyspnea and fatigue develop with characteristic physical findings of PAH and cor pulmonale. In plexogenic pulmonary arteriopathy, pulmonary perfusion scans typically show normal perfusion or small, nonsegmental peripheral perfusion defects, allowing distinction from large-vessel thromboembolic disease. Microembolic disease is

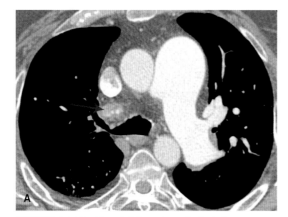
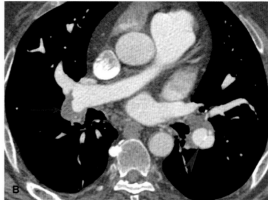

FIGURE 14.16. Chronic Thromboembolic Pulmonary Hypertension. A. Enhanced CT scan at the level of the main pulmonary artery shows dilated main and left pulmonary arteries, with thrombosis of the truncus anterior branch of the right pulmonary artery (*arrow*). **B.** At the level of the hila, there is an eccentric filling defect (*arrow*) in the right interlobar artery and a weblike filling defect (*arrowhead*) containing calcification in the left interlobar artery. These findings are characteristic of chronic unresolved emboli.

clinically and radiographically indistinguishable from plexo-genic arteriopathy. In this entity, plexogenic lesions within arterioles are absent. Perfusion scans are more likely to show small perfusion defects in this disorder. The presence of small microemboli histologically is not a distinguishing feature, because in situ thrombosis within diseased arterioles can have a similar appearance. In PVOD, the obliteration of small intra-pulmonary venules results in interstitial pulmonary edema. A condition related to PVOD is *pulmonary capillary hemangio-matosis* (PCH), which is characterized by the proliferation of capillaries throughout the pulmonary interstitium, resulting in venular obstruction. The transmission of increased pressure to the arterial side leads to medial hypertrophy and oblit-eration of vessel lumina with resultant arterial hypertension. Chest radiographs often show interstitial or airspace pulmo-nary edema with a normal heart size. Perfusion lung scanning is usually normal or shows small peripheral nonsegmental defects. The combination of pulmonary edema with a normal heart size, absent findings for PVH, normal PCWP, and the insidious onset of dyspnea should suggest this diagnosis rather than left heart failure, mitral valve disease, or large-vessel pul-monary venous occlusion. Thin-section CT features of PVOD and PCH are those of PVH and include interlobular septal thickening, centrilobular nodular ground-glass opacities, and pleural effusions (10). A definitive diagnosis can only be made by characteristic findings on open lung biopsy. The prognosis is universally poor, with most patients succumbing to their dis-ease within 2 years of diagnosis.

References

1. Pistolesi M, Miniati M, Milne ENC, Giuntini C. The chest roentgenogram in pulmonary edema. Clin Chest Med 1985;6:315–344.
2. Ketai L, Godwin D. A new view of pulmonary edema and acute respira-tory distress syndrome. J Thorac Imaging 1998;13:147–171.
3. Milne ENC, Pistolesi M, Miniati M, Giuntini C. The radiologic distinc-tion of cardiogenic and noncardiogenic edema. AJR Am J Roentgenol 1985;144:879–894.
4. Albelda SM, Gefter WB, Epstein DM, Miller WT. Diffuse pulmonary hemorrhage: a review and classification. Radiology 1985;154:289–297.
5. The PIOPED investigators. Value of the ventilation/perfusion scan in acute pulmonary embolism: results of the prospective investigation of pulmo-nary embolism diagnosis (PIOPED). JAMA 1990;263:2753–2759.
6. Buckner CB, Walker CW, Purnell GL. Pulmonary embolism: chest radio-graphic abnormalities. J Thorac Imaging 1989;4:23–27.
7. Schoepf UJ, Costello P. CT angiography for diagnosis of pulmonary embo-lism: state of the art. Radiology 2004;230:329–337.
8. Stein PD, Athanasoulis C, Alavi A, et al. Complications and validity of pulmonary angiography in acute pulmonary embolism. Circulation 1992;85:462–468.
9. Ng CS, Wells AU, Padley SPG. A CT sign of chronic pulmonary arterial hypertension: the ratio of the main pulmonary artery to aortic diameter. J Thorac Imaging 1999;14:270–278.
10. Hansell DM. Small-vessel diseases of the lung: CT-pathologic correlates. Radiology 2002;225:639–653.

CHAPTER 15 ■ PULMONARY NEOPLASMS

JEFFREY S. KLEIN

The Solitary Pulmonary Nodule Lesions Presenting as SPNs **Bronchogenic Carcinoma** Cytologic and Pathologic Features Radiologic Staging of Lung Cancer	**Tracheal and Bronchial Masses** **Metastatic Disease to the Thorax** **Nonepithelial Parenchymal Malignancies and** **Neoplastic-Like Conditions**

THE SOLITARY PULMONARY NODULE

The radiologic evaluation of a solitary pulmonary nodule (SPN) remains one of the most common and most difficult diagnostic dilemmas in thoracic radiology (1). The prevalence of SPNs has increased recently as a result of the growing use of MDCT. Before embarking on a detailed diagnostic evaluation of an SPN, one must determine whether a focal opacity seen on the chest radiograph is real or artifactual. When a focal opacity is detected radiographically, efforts should be made to ascertain whether it is truly intrathoracic, which should begin with a careful review of a lateral radiograph to localize the opacity. Densities seen on only a single view may reflect artifacts, skin, chest wall or pleural lesions, or true intrapulmonary nodules. Occasionally, physical examination can reveal a skin lesion that accounts for the opacity. Chest fluoroscopy can be useful to help localize an opacity seen on only a single radiographic projection and can identify the opacity as within the chest wall or alternatively in the lung. If available, dual energy chest radiography with review of the bone image can be used as a problem-solving tool to identify calcified lesions such as healed rib fractures or bone islands, calcified granulomas of lung, or calcified pleural plaques that may produce a nodular opacity on frontal radiographs. Often a limited chest CT focused on the area in question on the chest radiograph is necessary to definitively delineate the location and nature of a focal nodular radiographic opacity.

Comparison chest radiographs, when available, should be reviewed to determine whether nodular opacities were evident previously. An opacity completely stable in size for more than 2 years is considered benign and further evaluation is unnecessary. If there is any concern that a nodule previously seen has enlarged, a chest CT should be obtained for further characterization.

Once a new or enlarging SPN has been identified, the radiologist should initiate a series of investigations to determine whether the nodule has features that are definitely benign, highly suspicious for malignancy, or lacking clear benign or malignant features and therefore indeterminate. This stepwise approach is summarized in Figure 15.1.

Clinical Factors. Before considering the radiologic features used to characterize a lung nodule, several important clinical factors may be helpful in making this distinction. In a patient younger than 35 years, particularly a nonsmoker without a history of malignancy, an SPN is invariably a granuloma,

hamartoma, or inflammatory lesion. These nodules can be followed with plain radiographs to confirm their benign nature. Patients older than 35 years, particularly those who are current or recent cigarette smokers, have a significant incidence of malignant SPNs: approximately 50% of radiographically detected noncalcified SPNs in patients older than 50 years are malignant at thoracotomy. Therefore, an SPN in a patient older than 35 years should never be followed radiographically without tissue confirmation unless a benign pattern of calcification or the presence of intralesional fat is identified on radiographs or thin-section CT, or there has been radiographically documented lack of growth over a minimum of 2 years. There are exceptions to this rule: a history of cigarette smoking, prior lung or head-and-neck cancer, or asbestos exposure raises the likelihood for malignancy in a patient with an SPN. Alternatively, if the patient is from an area where histoplasmosis or tuberculosis is endemic, the likelihood of a granuloma is greater; in such patients, a conservative approach may be warranted. Finally, the finding of an SPN in a patient with an extrathoracic malignancy raises the possibility of a solitary pulmonary metastasis. An SPN that arises more than 2 years after the diagnosis of an extrathoracic malignancy is almost always a primary lung tumor rather than a metastasis; breast carcinoma and melanoma are notable exceptions to this rule.

Growth Pattern. Pulmonary malignancies grow at a relatively predictable rate. The growth rate of an SPN is usually expressed as the *doubling time*, or the time it takes for a nodule to double its volume. For a sphere, this corresponds to a 25% increase in diameter. Although some benign lesions (mostly hamartomas and histoplasmomas) may exhibit a growth rate similar to that of malignant lesions, the absence of growth or an extraordinarily slow or rapid rate of growth of a solid nodule is reliable evidence that an SPN is benign. Studies have shown that bronchogenic carcinoma presenting as a solid SPN has a doubling time of approximately 180 days. Therefore, a doubling time of less than 1 month or greater than 2 years reliably characterizes a solid lesion as benign. Infectious lesions and rapidly growing metastases from choriocarcinoma, seminoma, or osteogenic sarcoma comprise the majority of rapidly growing solitary nodules, whereas lack of growth or a doubling time exceeding 2 years is seen in hamartomas and histoplasmomas. However, there are exceptions to this rule. Giant cell carcinoma, a subtype of large cell carcinoma, and pulmonary carcinosarcomas and blastomas may have a doubling time of less than 1 month. Conversely, malignancies such as some well-differentiated adenocarcinomas or carcinoid tumors may

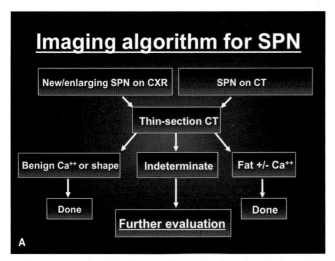
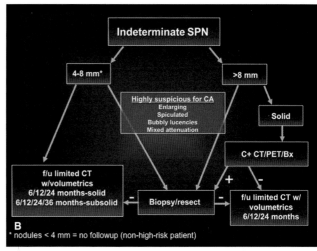

FIGURE 15.1. **Algorithm for Imaging Evaluation of the Solitary Pulmonary Nodule.** SPN, solitary pulmonary nodule; CT, computed tomography; Ca++, calcification; PET, positron emission tomography with 18F-fluorodeoxyglucose (FDG); TNB, transthoracic needle biopsy; CXR, chest x-ray; Bx, biopsy; F/U, follow-up.

have a doubling time of greater than 2 years, particularly if they are subsolid (i.e., ground-glass or mixed soft tissue/ground-glass attenuation).

In patients with clinical and imaging characteristics suggesting an indeterminate SPN, particularly lesions smaller than 8 mm in diameter, thin-section CT analysis of nodule volume appears to provide a noninvasive method of assessing nodule growth and determining which lesions require biopsy or resection. Published studies have shown that this technique is more accurate than cross-sectional measurements in determining nodule volume and distinguishing between growing malignant SPNs and stable benign lesions (Fig. 15.2). If a decision is made to simply follow an SPN radiologically, either because of a high likelihood of benignity or because the patient cannot tolerate or refuses an invasive diagnostic procedure, the lesion should be followed by limited thin-section CT. The frequency of thin-section CT follow-up of solid lesions 4 to 8 mm in diameter is inversely proportional to the clinical likelihood for malignancy and the lesion diameter. In other words, the larger the lesion and the greater the clinical concern for malignancy, the shorter the follow-up. Recommendations from the Fleischner Society for the follow-up

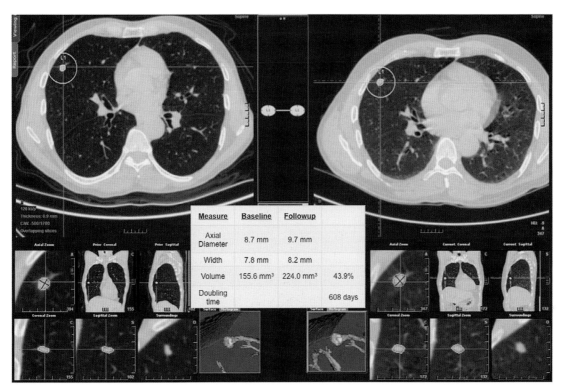

FIGURE 15.2. **Computer-Aided Two- and Three-Dimensional and Volumetric CT Analysis of Solitary Pulmonary Nodule.**

TABLE 15.1

FLEISCHNER SOCIETY GUIDELINES FOR THE MANAGEMENT OF SMALL (≤8 mm) INCIDENTAL LUNG NODULES ON CT

Management of incidental SPNs < or = 8 mm		
■ NODULE SIZE	■ LOW RISK PATIENT	■ HIGH RISK PATIENT
< or = 4 mm	No followup needed	Followup at 12 months
>4–6 mm	Followup CT @ 12 months	Followup CT at 6–12 months; the 18–24 months
>6–8 mm	Followup CT @ 6–12 months; then @ 18–24 months	Followup CT @ 3–6 months; then @ 9–12 and @ 24 months
Macmahon H et al. Radiology 2005;237:395–400.		

Adapted from Macmahon H, Austin JH, Gamsu G, et al. Guidelines for management of small pulmonary nodules detected on CT scans: a statement from the Fleischner Society. Radiology 2005;237: 395–400.

of incidentally detected small (4 to 8 mm) lung nodules have been published and provide a reasonable guideline for the frequency and length of follow-up (Table 15.1). The only exception to the published recommendations is for subsolid (i.e., ground-glass or mixed solid/ground-glass attenuation) nodules for which a greater than 2-year follow-up is likely necessary given the indolent nature and more typical slow growth of subsolid malignancies.

Size. Although size does not reliably discriminate benign from malignant SPNs, the larger the lesion, the greater the likelihood of malignancy. Masses exceeding 4 cm in diameter are usually malignant. However, the converse does not hold true; many pulmonary malignancies are less than 2 cm in diameter at the time of diagnosis, particularly if detected by screening chest CT. In patients with SPNs screened for lung cancer using low-dose CT, nodules <4 mm in diameter have a less than 1% likelihood of malignancy, and therefore most radiologists will not recommend routine follow-up of such lesions unless there is a very high clinical likelihood of malignancy.

Border (Margin, Edge) Characteristics. The appearance of the margin or edge of an SPN is a helpful sign in determining the nature of the lesion. The edge characteristics are best evaluated on thin-section CT, as this technique is considerably more accurate than plain radiographs. A round, smooth nodule is most likely a granuloma or hamartoma, although a rare primary pulmonary malignancy such as a carcinoid tumor, adenocarcinoma, or a solitary metastasis may have a perfectly smooth margin. A notched or lobulated contour may be seen in hamartomas, but malignant lesions including carcinoid tumors and some bronchogenic carcinomas will have a lobulated border. Pathologic examination has shown that the lobulated edge of a malignant nodule represents mounds of tumor extending into the adjacent lung. A spiculated margin is highly suspicious for malignancy (Fig. 15.3). The term *corona radiata* has been used to describe this appearance, in which linear densities radiate from the edge of a nodule into the adjacent lung. Pathologically, these linear radiations represent reoriented connective tissue (interlobular) septa drawn into the tumor by the cicatrizing (scarring) nature of many

malignant lung tumors (Fig. 15.3C). Tumor extension from the nodule, or fibrosis and edema of these connective tissue septa, may thicken these linear densities. However, it has been shown that spiculation is not specific for malignancy, because benign processes that produce cicatrization can have an identical appearance. Benign lesions that may show a spiculated border include lipoid pneumonia, organizing pneumonia, tuberculomas, and the mass lesions of progressive massive fibrosis in complicated silicosis. A peripherally situated pulmonary nodule may contact the costal pleura or interlobar fissure via a linear opacity known as a "pleural tail." As with the corona radiata, the recognition of this line, while suggestive of malignancy (particularly bronchioloalveolar cell carcinoma), is not specific and may be seen in peripheral granulomas.

There are additional characteristics of the border of an SPN which help identify the nature of the lesion. The presence of small "satellite" nodules around the periphery of a dominant nodule is strongly suggestive of benign disease, particularly granulomatous infection. The identification of feeding and draining vessels emanating from the hilar aspect of an SPN is pathognomonic of a pulmonary arteriovenous malformation (AVM). Contrast-enhanced helical CT scanning through the nodule or MR is diagnostic. A posttraumatic PA pseudoaneurysm will show marked contrast enhancement and contiguity with the feeding artery on CT. The presence of a halo of ground-glass opacity encircling an SPN in an immunocompromised, neutropenic patient should suggest the diagnosis of invasive pulmonary aspergillosis. Finally, a nodule or mass adjacent to an area of pleural thickening, with a "comet tail" of bronchi and vessels entering the hilar aspect of the mass, and associated with lobar volume loss is characteristic of round atelectasis.

Density. The internal density of an SPN is probably the single most important factor in characterizing the lesion as benign or indeterminate. In general, lesions that are calcified are benign. There are five patterns of calcification that reliably indicate the benignity of an SPN. These patterns can be identified on plain chest radiographs, but thin-section

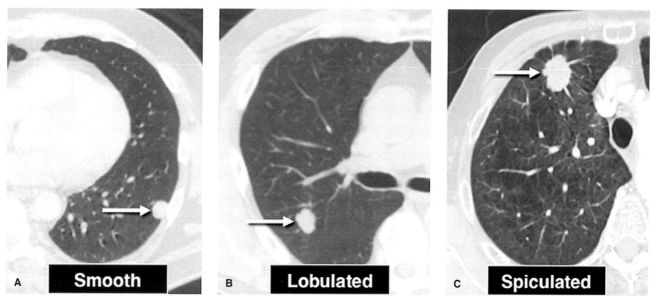

FIGURE 15.3. Edge or Marginal Characteristics of Solitary Pulmonary Nodules. A. Smooth borders in a granuloma. **B.** Lobulated contour of a hamartoma. **C.** Spiculated border in bronchogenic carcinoma.

CT is often necessary to detect and characterize the calcification. *Complete* or *central calcification* within an SPN is specific for a healed granuloma from tuberculosis or histoplasmosis. *Concentric* or *laminated calcification* indicates a granuloma and allows confident exclusion of neoplasm. *Popcorn calcification* within a nodule is diagnostic of a pulmonary hamartoma in which the cartilaginous component has calcified.

It is important to remember that calcification within an SPN is synonymous with a benign lesion only if the calcification follows one of the five patterns of benign calcification shown in Figure 15.4. Approximately 10% of malignant nodules contain calcification on CT. A bronchogenic carcinoma that arises in an area of previous granulomatous infection may engulf a preexisting calcified granuloma as it enlarges. In this situation, the calcification will be eccentric in the nodule, allowing distinction

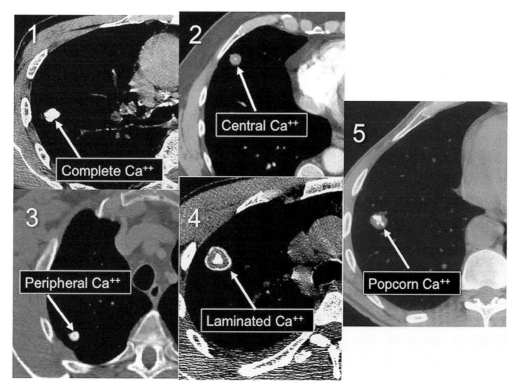

FIGURE 15.4. Patterns of Benign Calcifications in Solitary Pulmonary Nodules. Ca^{++}, calcification.

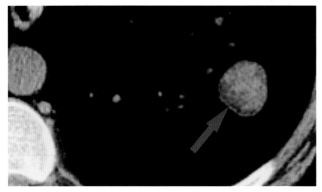

FIGURE 15.5. Fat in Pulmonary Hamartoma. Cone-down view of unenhanced thin-section CT through left lower lobe nodule shows fat in medial aspect of lesion (*arrow*), diagnostic of a hamartoma.

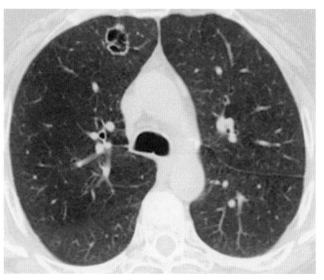

FIGURE 15.6. Cystic ("Bubbly") Lucencies in Adenocarcinoma. CT scan at lung windows through the tracheal carina shows a thin-walled irregular lesion with cystic lucencies (*arrow*) in the anterior segment of the right upper lobe. Note the presence of smoking-related respiratory bronchiolitis seen as upper lobe ground-glass opacity. PET scan (not shown) showed increased activity within the lesion. Resection revealed adenocarcinoma.

from a centrally calcified granuloma. Malignant pulmonary neoplasms may demonstrate small or microscopic foci of calcification, particularly adenocarcinomas that produce mucin or psammoma bodies. The rare solitary pulmonary metastasis from osteosarcoma or chondrosarcoma may contain calcium, but the diagnosis in these patients will usually be obvious clinically.

The identification of fat within an SPN is diagnostic of a pulmonary hamartoma (Fig. 15.5). A discussion of the radiographic and CT features of a pulmonary hamartoma can be found in the section "Lesions Presenting as SPNs."

It is important to remember that not all SPNs can be reliably characterized by their internal attenuation characteristics. A lesion with a diameter greater than 3 cm (termed a "mass"), those showing lobulated or spiculated margins, and thick-walled cavitary lesions have a high likelihood of malignancy, regardless of internal density, and almost invariably require tissue diagnosis when detected. Likewise, the demonstration of an air bronchogram or bubbly lucencies within an SPN is highly suspicious for adenocarcinoma (Fig. 15.6), particularly bronchioloalveolar cell subtypes.

Contrast-Enhanced CT. Several studies have demonstrated the utility of dynamic, contrast-enhanced CT in the evaluation of SPNs, with virtually all malignant lesions demonstrating an increase in attenuation of greater than 15 H after contrast administration (Fig. 15.7) (2). Therefore, lack of significant (>15 H) enhancement of a solid nodule 6 to 30 mm in diameter after IV iodinated contrast effectively excludes malignancy (sensitivity 98%).

PET. PET using fluorine-18-labeled fluorodeoxyglucose (FDG) has shown a high accuracy in the distinction between benign and malignant SPNs (Fig. 15.8) (3). For lesions larger than 10 mm in diameter, the sensitivity and specificity of FDG-PET is 97%, with a specificity of 78%, mostly as a result of inflammatory lesions such as active granulomas that are FDG-avid. False-negative PET studies are seen in patients with lesions smaller than 10 mm in diameter and metabolically hypoactive

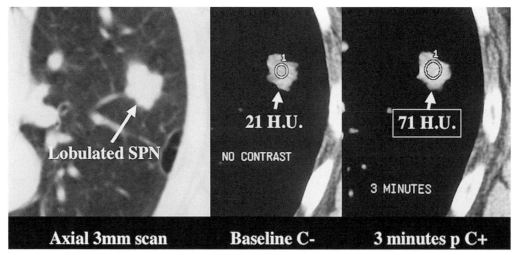

FIGURE 15.7. Contrast CT in Malignant Solitary Pulmonary Nodule. Thin-collimation (3-mm) CT scans through left upper lobe nodule in a 62-year-old woman with biopsy-proven lung cancer shows a lobulated contour with positive enhancement of 50 H after contrast administration. C–, prior to contrast administration; C+, following contrast administration.

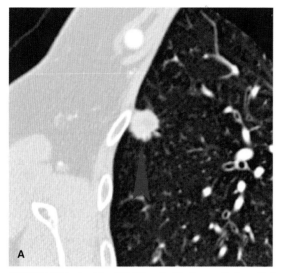 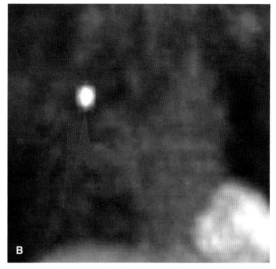

FIGURE 15.8. Positive PET Scan in Malignant Solitary Pulmonary Nodule (SPN). A. Cone-down thin-section CT of right upper lobe in a 72-year-old man shows a peripheral spiculated SPN (*arrowhead*). **B.** Coronal maximum intensity projection of PET demonstrates marked increased uptake in the lesion (*arrowhead*). Biopsy showed a squamous cell carcinoma.

lesions such as carcinoid tumor and bronchioloalveolar cell carcinoma. Dual-time point PET, in which images are obtained at both the standard 1 hour and then 2 hours after FDG administration, can improve the sensitivity of PET for nodules with an initial standardized uptake value (SUV) <2.5 (i.e., negative uptake) by showing an increase in SUV on the delayed as compared to the baseline images.

Management Decisions (Fig. 15.1). Patients with indeterminate SPNs should either have PET, radiologic follow-up or undergo transthoracic biopsy or resection. When the lesion is very likely to be malignant, it is reasonable to forgo biopsy and proceed directly to thoracotomy and resection. However, there are several reasons to perform a preoperative biopsy on an indeterminate SPN. The primary reason to biopsy an indeterminate SPN is to make the diagnosis of a benign lesion, thereby avoiding an unnecessary thoracoscopy or thoracotomy. This would most benefit the patient with a reasonable likelihood of having a benign lesion. Factors suggesting benignity include: age under 35, nonsmoker, patient from an area endemic for tuberculosis or histoplasmosis, nodule smaller than 2 cm with smooth margins, recent symptoms of a lower respiratory infection, and a doubling time of less than 30 days or greater than 2 years. The other major indication for the biopsy of an indeterminate but suspicious SPN is a patient with limited pulmonary reserve who is a poor surgical candidate for pulmonary resection. In these patients, a biopsy can provide a diagnosis and guide nonoperative therapy. Because most SPNs are peripherally situated in the lung, transthoracic needle biopsy (TNB) is the procedure of choice for tissue sampling. Peripheral lesions requiring biopsy that are too small for successful transthoracic needle biopsy (i.e., lesions <5 mm in diameter) can be sampled with video-assisted thoracoscopic surgery (VATS). Patients with SPNs that are centrally situated, with a large bronchus entering the lesion, should undergo transbronchoscopic biopsy.

An SPN that is judged to be benign on the basis of patient age, growth rate, presence of benign calcification, or those with a specific benign diagnosis provided by TNB should be followed with radiographs or CT for a minimum of 2 and preferably 3 years to confirm their benign nature. The radiographic follow-up consists of posteroanterior and lateral chest radiographs if the lesions are radiographically apparent, or limited thin-section CT at 6-month intervals.

Lesions Presenting as SPNs

The differential diagnosis of an SPN is shown in Table 15.2. In addition to bronchogenic carcinoma (particularly adenocarcinoma) and granulomas (e.g., tuberculosis and histoplasmosis), there are a number of entities that may produce an SPN. Many of these entities are discussed elsewhere in the text.

Carcinoid Tumors. While carcinoid tumors may present as SPNs, the majority (80%) are central endobronchial lesions that present with wheezing, atelectasis, or obstructive pneumonitis. A detailed discussion of carcinoid tumors can be found in the section on malignant pulmonary neoplasms.

Pulmonary hamartoma is a misnomer and actually reflects a benign neoplasm composed of an abnormal arrangement of the mesenchymal and epithelial elements found in normal lung. Histologically, these lesions contain cartilage surrounded by fibrous connective tissue, with variable amounts of fat, smooth muscle, and seromucous glands; calcification and ossification are seen in 30%. These tumors are seen most commonly in the fourth and fifth decades of life. Approximately 90% of hamartomas arise within the pulmonary parenchyma, accounting for approximately 5% of all SPNs.

These lesions usually present as incidental findings on chest radiographs. While the diagnosis is often suggested on plain radiographs, CT is obtained in most patients. A confident diagnosis of hamartoma can be made when HRCT shows a nodule smaller than 2.5 cm in diameter demonstrating a smooth or lobulated border and containing focal fat (Fig. 15.5). Calcification, when present, is in the form of multiple clumps of calcium dispersed throughout the lesion ("popcorn" calcification) (Fig. 15.4). As a rule, hamartomas that contain calcium also contain fat. While hamartomas tend to grow slowly, the presence of characteristic thin-section CT findings allows for observation alone. Rapid growth, pulmonary symptoms, or a size larger than 2.5 cm warrants transthoracic biopsy or resection.

Non-Hodgkin Lymphoma. Primary pulmonary lymphomas arising from the bronchus-associated lymphoid tissue (BALT) are low-grade B-cell lymphomas that present in adults

TABLE 15.2

SOLITARY PULMONARY NODULE OR MASS

Neoplasm	Bronchogenic carcinoma
	Hamartoma
	Carcinoid tumor
	Granular cell tumor
	Sclerosing hemangioma
	Mesenchymal neoplasms
	Leiomyoma/leiomyosarcoma
	Fibroma
	Lipoma
	Neurofibroma
	Lymphoma
	Solitary metastasis
	Colon carcinoma
Infection	Septic embolus
	Staphylococcus
	Round pneumonia
	Pneumococcus
	Legionella
	Nocardia
	Fungi
	Lung abscess
	Infectious granuloma
	Tuberculosis
	Histoplasmosis
	Coccidioidomycosis
	Cryptococcosis
	Parasitic
	Echinococcal cyst
	Amebic abscess
Collagen vascular disease	Necrobiotic nodule (rheumatoid lung)
	Wegener granulomatosis
Vascular	Infarct
	Arteriovenous malformation
	PA aneurysm
	Hematoma
Airways	Congenital foregut malformations
	Bronchogenic cyst
	Sequestration
	Mucocele
Trauma	Hematoma/traumatic lung cyst
	Infected bulla
Miscellaneous	Amyloidoma
	Rounded atelectasis

in their fifties. The most common radiographic finding is an SPN or focal airspace opacity. The diagnosis is made by immunohistochemistry and flow cytometry of resected specimens or of aspirated cells obtained by TNB.

Granular cell tumor (granular cell myoblastoma) is a benign neoplasm arising from neural elements in the central airways or parenchyma. The skin is the most common site for these tumors. These tumors may present as SPNs but are more commonly seen as endobronchial masses; half of lung lesions present with obstructive pneumonitis because of their endobronchial location (see "Tracheal and Bronchial Masses" section).

Sclerosing Hemangioma. This is a benign epithelial neoplasm that typically affects females and presents as a solitary, smoothly marginated juxtapleural nodule that enhances densely because of its vascular nature. The lesion may contain foci of low attenuation and may be calcified on thin-section CT analysis.

Leiomyoma/Leiomyosarcoma, Fibroma, Neurofibroma. Arising from the smooth muscle of the airways or pulmonary vessels, leiomyomas and leiomyosarcomas are rare neoplasms that present as endobronchial or intrapulmonary lesions with equal frequency. Radiographically, the parenchymal lesions are sharply marginated, smooth or lobulated nodules or masses. The histologic distinction of benign from malignant lesions is difficult. Similarly, fibromas and neurofibromas appearing as SPNs lack distinguishing radiographic features.

Lipomas are rare intrapulmonary lesions that arise more commonly within the tracheobronchial tree to produce atelectasis. The demonstration of fat attenuation on CT is diagnostic.

Hemangiopericytoma is a connective tissue tumor that arises within the lung from the pericyte, a cell associated with the arteriolar and capillary endothelium. On chest radiographs, these lesions are seen as SPNs and are indistinguishable from bronchogenic carcinoma.

Inflammatory myofibroblastic tumor (plasma cell granuloma, inflammatory pseudotumor) of lung refers to a localized chronic inflammatory response to an unknown agent in the lung. It is characterized histologically by an abundance of plasma cells. There are no distinguishing radiographic features.

Lipoid Pneumonia. The inadvertent aspiration of mineral oils ingested by elderly patients to treat constipation may produce a localized pulmonary lesion. Patients with gastroesophageal reflux or disordered swallowing mechanisms are at particular risk. Radiographically, a focal area of airspace opacification or a solid mass may be seen in the lower lobes. A spiculated appearance to the edge of the mass is not uncommon, as the oil may produce a chronic inflammatory reaction in the surrounding lung that leads to fibrosis. While CT can demonstrate fat within the lesion, most patients with the mass-like form of this entity require resection for definitive diagnosis (see Fig. 19.40).

Bronchogenic Cyst. Fluid-filled cystic lesions of the lung may produce an SPN. Intrapulmonary bronchogenic cysts are uncommon causes of SPNs; 90% of these lesions are found in the middle mediastinum. The characteristic finding is a sharply marginated cyst on CT or MR in a young patient, although distinction from an infected bulla, solitary echinococcal cyst, mucocele, or thin-walled lung abscess may be impossible. Superinfection of a lung bulla may produce an SPN or mass. In such patients, the radiographic or CT appearance of an intraparenchymal air-fluid level within a thin-walled localized air collection (usually in an upper lobe), with typical bullous changes in other portions of lung, usually allows for the proper diagnosis.

Focal Organizing Pneumonia. Occasionally, patients who have a resolving pneumonia or even those with a focal mass-like form of cryptogenic organizing pneumonia will have an SPN detected on radiographs or CT. These lesions often show irregular margins and may be PET-positive, thereby showing a significant overlap of findings with those of bronchogenic carcinoma. Sometimes a history of recent lower respiratory tract infection will be present. Radiologic follow-up, perhaps after empiric antibiotic therapy, will allow distinction from malignancy in most patients, although a minority will require surgical resection for definitive diagnosis.

Hematoma/Traumatic Lung Cyst. Blunt or penetrating chest trauma can result in the formation of traumatic lung cysts or hematomas, seen as round opacities often containing air or an air-fluid level.

BRONCHOGENIC CARCINOMA

Bronchogenic carcinoma is one of several neoplasms that may arise within the lung (Table 15.3). It is now the leading cause of death from malignancy in the United States and most

TABLE 15.3

PULMONARY NEOPLASMS

Benign
  Epithelial
    Squamous cell papilloma
    Pleomorphic adenoma (benign mixed tumor)
  Mesenchymal
    Hamartoma
    Lipoma
    Neurofibroma
    Leiomyoma
    Granular cell tumor
    Hemangiopericytoma

Malignant
  Epithelial
    Bronchogenic carcinoma
    Carcinoid tumor
    Bronchial gland carcinoma
      Mucoepidermoid carcinoma
      Adenoid cystic carcinoma (cylindroma)
  Epithelial/mesenchymal
    Pulmonary blastoma
    Carcinosarcoma
  Lymphoid
    Non-Hodgkin lymphoma
    Hodgkin lymphoma
    Primary melanoma of lung

industrialized countries for both men and women, having surpassed breast cancer in women in recent years. Although survival rates for lung cancer are poor, radiology plays a central role in diagnosis and management. This section will review the key pathologic, epidemiologic, and radiologic features of bronchogenic carcinoma with an emphasis on the radiologic staging of this disease.

Cytologic and Pathologic Features

Bronchogenic carcinoma is a malignant neoplasm that arises from the bronchial or alveolar epithelium. Ninety-nine percent of malignant epithelial neoplasms of the lung arise from the bronchi or lung, whereas fewer than 0.5% arise from the trachea. Bronchogenic carcinoma is divided into four main histologic subtypes on the basis of their gross and microscopic features: adenocarcinoma, squamous cell carcinoma, small cell carcinoma, and large cell carcinoma (Table 15.4) (Fig. 15.9).

Adenocarcinoma is the most common type of lung cancer, accounting for approximately one-third of all bronchogenic carcinomas. It is the most common subtype of lung cancer in nonsmokers. Whereas these tumors were once found to occur overwhelmingly in the lung periphery, they are now found in the central portions of the lungs in about one-fourth of cases. These tumors arise from the bronchiolar or alveolar epithelium and have an irregular or spiculated appearance where they invade adjacent lung. Fibrosis in and about the tumor is common. These gross features usually produce an ill-defined pulmonary nodule or mass on chest radiographs (Figs. 15.3C, 15.8B). Histologically, adenocarcinoma demonstrates gland formation and mucin production. A subtype of adenocarcinoma, newly termed adenocarcinoma-in-situ (AIS), previously called *bronchioloalveolar cell carcinoma* (BAC), has unique pathologic features. This tumor is characterized by growth along preexisting bronchiolar and alveolar walls ("lepidic growth") without invasion or distortion of alveolar walls, blood vessels, or lymphatics. When localized, AIS appears as a SPN or as a focal area of ground-glass opacity on CT scans (Fig. 15.9A). Diffuse disease, which represents transbronchial (i.e., aerogenous) spread of tumor, may present as airspace opacification simulating pneumonia or as diffuse bilateral nodular airspace opacities.

Squamous cell carcinoma is the second most common subtype of bronchogenic carcinoma, accounting for approximately one-fourth of all cases. This tumor arises centrally within a lobar or segmental bronchus. Grossly, these tumors are polypoid masses that grow into the bronchial lumen while simultaneously invading the bronchial wall. The central location and endobronchial component of the tumor account for the presenting symptoms of cough and hemoptysis and for the common radiographic findings of a hilar mass with or without obstructive pneumonitis or atelectasis. Central necrosis is common in large tumors; cavitation may be seen if communication has occurred between the central portion of the mass and the bronchial lumen (Fig. 15.9C). Histologically, squamous cell carcinoma is characterized by invasion of the bronchial wall by nests of malignant cells with abundant cytoplasm. The formation of keratin pearls and intercellular bridges, seen in well-differentiated tumors, is specific for this tumor.

Small cell carcinoma accounts for 25% of bronchogenic carcinomas and arises centrally within main or lobar bronchi. These tumors are the most malignant neoplasms arising from bronchial neuroendocrine (Kulchitsky) cells and are alternatively referred to as Kulchitsky cell cancers or KCC-3. Typical carcinoid tumors (KCC-1) represent the least malignant type, and atypical carcinoid tumors (KCC-2) are intermediate

TABLE 15.4

SUBTYPES OF BRONCHOGENIC CARCINOMA

■ TYPE	■ INCIDENCE	■ RADIOLOGIC FEATURES	■ TREATMENT	■ FIVE-YEAR SURVIVAL
Adenocarcinoma	35%	Peripheral nodule Peripheral mass	I–III = surgery III–IV = XRT/chemotherapy	17%
Squamous cell	25%	Hilar mass Atelectasis	I–III = surgery III–IV = XRT/chemotherapy	15%
Small cell	25%	Hilar mass Mediastinal mass	Chemotherapy	5%
Large cell	15%	Large peripheral mass	I–III = surgery III–IV = XRT/chemotherapy	11%

XRT, radiation therapy.

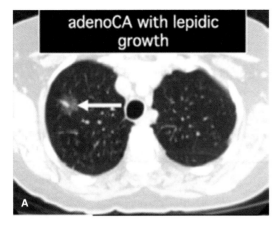

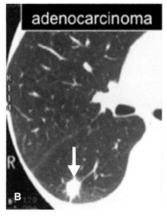

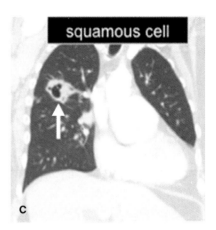

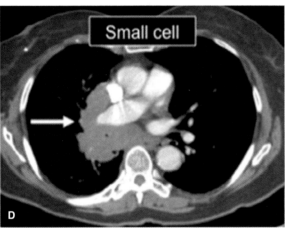

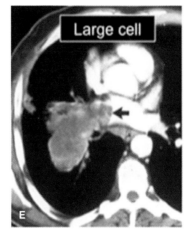

FIGURE 15.9. Typical CT Appearances of the Subtypes of Bronchogenic Carcinoma. A. Subsolid (mixed solid/ground-glass attenuation) solitary nodule (*arrow*). B. Spiculated peripheral solitary pulmonary nodule (*arrow*). C. Cavitary mass (*arrow*). D. Large right hilar mass (*arrow*). E. Large mass with left atrial invasion (*arrow*).

in aggressiveness. Small cell carcinomas exhibit a small endobronchial component, invading the bronchial wall and peribronchial tissues early in the course of disease. This produces a hilar or mediastinal mass with extrinsic bronchial compression and obstruction. Invasion of the submucosal and peribronchial lymphatics leads to local lymph node enlargement (Fig. 15.9D) and hematogenous dissemination, which are almost invariable at the time of presentation. Microscopically, these malignant cells are tightly clustered, with nuclei molded together because of the scant amount of cytoplasm. This lesion is distinguished from carcinoid tumor histologically by the presence of mitoses. Electron microscopy demonstrates the presence of intracytoplasmic neurosecretory granules.

Large cell carcinoma accounts for 15% of bronchogenic carcinomas and is occasionally diagnosed when a non-small cell bronchogenic carcinoma lacks the histologic characteristics of squamous cell carcinoma or adenocarcinoma. Histologic features include large cells with abundant cytoplasm and prominent nucleoli. This tumor tends to arise peripherally as a solitary mass and is often large at the time of presentation (Fig. 15.9E).

Epidemiology. The majority of patients with bronchogenic carcinoma are cigarette smokers who are over 40 years of age. Men are most commonly affected, although the percentage of female lung cancer patients has risen steadily in parallel with the increased prevalence of heavy cigarette smoking among women. The overall 5-year survival rate for all patients with lung cancer is 10% to 15%.

In addition to cigarette smoke, well-recognized risk factors for the development of bronchogenic carcinoma include asbestos exposure, previous Hodgkin lymphoma, radon exposure, viral infection, and diffuse interstitial or localized lung fibrosis. Cigarette smoke is by far the leading cause of lung cancer, with approximately 87% of cases attributed to smoking. The

relationship between cigarette smoke and bronchogenic carcinoma is irrefutable, with the intensity of smoking (number of pack-years) showing the greatest positive correlation with development rates of malignancy. Lung cancer is uncommon in nonsmokers, and cigarette smoking is associated with a 10- to 30-fold increase in the incidence of bronchogenic carcinoma as compared to nonsmokers. Cessation of smoking decreases the risk of developing lung cancer, with the greatest decline found in those with the longest smoking cessation interval. Carcinogens in cigarette smoke produce cellular atypia and squamous metaplasia of the bronchiolar epithelium that may precede malignant transformation. Small cell carcinoma and squamous cell carcinoma are the two histologic subtypes with the strongest association with cigarette smoking in men, whereas cigarette smoking in women is associated with an increased incidence of all histologic subtypes.

A subset of cigarette smokers is at particular risk of developing lung cancer. Young adult smokers with bullous lung disease tend to develop their lung cancers at an earlier age than the general population of smokers. Proposed theories include greater susceptibility of the lining of the bulla to metaplastic transformation and impaired ventilation within the bulla leading to prolonged exposure to the carcinogens in cigarette smoke.

Asbestos exposure is associated with an increased incidence of bronchogenic carcinoma, malignant pleural mesothelioma, laryngeal carcinoma, and esophagogastric carcinoma. Bronchogenic carcinoma may follow prolonged exposure (usually 20 years or greater in duration) from the mining or processing of asbestos fibers. A long latency period from the initial asbestos exposure, generally 35 years or longer, is necessary for the development of bronchogenic carcinoma. While asbestos exposure alone is associated with a fourfold increase in the incidence of bronchogenic carcinoma, concomitant cigarette smoking, perhaps by acting as a cocarcinogen, is

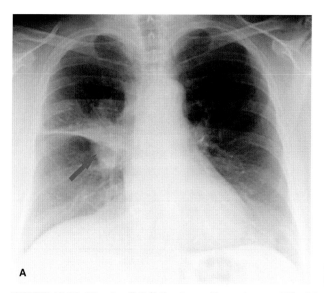 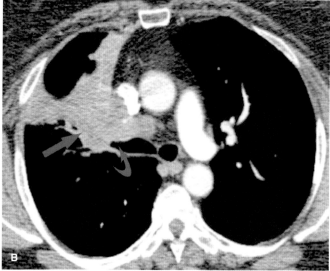

FIGURE 15.10. **Non-Small Cell Carcinoma Presenting as a Hilar Mass. A.** Chest radiograph shows a right hilar mass (*arrow*) with anterior segment right upper lobe atelectasis (*arrowhead*). **B.** CT confirms a right hilar mass (*straight arrow*) obstructing the right upper lobe bronchus (*curved arrow*). Diagnosis was confirmed bronchoscopically.

associated with a 40- to 50-fold increase in the incidence as compared to the nonexposed, nonsmoking individual.

Patients previously treated for mediastinal Hodgkin disease with radiation, chemotherapy, or a combination of the two have an eightfold increase in lung cancer beginning 10 years after treatment. Exposure to inhaled radioactive material, particularly radon, is associated with the development of small cell carcinoma of lung 20 years or more after the exposure.

The link between viral infection and bronchogenic carcinoma comes chiefly from the study of jaagsiekte, a disease of sheep that closely resembles BAC of the lung in humans. This disease is caused by a retroviral infection, leading to speculation that a similar pathogenesis exists in humans with this subtype of adenocarcinoma.

Diffuse interstitial fibrosis in patients with usual interstitial pneumonitis due to scleroderma, rheumatoid lung disease, or idiopathic pulmonary fibrosis has been associated with an increased incidence of bronchogenic carcinoma, particularly adenocarcinoma.

Radiographic findings in bronchogenic carcinoma depend on the subtype of cancer (4) and the stage of disease at the time of diagnosis. The two most common findings are an SPN (size between 2 mm and 3 cm) or mass (3 cm or larger in size) and a hilar mass with or without bronchial obstruction. All cell types can present with a pulmonary nodule. Because squamous and small cell carcinoma arise from the central bronchi, the majority of these types of bronchogenic carcinoma produce a hilar mass (Figs. 15.9D, 15.10). The hilar mass represents either the extraluminal portion of the bronchial tumor or hilar lymph node enlargement from metastatic disease. Extension of the hilar lesion into the mediastinum or the presence of mediastinal nodal metastases can produce a smooth or lobulated mediastinal mass. Marked mediastinal nodal enlargement producing a lobulated mediastinal contour is characteristic of small cell carcinoma. Extensive replacement of the mediastinal fat by either primary tumor or extracapsular nodal extension may produce diffuse mediastinal widening, with loss of the mediastinal fat planes and compression or invasion of the trachea or central bronchi, esophagus, and mediastinal vascular structures, as seen on contrast-enhanced CT or MR.

Obstruction of the bronchial lumen by the endobronchial component of a tumor can result in several different radiographic findings. The most common finding is resorptive

atelectasis (Fig. 15.11) or obstructive pneumonitis of lung distal to the obstructing lesion. Resorptive atelectasis is recognized by the classic findings of lobar or whole lung collapse, whereas obstructive pneumonitis results in minimal or no atelectasis or occasionally an increase in the volume of the affected portion of lung. An abnormal increase in lobar or whole lung volume is recognized radiographically by a bulging interlobar fissure marginating the obstructed lobe or by mediastinal shift, respectively, and is termed "drowned lung." Occasionally, the mass producing the lobar atelectasis creates a central convexity in the normally concave contour of the collapsed lobe, producing the S sign of Golden (Fig. 15.11A). Most commonly, the opacity of the obstructed lung obscures the underlying central lesion. The lung with obstructive pneumonitis is not infected but rather shows a chronic inflammatory infiltrate and alveolar filling with lipid-laden macrophages; the latter finding accounts for the descriptive terms "golden" or "endogenous lipoid pneumonia."

Additional radiographic features of atelectasis that should suggest obstruction by tumor include obliteration of the main or proximal lobar bronchial air column, hilar mass, combined middle and lower lobe atelectasis, and atelectasis or opacification that persists beyond 3 to 4 weeks. CT confirms the presence of lobar atelectasis and typically demonstrates mucus bronchograms within the lung distal to the obstructing lesion. The central mass is readily distinguished from vascular structures, with narrowing or occlusion of the bronchial lumen best seen on images viewed at lung windows. The central tumor is usually distinguished from atelectatic lung by the contrast between the perfused but nonventilated enhancing lung and the low-attenuation, nonenhancing central mass. An uncommon manifestation of bronchial obstruction by bronchogenic carcinoma is the development of mucoid impaction (mucocele). This represents mucus within dilated segmental bronchi distal to the obstructing neoplasm. The appearance has been likened to a gloved hand, with the dilated bronchi representing the fingers of the glove. Radiographic visualization of the mucocele requires collateral ventilation to the obstructed lobe or segment.

Tumors that arise from the bronchiolar or alveolar epithelium—namely, adenocarcinoma and large cell carcinoma—commonly produce an SPN or mass on chest radiography. The radiographic evaluation of the SPN, in particular the size, growth rate, shape, margins, and internal density, has been

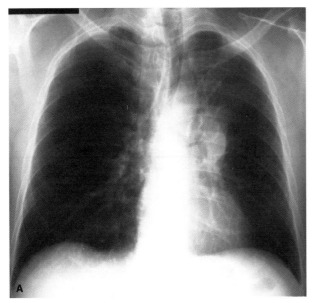
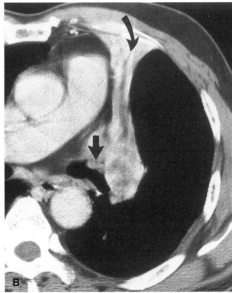

FIGURE 15.11. Hilar Mass Due to Squamous Cell Carcinoma. A. Posteroanterior chest film in a 58-year-old male smoker with hemoptysis shows a left hilar mass with left upper lobe atelectasis. **B.** Enhanced CT scan shows the left hilar mass occluding the left upper lobe bronchus with an endobronchial component (*straight arrow*). Note the presence of mucus bronchograms within the atelectatic lung (*curved arrow*).

reviewed in detail earlier in this chapter. A notched, lobulated, or spiculated margin to the nodule is common in bronchogenic carcinoma (Fig. 15.3C). The radially spiculated appearance of a peripheral nodule has been termed "corona radiata." While it was initially thought to be pathognomonic for malignancy, the finding of a corona radiata is nonspecific and can be seen in granulomas. The edge characteristics of an SPN are best appreciated on thin-section HRCT images through the lesion.

Cavitation of solitary malignant nodules is uncommon, but is most often seen in squamous cell carcinomas. The walls of cavitating neoplasms tend to be thicker and more nodular than those of inflammatory lesions. The presence of air bronchograms or bubbly lucencies within a nodule or mass (Fig. 15.6) or mixed solid/ground-glass attenuation is highly suggestive of an adenocarcinoma, particularly BAC (Fig. 15.9A). Eccentric

calcification within nodules may represent dystrophic calcification of necrotic regions, granulomas engulfed by an enlarging tumor, or calcification of mucin or psammoma bodies secreted by tumor cells in adenocarcinomas.

The size and growth pattern of an SPN are important characteristics. Masses larger than 3 cm in diameter seen in adults older than 35 years of age are most often malignant. The volume-doubling time (equivalent to a 25% increase in diameter) for a malignant nodule usually ranges from 1 month (some squamous cell and large cell carcinomas) to nearly 5 years (certain BACs).

Pancoast (superior sulcus) tumor is a peripheral neoplasm arising in that portion of the lung apex indented superiorly by the subclavian artery. Although they can be of any cell type, the majority of these lesions are squamous cell carcinomas or

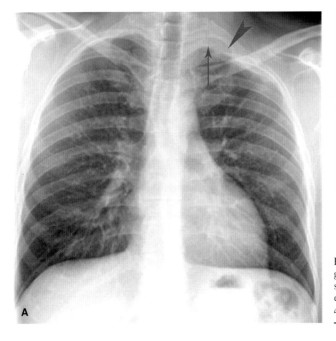

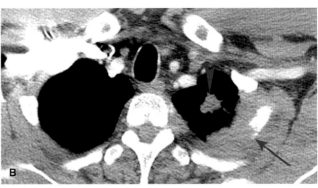

FIGURE 15.12. Superior Sulcus (Pancoast) Tumor. A. Frontal radiograph shows a left apical mass (*arrowhead*) with loss of the medial left second rib (*long arrow*). **B.** CT scan shows a nodule (*arrowhead*) with extension to the pleura and destruction of the left second rib (*long arrow*). Diagnosis was non-small cell carcinoma.

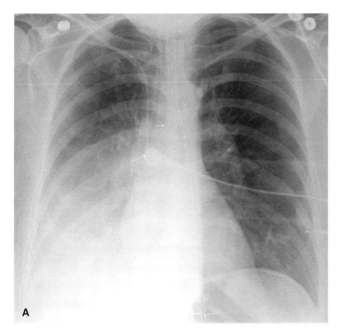

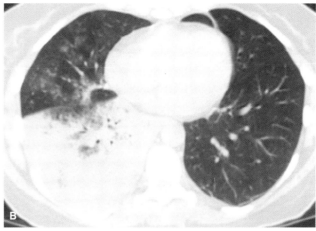

FIGURE 15.13. Bronchioloalveolar Cell Carcinoma (BAC). A. Chest radiograph shows dense consolidation of the right lower lobe. **B.** CT confirms airspace consolidation in the lower lobe with additional areas of ground-glass opacity in the middle lobe. Biopsy showed BAC.

adenocarcinomas. The presenting symptoms are related to invasion of adjacent structures, with arm pain and muscular atrophy attributable to brachial plexus involvement, Horner syndrome from involvement of the sympathetic chain, and shoulder pain from chest wall invasion (Fig. 15.12). The chest radiographic finding of an apical density may be mistaken for a pleuroparenchymal fibrous cap, which is a common finding in older individuals. Apical thickness exceeding 5 mm, asymmetry of the apical opacities of more than 5 mm, enlargement on serial radiographs, or evidence of rib destruction should prompt further evaluation with helical CT or MR. The presence of a mass with an inferior convex margin toward the lung and/or the presence of rib or vertebral body destruction are uncommon plain film findings. MDCT demonstrates the apical region to better advantage and is best for determining the extent of chest wall and vertebral invasion. Coronal and sagittal MR is useful for determining the relationship of the mass to the subclavian artery, brachial plexus, and spinal canal.

Airspace opacification caused by bronchogenic carcinoma is an uncommon radiographic finding in the absence of an obstructing endobronchial lesion. BAC may produce airspace opacification as malignant cells grow along the preexisting parenchymal lattice while producing large amounts of mucus. The majority (60% to 90%) of BACs are localized and appear as SPNs. CT often shows air-filled bronchi within the lesion and a pleural tail extending from the tumor toward the pleural surface. The diffuse form may present as lobar or multilobar airspace opacification (Fig. 15.13) or as diffuse bilateral airspace nodules. These latter appearances may be indistinguishable from pneumonia or edema, although the clinical findings, chronicity of the process, and cytologic examination of sputum and bronchoalveolar lavage specimens should provide the correct diagnosis. The production of copious amounts of mucus by these tumors may be an occasional clinical feature. An additional finding on contrast-enhanced CT in patients with the diffuse form of BAC is the so-called "CT angiogram" sign within consolidated areas. In these patients, filling of the airspaces with mucoid material produced by the malignant cells creates low-density airspace opacification surrounding the enhanced PAs that traverses the consolidated regions. However, the CT angiogram sign is not specific for BAC and may be seen in other airspace-filling diseases, including bacterial pneumonia, lymphoma, and lipoid pneumonia.

Superior vena cava (SVC) syndrome results from obstruction of the SVC from compression or invasion by mediastinal tumor, particularly small cell carcinoma or lymphoma. Lung cancer is the most common cause of SVC syndrome (Fig. 15.14).

A malignant pleural effusion is an exudative fluid collection in a patient with proven malignancy that shows malignant cytology on thoracentesis or tumor on pleural biopsy. The detection of a malignant pleural effusion has been upstaged in the most recent lung cancer staging classification to M1a or Stage IVa lung cancer, because of its worse prognosis relative to the presence of nodal metastases. Although the presence of a pleural effusion in patients with bronchogenic carcinoma is associated with a poor prognosis, it is not synonymous with malignant pleural involvement, because central lymphatic obstruction and postobstructive infection can produce benign effusions in patients with malignancy. Smooth or lobulated pleural thickening or a discrete pleural mass suggests malignant pleural involvement. Contrast-enhanced CT may

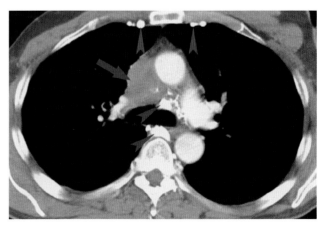

FIGURE 15.14. Superior Vena Cava (SVC) Syndrome in Small Cell Carcinoma. Contrast-enhanced CT at the level of the tracheal carina reveals a right paratracheal mass (*arrow*) that obliterates the SVC. Note the associated mediastinal venous collaterals (*red arrowheads*) and dilated internal mammary veins (*blue arrowheads*).

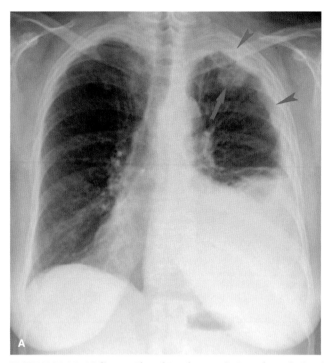
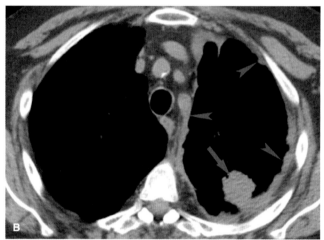

FIGURE 15.15. Malignant Pleural Involvement in Bronchogenic Carcinoma. A. Frontal chest radiograph shows a left apical lesion (*arrow*) with a moderate left pleural effusion and associated lobulated left pleural thickening (*arrowheads*). **B.** Non-contrast-enhanced CT through the upper lobes reveals an irregular left upper lobe lesion (*arrow*) with circumferential irregular left pleural thickening (*arrowheads*). Analysis of pleural fluid cytology revealed adenocarcinoma.

demonstrate pleural thickening or mass with associated pleural fluid on plain radiographs (Fig. 15.15). The utility of CT in the diagnosis of pleural and chest wall invasion is discussed in the section on lung cancer staging. Chest wall invasion is detected radiographically by the presence of an extrathoracic soft tissue mass or rib destruction. CT is more sensitive in detecting subtle bone destruction, whereas MR is better for detecting invasion of chest wall fat or muscle, particularly in superior sulcus tumors. Diaphragmatic elevation and paralysis may be seen with malignant invasion of the phrenic nerve. Progressive enlargement of the cardiac silhouette may be seen

in patients with a malignant pericardial effusion; echocardiography and pericardiocentesis are diagnostic.

Lymphangitic carcinomatosis represents invasion of the lymphatic channels of the lung by tumor. Invasion of lymphatics or neoplastic involvement of hilar and mediastinal nodes leads to retrograde (centrifugal) lymphatic flow with dilatation of lymphatic channels, interstitial deposits of tumor, and fibrosis. Radiographically, the typical findings are linear and reticulonodular opacities with peribronchial cuffing and subpleural edema or pleural effusion. In bronchogenic carcinoma, invasion and obstruction of lymphatics at the site of tumor may

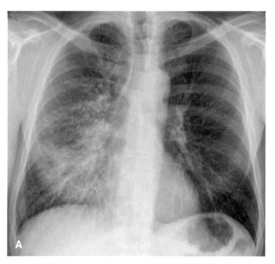
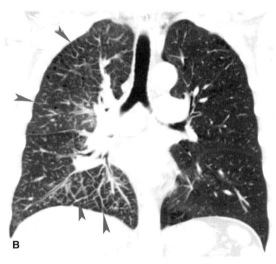

FIGURE 15.16. Lymphangitic Carcinomatosis (LC) From Lung Cancer. A. Chest radiograph in a 57-year-old female with cough shows unilateral right-sided linear interstitial opacities associated with a right hilar mass (*arrow*). **B.** Coronal-reformatted CT through the level of the hila at lung windows shows smooth thickening of the interlobular septa (*arrowheads*) representing LC.

produce a segmental or lobar distribution of opacities. Lymphangitic spread to hilar and mediastinal lymph nodes produces unilateral lymph node enlargement with interstitial opacities, whereas hematogenous dissemination of tumor to the pulmonary capillaries with secondary lymphatic invasion leads to bilateral interstitial abnormalities. Unilateral or asymmetric involvement of the lungs by lymphangitic tumor suggests lung cancer rather than an extrapulmonary site (Fig. 15.16). HRCT best demonstrates the characteristic smooth or beaded thickening of the interlobular septa and bronchovascular interstitium.

Diagnostic Evaluation. While prevention of lung cancer is the best and most cost-effective solution to the problem of lung cancer mortality, this is not achievable as long as the addictive habit of cigarette smoking is not entirely eliminated. Early detection and treatment have the potential to improve survival rates from this deadly disease. Screening with periodic chest radiographs in high-risk patients has not been shown to be effective because chest radiographs detect only lesions exceeding 1 cm in diameter. As a result of its cross-sectional format and volumetric data acquisition, MDCT is capable of routinely detecting lesions as small as 1 to 2 mm in diameter. Several nonrandomized observational studies have demonstrated promising results for lung cancer detection using low-dose spiral CT techniques. Preliminary results of the largest randomized study of low-dose CT for lung cancer screening, the National Lung Screening Trial (NLST), show 20% fewer lung cancer deaths among trial participants screened with low-dose helical CT. The increased radiation exposure with CT as compared to chest radiography for lung cancer screening has been minimized by reducing CT exposure factors (30 to 50 mA vs. 120 mA), with effective doses for screening chest CT studies routinely less than 1 mSv (millisievert). Whether the use of CT in screening high-risk individuals actually reduces lung cancer mortality remains undetermined. The relatively high cost of screening chest CT, the cost and potential morbidity of subsequent studies and procedures resulting from a false-positive screen, difficulties in CT interpretation, and quality of life issues associated with a false-positive screening result are additional considerations.

FDG-PET scans have been shown to have a very high sensitivity and moderately high specificity in detecting malignant tumors. FDG is a glucose precursor that is incorporated into metabolically active cells but is not further metabolized. Because malignant tumors have a higher rate of glucose metabolism than most benign processes, increased FDG uptake is suggestive of malignancy. The current threshold for lung cancer detection appears to be a lesion size of 1 cm. This technique is not limited to primary tumor detection. PET scans using FDG can reliably discriminate between malignant and benign lymph nodes exceeding 1 cm in diameter. Sensitivities and specificities of approximately 90% and 80%, respectively, have been reported for lymph node staging using this technique (5). In particular, integrated PET-CT has improved the accuracy of PET imaging of lung cancer and should be considered in all patients for nodal staging. This is in contrast to CT and MR, where the accuracy for lymph node metastases is 60% to 70%.

Efforts to diagnose lung cancer should also attempt to stage the patient whenever possible so that management decisions, particularly regarding resectability, can be made expeditiously. Cytologic examination of sputum or bronchoalveolar lavage fluid is simple and inexpensive and is most useful in central tumors. Bronchoscopy with endobronchial biopsy is useful for the visualization and biopsy of main or lobar bronchial lesions, with endobronchial ultrasound (EBUS)-guided needle biopsy used to sample subcarinal masses. Endoscopic ultrasound (EUS) is useful in mediastinal nodal sampling of periesophageal lymph nodes in patients with lung cancer. CT- or fluoroscopically guided transthoracic biopsy of peripheral masses can establish a diagnosis in over 90% of patients with lung cancer. Where available, FDG-PET scans may complement CT and decrease the need for more invasive staging procedures.

CT is obtained in all patients with possible bronchogenic carcinoma to guide efforts at tissue sampling. The detection of distal lesions in the adrenal gland, liver, or bones with biopsy of accessible lesions can provide both diagnostic and staging information. The relationship of the tumor to the central airways determines the utility of transbronchoscopic endobronchial or endotracheal biopsy, whereas the detection of large subcarinal nodes can direct transcarinal biopsy using endobronchial ultrasound guidance. The pleura may be evaluated for thickening, masses, or effusions, suggesting that thoracentesis or closed pleural biopsy is the appropriate initial diagnostic procedure. Thoracotomy with resection of a peripheral lesion is appropriate for suspicious solitary lesions lacking clinical or CT evidence of unresectable nodal, mediastinal, pleural, or extrathoracic metastases. In some cases, patients with peripheral lesions may benefit from more limited surgery using VATS. Radiology may occasionally play a role in VATS by guiding placement of localizing needles and wires preoperatively using CT or intraoperative sonographic guidance.

Radiologic Staging of Lung Cancer

The primary role of the radiologist in imaging the patient with bronchogenic carcinoma is to determine the anatomic extent or stage of the tumor (6). This has prognostic importance and determines the resectability of the lesion. The staging of non-small cell bronchogenic carcinoma is based on the extent of the primary tumor (T), the presence of nodal involvement (N), and evidence of distant metastases (M). Using this TNM classification, lung cancer is divided into four stages. This scheme was modified in 2009, representing the seventh edition of the TNM staging system (Table 15.5) (7). Patients with small cell carcinoma, which is almost invariably not a surgically curable disease, have been traditionally divided into two groups: those with disease limited to one hemithorax (limited disease) and those with contralateral lung or extrathoracic spread (extensive disease). However, the new edition of the TNM lung cancer staging system will be applied to the staging of both non-small cell and small cell lung cancer as well as typical and atypical carcinoid tumors.

The major distinction in lung cancer staging is the division of patients with stage I to II (resectable) from those with stage III and IV (unresectable) disease (Tables 15.4, 15.6). Stage IIIa disease represents T3 disease (i.e., localized tumor invasion of the pleura, chest wall, diaphragm, or pericardium or tumor extending into the proximal main bronchus with sparing of the tracheal carina) associated with ipsilateral hilar nodal involvement (N1) or a T1 or T2 lesion associated with mediastinal or subcarinal nodal involvement (N2). The surgical techniques used for stage IIIa disease include en bloc resection of locally invaded chest wall, pleura, or pericardium; resection of proximal main bronchial tumors by resecting distal trachea and reimplanting the contralateral main bronchus into the proximal trachea; and mediastinal and subcarinal lymph node dissection with resection of the lung. Stage IIIb disease represents invasion of tracheal carina, mediastinum, major cardiovascular structures, esophagus, or vertebral body (T4); separate tumor nodules in the same lung but different lobes (T4); or contralateral hilar, mediastinal, scalene, or supraclavicular nodal involvement (N3). The presence of malignant pleural or pericardial effusion or tumor nodules in different lungs is now classified as M1a or stage IV disease. Distant metastases is classified as M1b or stage IV disease.

Primary Tumor (T). The new TNM classification has subdivided the T designation of the primary tumor to better reflect

TABLE 15.5

TNM CLASSIFICATION OF LUNG CANCER

Primary tumor (T)

Tx	Malignant cells in sputum without identifiable tumor
T0	No evidence of primary tumor
T1a	Tumor ≤2 cm in diameter, surrounded by lung or visceral pleura, arising distal to a main bronchus
T1b	Tumor >2 but ≤3 cm in diameter
T2a	Tumor >3 but ≤5 cm in diameter; any tumor invading the visceral pleura; any tumor with atelectasis or obstructive pneumonitis of less than an entire lung; tumor must be >2 cm from the tracheal carina
T2b	Tumor >5 but ≤7 cm
T3	Tumor >7 cm in diameter; any tumor with localized chest wall, diaphragmatic, mediastinal pleural, or pericardial invasion; phrenic nerve invasion; satellite nodules in the same lobe; the tumor may be <2 cm from the carina but cannot involve the carina
T4	Any tumor that invades the mediastinum or vital mediastinal structures including the heart, great vessels, trachea, carina, recurrent laryngeal nerve, or vertebral body; satellite tumor nodules in the same lung but different lobes

Nodal metastases (N)

N0	No evidence of nodal metastases
N1	Metastasis to ipsilateral peribronchial or hilar nodes, including involvement by contiguous spread of tumor
N2	Metastasis to ipsilateral mediastinal or subcarinal nodes
N3	Metastasis to contralateral mediastinal or hilar nodes or scalene or supraclavicular nodes

Distant metastases (M)

M0	No evidence of distant metastases
M1a	Contralateral lung metastases; pleural or pericardial tumor nodules; malignant pleural or pericardial effusion
M1b	Distant metastases; separate tumor nodules in different lobes

TABLE 15.6

CLINICAL STAGING OF LUNG CANCER BASED ON TNM CLASSIFICATION

■ STAGE	■ TNM
Ia	T1a, or b N0 M0
Ib	T2a N0 M0
IIa	T1a, or b N1 M0 T2a N1 M0 T2b N0 M0
IIb	T2a N1 M0 T3 N0 M0
IIIa	T1 or T2 N2 M0 T3 N1 or N2 M0 T4 N0 or N1 M0
IIIb	T4 N2 M0 Any T N3 M0
IV	Any T Any N M1a or M1b

survival statistics based on the long-axis diameter of the tumor and improvements in surgical resection of patients with multiple nodules in the same lobe or lung. Therefore there is now subdivision of tumors by size into T1a, T1b, T2a, T2b, and T3 designations (Table 15.5). Whereas multiple nodules in the same lobe had been designated as T4 disease, in the new staging system this is now T3 disease. Similarly, with multiple nodules in different lobes of the same lung, the new T designation is T4, as improved surgical and radiation therapy treatments for such lesions have resulted in improved survival for such patients.

Chest Wall Invasion. Tumors invading the chest wall (including the superior pulmonary sulcus), diaphragm, mediastinal pleura, pericardium, or proximal main bronchus are considered resectable by many surgeons and are classified as T3 lesions. In patients with superior sulcus tumors, vertebral body or mediastinal invasion or involvement of the brachial plexus or subclavian artery above the lung apex precludes surgical resection. Lower grade superior sulcus tumors can be treated by local irradiation followed by en bloc resection of the tumor and chest wall with reasonable survival rates.

Rib destruction or presence of an extrathoracic soft tissue mass are the only plain film findings specific for chest wall invasion; pleural thickening adjacent to a lung mass is nonspecific and need not indicate chest wall invasion. The CT diagnosis of chest wall invasion can be difficult, although CT should be obtained if this is suspected. CT findings suggestive of chest wall invasion are obtuse angles at the point of contact of the tumor and pleura, greater than 3 cm of contact between tumor and pleura, pleural thickening adjacent to the mass, and infiltration of extrapleural fat. Extrathoracic extension of the mass or rib destruction are specific but insensitive CT findings for chest wall invasion. Additional techniques that have been described to assess parietal pleural invasion by tumor include assessment of respiratory movement on dynamic expiratory CT and the use of diagnostic pneumothorax.

MR is equal to CT in its ability to diagnose chest wall invasion. Coronal MR images are useful in superior sulcus tumors to determine chest wall, brachial plexus, or subclavian artery involvement.

Mediastinal Invasion. Tumor invasion of the mediastinum with involvement of the heart, great vessels, trachea, or esophagus (T4 tumor) precludes resection. Localized invasion of the mediastinal pleura or pericardium (T3 tumor) does not prevent resection, although extensive invasion with replacement of mediastinal fat does.

On conventional radiographs, a mediastinal mass, mediastinal widening, or diaphragmatic elevation (from phrenic nerve involvement) suggests invasion. As with the diagnosis of chest wall invasion, CT demonstration of tumor mass in contiguity with the mediastinal pleura or thickening of the mediastinal pleura does not necessarily indicate mediastinal extension or unresectability. However, a significant mediastinal mass that is contiguous with a lung tumor, compresses mediastinal vessels or esophagus, or replaces mediastinal fat strongly suggests this diagnosis. Other findings that may suggest mediastinal

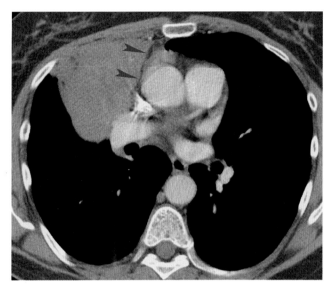

FIGURE 15.17. CT to Assess Mediastinal Invasion of Lung Cancer. In a patient with a medial segment, middle lobe, non-small cell carcinoma, CT scan shows a fat plane (*arrowheads*) between the lesion and the heart. Surgical resection confirmed the absence of pericardial or mediastinal invasion.

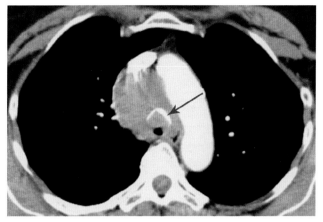

FIGURE 15.18. Tracheal Involvement by Non-Small Cell Carcinoma. Contrast-enhanced CT through the level of the distal trachea in a patient with hemoptysis shows a soft tissue mass involving the trachea (*arrow*) with a large extraluminal component. Biopsy revealed non-small cell carcinoma.

invasion include (1) obliteration of the fat plane adjacent to the descending aorta or other mediastinal vessels, (2) tumor contacting more than one-fourth of the circumference of the aortic wall, or (3) tumor contacting more than 3 cm of the mediastinum. If none of these findings are present, the tumor is potentially resectable (Fig. 15.17), even though 29% of resectable lesions lacking any of these findings are found to invade the mediastinum locally (8).

As with CT, MR is incapable of accurately demonstrating mediastinal pleural invasion or minimal invasion of mediastinal fat. Mediastinal invasion can be diagnosed with a reasonable degree of accuracy when there is significant obliteration of fat planes or compression or displacement of mediastinal vessels. In one study, MR was found to be significantly more accurate than CT in diagnosing mediastinal invasion, but this result was based on a small number of patients who had invasion, and the study predated the advent of isotropic MDCT (8). Other studies have shown no significant advantage of MR over CT for this purpose. MR is occasionally performed when vascular invasion is suspected and is likely more accurate than CT in this regard.

Central Airway Involvement. Tumors that extend into a main bronchus within 2 cm of the tracheal carina (T3 tumors) are resectable. Although tracheal or tracheal carinal involvement (T4 tumor) can be treated by carinal resection with end-to-side anastomosis of the remaining bronchus to the tracheal stump ("sleeve pneumonectomy"), most surgeons would consider this an unresectable tumor. Although plain films can occasionally demonstrate a mass within the main bronchus or trachea, CT is more accurate in assessing the relationship of the mass to the trachea and tracheal carina (Fig. 15.18). However, CT is known to underestimate the mucosal or submucosal extent of tumor as seen bronchoscopically. Therefore, any patient with a central lesion should undergo bronchoscopy to determine the proximal extent of the tumor, unless CT shows obvious carinal or tracheal invasion.

Multiple Tumor Nodules in the Same Lobe. The recent update to the staging system for non-small cell lung cancer classifies cases of satellite tumor nodules in the same lobe as the primary tumor as T3 disease, based on prognosis. In the absence of mediastinal nodal (i.e., N2) disease and distant metastases, most patients with multiple nodules in the same lobe with adequate pulmonary reserve will undergo attempt at curative resection.

Pleural Effusion. Malignant pleural effusion (now M1a disease) precludes curative resection of a tumor. In a patient with bronchogenic carcinoma, pleural effusion can occur for a variety of reasons, including pleural invasion, obstructive pneumonia, and lymphatic or pulmonary venous obstruction by tumor. Although the presence of effusion associated with lung cancer indicates a poor prognosis, only those patients with tumor cells in the pleural fluid or on pleural biopsy are considered unresectable. Other patients with effusion are considered to have "resectable" lesions, despite their poor prognosis. Usually plain radiographs, including decubitus films, are sufficient to diagnose a pleural effusion. Thoracentesis with cytologic examination and/or pleural biopsy is necessary for definitive diagnosis of malignant pleural involvement. Pleural thickening of more than 1 cm, lobulated pleural thickening, or circumferential pleural thickening (i.e., involvement of the mediastinal pleura) on CT or MR strongly suggests pleural invasion (Fig. 15.15). While PET can be useful in characterizing pleural effusions in patients with lung cancer as malignant, caution is advised in patients who have undergone prior pleurodesis, as focal plaques from intrapleural talc administration can be FDG avid on PET.

Lymph Node Metastases (N). While selected patients with ipsilateral mediastinal or subcarinal node metastases (N2 disease) are considered potentially resectable, most patients with N2 nodal disease based on preoperative imaging or nodal biopsy have a poor prognosis and are usually offered neoadjuvant therapy. Those patients with pathologic N2 disease from nonbulky intracapsular nodal metastases limited to one mediastinal nodal station that are detected microscopically following surgical resection have a better survival and therefore resection may be appropriate. Contralateral hilar or mediastinal, supraclavicular or infraclavicular nodal metastases represent N3 disease and are unresectable (Fig. 15.19).

While the previous N0–N3 designation was based on groupings from 14 nodal stations or zones, a new 7-zone system has been proposed (Fig. 15.20). This new nodal chart is essentially a slightly simplified version of the previous nodal stations for patients with lung cancer with no change in prognostic significance.

The detection of a large mediastinal mass on chest radiograph in a patient with lung cancer requires mediastinoscopic or transthoracic biopsy confirmation of tumor invasion before deeming the patient unresectable. A normal chest radiograph

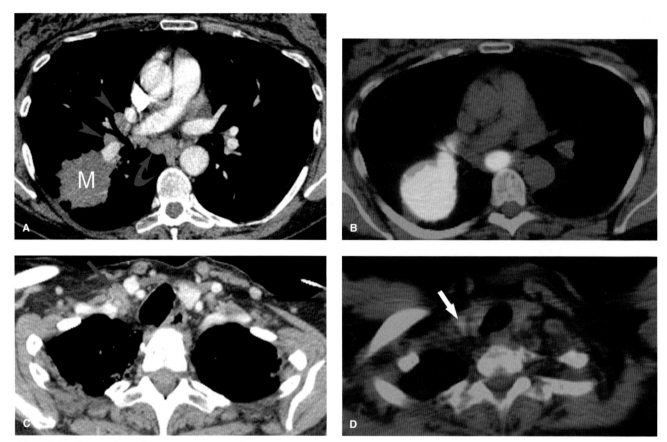

FIGURE 15.19. Lymph Node Metastases in Bronchogenic Carcinoma. A. Contrast-enhanced CT scan through the mid lungs at the level of the middle lobe bronchus shows a right lower lobe mass (*M*) with enlarged right hilar-interlobar (*arrowheads*) (N1 disease) and subcarinal (*curved arrow*) (N2 disease) nodes. **B.** Fused axial PET-CT at same level shows marked increased FDG activity in the mass and nodes. **C.** Scan at the lung apices shows an enlarged right supraclavicular node (*arrow*) (N3 disease). **D.** Fused axial PET-CT at same level shows marked increased FDG activity in the supraclavicular node (*arrow*). Biopsy of the supraclavicular node showed metastatic adenocarcinoma.

or the suggestion of hilar or mediastinal adenopathy should prompt a chest CT to assess the status of the lymph nodes. No single measurement allows completely accurate distinction of normal nodes from malignant ones. This is because malignant involvement does not always enlarge the lymph node (producing false-negative findings and reducing sensitivity), whereas enlarged nodes in patients with lung cancer may represent reactive hyperplasia rather than tumor replacement (producing false-positive findings and reducing specificity). If a small nodal diameter (5 mm) is used as the dividing point between benign and malignant, sensitivity will be excellent but specificity will be low. However, choosing a large nodal diameter (2 cm) increases specificity but decreases sensitivity. Most radiologists use a short-axis nodal diameter of 1 cm because this value achieves the best compromise of sensitivity and specificity.

CT is relatively inaccurate in determining the nodal status of a patient with lung cancer. Both sensitivity and specificity for nodal metastases, when a short-axis diameter of 1 cm or greater is used as abnormal, are approximately 60% to 65% on a patient-by-patient basis and may be even lower when looking at individual nodal stations (9). Although CT cannot be considered accurate enough to determine with certainty whether mediastinal lymph nodes are involved by tumor, it can provide information of value in guiding invasive staging procedures such as mediastinoscopy, transcarinal Wang biopsy, endoscopic US-guided biopsy, and transthoracic or open biopsy. As discussed earlier, integrated PET-CT provides superior accuracy in the nodal staging of lung cancer (10).

In select institutions, mediastinoscopy and endoscopic techniques complement CT in the nodal staging of lung cancer.

Most patients with lung cancer who have PET-positive and/or enlarged mediastinal nodes on CT that are accessible to mediastinoscopy (i.e., pretracheal, anterior subcarinal, and right tracheobronchial nodes), endobronchial ultrasound (pretracheal, paratracheal, subcarinal, hilar, and interlobar nodes) or endoscopic ultrasound (subcarinal, paraesophageal, inferior pulmonary ligament) should have nodal sampling. The decision of whether patients with negative PET or CT studies for nodal enlargement should undergo empiric nodal sampling remains controversial (11). Patients with borderline pulmonary function benefit most from preoperative nodal sampling, because a positive mediastinoscopic biopsy almost certainly precludes any attempt at resection.

Metastatic Disease (M). Each patient with proven lung cancer should be carefully evaluated for the presence of distant metastases (M1). Unequivocal evidence of metastases can obviate an unnecessary thoracotomy. Common sites of extrathoracic spread in patients with lung cancer include lymph nodes, liver, adrenal gland, bone, and brain. Metastases to lobes outside the primary lobe or to the other lung, although intrathoracic, are also considered M1 disease. Involvement of these sites probably represents hematogenous spread of tumor from the lung.

CT of the chest and upper abdomen is part of the initial evaluation in virtually all patients evaluated for bronchogenic carcinoma. This is adequate for assessing the liver, spleen, adrenal glands, and upper abdominal lymph nodes for evidence of metastases. US or MR may be used to distinguish soft tissue hepatic masses from incidental cysts. Technetium-99 m-methylene diphosphonate radionuclide bone scanning or whole-body FDG-PET imaging is used to detect bone

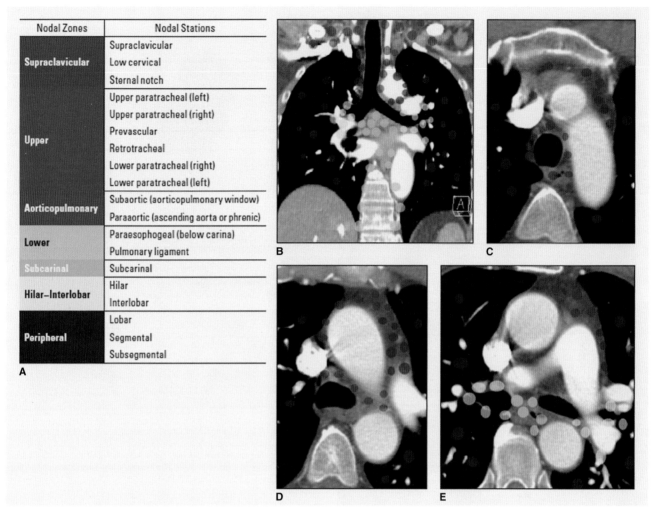

Nodal Zones	Nodal Stations
Supraclavicular	Supraclavicular
	Low cervical
	Sternal notch
Upper	Upper paratracheal (left)
	Upper paratracheal (right)
	Prevascular
	Retrotracheal
	Lower paratracheal (right)
	Lower paratracheal (left)
Aorticopulmonary	Subaortic (aorticopulmonary window)
	Paraaortic (ascending aorta or phrenic)
Lower	Paraesophogeal (below carina)
	Pulmonary ligament
Subcarinal	Subcarinal
Hilar–Interlobar	Hilar
	Interlobar
Peripheral	Lobar
	Segmental
	Subsegmental

FIGURE 15.20. Proposed New Nodal Zones for Lung Cancer Staging. International Association for the Study of Lung Cancer nodal zones in revised staging system for lung cancer. **A.** Comparison of seven new lymph node zones (*colored rows*) compared with lymph node stations in Mountain-Dressier classification used in prior system. **B–E.** Single coronal and three axial CT images through modiastinum show imaging-based map of location of seven new lymph node zones (*colored circles*) in revised classification.

metastases, with studies suggesting that PET is as sensitive but more specific than bone scanning (12). Plain films are obtained to assess specific foci of abnormally increased bone tracer uptake or to evaluate localized bone pain.

Imaging of the brain is routinely performed in patients with symptoms or signs suggesting intracranial metastases. This usually involves MR. Head scanning in patients without clinical evidence of CNS involvement is somewhat more controversial. Because virtually all patients with isolated or asymptomatic brain metastases are found to have adenocarcinoma or large cell carcinoma, patients with these subtypes of bronchogenic carcinoma should have head CT scans, regardless of the clinical findings, to identify silent metastases. Patients with positive findings can be spared an unnecessary thoracotomy.

Approximately 60% to 65% of patients with small cell carcinoma have metastatic disease at the time of diagnosis. Because it is likely that all patients with small cell carcinoma have gross or microscopic metastatic foci at presentation, these patients are generally not candidates for curative surgical resection. However, accurate staging of these patients for extrathoracic involvement determines prognosis and allows for proper assessment of response to chemotherapy. An additional reason for extrathoracic staging of small cell carcinoma is the ability to manage localized bone or soft tissue involvement with radiation or resection.

Adrenal masses are seen in approximately 10% of patients undergoing staging CT examinations for bronchogenic carcinoma. However, approximately 5% of normal individuals are known to have benign adrenal cortical adenomas. In fact, isolated adrenal masses in patients with non-small cell bronchogenic carcinoma are twice as likely to be adenomas than metastases. In many patients, the adrenal mass is the only extrathoracic site of abnormality, making accurate diagnosis of the adrenal mass crucial in determining management.

Methods used to distinguish adenomas from malignant (primary or metastatic) adrenal lesions include CT, chemical-shift MR, FDG-PET, and fine-needle aspiration biopsy (see Chapter 33). The combined ability of unenhanced CT to detect lipid-rich adenomas (≤10 H) and delayed enhanced CT to detect lipid-poor adenomas (≥60% relative washout at 15 minutes) has been used with high accuracy to distinguish between adenomas and malignant adrenal lesions. Chemical-shift MR is rarely used nowadays to characterize adrenal lesions. PET has a sensitivity approaching 100% for detecting adrenal metastases, such that a negative study effectively excludes this possibility. However, adenomas can be FDG avid and produce false-positive studies; therefore, isolated, FDG-positive adrenal lesions may require biopsy for definitive characterization (Fig. 15.21).

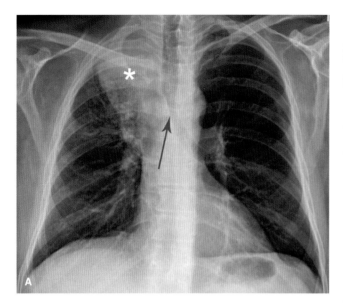

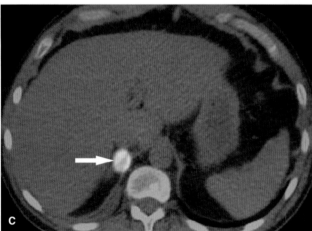

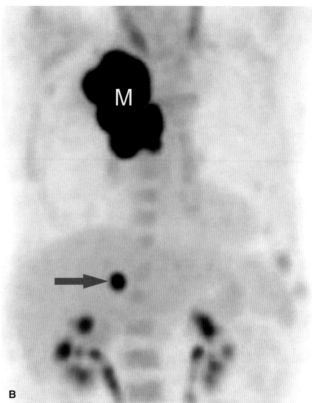

FIGURE 15.21. Adrenal Metastasis From Bronchogenic Carcinoma. **A.** Frontal chest radiograph shows right upper lobe atelectasis (*asterisk*) and a right hilar mass (*arrowhead*) with narrowing of the distal trachea/ right main bronchus (*long arrow*). **B.** Coronal maximum intensity projection image from a PET shows marked increased radiotracer activity in the mass (*M*) which replaces the right upper lobe. There is a focus of increased activity in the right upper abdomen (*arrow*). **C.** Fused axial image from PET-CT shows the focal uptake within the right adrenal gland (*arrow*).

TRACHEAL AND BRONCHIAL MASSES

Tracheal Neoplasms. Intratracheal masses may be divided into neoplastic (13) and nonneoplastic masses. Primary tracheal tumors are rare; however, 90% of all primary tracheal tumors in adults are malignant. The majority of primary tracheal malignancies arise from tracheal epithelium or mucous glands (90%); the remainder arise from the mesenchymal elements of the tracheal wall (10%). Squamous cell carcinoma is the most common primary tracheal malignancy, accounting for at least 50% of all malignant tracheal neoplasms (Fig. 15.22). These tumors affect middle-aged male smokers and are associated with laryngeal, bronchogenic, or esophageal malignancies in up to 25% of cases. The majority arise in the distal trachea within 3 to 4 cm of the tracheal carina, with the cervical trachea the next most common site. Cough, hemoptysis, dyspnea, and wheezing are common presenting symptoms. Patients may be mistakenly treated for asthma before the correct diagnosis is made. Adenoid cystic carcinoma (formerly called cylindroma) is a malignant neoplasm that arises from the tracheal salivary glands and accounts for 40% of primary tracheal malignancies. This neoplasm tends to involve the posterolateral wall of the distal two-thirds of the trachea or main or lobar bronchi (14).

The diagnosis of a primary tracheal malignancy is rarely made prospectively on chest radiographs, although well-penetrated radiographs can demonstrate distortion of the tracheal air column by a mass. CT typically shows a lobulated or irregular soft tissue mass that eccentrically narrows the tracheal lumen and has a variable extraluminal component (Fig. 15.20). Masses larger than 2 cm in diameter are likely to be malignant, whereas those smaller than 2 cm are more likely benign. Calcification is uncommon. Resectability of these lesions depends on the length of tracheal involvement and the extent of mediastinal invasion at the time of diagnosis. CT is particularly well suited for determining mediastinal involvement and has become the modality of choice for imaging tracheal neoplasms. The prognosis in patients with squamous cell carcinoma is poor, as up to 50% of patients have mediastinal extension of tumor at the time of diagnosis. While adenoid cystic carcinoma has a better prognosis, these slow-growing lesions are locally invasive with a tendency toward late recurrence and metastases.

A variety of other lesions comprise the remainder of primary tracheal malignancies and include mucoepidermoid carcinoma, carcinoid tumor, adenocarcinoma, lymphoma, small cell carcinoma, leiomyosarcoma, fibrosarcoma, and chondrosarcoma. Chondrosarcoma arises from tracheal cartilage and is identified by the presence of calcified chondroid matrix within the tumor. The trachea may be secondarily involved by malignancy, either by direct invasion or by hematogenous

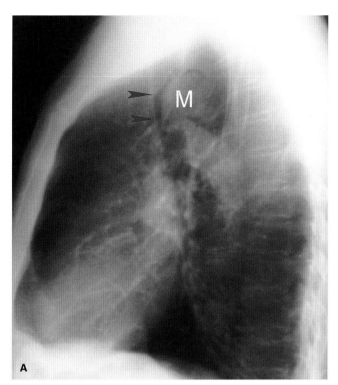
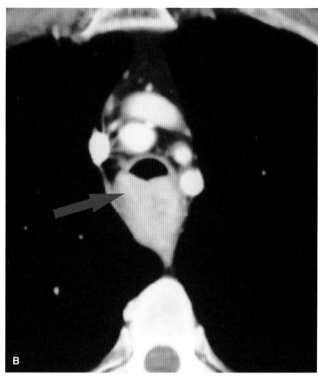

FIGURE 15.22. **Squamous Cell Carcinoma of the Trachea. A.** Lateral chest radiograph in a 68-year-old man shows a mass (*M*) narrowing the mid trachea (*arrowheads*). **B.** CT scan shows an enhancing mass (*arrow*) in the posterior trachea with narrowing of the tracheal lumen. Bronchoscopic biopsy showed squamous cell carcinoma.

spread. Laryngeal carcinoma may extend below the vocal cords to involve the cervical trachea. There is also a tendency for tumor to recur at the tracheostomy site in patients who have undergone total laryngectomies for carcinoma. Papillary and follicular carcinoma are the most common types of thyroid malignancy to invade the trachea. Squamous cell carcinoma of the upper third of the esophagus can invade the posterior tracheal wall and may produce a tracheoesophageal fistula. Bronchogenic carcinoma may involve the trachea by direct proximal extension from central bronchi, by extranodal spread of tumor from metastatic pretracheal or paratracheal lymph nodes, or by direct invasion of large right upper lobe tumors. CT is best at demonstrating tumor invasion of the tracheal wall and the extent of intraluminal mass. The extrathoracic primary tumors that are most often associated with hematogenous endotracheal metastases are carcinomas of the breast, kidney, and colon and melanoma. These lesions may appear on CT as irregular thickening of the tracheal wall or as well-defined, localized masses that are indistinguishable from benign tracheal tumors.

Chondroma, fibroma, squamous cell papilloma, hemangioma, and granular cell tumors are the most common benign tracheal tumors in adults. A *chondroma* arises from the tracheal cartilage and produces a well-circumscribed endoluminal mass. CT may demonstrate stippled cartilaginous calcification within the mass. *Fibromas* are sessile or pedunculated fibrous masses arising in the cervical trachea. *Squamous cell papilloma* is a mucosal lesion caused by infection with human papilloma virus. This disease typically produces multiple laryngeal masses in children born to women with venereal warts (condylomata acuminata). The trachea, bronchi, and lungs may become involved over time. These lesions usually regress by adolescence and therefore are uncommon causes of a solitary tracheal lesion in adults. *Hemangiomas* are seen in the cervical trachea almost exclusively in infants and young children;

they appear as focal masses on CT. *Granular cell tumor* is a neoplasm that arises from neural elements in the tracheal or bronchial wall (Fig. 15.23). These lesions usually involve the cervical trachea or main bronchi. CT shows a broad-based or pedunculated soft tissue mass that may invade the tracheal wall. This neoplasm has a tendency toward local recurrence.

Nonneoplastic intratracheal masses from ectopic intratracheal thyroid or thymic tissue have been reported and are

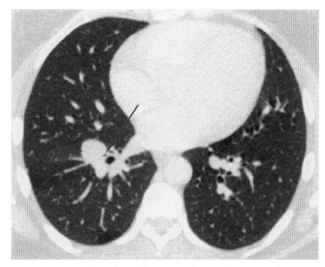

FIGURE 15.23. **Granular Cell Tumor of Lung.** CT scan at lung windows through the lower lobes shows a smoothly bordered mass (*arrowhead*) that narrows the anterior basal segmental bronchus (*arrow*). Surgical lobectomy revealed a granular cell tumor arising from the segmental bronchus.

radiographically indistinguishable from intratracheal neoplasms. Intratracheal thyroid is seen in women with extratracheal goiters. The intratracheal tissue is likewise goitrous and most commonly found in the posterolateral wall of the cervical trachea, although any portion of the trachea may be involved. Mucus plugs may appear as intratracheal masses in patients with excess sputum production or diminished clearance mechanisms. They are typically low-attenuation masses on CT which change position or disappear after an effective cough.

Primary malignant neoplasms of the central bronchi include carcinoma, carcinoid tumor, and bronchial gland tumors (adenoid cystic carcinoma and mucoepidermoid carcinoma) (14). Carcinoid and bronchial gland tumors account for approximately 2% of all tracheobronchial neoplasms; 90% of these lesions arise in a bronchus or lung, whereas the remainder arise within the trachea. Carcinoid tumor accounts for nearly 90%, adenoid cystic carcinoma 8%, and mucoepidermoid 2% of these lesions. However, adenoid cystic carcinoma accounts for 90% and carcinoid 10% of all malignant tracheal neoplasms excluding bronchogenic carcinoma.

Carcinoid tumors arise from neuroendocrine (amine precursor uptake and decarboxylation or Kulchitsky) cells within the airways. There is a spectrum of histologic differentiation and malignant behavior in tumors of Kulchitsky cell origin, ranging from the low-grade malignant typical carcinoid (KCC-1) to atypical carcinoid (KCC-2) to the highly malignant small cell carcinoma (KCC-3). Eighty percent of bronchial carcinoid tumors arise within the central bronchi, and patients present with cough, dyspnea, wheezing, recurrent episodes of atelectasis or pneumonia, or hemoptysis (Fig. 15.24). The hemoptysis may be massive and is attributable to the highly vascular nature of these lesions. The average age at diagnosis is 50. Histologically, these tumors show sheets or trabeculae of uniform cells separated by a fibrovascular stroma. The cells may contain intracytoplasmic inclusions; immunohistochemistry will reveal a variety of neuroendocrine products, including

serotonin, vasoactive intestinal polypeptide, adrenocorticotropic hormone, and antidiuretic hormone. Carcinoid syndrome is seen in fewer than 3% of cases.

Radiologically, central bronchial carcinoids present with atelectasis or pneumonia secondary to large airway obstruction. A hyperlucent lobe or lung of diminished volume may result from incomplete obstruction or collateral airflow with reflex hypoxic vasoconstriction; this finding is also rarely seen in bronchogenic carcinoma. Carcinoids arising within the lung have a propensity to involve the right upper and middle lobes and appear as well-defined, smooth or lobulated nodules or masses. Calcification or ossification is seen in 10% of pathologic specimens but is rarely visualized on plain radiographs. CT is ideally suited to demonstrate the relationship of the mass to the central airways. The typical appearance on CT is a smooth or lobulated soft tissue mass within a main or lobar bronchus (Fig. 15.24). The presence of a small intraluminal and large extraluminal soft tissue component has given rise to the descriptive term "iceberg tumor." Atypical carcinoids tend to have more irregular margins and inhomogeneous contrast enhancement and are much more likely to be associated with hilar and mediastinal lymph node metastases. In some cases, the presence of small punctate peripheral calcifications or marked contrast enhancement on CT may allow distinction from bronchogenic carcinoma. Indium-labeled octreotide nuclear imaging has proven useful in the staging of carcinoid tumors, particularly the preoperative assessment of nodal or distant metastases. Given the relatively high false-negative rate of FDG-PET for typical carcinoid tumors, octreotide scanning for TNM staging should be considered in all patients with known or suspected carcinoid tumors.

The prognosis for patients with typical bronchial carcinoid is excellent, with a 5-year survival rate of 90%. Regional lymph node metastases, seen in approximately 5% of operative specimens, lower the 5-year survival rate to 70%. Atypical carcinoids are associated with metastases in up to 70% of cases, although these may appear many years after discovery

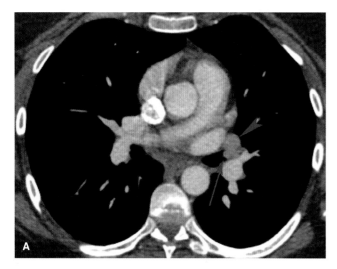

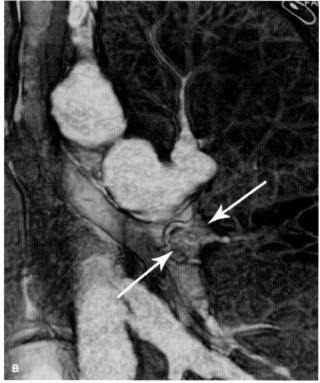

FIGURE 15.24. **Carcinoid Tumor Left Upper Lobe Bronchus.** **A.** Contrast-enhanced axial CT scan through the mid chest shows a lobulated soft tissue mass (*arrowhead*) in the left hilum with an endoluminal component in the left upper lobe bronchus (*arrow*). **B.** Coronal volume-rendered CT reconstruction through the left hilum shows the mass (*arrows*) within the left upper lobe bronchus. Bronchoscopic biopsy revealed typical carcinoid tumor.

of the primary tumor. The 5-year survival rate in these patients is less than 50%.

Pulmonary hamartoma is actually not a congenital lesion but rather a benign neoplasm comprising disorganized epithelial and mesenchymal elements normally found in the bronchus or lung. Histologically, these lesions contain cartilage surrounded by fibrous connective tissue, with variable amounts of fat, smooth muscle, and seromucous glands; calcification and ossification are seen in 30% of cases. Ninety percent of these lesions arise within the pulmonary parenchyma (Figs. 15.4E, 15.5); fewer than 10% are endobronchial. Endobronchial hamartomas are usually pedunculated lesions with fatty centers covered by fibrous tissue that contain little cartilage. Patients are usually diagnosed in the fifth decade. Central bronchial hamartomas present with cough or upper airway obstruction. CT shows a soft tissue mass that is usually indistinguishable from a bronchial carcinoid.

METASTATIC DISEASE TO THE THORAX

The spread of extrapulmonary neoplasm to the lung may occur by direct invasion of the pulmonary parenchyma or as a result of hematogenous dissemination, with the latter mechanism much more common. Rarely, a tumor can disseminate throughout the lungs via the tracheobronchial tree, as in laryngotracheal papillomatosis and some cases of BAC. Transpleural spread of tumor can be seen in cases of invasive thymoma (15).

Direct invasion of the lung may occur with mediastinal, pleural, or chest wall malignancies. The most common mediastinal malignancies to invade the lung are esophageal carcinoma, lymphoma, and malignant germ cell tumors, or any malignancy metastasizing to mediastinal or hilar lymph nodes. Malignant mesothelioma and metastases to the pleura or chest wall can extend through the pleura to invade the adjacent lung.

Hematogenous metastases to the lung may be seen with any tumor that gains access to the SVC, inferior vena cava, or thoracic duct, because the PA is the final common pathway for these channels. Although only a minority of tumor emboli survive within the pulmonary interstitium, those that do produce one of two morphologic and radiographic appearances: pulmonary nodules or lymphangitic carcinomatosis.

Pulmonary nodules are the most common manifestation of hematogenous metastases to the lung. They are most commonly seen in carcinomas of the lung, breast, kidney, thyroid, colon, uterus, and head and neck. Although most patients have multiple nodules, metastases can present as SPNs. SPNs caused by metastasis are typically smooth in contour, whereas primary bronchogenic tumors tend to be lobulated or spiculated. The likelihood that an SPN represents a solitary metastasis in a patient with a synchronous extrathoracic malignancy is slightly less than 50%, whereas SPNs in patients with prior malignancies are almost always primary bronchogenic tumors or granulomas. However, the site of the primary tumor may affect the likelihood that an SPN is a metastasis. Carcinomas of the rectosigmoid colon, osteogenic sarcoma, renal cell carcinoma, and melanoma are more likely to result in solitary pulmonary metastases. It should be cautioned that what may appear as a solitary metastasis on plain radiographs may be only one of multiple pulmonary nodules as shown by chest CT.

Nodular pulmonary metastases are usually smooth or lobulated lesions that are found in greater numbers in the peripheral portions of the lower lobes because of the greater pulmonary blood flow to these regions. Helical CT is the modality of choice for the evaluation of pulmonary metastases because it is considerably more sensitive than plain

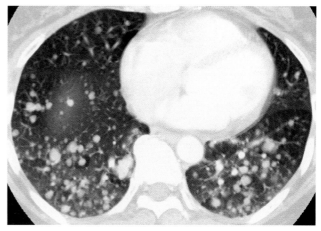

FIGURE 15.25. **Nodular Pulmonary Metastases.** CT scan through the lower lobes in a 50-year-old woman with metastatic papillary carcinoma of the thyroid shows multiple smooth nodules, reflecting hematogenous pulmonary metastases.

radiographs, conventional whole lung tomography, and incremental CT in detecting lung nodules (Fig. 15.25). There are no characteristic features of nodular metastases that allow distinction among different primary neoplasms. Similarly, the distinction between metastases and granulomas is usually impossible. The demonstration of calcification within multiple pulmonary nodules, in the absence of a history of a primary bone-forming neoplasm such as osteogenic sarcoma or chondrosarcoma, is diagnostic of granulomatous disease. Although primary mucinous adenocarcinomas of the colon and ovary may rarely produce calcification within pulmonary metastases, these microscopic calcifications are usually too small to be detected, even on CT. Additionally, in patients with miliary nodular opacities, the presence of one or more larger nodules interspersed with uniformly sized miliary nodules is highly suggestive of metastases from melanoma or carcinoma of the lung, thyroid, or kidney.

The diagnosis of nodular pulmonary metastases is usually presumptive. It is based on the demonstration of multiple pulmonary nodules in a patient with a known malignancy that has a propensity for lung metastases who lacks evidence of a granulomatous process. In some patients, particularly those with SPNs and no evidence of additional sites of metastases, or those with a history of a prior localized malignancy, a biopsy of the nodule should be performed. Although most patients with extrathoracic malignancy who have malignant SPNs have primary bronchogenic carcinoma, patients with an SPN and a history of melanoma, seminoma, or sarcoma are more likely to have a solitary metastasis. In selected patients, resection of a solitary pulmonary metastasis or several peripheral metastases may be undertaken. CT is the best imaging modality to follow the response of metastases to chemotherapy, with resolution of nodules indicating a positive response. An important caveat is that persistent nodular opacities representing sterilized tumor deposits may be seen following successful treatment of metastatic choriocarcinoma or seminoma. In these patients, follow-up CT scans will demonstrate a lack of growth of these "sterile" nodules.

Lymphangitic Carcinomatosis (LC). While direct parenchymal lymphatic invasion and obstruction of hilar and mediastinal lymph nodes by bronchogenic carcinoma is the most common cause of unilateral LC, extrapulmonary malignancies may invade pulmonary lymphatics after hematogenous dissemination to both lungs to produce interstitial deposits of tumor. In LC, the tumor cells invade the lymphatics within the peribronchovascular and peripheral interstitium, resulting in lymphatic dilatation, interstitial edema, and fibrosis. The most common extrathoracic malignancies to produce LC are carcinomas of the breast, stomach, pancreas, and prostate. Occasionally, LC will present in a patient without a known primary malignancy. Most patients with LC have slowly progressive dyspnea and a nonproductive cough.

The chest radiographic findings in LC complicating extrathoracic malignancy correlate with the involvement of the peribronchovascular and peripheral interstitium seen pathologically. Peribronchial cuffing and linear opacities, particularly Kerley B lines, are characteristically seen. Coarse reticulonodular opacities may also be present. Concomitant hilar and mediastinal lymph node enlargement need not be present.

The predominant HRCT findings in LC are thickening of interlobular septa and the subpleural interstitium (Fig. 15.16, see Fig. 17.4). While nodular thickening of the septa, reflecting tumor nodules, is characteristic of LC, it is seen in only a minority of patients. The thickened septal lines do not distort the pulmonary lobule, a feature that helps distinguish LC from interstitial fibrosis, which characteristically distorts the normal lobular shape. Visibility of the intralobular bronchioles or prominence of the centrilobular vessel is frequently seen, as is thickening of the peribronchovascular interstitium within the central (parahilar) portions of the lung. The findings may be unilateral or even limited to one lobe, particularly when LC occurs secondary to bronchogenic carcinoma. Because most patients with LC have pathologic involvement of the peribronchovascular interstitium, the diagnosis is best made by transbronchial biopsy. In a patient with the appropriate history, the HRCT appearance of lymphangitic spread may be specific enough to obviate the need for transbronchial biopsy. Occasionally, the HRCT study will demonstrate the typical findings of LC when the conventional radiograph is normal or equivocal.

NONEPITHELIAL PARENCHYMAL MALIGNANCIES AND NEOPLASTIC-LIKE CONDITIONS

Lymphoma. Parenchymal involvement in Hodgkin disease is two to three times more common than in non-Hodgkin lymphoma. Parenchymal abnormalities in Hodgkin lymphoma usually produce linear and coarse reticulonodular opacities that extend directly into the lung from enlarged hilar lymph nodes. Extensive areas of parenchymal involvement can produce mass-like opacities and areas of airspace opacification. Atelectasis in Hodgkin disease is rarely caused by extrinsic nodal compression of the bronchi, but rather develops from an obstructing endobronchial tumor. Extension into the subpleural lymphatics may produce subpleural plaques or masses that are visible only by CT. While parenchymal involvement in Hodgkin disease does not occur in the absence of hilar and mediastinal nodal disease (excluding patients who have undergone mediastinal irradiation), non-Hodgkin lymphoma may involve the parenchyma without concomitant nodal disease in up to 50%. The parenchymal involvement most often appears as masses or airspace opacities (Fig. 15.26); the latter may simulate lobar pneumonia. Coarse reticulonodular or tree-in-bud opacities are uncommon, and rarely an SPN is the sole manifestation of intrathoracic disease. Most cases of primary pulmonary non-Hodgkin lymphoma arise from the BALT and represent low-grade B-cell lymphomas.

Nodular Lymphoid Hyperplasia. This entity, previously termed *pseudolymphoma,* is used to describe a localized nonneoplastic reactive proliferation of lymphocytes in the lung. Histologically, the distinction from well-differentiated lymphoma may be difficult; the demonstration of a polyclonal population of lymphocytes with multiple germinal centers and the absence of lymph node enlargement are necessary for the diagnosis. This condition produces a sharply marginated pulmonary nodule or mass. The mass may contain air bronchograms as alveoli are compressed by large numbers of interstitial lymphocytes. Nodular lymphoid hyperplasia is usually associated with a good prognosis, although it may develop into lymphoma in patients with Sjögren syndrome.

Lymphocytic interstitial pneumonitis or diffuse lymphoid hyperplasia is an infiltration of the pulmonary interstitium by mature lymphocytes that is histologically indistinguishable from nodular lymphoid hyperplasia. Patients with Sjögren syndrome, hypogammaglobulinemia, multicentric Castleman disease, and AIDS are at particular risk for this condition. Radiographically, a predominantly lower lobe reticulonodular and linear pattern of disease is seen, often with intermixed areas of airspace opacification. CT findings

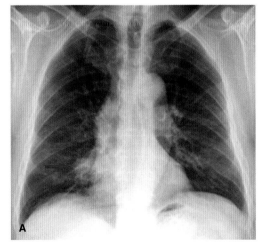
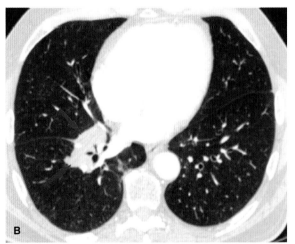

FIGURE 15.26. Primary Pulmonary Lymphoma. A. Chest radiograph shows a mass in the right lower lobe (*arrow*). **B.** CT scan at lung windows through the level of the right inferior pulmonary vein shows a lobulated mass in the middle and right lower lobes (*arrows*) surrounding but not occluding the basal segmental bronchi. Biopsy revealed non-Hodgkin B-cell lymphoma.

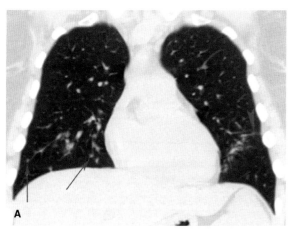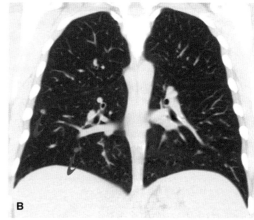

FIGURE 15.27. **Lymphocytic Interstitial Pneumonitis.** Coronal reformatted CT scans at lung windows through the anterior (**A**) and mid (**B**) thorax in a patient with immunodeficiency show ill-defined centrilobular nodules (*arrows*), reticular opacities (*arrowhead*), and cystic lesions (*curved arrows*), indicative of lymphocytic interstitial pneumonitis.

include diffuse ground-glass opacity, poorly defined centrilobular nodules, and thin-walled cysts (Fig. 15.27); lymph node enlargement may be an associated finding. Some patients with this disorder develop frank pulmonary lymphoma or interstitial fibrosis; others resolve with the administration of corticosteroid treatment. In children with AIDS, the course of lymphocytic interstitial pneumonitis is often indolent.

Posttransplant lymphoproliferative disorder represents a spectrum of entities ranging from benign polyclonal lymphoid proliferation to aggressive non-Hodgkin lymphoma which develop in a small percentage of transplant patients, with lung transplant recipients most commonly affected. Infection with Epstein–Barr virus is responsible for most cases. The disease often presents with extranodal disease, with the lung commonly involved. The most common imaging finding is that of solitary or multiple sharply marginated nodules or masses. Treatment varies, but for indolent forms of disease, reduction in immunosuppression is effective.

Lymphomatoid granulomatosis was originally thought to represent a distinct histologic entity but has recently been reclassified as a form of pulmonary lymphoma. Histologically, there are multiple round nodules containing lymphocytes that infiltrate small vessels to produce an obliterative vasculitis. These findings are similar to Wegener granulomatosis, although well-formed granulomas are rare in lymphomatoid granulomatosis. CNS and skin involvement are common, but renal failure is not present. Radiographically, there are multiple nodular opacities with a lower lobe predilection. Cavitation is common and results from ischemic necrosis. This condition is a lymphatic malignancy and is treated with chemotherapy. The prognosis is poor, with 50% of patients developing frank lymphoma. The overall 5-year survival rate is approximately 20%.

Leukemia. While leukemic involvement of the lung is found in approximately one-third of patients at autopsy, clinical or radiographic evidence of parenchymal infiltration is uncommon during life. The majority of pulmonary disease in leukemic patients is caused by pneumonia complicating immunosuppression, edema from cardiac disease, or hemorrhage owing to thrombocytopenia. Parenchymal involvement in leukemia usually takes the form of interstitial infiltration by leukemic cells, with resultant peribronchial cuffing and reticulonodular opacities on chest radiograph. Focal accumulation of leukemic cells can produce a chloroma and the radiographic appearance of an SPN. An unusual pulmonary manifesta-

tion of leukemia is *pulmonary leukostasis*, which is seen in acute leukemia or those in blast crisis in whom the peripheral white blood cell count exceeds 100,000 to 200,000/cm^3. In this condition, the white cell blasts clump within the pulmonary microvasculature to produce dyspnea. Approximately half of affected patients have normal radiographs, whereas the remainder demonstrate a diffuse reticulonodular pattern of disease.

Kaposi sarcoma (KS) of the lung is a common complication of AIDS. Pulmonary involvement almost invariably follows skin, oropharyngeal, and/or visceral involvement. The histologic features are characteristic: clusters of spindle cells with numerous mitotic figures are separated by thin-walled vascular channels containing red blood cells. The tumor involves the tracheobronchial mucosa and the peribronchovascular, alveolar, and subpleural interstitium of the lung. KS produces small to medium, poorly marginated nodular and coarse linear opacities that extend from the hilum into the mid lung and lower lung. CT shows the typical peribronchovascular location of the opacities and may demonstrate air bronchograms traversing mass-like areas of confluent disease. A bloody pleural effusion is present in up to 50% of patients; this is attributed to lesions within the subpleural interstitium of the lung. Hilar and mediastinal lymph node enlargement is found in 20% of patients. Important diagnostic features of pulmonary KS are the slow rate of progression of disease (usually over many months) and the absence of fever or pulmonary symptoms despite extensive parenchymal disease. Bleeding from endobronchial or parenchymal lesions may produce focal or diffuse airspace opacities that are difficult to distinguish from complicating bacterial pneumonia or *Pneumocystis carinii* infection.

The diagnosis of pulmonary KS is usually made indirectly, by the visualization of typical endobronchial lesions in a patient with characteristic chest radiographic findings. Combined thallium and gallium lung scanning has been used successfully to distinguish KS from pneumonia and non-Hodgkin lymphoma. While pneumonia is both gallium and thallium avid, lymphoma is gallium avid only and KS is thallium avid only.

Pulmonary blastoma is a rare malignant tumor affecting children and young adults. The tumors comprise both mesenchymal and glandular elements of lung, with an appearance that simulates fetal lung at 10 to 16 weeks' gestation. Those tumors composed predominantly of glandular elements are also called *fetal adenocarcinomas*, while tumors

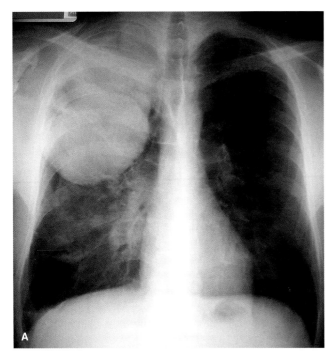

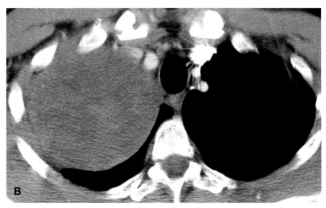

FIGURE 15.28. Pulmonary Blastoma. A. Posteroanterior radiograph in a 29-year-old man with hemoptysis shows a large right upper lobe mass. **B.** Enhanced CT scan shows a large mass that occupies much of the right upper lobe. Pathologic examination of the pneumonectomy specimen revealed pulmonary blastoma.

with malignant mesenchyme alone are referred to as *cystic and pleuropulmonary blastomas of childhood.* Tumors with mixed malignant epithelial and mesenchymal components are termed *biphasic blastomas.* Pulmonary blastomas are difficult to distinguish histologically from carcinosarcomas. These tumors tend to be extremely large at presentation (Fig. 15.28). Diagnosis is made by resection of the lesion. The prognosis is poor because many lesions have metastasized at the time of diagnosis.

References

1. Klein JS, Braff S. Imaging evaluation of the solitary pulmonary nodule. Clin Chest Med 2008;29:15–38.
2. Swensen SJ, Viggiano RW, Midthun DE, et al. Lung nodule enhancement at CT: multicenter study. Radiology 2000;214:73–80.
3. Gould MK, Maclean CC, Kuschner WG, et al. Accuracy of positron emission tomography for diagnosis of pulmonary nodules and mass lesions: a meta-analysis. JAMA 2001;285:914–924.
4. Klein JS, Febles A. Lung cancer: radiologic manifestations and diagnosis. In: Müller NL, Silva CIS, eds. Imaging of the Chest. Philadelphia, PA: WB Saunders, Philadelphia. 2008:494–516.
5. Gould MK, Kuschner WG, Rydzak CE, et al. Test performance of positron emission tomography and computed tomography for mediastinal staging in patients with non-small-cell lung cancer. Ann Intern Med 2003;139:879–892.
6. Ravenel JG. Lung cancer staging. Semin Roentgenol 2004;39:373–385.
7. Kligerman S, Abbott G. A radiologic review of the new TNM classification for lung cancer. AJR Am J Roentgenol 2010;194:562–573.
8. Glazer HS, Kaiser LR, Anderson DJ, et al. Indeterminate mediastinal invasion in bronchogenic carcinoma: CT evaluation. Radiology 1989;173:37–42.
9. McLoud TC, Bourgouin PM, Greenberg RW, et al. Bronchogenic carcinoma: analysis of staging in the mediastinum with CT by correlative lymph node mapping and sampling. Radiology 1992;182:319–323.
10. Lardinois D, Weder W, Hany TF, et al. Staging of non-small-cell lung cancer with integrated positron emission tomography and computed tomography. N Engl J Med 2004;25:2500–2507.
11. Fischer B, Lassen U, Mortensen J, et al. Preoperative staging of lung cancer with combined PET-CT. N Engl J Med 2009;361:32–39.
12. Songa JW, Oha YM, Shiwa TS, et al. Efficacy comparison between 18F-FDG PET/CT and bone scintigraphy in detecting bony metastases of non-small cell lung cancer. Lung Cancer 2009;65:333–338.
13. Marom EM, Goodman PC, McAdams HP. Focal abnormalities of the trachea and main bronchi. AJR Am J Roentgenol 2001;176:707–711.
14. Henning AG, Mark EJ. Tracheobronchial gland tumors. Cancer Control 2006;13:286–294.
15. Aquino SL. Metastatic disease to the thorax. Radiol Clin North Am 2005;43:481–495.

CHAPTER 16 ■ **PULMONARY INFECTION**

JEFFREY S. KLEIN

Infection in the Normal Host
  Bacterial Pneumonia
  Viral Pneumonia
  Fungal Pneumonia
  Parasitic Infection
  Complications of Pulmonary Infection

**Infection in the Immunocompromised Host
and in Persons with AIDS**

INFECTION IN THE NORMAL HOST

The bronchopulmonary system is open to the atmosphere and therefore is relatively accessible to airborne microorganisms. Multiple host defense mechanisms exist at the level of the pharynx, trachea, and central bronchi. When these mechanisms fail, pathogenic organisms can penetrate to the small distal bronchi and the pulmonary parenchyma. Once the invading organisms penetrate the parenchyma, there is activation of both the cellular and humoral immune systems. This response may manifest clinically and radiographically as pneumonia, and in a normal host it will often lead to eradication or at least suppression of the infecting organisms. If the immune response is impaired, a lower respiratory tract infection may lead to a very severe illness and often death, despite appropriate antibiotic therapy.

Mechanisms of Disease and Radiographic Patterns. Microorganisms responsible for producing pneumonia enter the lung and cause infection by three potential routes: via the tracheobronchial tree, via the pulmonary vasculature, or via direct spread from infection in the mediastinum, chest wall, or upper abdomen.

Infection via the tracheobronchial tree is generally secondary to inhalation or aspiration of infectious microorganisms and can be divided into three subtypes on the basis of gross pathologic appearance and radiographic patterns: lobar pneumonia, lobular or bronchopneumonia, and interstitial pneumonia (1). As will be discussed in later sections, certain organisms will typically produce one of these three patterns, although there is considerable overlap.

Lobar pneumonia is typical of pneumococcal pulmonary infection. In this pattern of disease, the inflammatory exudate begins within the distal airspaces. The inflammatory process spreads via the pores of Kohn and canals of Lambert to produce nonsegmental consolidation. If untreated, the inflammation may eventually involve an entire lobe (Fig. 16.1). Because the airways are usually spared, air bronchograms are common and significant volume loss is unusual (see Table 12.7).

Lobular or *bronchopneumonia* is the most common pattern of disease and is most typical of staphylococcal pneumonia. In the early stages of bronchopneumonia, the inflammation is centered primarily in and around lobular bronchi. As the inflammation progresses, exudative fluid extends peripherally along the bronchus to involve the entire pulmonary lobule. Radiographically, multifocal opacities that are roughly lobular in configuration produce a "patchwork quilt" appearance because of the interspersion of normal and diseased lobules (Fig. 16.2). While bronchopneumonia is the most common cause of multifocal patchy airspace opacities, there is a broad list of differential diagnostic considerations (see Table 12.9). Exudate within the bronchi accounts for the absence of air bronchograms in bronchopneumonia. With coalescence of affected areas, the pattern may resemble lobar pneumonia.

In *atypical pneumonia,* as in viral and mycoplasma infection, there is inflammatory thickening of bronchial and bronchiolar walls and the pulmonary interstitium. This results in a radiographic pattern of airways thickening and reticulonodular opacities (see Table 12.12). Air bronchograms are absent because the alveolar spaces remain aerated. Segmental and subsegmental atelectasis from small airways obstruction is common.

The spread of infection to the lung via the pulmonary vasculature usually occurs in the setting of systemic sepsis. The pattern of parenchymal involvement is patchy and bilateral. The lung bases are most severely involved because blood flow is greatest in the dependent portions of the lungs. Pulmonary infection from direct spread usually results in a localized parenchymal process adjacent to an extrapulmonary source of infection. If an organism causes extensive parenchymal necrosis, an abscess may form.

Bacterial Pneumonia

Community-acquired bacterial pneumonia accounts for between 0.5 million and 1 million hospitalizations in the United States annually and is most often due to infection by *Streptococcus pneumoniae, Mycoplasma pneumoniae, Chlamydia pneumoniae,* and *Legionella pneumophila.*

Gram-Positive Bacteria. *S pneumoniae (pneumococcus)* is a gram-positive organism that may cause infection in healthy individuals but is much more commonly seen in the

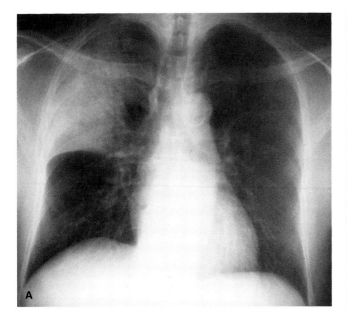

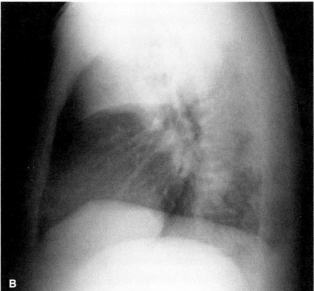

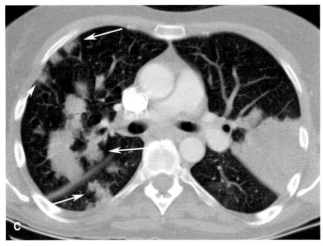

FIGURE 16.1. Pneumococcal Pneumonia. Posteroanterior (**A**) and lateral (**B**) radiographs of a 57-year-old man with fever, chills, and productive cough show airspace opacification in the right upper lobe with air bronchograms. Sputum culture was positive for *Streptococcus pneumonia*. CT scan in another patient with pneumococcal pneumonia (**C**) shows dense multifocal segmental airspace opacification in the upper lobes. Note the lobular pattern of consolidation in the right upper lobe and superior segment of the right lower lobe (*arrows*), reflecting bronchopneumonia.

elderly, alcoholics, and other compromised hosts. Patients with sickle cell disease or those who have undergone splenectomy are at particular risk for severe pneumococcal pneumonia.

Pneumococcal pneumonia tends to begin in the lower lobes or the posterior segments of the upper lobes. Initially there is involvement of the terminal airways, but rather than remaining localized to this site, there is rapid development of an airspace inflammatory exudate. The spread of infection to contiguous airspaces via interalveolar connections accounts for the nonsegmental distribution and homogeneity of the resultant consolidation.

The typical radiographic appearance of acute pneumococcal pneumonia is lobar consolidation (Fig. 16.1). Air bronchograms are usually evident. Cavitation in pneumococcal pneumonia is rare, with the exception of infections caused by serotype 3. Uncomplicated parapneumonic effusion or empyema may be seen in up to 50% of patients. With appropriate therapy, complete clearing may be seen in 10 to 14 days. In older patients or those with underlying disease, complete resolution may take 8 to 10 weeks.

Patients with pneumococcal pneumonia occasionally present with atypical radiographic patterns of disease. Patchy lobular opacities similar to those seen with bronchopneumonia (Fig. 16.1C), or rarely, a reticulonodular pattern, may be seen. In some patients, the atypical appearance may relate to the presence of preexisting lung disease (e.g., emphysema), partial treatment, or an impaired immune response (e.g., AIDS). In children, pneumococcal pneumonia may present as a spherical opacity ("round pneumonia") simulating a parenchymal mass.

Staphylococcus aureus pneumonia is most common in hospitalized and debilitated patients. It may also develop following hematogenous spread to the lung in patients with endocarditis or indwelling catheters and in intravenous drug users. Community-acquired infection may complicate influenza or other viral pneumonias.

S aureus typically produces a bronchopneumonia and appears radiographically as patchy opacities (Fig. 16.3). In severe cases, the opacities may become confluent to produce lobar opacification. Because the inflammatory exudate fills the airways, air bronchograms are rarely seen. In adults, the process is often bilateral and may be complicated by abscess formation in 25% to 75% of patients. In patients who develop pulmonary infection from hematogenous seeding, one sees multiple bilateral poorly defined nodular opacities that eventually become more sharply defined and cavitate. Parapneumonic effusion and empyema are common. Pneumatocele formation is common in children and may lead to pneumothorax. Pneumatoceles may be distinguished from abscesses by their thin walls, rapid change in size, and tendency to develop during the late phase of infection.

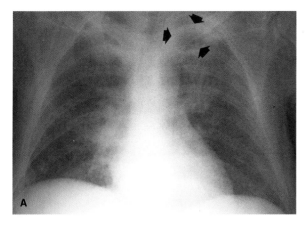

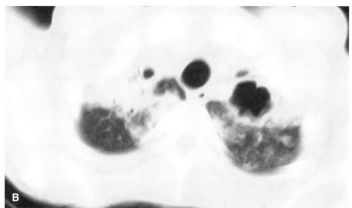

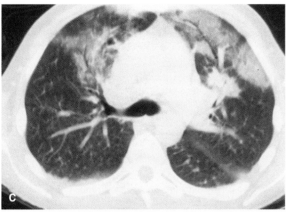

FIGURE 16.2. *Pseudomonas aeruginosa* Pneumonia. **A.** Frontal radiograph of an HIV-positive man with fever and progressive respiratory symptoms shows multifocal airspace opacities with dense apical opacification with cavitation (*arrows*). **B.** A CT scan through the apices shows airspace opacification with left apical cavitation. **C.** A scan at the level of the tracheal carina shows airspace disease in the anterior segments of right and left upper lobes with sparing of the dependent portions of lung. Bronchoscopy revealed *Pseudomonas*.

Streptococcus pyogenes. Acute streptococcal pneumonia is rarely seen today, though it can occasionally complicate viral infection or streptococcal pharyngitis. Its radiographic appearance is similar to that of staphylococcal pneumonia, with lobular or segmental lower lobe opacities. The process may be complicated by abscess formation and cavitation; empyema is relatively common.

Bacillus anthracis. Anthrax is caused by a sporulating gram-positive bacillus that is distributed worldwide. Naturally occurring inhalational anthrax is rare; however, anthrax has been used as an agent of bioterrorism in the United States. The primary radiographic manifestations of inhalational anthrax

are related to the underlying pathology of hemorrhagic lymphadenitis and mediastinitis accompanied by hemorrhagic pleural effusions. Conventional radiographs demonstrate mediastinal widening, hilar enlargement, and often pleural effusion. Frank areas of consolidation are not usually present but peribronchial opacities may be seen. CT scans of recent bioterrorism victims, performed in 2001 without intravenous contrast, demonstrated high-attenuation lymphadenopathy and pleural effusions secondary to hemorrhage. CT scans may show extensive adenopathy in the setting of normal radiographs and should be obtained if the suspicion of anthrax is high (2).

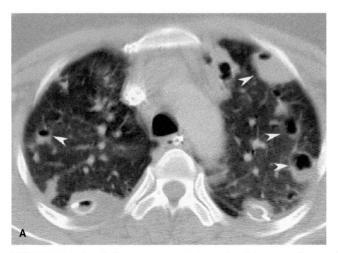

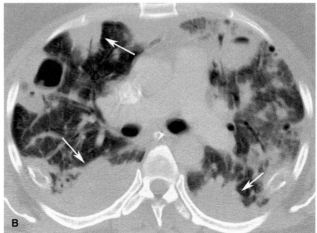

FIGURE 16.3. *Staphylococcus aureus* Pneumonia. CT scans at the top of the aortic arch (**A**) and central pulmonary arteries (**B**) show a combination of abscess and cavity formation (*arrowheads*) and lobular consolidation (*arrows*). Sputum cultures showed *S aureus* pneumonia.

Gram-Negative Bacteria. Gram-negative bacteria are increasingly important causes of pneumonia in hospitalized patients, accounting for more than 50% of nosocomial pulmonary infections. While gram-negative organisms may be isolated from only a small percentage of healthy individuals, the isolation rate in hospitalized and severely ill patients ranges from 40% to 75%. The organisms most often responsible for pneumonia include members of the Enterobacteriaceae family (*Klebsiella*, *Escherichia coli*, and *Proteus*), *Pseudomonas aeruginosa*, *Haemophilus influenzae*, and *L pneumophila* (3).

The radiographic appearance of gram-negative bacterial pneumonia varies from small ill-defined nodules to patchy areas of opacification that may become confluent and resemble lobar pneumonia. Involvement is usually bilateral and multifocal, and the lower lobes are most frequently affected. Abscess formation and cavitation are relatively common. Parapneumonic effusion is common and is often complicated by empyema formation.

Klebsiella pneumoniae. *Klebsiella* pneumonia occurs predominantly in older alcoholic men and debilitated hospitalized patients. Radiographically it appears as a homogeneous lobar opacification containing air bronchograms. Three features help distinguish it radiographically from pneumococcal pneumonia: (1) the volume of the involved lobe may be increased by the exuberant inflammatory exudate, producing a bulging interlobar fissure; (2) an abscess may develop, with cavity formation, which is uncommon in pneumococcal pneumonia; and (3) the incidence of pleural effusion and empyema is higher. Pulmonary gangrene may be seen but is uncommon.

H influenzae. In adults, *H influenzae* infection is most common among patients with chronic obstructive pulmonary disease (COPD), alcoholism, and diabetes mellitus as well as those with an anatomic or functional splenectomy. It most often causes bronchitis, although it may extend to produce bilateral lower lobe bronchopneumonia.

P aeruginosa pneumonia most often affects debilitated patients, particularly those requiring mechanical ventilation. There is a high mortality associated with the disease. The radiographic pattern of parenchymal involvement depends upon the method by which the organisms reach the lung. Patchy opacities with abscess formation, which mimic staphylococcal pneumonia, are common when the infection reaches the lung via the tracheobronchial tree (Fig. 16.2). Diffuse, bilateral, ill-defined nodular opacities usually reflect hematogenous dissemination. Pleural effusions are common and are usually small.

L pneumophila. Legionnaires disease is caused by infection with *L pneumophila*, a gram-negative bacillus commonly found in air conditioning and humidifier systems. This infection tends to affect older men. Community-acquired infection is seen in patients with COPD or malignancy, whereas nosocomial infection primarily affects immunocompromised patients or those with renal failure or malignancy.

The characteristic radiographic pattern is airspace opacification, which is initially peripheral and sublobar. In some patients, the airspace opacities appear as a round pneumonia. The infection progresses to lobar or multilobar involvement despite the initiation of antibiotic therapy. At the peak of disease, the parenchymal involvement is usually bilateral. Pleural effusions are seen in approximately 30% of patients. Cavitation is not seen except in the immunocompromised patient (Fig. 16.4). The radiographic resolution of pneumonia is often prolonged and may lag behind symptomatic improvement.

Anaerobic Bacterial Infections. The majority of anaerobic lung infections arise from aspiration of infected oropharyngeal

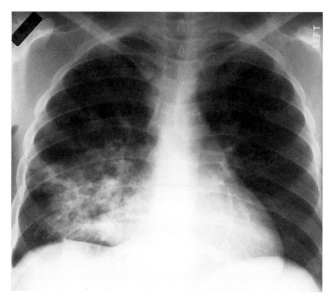

FIGURE 16.4. *Legionella* Pneumonia in an Immunocompromised Patient. Frontal chest radiograph in a 35-year-old man with AIDS shows a middle lobe airspace opacification with areas of cavitation. Bronchoscopy showed *Legionella pneumophila* pneumonia.

contents (4). Approximately 25% of patients give a history of impaired consciousness and many are alcoholic. The most common organisms responsible are the gram-negative bacilli *Bacteroides* and *Fusobacterium*, although the majority of pulmonary infections are polymicrobial. All anaerobic pulmonary infections produce a similar radiographic appearance. The distribution of parenchymal opacities reflects the gravitational flow of aspirated material. When aspiration occurs in the supine position, it is the posterior segments of the upper lobes and superior segments of the lower lobes that are predominantly involved, whereas aspiration in the erect position leads to involvement of basal segments of the lower lobes. The typical radiographic appearance is peripheral lobular and segmental airspace opacities. Cavitation within the areas of consolidation is relatively common, and discrete lung abscesses may be seen in up to 50% of patients. Hilar and/or mediastinal lymph node enlargement may be seen in those with lung abscesses. Empyema, with or without bronchopleural fistula formation, is a common complication and is seen in up to 50% of patients.

Atypical Bacterial Infections. *Actinomycosis.* *Actinomyces israelii* is an anaerobic gram-positive filamentous bacterium that is a normal inhabitant of the human oropharynx. It causes disease when it gains access to devitalized or infected tissues that facilitate its growth. Actinomycosis most commonly follows dental extractions, manifesting as mandibular osteomyelitis or a soft tissue abscess. The lungs may be infected by aspiration of infectious oral debris or, less commonly, by direct extension from the primary site of disease.

The radiographic pattern of actinomycosis is often indistinguishable from that of nocardiosis. Findings consist of nonsegmental airspace opacities in the periphery of the lower lobes. In some cases, the infection manifests as a localized mass-like opacity that mimics bronchogenic carcinoma (Fig. 16.5). If therapy is not instituted, a lung abscess may develop. Thoracic actinomycosis is characterized by its ability to spread to contiguous tissues without regard for normal anatomic barriers. Extension into the pleura will cause empyema, whereas chest wall involvement is characterized by osteomyelitis of the ribs

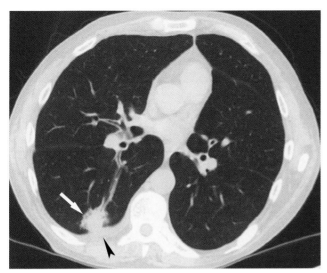

FIGURE 16.5. *Actinomyces Pulmonary Infection.* CT scan at lung windows of a 52-year-old smoker shows an irregular nodule in the superior segment of the right lower lobe posteriorly (*arrow*). Note the associated localized posterior pleural thickening (*arrowhead*). CT-guided transthoracic biopsy revealed *Actinomyces israelii* infection.

and chest wall abscess. Involvement of the ribs is seen as wavy periosteal reaction or lytic rib destruction (5). If the pleuropulmonary disease becomes chronic, extensive fibrosis may be seen. Rarely, the disease is disseminated and a miliary pattern is seen.

Mycoplasma pneumonia displays both bacterial and viral characteristics and is considered as a separate group (6). It is probably the most common atypical pneumonia and accounts for 10% to 30% of all community-acquired pneumonia. Affected patients usually have a subacute illness of 2 to 3 weeks' duration. Symptoms include fever, nonproductive cough, headache, and malaise. Unusual physical findings include bullous myringitis and rash.

In the early stages of infection, interstitial inflammation leads to a fine reticular pattern on the chest radiograph. This may progress to patchy segmental airspace opacities (Fig. 16.6),

which may coalesce to produce lobar consolidation. CT scan of mycoplasma pneumonia usually appears as patchy airspace opacities with a tree-in-bud appearance that reflects infectious bronchiolitis (Fig. 16.7). The process is often unilateral and tends to involve the lower lobes. Pleural effusion may be seen in the consolidative form of disease and occurs most commonly in children. Lymph node enlargement is uncommon but may be seen in children. Radiographic resolution may require 4 to 6 weeks.

Mycobacterial Infections. *Mycobacterium tuberculosis* is an aerobic acid-fast bacillus. Two principal forms of tuberculous pulmonary disease are recognized clinically and radiographically: primary tuberculosis (TB) and "reactivation" or postprimary disease. The inflammatory response to *M tuberculosis* differs from the normal response to bacterial organisms in that it involves cell-mediated immunity (delayed hypersensitivity). Initially, droplet nuclei laden with bacilli are inhaled and implanted in a subpleural location. In most patients, the bacilli are phagocytized and killed by alveolar macrophages. If the bacilli overcome the immune response of the host, an inflammatory focus is established. The macrophages are then transformed into epithelioid cells, which aggregate to form granulomas. The granulomas are usually well-formed by 1 to 3 weeks, coinciding with the development of delayed hypersensitivity. The granulomas typically demonstrate central caseous necrosis, thereby distinguishing them from the granulomas seen in sarcoidosis. Inflammation and enlargement of draining hilar and mediastinal lymph nodes is common in primary disease, particularly in children and immunocompromised patients.

In primary infection, the parenchymal disease and adenopathy may completely resolve, or there may be a residual focus of scarring or calcification. In some situations, usually in infants younger than 1 year, local parenchymal disease progresses and is termed *progressive primary TB*. More commonly, the disease will be contained by the granulomatous response and recur years later (reactivation or postprimary TB) in the setting of weakened host defenses from aging, alcoholism, diabetes, cancer, or HIV infection. Postprimary TB develops under the influence of hypersensitivity, with caseous necrosis seen histologically.

Primary TB has classically been a disease of childhood, although the incidence of primary disease has increased

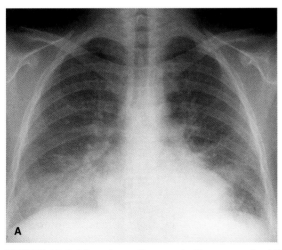

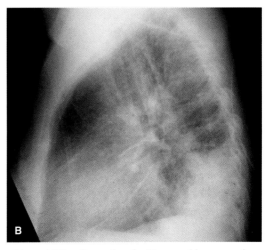

FIGURE 16.6. *Mycoplasma* Pneumonia. Posteroanterior (A) and lateral (B) radiographs of a 21-year-old woman show mixed diffuse interstitial and bibasilar airspace opacities. Immunofluorescent staining of induced sputum samples revealed *Mycoplasma pneumoniae*.

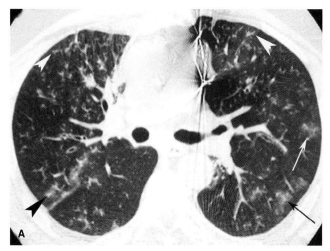 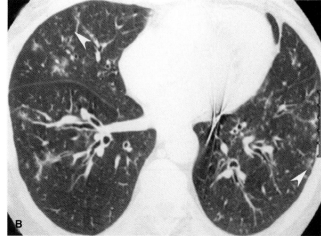

FIGURE 16.7. CT of *Mycoplasma* Pneumonia. Thin-section CT scans through the upper (**A**) and lower (**B**) lungs in a patient with mycoplasma pneumonia show patchy ground glass opacities (*arrows*) with scattered tree-in-bud opacities (*arrowheads*).

because of the HIV epidemic. Most patients with primary TB are asymptomatic and have no radiographic sequelae of infection. In some patients a Ranke complex, consisting of a calcified parenchymal focus (the Ghon lesion) and nodal calcification, is seen. If the patient is symptomatic, a nonspecific focal pneumonitis occurs and is seen as small, ill-defined areas of segmental or lobar opacification (Fig. 16.8). The parenchymal consolidation may mimic a bacterial pneumonia, but the clinical and radiographic course is much more indolent. Cavitation is relatively uncommon in the immunocompetent patient (7). The pulmonary focus may resolve completely or persist as a Ghon lesion or a Ranke complex. *Tuberculomas* are discrete nodular opacities that may develop in primary TB but are much more common in postprimary TB Unilateral pleural effusions are seen in 25% of cases and are usually associated with parenchymal disease. If a tuberculous empyema develops,

it may break through the parietal pleura to form an extrapleural collection (empyema necessitatis). Unilateral hilar or mediastinal lymph node enlargement is common, particularly in children, and may be the sole radiographic manifestation of infection. Bilateral hilar or mediastinal lymph node enlargement may be seen, but this is uncommon and is almost invariably asymmetric in distinction to lymph node enlargement in sarcoidosis. During the primary tuberculous infection, there is hematogenous dissemination of the organism to regions with a high partial pressure of oxygen; these include the lung apices, renal medullae, and bone marrow. These microscopic foci are clinically silent and serve as a source of reactivation disease.

Post-primary TB patientsoften present with cough and constitutional symptoms, including chills, night sweats, and weight loss. Reactivation tends to occur in the apical and posterior segments of the upper lobes and the superior segments of the lower lobes. Ill-defined patchy and nodular opacities are commonly seen. Cavitation is an important radiographic feature of postprimary TB and usually indicates active and transmissible disease (Fig. 16.9). The cavitary focus may lead to transbronchial spread of organisms and result in multifocal bronchopneumonia. Erosion of a cavitary focus into a branch of the pulmonary artery can produce an aneurysm (Rasmussen aneurysm) and cause hemoptysis. With appropriate antimicrobial treatment, the disease is usually controlled by a granulomatous response. Parenchymal healing is associated with fibrosis, bronchiectasis, and volume loss (cicatrizing atelectasis) in the upper lobes.

There are several late complications of pulmonary TB. Interstitial fibrosis can cause pulmonary insufficiency and secondary pulmonary arterial hypertension. Hemoptysis may be secondary to bronchiectasis, mycetoma formation in an old tuberculous cavity, or erosion of a calcified peribronchial lymph node (broncholith) into a bronchus. Bronchostenosis is a result of healed endobronchial TB.

Miliary TB may complicate either primary or reactivation disease. It results from hematogenous dissemination of tubercle bacilli and produces diffuse bilateral 2- to 3-mm pulmonary nodules (Fig. 16.10). Miliary disease is associated with a high mortality and requires prompt therapy.

Atypical Mycobacterial Infections. There are several nontuberculous mycobacteria that may cause pulmonary disease (8). The most common organism responsible for pulmonary disease is *Mycobacterium avium-intracellulare* (MAI) or *M kansasii.* Disease in nonimmunocompromised patients typically

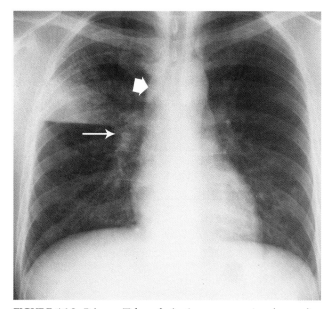

FIGURE 16.8. Primary Tuberculosis. A posteroanterior chest radiograph in a 32-year-old homeless man shows airspace disease within the anterior segment of the right upper lobe, with right hilar (*skinny arrow*) and paratracheal (*fat arrow*) lymph node enlargement. Sputum stains and cultures revealed *Mycobacterium tuberculosis.*

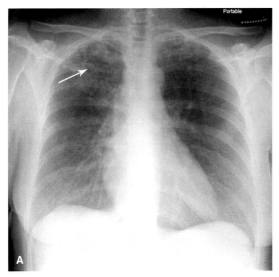

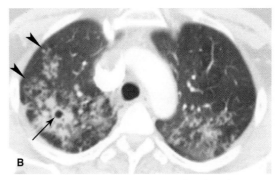

FIGURE 16.9. **Postprimary (Reactivation) Tuberculosis. A.** Frontal chest radiograph in a 49-year-old female with a cough and hemoptysis shows bilateral upper lobe reticulonodular opacities with a right upper lobe cavity (*arrow*). **B.** CT scan through the upper lobes at lung windows confirms the presence of a cavity (*arrow*) and bilateral upper lobe tree-in-bud opacities (*arrowheads*) that reflect endobronchial spread of disease. Sputum cultures were positive for *Mycobacterium tuberculosis*.

affects those with underlying COPD. The radiographic features are often indistinguishable from those of reactivation TB, with chronic fibrocavitary opacities involving the upper lobes. While cavitation is common, pleural effusion, lymph node enlargement, and miliary spread are distinctly unusual. A second pattern of disease with MAI has recently been described in middle-aged and elderly women, with small peribronchial nodules and bronchiectasis seen in a middle lobe and lingular distribution (Fig. 16.11). Although the disease caused by nontuberculous mycobacteria tends to be more indolent than that seen with *M tuberculosis*, it is often difficult to treat effectively.

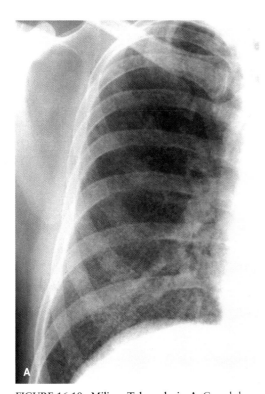

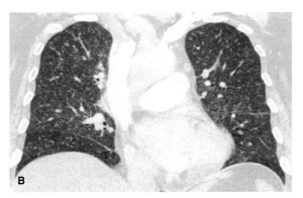

FIGURE 16.10. **Miliary Tuberculosis. A.** Coned-down view of a frontal radiograph demonstrates innumerable micronodular opacities characteristic of micronodular (miliary) interstitial disease. Transbronchial biopsy demonstrated caseating granulomas containing acid-fast bacilli. **B.** Coronal reformation at lung windows of a CT scan in another patient with proven military tuberculosis shows innumerable randomly distributed small lung nodules.

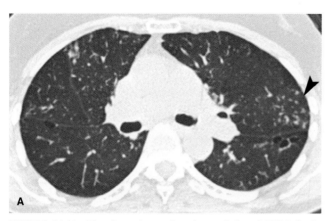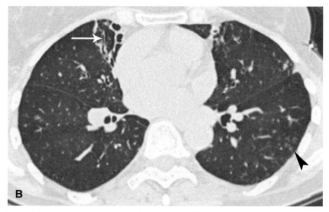

FIGURE 16.11. *Mycobacterium avium-intracellulare* **(MAI) Infection. A, B.** Thin-section CT scans through mid lungs in a patient with MAI pulmonary infection show scattered nodules, middle lobe bronchiectasis (*arrow* in B), and tree-in-bud opacities (*arrowheads*).

Viral Pneumonia

Viruses are a major cause of upper respiratory tract and airways infection, although pneumonia is relatively uncommon. The diagnosis of viral pneumonia is often one of exclusion. Chest radiographic features are nonspecific and usually demonstrate a pattern of bronchopneumonia or interstitial opacities (9). Resolution is usually complete, but permanent sequelae may be seen, including bronchiectasis, bronchiolitis obliterans (which may produce a unilateral hyperlucent lung or Swyer-James syndrome), and interstitial fibrosis.

Influenza is the most common cause of viral pneumonia in adults. Outbreaks of influenza can occur in pandemics, epidemics, or sporadically. In most patients, the disease is confined to the upper respiratory tract, but in elderly persons, those with underlying cardiopulmonary disease or those who are immunocompromised, and pregnant women, a severe hemorrhagic pneumonia may develop. In adults with influenzal pneumonia, there is often bilateral lower lobe patchy airspace opacification. In children, a diffuse interstitial reticulonodular pattern is more commonly seen. Bacterial superinfection with *Streptococcus* or *Staphylococcus* organisms contributes to a fulminating course that may result in death. The development of lobar consolidation, pleural effusion, or cavitation suggests bacterial superinfection.

Infection due to H1N1 influenza or swine flu was first described in 2009 and has produced a spectrum of illness from self-limited disease to fatal pneumonia. Typical radiographic and CT findings in swine flu pneumonia include patchy ground glass or airspace consolidation involving the central and lower lungs (Fig. 16.12), with progression to confluent bilateral airspace consolidation in the most severely affected patients (10).

Respiratory syncytial virus and parainfluenza virus are common causes of epidemic viral pneumonia in children. When seen in adults, the disease is usually in the setting of a debilitated or immunocompromised patient (Fig. 16.13). Findings are similar to other viral pneumonias: patchy airspace opacities, bronchial wall thickening, and tree-in-bud opacities.

Varicella-zoster virus, which causes chickenpox and shingles, may produce a severe pneumonia in adults. Patients on immunosuppressive therapy or with lymphoma are at greatest risk. Chest radiographs characteristically show diffuse bilateral ill-defined nodular opacities 5 to 10 mm in diameter. These opacities usually resolve completely; however, in some patients these opacities involute and calcify to produce innumerable small (2 to 3 mm) calcified nodules (Fig. 16.14).

Adenovirus is a frequent cause of upper and, occasionally, lower respiratory tract infection. Overinflation and bronchopneumonia accompanied by lobar atelectasis are the most frequent radiographic manifestations of adenovirus pneumonia; however, adenovirus in children may present as lobar or segmental consolidation.

SARS-Associated Coronavirus (SARS-CoV). Severe acute respiratory syndrome (SARS) is a recently described respiratory illness caused by a new coronavirus, SARS-CoV, not previously seen in humans. The disease appears to have originated in southern China and rapidly spread to other areas of the world, causing more than 8000 reported cases in late 2002 and early 2003. The clinical symptoms and signs as well as the radiographic manifestations of SARS are nonspecific. Unilateral or bilateral areas of airspace opacity are seen on initial radiographs in the majority of affected patients. The opacities are typically peripheral and lower zone in location, progressively involving the central lungs. Occasionally, initial radiographs are negative; CT demonstrates areas of ground glass opacity and/or consolidation. Lymphadenopathy and pleural effusions are not characteristic.

Fungal Pneumonia

Fungal infections are now seen with increased frequency because of an increase in the incidence of disease caused by

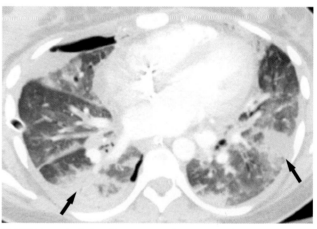

FIGURE 16.12. Swine Flu (H1N1 Influenza) Pneumonia. CT scan at lung windows of a young female with H1N1 influenza shows multifocal subsegmental consolidation (*arrows*). Note the presence of a right chest tube placed for a right pneumothorax complicating mechanical ventilation.

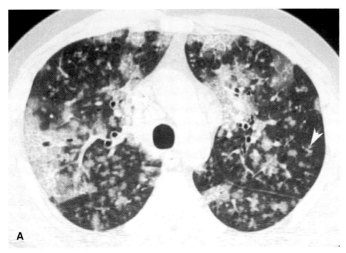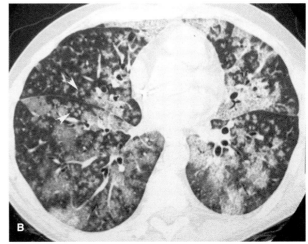

FIGURE 16.13. Parainfluenza Virus Pneumonia. CT scans through upper lungs (**A**) and mid lungs (**B**) in a patient with acute myelogenous leukemia show striking bronchopneumonia and bronchiolitis (*arrowheads*). Parainfluenza virus was isolated from bronchoalveolar lavage fluid.

pathogenic fungi in healthy hosts and the emergence of opportunistic species in immunocompromised hosts. Fungi can cause pulmonary disease by several mechanisms. Some fungi, including *Histoplasma capsulatum*, *Coccidioides immitis*, and *Blastomyces dermatitidis*, are primary pathogens and most commonly infect normal hosts (11). Other fungi, most notably *Aspergillus*, *Candida*, and *Cryptococcus*, are opportunistic pathogens in immunocompromised individuals. In all cases, the fungi elicit a necrotizing granulomatous reaction. The high mortality among patients with untreated invasive infection and the availability of effective antifungal therapy with intravenous amphotericin B and the oral azoles (e.g., fluconazole, itraconazole) have made the early and accurate diagnosis of fungal infection imperative. A number of serologic assays

(complement fixation and immunodiffusion) and histologic methods are available for the accurate diagnosis of this fungal infection.

Histoplasmosis. *H capsulatum* is endemic to certain areas of North America, most notably the Ohio, Mississippi, St. Lawrence River valleys, and Mexico. The overwhelming majority (95% to 99%) of infections caused by *H capsulatum* are asymptomatic. A routine chest film demonstrating multiple well-defined calcified nodules less than 1 cm in size, with or without calcified hilar or mediastinal lymph nodes, may be the only indication of prior infection.

Acute histoplasma infection most often presents with the abrupt onset of flu-like symptoms. The chest radiograph in such patients may be normal or may show nonspecific changes, including subsegmental airspace opacities with or without associated hilar lymph enlargement. If the patient inhales a large inoculum of organisms, widespread, fairly discrete nodular opacities 3 to 4 mm in diameter are seen with hilar adenopathy. Alternatively, acute histoplasmosis may result in a solitary, sharply defined nodule <3 cm in diameter, termed as *histoplasmoma* (Fig. 16.15). Histoplasmomas are most common in the lower lobes and frequently calcify.

FIGURE 16.14. Healed Varicella Pneumonia. Coronal maximum intensity projection reformation of a CT scan in a patient with a history of varicella pneumonia shows multiple scattered calcified nodules (*arrowheads*).

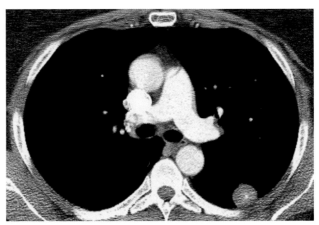

FIGURE 16.15. Histoplasmoma. Contrast-enhanced CT scan through the midthorax shows a nodule in the lower lobe posteriorly with central calcification, characteristic of a histoplasmoma.

H capsulatum can also cause chronic pulmonary disease, usually in patients with underlying emphysema. Unilateral or bilateral upper lobe cicatrizing atelectasis with marked hilar retraction may mimic the radiographic findings seen in postprimary TB. Similarly, chronic upper lobe fibrocavitary disease may be seen. Involvement of the mediastinum by chronic granulomatous inflammation may lead to fibrosing mediastinitis, while endobronchial disease can produce bronchostenosis.

Asymptomatic blood-borne dissemination of *H capsulatum* is common, as judged by the frequency of calcified splenic granulomas in residents of endemic areas. Clinically apparent disseminated histoplasmosis, however, is extremely rare and is usually seen in infants or immunocompromised adults. The chest film most commonly shows widespread 2- to 3-mm nodules that are indistinguishable from those of miliary TB, although reticular opacities and patchy areas of consolidations may also be seen.

Coccidioidomycosis. *C immitis* is endemic to the southwestern United States and the San Joaquin Valley of California. There are four types of clinical and radiographic coccidioidal pulmonary infections: acute, persistent, chronic progressive, and disseminated coccidioidomycosis. Acute coccidioidomycosis develops in 40% of infected adults. These patients develop a self-limiting viral-type illness, which is referred to as "valley fever" when associated with erythema nodosum and arthralgias. The chest radiograph may be normal or show focal or multifocal segmental airspace opacities that resolve over several months. Hilar and mediastinal adenopathy and pleural effusions may be seen in association with parenchymal disease (Fig. 16.16).

Patients whose symptoms or radiographic abnormalities persist beyond 6 to 8 weeks are considered to have persistent coccidioidomycosis. The radiographic features of persistent pulmonary disease include coccidioidal nodules or masses (coccidioidomas), persistent areas of consolidation, and miliary nodules. Coccidioidal nodules are areas of round pneumonia, usually located in the subpleural regions of the upper lobes. These nodules tend to cavitate rapidly and produce characteristic thin-walled cavities. In chronic progressive disease, upper lobe fibrocavitary disease (similar to postprimary TB and histoplasmosis) is seen. Disseminated (miliary) coccidioidomycosis is relatively rare and usually affects immunocompromised patients and non-Caucasians.

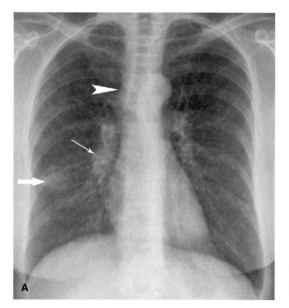

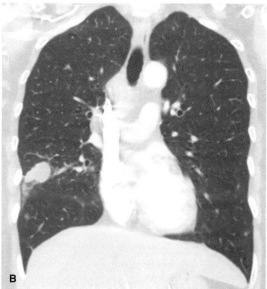

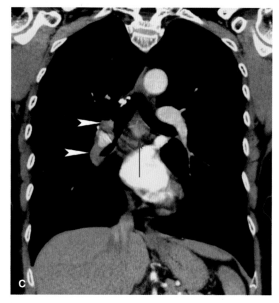

FIGURE 16.16. Primary *Coccidioides* Infection. A. Frontal radiograph of a 63-year-old woman with a clinical diagnosis of Valley fever reveals a mass-like opacity in the right lower lung (*large arrow*) with enlarged right hilar (*skinny arrow*) and paratracheal (*arrowhead*) nodes. **B.** Coronal reformatted CT scan confirms a right middle lobe nodule. **C.** Contrast-enhanced coronal reformatted CT scan through the carina shows enlarged right hilar (*arrowheads*) and subcarinal nodes (*red arrow*). CT-guided transthoracic biopsy of the peripheral lung lesion revealed coccidioidomycosis.

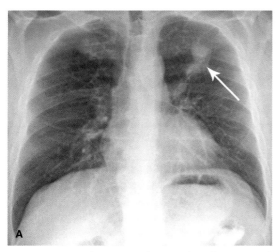
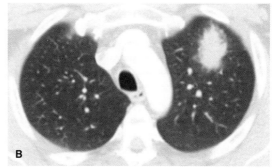

FIGURE 16.17. *Blastomyces dermatitidis* Infection. A. Chest radiograph in a 39-year-old man shows an ill-defined mass in the left upper lobe (*arrow*). B. CT scan through the upper lobes shows an irregular mass in the left upper lobe with surrounding ground glass opacity. Biopsy revealed *Blastomyces dermatitidis* infection.

Blastomycosis. North American blastomycosis, caused by *B. dermatitidis,* is a chronic systemic disease primarily affecting the lungs and the skin. Its geographic distribution overlaps that of histoplasmosis but extends farther to the east and the north. The pulmonary infection is often asymptomatic. Symptomatic infection resembles that of an acute bacterial pneumonia. The radiographic findings in pulmonary blastomycosis are nonspecific. The most common manifestation of disease is homogeneous nonsegmental airspace opacification with a propensity for the upper lobes. A less common presentation is single or multiple masses (Fig. 16.17), which cavitate in 15% of cases. Pulmonary masses tend to occur in patients with prolonged symptoms (>1 month) and may mimic bronchogenic carcinoma. A third pattern of disease is diffuse reticulonodular opacities. Pleural effusion and lymph node enlargement are uncommon. A disseminated miliary form may be seen in immunocompromised hosts.

Aspergillus species are responsible for a spectrum of pulmonary diseases in humans. These include aspergilloma or mycetoma formation within preexisting cavities, semi-invasive (chronic necrotizing) aspergillosis in patients with mildly impaired immunity, invasive pulmonary aspergillosis in the neutropenic lymphoma or leukemia patient, and allergic bronchopulmonary aspergillosis in the hyperimmune patient.

An aspergilloma (mycetoma, also known as a fungus ball) is a ball of hyphae, mucus, and cellular debris that colonizes a preexisting bulla or a parenchymal cavity created by some other pathogen or destructive process. Invasion into adjacent lung parenchyma does not occur unless host defense mechanisms are compromised. The mycetoma is usually asymptomatic but may cause hemoptysis, which may be massive (>350 mL/24 h). An aspergilloma is seen as a solid round mass within an upper lobe cavity, with an "air crescent" separating the mycetoma from the cavity wall (Fig. 16.18). The mycetoma is usually free within the cavity and can be seen to roll dependently on decubitus radiographs or CT scans. Progressive apical pleural thickening adjacent to a cavity is a common radiographic finding and should prompt a search for a complicating mycetoma.

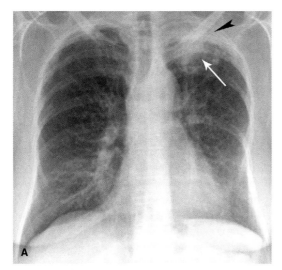
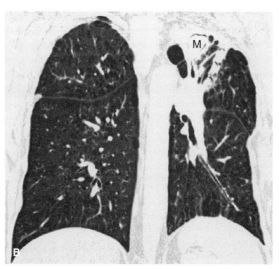

FIGURE 16.18. Aspergilloma. A. Chest radiograph in a 67-year-old woman with hemoptysis reveals left upper lobe volume loss, a left upper lobe mass (*arrow*) with associated apical pleural thickening (*arrowhead*). Note the changes from prior left thoracotomy for bullectomy. B. Coronal reformatted CT scan reveals left apical scarring and a mass (M) within a bulla. There are emphysematous changes bilaterally.

Semi-invasive and invasive aspergilloses are discussed later in this chapter, whereas allergic bronchopulmonary aspergillosis is reviewed in Chapter 18.

Parasitic Infection

Parasitic infections of the lung are relatively uncommon in the United States. However, it is important to be familiar with the radiologic appearances of parasitic infections as the incidence of disease has increased owing to increased travel to countries where parasites are endemic and due to a growing population of immunocompromised patients at risk for these infections. In general, parasitic diseases of the thorax are manifested by either a direct invasion of lungs and pleura or, less commonly, a hypersensitivity reaction (12).

Amebiasis. Symptomatic infection with *Entamoeba histolytica* is usually confined to the GI tract and the liver. If the infection remains confined to the subphrenic space, a right pleural effusion and basilar atelectasis may result from local diaphragmatic inflammation. The most common method of pleuropulmonary involvement by amebiasis is by the direct intrathoracic extension of infection from a hepatic abscess. This transdiaphragmatic spread of organisms may extend into the right pleural space to produce an empyema or may involve the right lower lobe to produce an amebic pneumonia or lung abscess.

Hydatid Disease (Echinococcosis) of the Lung. Echinococcus granulosus is the cause of most cases of human hydatid disease. The disease is endemic in sheep-raising areas and is relatively uncommon in the United States. Dogs are the usual definitive hosts, with sheep acting as intermediate hosts. When a human becomes an accidental intermediate host, disease may result. The larval organisms travel to the liver and the lungs and, if they survive host defenses, encyst and gradually enlarge. Pulmonary echinococcal cysts are composed of three layers: an exocyst (chitinous layer), which is a protective membrane; an inner endocyst, which produces the "daughter cysts"; and a surrounding capsule of compressed, fibrotic lung known as the "pericyst."

Pulmonary echinococcal cysts characteristically present as well-circumscribed, spherical soft tissue masses. In distinction to hepatic cysts, lung cysts do not have calcified walls. The cysts range in size from 1 to 20 cm, with a predilection for the lower lobes and the right side. While most cysts remain asymptomatic, patients may present when the cyst develops a communication with the bronchial tree. If the pericyst ruptures, a thin crescent of air will be seen around the periphery of the cyst, producing the "meniscus" or "crescent" sign. If the cyst itself ruptures, the contents of the cyst are expelled into the airways, producing an air–fluid level. On occasion, the cyst wall may be seen crumpled and floating within an uncollapsed pericyst, producing the pathognomonic "sign of the camalote" or "water lily" sign. Rarely, a cyst will rupture into the pleural space, producing a large pleural effusion.

Paragonimiasis results from infection with the lung fluke *Paragonimus westermani*. The organism is found predominantly in eastern Asia and is usually acquired by eating raw crabs or snails. Infestation of the lung may be asymptomatic, or a patient may present with cough, hemoptysis, dyspnea, and fever. In 20% of affected patients, the chest radiograph is normal. The most common radiographic finding is multiple cysts with variable wall thickness. These cystic opacities may become confluent and are often associated with focal atelectasis and subsegmental consolidation. Dense linear opacities representing the burrows of the organisms may be identified. Because the flukes penetrate the pleura, effusions are common and may be massive.

Schistosomiasis. Human schistosomiasis is caused by three blood flukes: *Schistosoma mansoni, S japonicum,* and *S haematobium.* It is one of the most important parasitic infestations of humans worldwide, although it is rarely acquired in the United States. The life cycle of the fluke is complex, with human infestation acquired through contact with infested water. The larvae penetrate the skin or oropharyngeal mucosa and travel via the venous circulation to the pulmonary capillaries. As the larvae pass through the lungs, an allergic response may develop, presenting radiographically as transient airspace opacities (eosinophilic pneumonia) that resolve spontaneously. The larvae then pass through the pulmonary capillaries into the systemic circulation. *S japonicum* and *S mansoni* eventually migrate to the mesenteric venules, while *S haematobium* migrates to the bladder venules. The mature flukes produce ova, which may embolize to the lungs, where they implant in and around small pulmonary arterioles. The organism induces granulomatous inflammation and fibrosis, which leads to an obliterative arteriolitis, resulting in pulmonary hypertension and cor pulmonale. Radiographically, a diffuse fine reticular pattern is most commonly seen in association with dilatation of the central pulmonary arteries. Small nodular opacities resembling miliary TB may be seen as granulomata forming around ova.

Complications of Pulmonary Infection

There are a number of acute and chronic complications of pulmonary infection that may produce characteristic radiological findings and therefore are important to be aware of (Table 16.1).

Parapneumonic Effusion. Pleural effusions associated with underlying pneumonia, termed "parapneumonic effusions,"

TABLE 16.1

COMPLICATIONS OF PULMONARY INFECTION

		■ SITE OF COMPLICATION		
	■ LUNG/AIRWAYS	■ PLEURA/CHEST WALL	■ VASCULAR	■ MEDIASTINUM
Acute	Abscess Gangrene Pneumatocele	Parapneumonic effusion/empyema	Mycotic aneurysm	
Chronic	Bronchiectasis Swyer-James syndrome Broncholithiasis Bronchial stenosis Interstitial fibrosis	Empyema necessitatis		Fibrosing mediastinitis

are the most common complication of pneumonia and is seen in up to 50% of patients. Complicated parapneumonic effusions and empyemas represent a spectrum from exudative effusions with low pH and elevated lactate dehydrogenase (LDH) and protein in the former to frank pus with loculations in the latter. A detailed discussion of the imaging features of parapneumonic effusions is given in Chapter 19.

Chest Wall Involvement. Uncommonly, a peripheral pulmonary infection will extend through the pleural membranes to invade the chest wall. When an empyema collection extends to create an infected subcutaneous collection in the chest wall, it is termed *empyema necessitates.* The organisms most often associated with this rare complication of pulmonary infection include TB, *A israelii,* fungus, and staphylococcal infection.

Lung abscess is most often the result of aspiration of mouth anaerobes with or without aerobes and is seen 10 to 14 days following aspiration. Risk factors for lung abscess formation include poor dental hygiene and conditions that predispose to aspiration such as alcoholism, seizures, altered consciousness, and drug overdose. Some lung abscesses develop as an embolic complication of septic thrombophlebitis or tricuspid endocarditis. Abscesses appear as nodules or masses typically with central necrosis with or without air–fluid levels and develop in the gravity-dependent portions of the lungs (posterior upper lobes, superior segment, and subpleural regions of the lower lobes).

Pulmonary gangrene is a rare complication of severe pulmonary infection when a portion of lung is sloughed. Imaging findings include a nodule or mass within a cavity with a crescent of air surrounding the sloughed portion of lung. Treatment can be medical or surgical.

Mycotic aneurysm is a rare complication of pulmonary infection or infective endocarditis. While a lung nodule or mass adjacent to a hilar vessel in a patient with endocarditis or pneumonia should suggest the diagnosis, contrast CT is the definitive diagnostic procedure as it demonstrates the relationship of the mass with the pulmonary arterial vasculature.

Bronchiectasis. While postinfectious bronchiectasis is now less common in industrialized nations, pulmonary infection due to viral pneumonia, atypical mycobacteria, bacterial infection, and fungal infection may result in localized bronchiectasis. Bronchiectasis is reviewed in more detail in Chapter 18.

Swyer-James Syndrome is an uncommon postinfectious form of constrictive bronchiolitis that typically results from a severe viral or mycoplasma infection in infancy or childhood. Typical radiologic findings include a hyperlucent lung with normal or small volume, attenuated vasculature, expiratory air trapping, and occasionally proximal bronchiectasis (see Fig. 18.13).

Bronchial Stenosis. This is a rare complication of infection and when seen is most often associated with endobronchial TB or fungal infection such as from histoplasmosis.

Broncholithiasis. This condition reflects the presence of an endobronchial calcified nodule, most often seen as a result of erosion of a calcified peribronchial lymph node resulting from histoplasmosis or TB. Imaging findings include the identification of an endobronchial calcified nodule, often with distal atelectasis, bronchiectasis, or mucoid impaction (see Fig. 18.9). Thin-section CT is the diagnostic imaging modality of choice.

Fibrosing Mediastinitis (Sclerosing Mediastinitis) is a rare condition that produces mediastinal fibrosis can develop in a small subset of patients with prior *Histoplasma* infection, perhaps as an immunologic reaction to fungal antigens. Other fungal infections, autoimmune disorders, drugs, and fibroinflammatory diseases have been associated with fibrosing mediastinitis. Pathologically, dense fibrous tissue is seen to infiltrate the mediastinum. Clinically, this condition presents with signs and symptoms related to the obstruction of central airways,

vessels, or of the esophagus. Radiologically, there is mediastinal widening with calcifications visible. A focal mediastinal mass can also be seen. CT typically demonstrates either a localized calcified right paratracheal or subcarinal mass or a soft-tissue infiltration of the middle mediastinum with compression or obliteration of structures (see Fig. 13.17). Secondary pulmonary parenchymal changes are the result of central airway and vascular compromise (12).

INFECTION IN THE IMMUNOCOMPROMISED HOST AND IN AIDS

Immunocompromise is defined as "a decrease in the normal host defense mechanisms that fight infection." Immunocompromised patients include those with HIV infection, underlying hematologic malignancy, and individuals receiving chemotherapeutic and immunosuppressive therapy. The types of pulmonary infection seen in the immunocompromised patients depend on the specific defect(s) in host defense mechanisms. While the majority of pulmonary complications in immunocompromised patients are infectious in nature, noninfectious complications of disease can account for up to 25% of lung disease in this population. The accurate identification of the predominant radiographic pattern of abnormality in the immunocompromised patients helps limit the differential diagnostic considerations (Tables 16.2 and 16.3) (13). With the advent of highly active antiretroviral therapy (HAART) and effective prophylaxis, the incidence of opportunistic infection in HIV/AIDS has decreased dramatically. Bacterial respiratory infections now account for most pulmonary

TABLE 16.2

RADIOGRAPHIC PATTERNS OF ABNORMALITY IN NON-HIV IMMUNOCOMPROMISED PATIENTS

■ PATTERN	■ POTENTIAL ETIOLOGY
Lobar/segmental consolidation	Gram-negative bacteria Gram-positive bacteria *Legionella*
Nodules ± cavitation	Fungi *Aspergillus* species *Coccidioides immitis* *Cryptococcus neoformans* *Mucor* species *Nocardia asteroides* *Legionella micdadei* Neoplasm Other
Diffuse lung disease	*Pneumocystis jiroveci* Viral pneumonia Fungi *Toxoplasma gondii* *Strongyloides stercoralis* Drug reaction Hemorrhage Radiation pneumonitis Nonspecific interstitial pneumonia Lymphangitic carcinomatosis

Modified from McLoud and Naidich (15); material used with permission.

TABLE 16.3

RADIOGRAPHIC PATTERNS OF ABNORMALITY IN
AIDS PATIENTS

■ PATTERN	■ POTENTIAL ETIOLOGY
Normal	*Pneumocystis jiroveci* pneumonia PCP Tuberculosis or fungal infection Nonspecific interstitial pneumonia (NSIP)
Focal lung disease	Bacterial pneumonia PCP Mycobacterial/fungal infection Non-Hodgkin lymphoma
Diffuse lung disease	PCP PCP + other infection (cytomegalovirus, *Mycobacterium avium-intracellulare*, miliary tuberculosis, and fungus) *Mycobacterium tuberculosis* Fungal infection NSIP Lymphocytic interstitial pneumonia (LIP) Kaposi sarcoma
Nodules	Non-Hodgkin lymphoma Kaposi sarcoma Septic emboli Mycobacterial/fungal infection
Adenopathy	Mycobacterial or fungal infection Kaposi sarcoma Non-Hodgkin lymphoma PCP (uncommon)
Pleural effusion	Kaposi sarcoma Mycobacterial/fungal infection Non-Hodgkin lymphoma Pyogenic empyema PCP (uncommon)

Modified from McLoud and Naidich (15); material used with permission.

infections in individuals living with HIV in the developed world (16,17).

Bacterial Pneumonia. Bacteria are the most common cause of pneumonia in immunocompromised hosts. In HIV-infected patients, bacterial pneumonia may occur early in the course of infection and has an incidence six times that seen in the normal population. The occurrence of two or more episodes of bacterial pneumonia within 1 year is categorized as an AIDS-defining illness for patients with HIV infection. The most common organisms causing pneumonia in HIV-infected patients are *S pneumoniae, H influenzae, S aureus, E coli,* and *P aeruginosa.* Uncommon causes of bacterial pneumonia in the AIDS population include *Nocardia asteroides, Rhodococcus equi, Bartonella henselae,* and *B quintana* (bacillary angiomatosis). In the non-HIV immunocompromised patient, *S aureus* and gram-negative aerobes including *Klebsiella, Proteus, E coli, Pseudomonas, Enterobacter,* and *Serratia* are the most common bacterial pathogens. Bacterial pneumonia is characterized by focal segmental or lobar airspace opacities. Cavitation is more frequent in the immunocompromised population than in normal individuals and

may occur as multiple microabscesses. Multilobar involvement and diffuse pneumonia may occur and are distinctly unusual in normal individuals. Pleural effusions and empyema are uncommon (16).

Renal transplant recipients and patients on high-dose corticosteroids are at increased risk of pneumonia caused by *Legionella pneumophila* and *L micdadei* (Pittsburgh agent). *L pneumophila* causes multilobar focal areas of consolidation (Fig. 16.4), sometimes with cavitation and pleural effusion. The Pittsburgh agent causes a characteristic appearance of multiple, well-circumscribed, centrally cavitating nodules.

Nocardia is a gram-positive, branching, filamentous bacillus that is weakly acid-fast. *N asteroides* is the most important cause of pulmonary disease. It is usually an opportunistic infection in patients on immunosuppressive therapy, those with lymphoma or leukemia, and those with alveolar proteinosis. The most frequent radiographic presentation is a homogeneous, nonsegmental airspace opacity or a mass. Cavitation is frequent (Fig. 16.19). Infection may extend into the pleural space and chest wall to produce empyema and osteomyelitis, respectively. Hilar lymph nodes may be enlarged. Treatment includes sulfur antibiotics.

Tuberculosis. The incidence of TB has increased considerably since the onset of the AIDS epidemic. Most cases are caused by reactivation of previously acquired disease. The diagnosis of TB in immunocompromised hosts is complicated because skin reactivity and sputum analysis are less sensitive in immunocompromised hosts and the yield of bronchoalveolar lavage is decreased in this patient population. The chest radiographic findings depend on the stage of HIV infection and the degree of immune dysfunction, which can be estimated by the CD4 count. In the early stages of AIDS (CD4 count >200 cells/mm^3), a postprimary pattern of upper lobe fibrocavitary disease indistinguishable from that seen in the immunocompetent patient is most common. Later in the course of AIDS (CD4 count 50 to 200 cells/mm^3), the radiographic features most often associated with primary disease are seen and include lobar consolidation, mediastinal and hilar lymphadenopathy, and pleural effusion (7). Rim-enhancing nodes with central necrosis on CT scans are a characteristic finding and should strongly suggest TB in a patient with AIDS. In advanced stages of AIDS (CD4 count <50 cells/mm^3), the radiographic findings are atypical and are characterized by diffuse reticular or nodular (miliary) opacities.

Mycobacterium Avium-Intracellulare infection is the most common nontuberculous mycobacterial infection in patients with AIDS. The disease primarily affects the GI tract, but disseminated disease can involve the chest. Lymphadenopathy is the major radiographic manifestation, but nonspecific focal airspace opacity or diffuse nodular opacities may be seen. Infection by *M kansasii* may produce a pattern identical to that of postprimary TB.

Viral pneumonia is uncommon in AIDS and other immunocompromised patients with defects in cell-mediated immunity (Fig. 16.11).

Cytomegalovirus is a common cause of viral pneumonia in patients with impaired cell-mediated immunity, specifically renal transplant recipients and patients with lymphoma. It is an uncommon cause of pneumonia in the AIDS population. Chest radiographs show diffuse bilateral reticular or nodular opacities in the lower lobes.

Aspergillosis. Invasive aspergillus infection usually occurs in severely immunocompromised patients with neutropenia, most commonly those with leukemia or those receiving chemotherapy or corticosteroids. It occurs less frequently in patients with AIDS, usually in the terminal stages of disease. The radiographic manifestations range from large nodular opacities to diffuse parenchymal consolidation (Fig. 16.20). The organism tends to invade blood vessels, causing infarction. Much of the

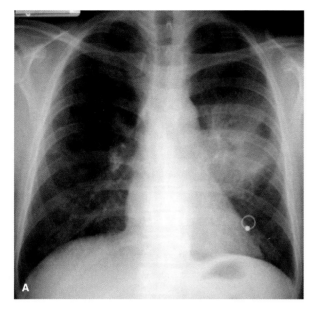

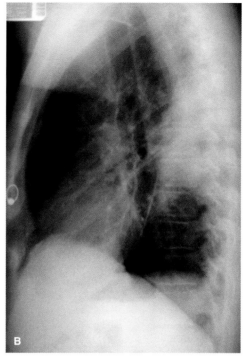

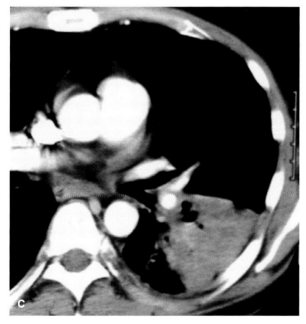

FIGURE 16.19. **Nocardiosis.** Posteroanterior (**A**) and lateral (**B**) chest radiographs of a 34-year-old man with AIDS show airspace opacification in the superior segment of the left lower lobe. **C.** CT scan shows consolidation with cavitation. Sputum stain and culture shows *Nocardia* infection.

observed opacity represents hemorrhage and edema. If pleural effusion develops, it usually indicates empyema. Cavitation, in the form of an air crescent, is not usually evident on chest films early in the course of disease, but it characteristically develops when the patient's complement of circulating neutrophils returns to a normal level. CT, particularly HRCT, is useful for the early diagnosis of invasive aspergillosis (11). The demonstration of a zone of relative decreased attenuation surrounding a dense, mass-like opacity has been termed the "CT halo sign" and is relatively specific for invasive aspergillosis in a neutropenic patient (Fig. 16.20B). The halo represents a region of edema and hemorrhage where an air crescent will develop, separating the region of infected, necrotic lung from normal parenchyma.

Semi-invasive aspergillosis is an unusual form of *Aspergillus* pulmonary infection seen in patients with mild degrees of immunosuppression. The organism invades previously diseased lung tissue, producing slowly progressive airspace opacification or chronic cavitary disease.

Coccidioidomycosis in AIDS and other immunocompromised hosts is usually manifested by disseminated infec-

tion rather than the localized granulomatous disease seen in normal hosts. Pulmonary involvement is usually diffuse and produces miliary nodules, diffuse nodules, or reticulonodular opacities. Hilar and mediastinal lymphadenopathy and pleural effusions are uncommon.

Cryptococcosis. *Cryptococcus neoformans* is a budding yeast commonly found in soil and bird droppings. *Cryptococcus* is the most common cause of fungal infection in the AIDS population but can affect any immunocompromised patient. In some patients, particularly those with AIDS, the organism disseminates from its portal of entry in the lung to involve the CNS, bones, and mucocutaneous tissues. Meningitis is the most serious consequence of infection. There are several chest radiographic patterns of disease: single or multiple nodules or masses (mimicking bronchogenic carcinoma) (Fig. 16.21), single or multiple patchy airspace opacities, and multiple small nodules (mimicking miliary TB). Cavitation, lymphadenopathy, and pleural effusion are more commonly seen in patients with AIDS than in normal hosts.

Candidiasis. *Candida albicans* is an unusual cause of pneumonia in the immunocompromised patients. Patients

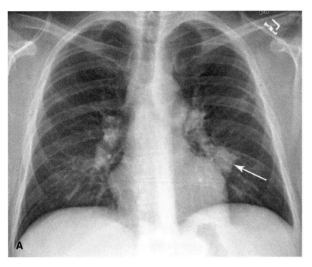

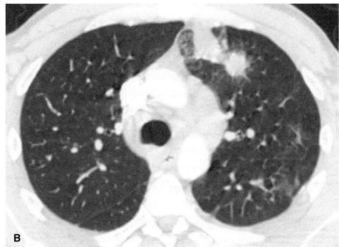

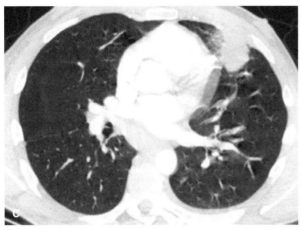

FIGURE 16.20. **Invasive Aspergillosis. A.** Posteroanterior radiograph in a pancytopenic patient with chronic lymphocytic leukemia and *Aspergillus* infection reveals a left lower lung mass (*arrow*) and additional small bilateral nodules. CT scans at lung windows through the upper (**B**) and mid (**C**) lungs show multiple ill-defined nodules with adjacent ground glass opacity.

with severe neutropenia caused by lymphoma or leukemia in the late stages of disease are most susceptible. The diagnosis is often difficult because *Candida* is a common colonizer in immunocompromised patients and its presence is often associated with other opportunistic infections.

Chest radiographs in patients with *Candida* pneumonia show diffuse, bilateral, nonsegmental airspace or interstitial opacities (Fig. 16.22). Miliary nodules may be seen, but cavitation, adenopathy, and pleural effusion are uncommon features.

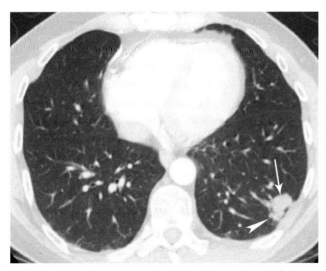

FIGURE 16.21. *Cryptococcus* in AIDS. CT scan through the lower lobes in a 45-year-old patient with AIDS shows a nodule (*arrow*) with adjacent satellite lesions (*arrowhead*). Stains of a transthoracic needle biopsy aspirate showed cryptococcal infection.

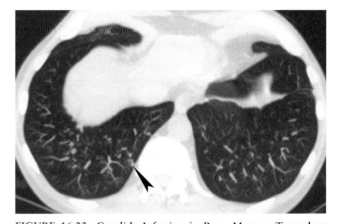

FIGURE 16.22. *Candida* Infection in Bone Marrow Transplant Recipient. Maximum intensity projection axial CT scan in an immunocompromised patient with myeloma and oral candidiasis demonstrates right lower lobe tree-in-bud (*arrowhead*) and nodular opacities indicative of bronchiolitis. Bronchoalveolar lavage revealed *Candida albicans* infection.

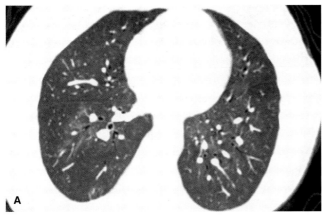 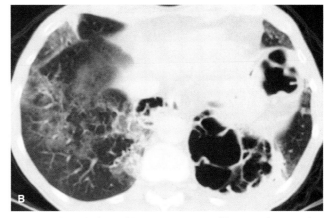

FIGURE 16.23. *Pneumocystis jiroveci* Pneumonia (PCP). **A.** Thin-section CT scan through the mid lungs in a 36-year-old man with HIV infection shows bilateral ground glass opacities. Stains of bronchioalveolar lavage fluid revealed *P jiroveci*. **B.** CT scan in another patient with PCP complicating AIDS shows bilateral multilobulated cysts reflecting pneumatoceles with associated ground glass opacities.

Mucormycosis is a rare cause of pneumonia in immunocompromised patients with lymphoma, leukemia, or diabetes. Pulmonary infection is commonly accompanied by paranasal sinus infection, which may extend to involve the brain or the meninges. Chest radiographic appearances include a solitary nodule or mass or focal airspace opacity, which may cavitate (11). Pleural effusion is uncommon.

***Pneumocystis jiroveci* Pneumonia (PCP).** *P jiroveci* (formerly *P carinii*) is a fungus commonly found in human lungs, although clinically significant pneumonia is seen only in immunocompromised individuals. PCP is most common in patients with AIDS, usually those in the late stages of HIV infection (CD4 count <200 cells/mm³) (17). With the advent of HAART, the incidence of PCP has decreased significantly in the developed world. PCP still occurs in patients with HIV infection who are undiagnosed, not taking or responding to HAART, and those failing or not taking prophylaxis with trimethoprim sulfamethoxazole. Despite HAART and prophylaxis, PCP remains the most common AIDS-defining opportunistic infection. Organ transplant recipients on immunosuppressive drugs (particularly corticosteroids) and patients with lymphoreticular malignancies are also at increased risk for infection.

The chest radiograph may be normal in the early phase of disease. In such patients, gallium scanning or HRCT of the lung may provide evidence of subradiographic disease. As the disease progresses, a fine reticular or ground glass pattern develops, particularly in the parahilar regions (Fig. 16.23). Progressive disease leads to confluent symmetric airspace opacification. Pleural effusion or lymph node enlargement isw distinctly uncommon (<5%) and should suggest an alternative or additional diagnosis. The diagnosis of PCP in AIDS is made by methenamine silver staining of induced sputum samples or bronchoalveolar lavage fluid specimens.

Several atypical radiographic features of PCP have been described. PCP may manifest as single or multiple pulmonary nodules, simulating fungal infection or such malignancies as Kaposi sarcoma. Thin-walled cysts or pneumatoceles may develop during the course of disease and are responsible for an increased incidence of spontaneous pneumothorax, complicating PCP (Fig. 16.23B). Patients receiving prophylaxis with inhaled aerosolized pentamidine are prone to develop predominantly upper lobe PCP, which simulates postprimary TB. Rare cases of miliary PCP simulating TB or disseminated fungal infection have been reported. Patients receiving systemic prophylaxis with co-trimoxazole are also at risk for extrapulmonary *Pneumocystis* infection. Systemic *Pneumocystis* infection

generally involves liver, spleen, kidney, and lymph nodes, and appears on CT or US as microabscesses or punctate calcifications.

Toxoplasmosis. *Toxoplasma gondii* is an obligate intracellular protozoan whose definitive host is the cat. Humans acquire the organism by ingestion of material contaminated by oocyst-containing stool. It has been estimated that toxoplasmosis exists in a chronic asymptomatic form in 50% of the population of the United States. The disease can be recognized in four clinicopathologic forms: congenital, ocular, lymphatic, and generalized. Pulmonary involvement is usually seen in the generalized form of the disease, which affects immunocompromised hosts, including those with AIDS, organ transplant recipients, and patients with leukemia or lymphoma.

The radiographic findings in pulmonary toxoplasmosis include diffuse reticular opacities that resemble those of acute viral pneumonia. Less commonly, airspace opacities with air

TABLE 16.4

PULMONARY COMPLICATIONS IN BONE MARROW TRANSPLANT RECIPIENTS

■ TIME PERIOD	■ COMPLICATION
Neutropenic phase (0–30 days)	Pulmonary edema Alveolar hemorrhage Fungal infection Drug reaction
Early phase (30–100 days)	Fungal infection Drug reaction Cytomegalovirus infection Upper respiratory virus infection Idiopathic pneumonia Acute graft-versus-host disease
Late phase (>100 days)	Bronchiolitis obliterans Bronchiolitis obliterans-organizing pneumonia Chronic graft-versus-host disease Upper respiratory virus (up to 6 months) Idiopathic pneumonia (up to 6 months)

Modified from Gosselin and Adams (18); material used with permission.

bronchograms may be seen. Hilar and mediastinal lymph node enlargement is common, whereas pleural effusion is rare. With generalized disease, most often seen in patients with AIDS, diffuse bilateral small nodular opacities may be seen.

Bone marrow transplant (BMT) recipients have a high (40% to 60%) incidence of pulmonary complications. Because of the predictable course of immunosuppression, a timeline of expected pulmonary complications can be constructed to help narrow the differential diagnosis for radiographic abnormalities in patients following BMT. The time following BMT can be divided into three phases: the neutropenic phase, the early phase, and the late phase. The neutropenic phase lasts for approximately the first 30 days, followed by the early phase (from 30 to 100 days), and finally the late phase (more than 100 days post-BMT). Complications can be infectious or noninfectious and are detailed according to time of presentation (see Table 16.4) (18).

References

1. Sharma S, Maycher B, Eschun G. Radiological imaging in pneumonia: recent innovations. Curr Opin Pulm Med 2007;13:159–169.
2. Krol CM, Uszynski M, Dillon EH, et al. Dynamic CT features of inhalational anthrax infection. AJR Am J Roentgenol 2002;178:1063–1066.
3. Vilar J, Domingo ML, Soto C, Cogolios J. Radiology of bacterial pneumonia. Eur J Radiol 2004;51(2):102–113.
4. Bartlett JG, Finegold SM. Anaerobic infections of the lung and pleural space. Am Rev Respir Dis 1974;110:56–77.
5. Cheon JE, Im JG, Kim MY, Lee JS, Choi GM, Yeon KM. Thoracic actinomycosis: CT findings. Radiology 1998;209(1):229–233.
6. Reittner P, Muller NL, Heyneman L, et al. Mycoplasma pneumoniae pneumonia: radiographic and high-resolution CT features in 28 patients. AJR Am J Roentgenol 2000;174:37–41.
7. Leung AL. Pulmonary tuberculosis: the essentials. Radiology 1999; 210:307–322.
8. Ellis SM, Hansell DM. Imaging of non-tuberculous (atypical) mycobacterial pulmonary infection. Clin Radiol 2002;57(8):661–669.
9. Kim EA, Lee KS, Primack SL, et al. Viral pneumonias in adults: radiologic and pathologic findings. Radiographics 2002;22:S137–S149.
10. Agarwal PP, Cinti S, Kazerooni EA. Chest radiographic and CT findings in novel swine-origin influenza A (H1N1) virus (S-OIV) infection. AJR Am J Roentgenol 2009;193:1488–1493.
11. Chong S, Lee KS, Yi CA, Chung MJ, Kim TS, Han J. Pulmonary fungal infection: imaging findings in immunocompetent and immunocompromised patients. Eur J Radiol 2006;59:371–383.
12. Rossi SE, McAdams HP, Rosado-de-Christensen ML, Franks TJ, Galvin JR. Fibrosing mediastinitis. Radiographics 2001;21:737–757.
13. Oh YW, Effmann EL, Godwin JD. Pulmonary infections in immunocompromised hosts: the importance of correlating the conventional radiologic appearance with the clinical setting. Radiology 2000;217:647–656.
14. Brecher CW, Aviram G, Boiselle P. CT and radiography of bacterial respiratory infections in AIDS patients. AJR Am J Roentgenol 2003;180:1203–1209.
15. McLoud TC, Naidich DP. Thoracic disease in the immunocompromised patient. Radiol Clin North Am 1992;30:525–554.
16. Morris A, Lundgren JD, Masur H, et al. Current epidemiology of *Pneumocystis* pneumonia. Emerg Infect Dis 2004;10:1713–1720.
17. Gosselin M, Adams R. Pulmonary complications in bone marrow transplantation. J Thorac Imaging 2002;17:132–144.

CHAPTER 17 ▪ DIFFUSE LUNG DISEASE

JEFFREY S. KLEIN AND CURTIS E. GREEN

Diffuse lung disease represents a broad spectrum of disorders that primarily affect the pulmonary interstitium (Table 17.1). These diseases present in a variety of manners, most typically with symptoms of progressive dyspnea. Some patients, however, present with minimal or no symptoms and interstitial lung disease is discovered either incidentally or during radiologic screening for interstitial disease associated with collagen vascular disease. Restrictive lung disease and hypoxemia on pulmonary function tests are characteristically present. The radiographic findings produced by interstitial disease are reviewed in Chapter 12. Thin-section CT has revolutionized the diagnosis of interstitial lung disease, and its role in the evaluation of interstitial disease is detailed in this chapter.

THIN-SECTION CT OF THE PULMONARY INTERSTITIUM

Normal Anatomy. Thin-section CT provides the most direct radiographic method for assessment of the pulmonary interstitium. The general utility of thin-section CT in the evaluation of chronic interstitial lung disease is outlined in Table 17.2 (1). The pulmonary interstitium is the scaffolding of the lung, providing support for the airways, gas-exchanging units, and vascular structures. It is a continuous network of connective tissue fibers that begins at the lung hilum and extends peripherally to the visceral pleura (see Fig. 12.10). The central interstitial compartment extending from the mediastinum peripherally and enveloping the bronchovascular bundles is termed the *axial* or *bronchovascular interstitium.* The axial interstitium is contiguous with the interstitium surrounding the small centrilobular arteriole and bronchiole within the secondary pulmonary lobule, where it is called the *centrilobular interstitium.* The most peripheral component of the intersti-

tium is the *subpleural* or *peripheral interstitium,* which lies between the visceral pleura and the lung surface. Invaginations of the subpleural interstitium into the lung parenchyma form the borders of the secondary pulmonary lobules and represent the interlobular septa. Extending between the centrilobular interstitium within the lobular core and the interlobular septal/subpleural interstitium in the lobular periphery is a fine network of connective tissue fibers that support the alveolar spaces called the *intralobular, parenchymal,* or *alveolar interstitium.*

The secondary pulmonary lobule is defined as that subsegment of lung supplied by three to five terminal bronchioles and separated from adjacent secondary lobules by intervening connective tissue (interlobular septa) (Fig. 17.1). Each terminal bronchiole further subdivides into respiratory bronchioles, alveolar ducts, alveolar sacs, and alveoli. The unit of lung subtended from a single terminal bronchiole is called a *pulmonary acinus.* The centrilobular artery and preterminal bronchiole are located in the center of the secondary lobule. Pulmonary veins and lymphatics run at the margins of lobules within the interlobular septa, with lymphatics and connective tissue found within the contiguous subpleural interstitium. The secondary pulmonary lobule is typically polyhedral in shape, with each side ranging from 1 to 2.5 cm in length. The interlobular septa are most prominent over the periphery of the lung, where they are readily seen on CT. At the surface of the lung, these septa are short structures that course perpendicular to the pleural surface and completely separate adjacent lobules. Within the parahilar portions of the lung, the interlobular septa are longer and more obliquely oriented and incompletely marginate the secondary lobules.

Normal Thin-Section CT Findings. Thin-section CT can demonstrate much of the normal anatomy of the secondary pulmonary lobule. Interlobular septa are normally 0.1 mm thick and can be seen in the lung periphery, particularly along

TABLE 17.1

THE ALPHABET SOUP OF INTERSTITIAL LUNG DISEASE

■ ABBREVIATION	■ DISEASE
AIP	Acute interstitial pneumonia
BOOP	Bronchiolitis obliterans with organizing pneumonia
COP	Cryptogenic organizing pneumonia
CWP	Coal worker's pneumoconiosis
DIP	Desquamative interstitial pneumonia
EG	Eosinophilic granuloma
IPF	Idiopathic pulmonary fibrosis
LIP	Lymphocytic interstitial pneumonitis
LAM	Lymphangioleiomyomatosis
LCH	Langerhans cell histiocytosis
NSIP	Nonspecific interstitial pneumonia
PAP	Pulmonary alveolar proteinosis
PMF	Progressive massive fibrosis
RB-ILD	Respiratory bronchiolitis-associated interstitial lung disease
SLE	Systemic lupus erythematosus
TS	Tuberous sclerosis
UIP	Usual interstitial pneumonia

TABLE 17.2

UTILITY OF THIN-SECTION CT IN THE EVALUATION OF CHRONIC INTERSTITIAL LUNG DISEASE

1. Detection of clinically suspected parenchymal abnormality when the chest radiograph is normal or shows questionable abnormality
2. Characterization of parenchymal abnormalities
3. Biopsy planning:
    Determination of route for biopsy, i.e., transbronchial, open lung, or bronchoalveolar lavage
    Targeting biopsy to area(s) of active disease and avoiding areas of end-stage fibrosis
4. Monitoring of response to therapy or progression of disease

Thin-Section CT Signs of Disease

The signs of interstitial lung disease on thin-section CT are illustrated in Fig. 17.3 and their differential diagnosis is listed in Table 17.3 (1).

Interlobular (Septal) Lines. Septal thickening is most often seen as thin, short, 1- to 2-cm lines oriented perpendicular to and intersecting the costal pleura. These lines are best visualized in the subpleural and juxtadiaphragmatic regions of the lung, where they outline the anterior and posterior margins of secondary lobules. In the central regions of the lung, the thickened septa can completely envelope lobules to produce polygonal structures. Although septa can be seen in normal individuals, these lines are thicker (>1 mm) and more numerous in patients with diseases primarily affecting the interlobular interstitium, such as interstitial pulmonary edema, idiopathic pulmonary fibrosis (IPF), and lymphangitic carcinomatosis (Fig. 17.4). Interlobular lines on thin-section CT are the equivalent of Kerley B lines seen in the inferolateral portions of the lungs on frontal radiographs. Within the central regions of the lung, long (2 to 6 cm) linear opacities representing obliquely

the superior and inferior pleural surfaces (Fig. 17.2). Centrilobular arteries (1 mm in diameter) are V- or Y-shaped structures on thin-section CT seen within 5 to 10 mm of the pleural surface. Normal intralobular (0.7 mm) and acinar (0.3 to 0.5 mm) arteries are commonly seen. Normal airways are visible only to within 3 cm of the pleura. The centrilobular bronchiole, with a diameter of 1 mm and a wall thickness of 0.15 mm, is not normally visible on thin-section CT. Pulmonary veins (0.5 cm) are occasionally seen as linear or dot-like structures within 1 to 2 cm of the pleura and, when visible, indicate the locations of interlobular septa. The peribronchovascular, centrilobular, and intralobular interstitial compartments are not normally visible on thin-section CT.

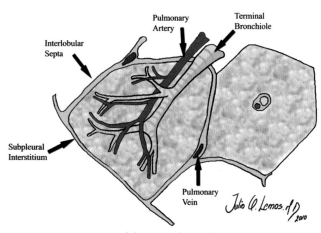

FIGURE 17.1. Diagram of the Normal Secondary Pulmonary Lobule.

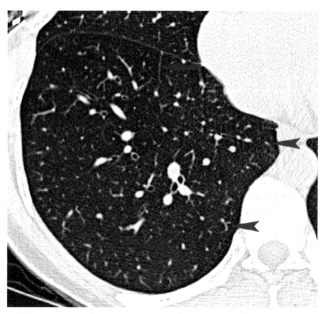

FIGURE 17.2. Thin-Section CT of Normal Lobular Anatomy. Normal interlobular septum (*blue arrowheads*) and centrilobular arteries (*red arrow*) are clearly visible.

TABLE 17.3

DIFFERENTIAL DIAGNOSTIC THIN-SECTION CT FEATURES IN INTERSTITIAL LUNG DISEASE

■ CT FINDING	■ DIFFERENTIAL DIAGNOSIS	■ CT FINDING	■ DIFFERENTIAL DIAGNOSIS
Interlobular (septal) lines	Interstitial edema Lymphangitic carcinomatosis Sarcoidosis UIP	Irregular lung interfaces	Neurofibromatosis (pneumatocele) (emphysema) Pulmonary edema UIP Sarcoidosis
Intralobular lines	UIP Alveolar proteinosis Hypersensitivity pneumonitis (chronic)	Micronodules, random distribution	Miliary tuberculosis or histoplasmosis Hematogenous metastases Silicosis/CWP EG
"Thickened" fissures	Pulmonary edema Sarcoidosis Lymphangitic carcinomatosis	Micronodules, perilymphatic distribution	Sarcoidosis Lymphangitic carcinomatosis Silicosis/CWP
Peribronchovascular interstitial thickening	Pulmonary edema (smooth) Sarcoidosis (nodular) Lymphangitic carcinomatosis (smooth or nodular)	Ground glass opacities	UIP Desquamative interstitial pneumonia AIP Hypersensitivity pneumonitis
Centrilobular nodules	Hypersensitivity pneumonitis BOOP/COP RB-ILD		BOOP/COP RB-ILD Hemorrhage Pneumocystis jiroveci pneumonia Cytomegalovirus pneumonia Alveolar proteinosis
Subpleural lines	Asbestosis IPF	Architectural distortion Traction bronchiectasis	UIP Sarcoidosis
Parenchymal bands	UIP Sarcoidosis	Conglomerate mass	Silicosis/CWP Sarcoidosis Silicosis
Honeycombing	UIP Hypersensitivity pneumonitis (chronic) Sarcoidosis	Consolidation	CWP Radiation fibrosis BOOP/COP Sarcoidosis
Thin-walled cysts	EG Lymphangioleiomyomatosis Tuberous sclerosis		AIP UIP

UIP, usual interstitial pneumonitis; CWP, coal worker's pneumoconiosis; EG, eosinophilic granuloma; AIP, acute interstitial pneumonia; BOOP, bronchiolitis obliterans with organizing pneumonia; COP, cryptogenic organizing pneumonia; RB-ILD, respiratory bronchiolitis-associated interstitial lung disease; IPF, idiopathic pulmonary fibrosis.

oriented connective tissue septa are the equivalent of radiographic Kerley A lines.

Intralobular Lines. In some patients, a lattice of fine lines is seen within the central portion of the pulmonary lobule radiating out toward the thickened lobular borders to produce a "spoke-and-wheel" or "spider web" appearance. These lines are not normally visible on thin-section CT and represent thickening of the intralobular or parenchymal interstitium. Thickened intralobular lines usually result from fibrosis and are most commonly seen in idiopathic pulmonary fibrosis (IPF) and other causes of usual interstitial pneumonitis (UIP). Thickened intralobular lines can also be seen in other infiltrative diseases such as pulmonary alveolar proteinosis (PAP).

"Thickened" Fissures. The apparent thickening of interlobar fissures in patients with interstitial lung disease is usually a direct extension of the thickening of interlobular septa to involve the subpleural interstitium of the lung. While such a process normally involves all pleural surfaces equally, the "thickening" is usually best appreciated on the fissures, where two layers of visceral pleura—and therefore two layers of subpleural interstitium—are seen outlined on either side by aerated lung. The fissural thickening can be smooth or nodular. Smooth fissural thickening is virtually indistinguishable from a small amount of pleural fluid within the fissure and is most commonly seen with pulmonary edema. Nodular fissural thickening is commonly seen in sarcoidosis and lymphangitic carcinomatosis (Fig. 17.4), where the nodules lie within the subpleural lymphatics.

Thickened bronchovascular structures of the lung result from thickening of the peribronchovascular interstitium. This produces apparent enlargement of perihilar vascular structures and thickening of bronchial walls, which are the thin-section CT equivalent of peribronchial cuffing and tram tracking seen radiographically. Pulmonary edema causes smooth thickening of the peribronchovascular interstitium, whereas sarcoidosis causes nodular thickening. Lymphangitic carcinomatosis can

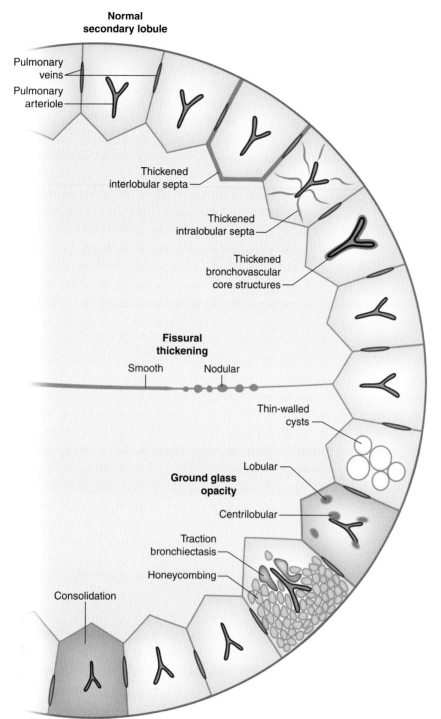

FIGURE 17.3. Thin-Section CT Findings in Interstitial Lung Disease (Adapted from The Radiologist, Baltimore: Williams & Wilkins, 1998, with permission).

result in either smooth or irregular peribronchovascular thickening (Fig. 17.6).

Centrilobular (Lobular Core) Abnormalities. Thickening of the axial interstitium within the lobular core produces an abnormal prominence of the "dot like" or branching centrilobular arteriole. Diseases that commonly produce this appearance include pulmonary edema, lymphangitic carcinomatosis, and UIP. The centrilobular bronchiole is not normally seen on thin-section CT but may be rendered visible as a result of luminal dilatation or thickening of the centrilobular interstitium. Small airways disease can produce centrilobular bronchiolar abnormalities, which are seen on thin-section CT as fluid-filled

dilated branching Y-shaped structures that produce a "tree-in-bud" appearance. Ill-defined centrilobular nodules represent disease of the bronchiole and adjacent parenchyma and are commonly present in subacute hypersensitivity pneumonitis (Fig. 17.7), cryptogenic organizing pneumonia (COP), RB-ILD, as well as other disorders.

Subpleural Lines. These 5- to 10-cm-long curvilinear opacities are found within 1 cm of the pleura and parallel the chest wall. They are most frequent in the posterior portions of the lower lobes and remain unchanged on prone scans. They probably represent an early phase of lung fibrosis and should be distinguished from a similar line that is seen as a result

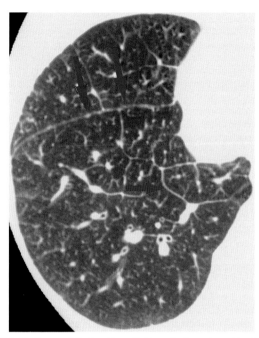

FIGURE 17.4. Interlobular (Septal) Lines in Lymphangitic Carcinomatosis. A thin-section CT scan through the upper lobes in a patient with lymphangitic carcinomatosis shows thickened interlobular septa (*blue arrow*). Note the presence of nodular fissural thickening (*red arrows*), another common finding in this entity.

of atelectasis in the dependent portion of the lungs in normal individuals. Subpleural lines are most often seen in patients with asbestosis and, less commonly, IPF.

Parenchymal bands are nontapering linear opacities, 2 to 5 cm in length, that extend from the lung to contact the pleural surface. These fibrotic bands can be distinguished from vessels and thickened septa by their length, thickness, course, absence of branching, and their association with regional parenchymal distortion. Parenchymal bands are frequently seen in asbestosis, IPF, and sarcoidosis.

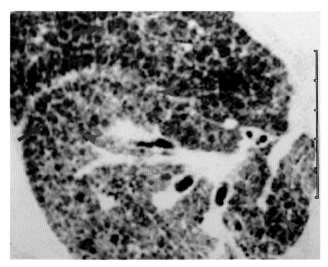

FIGURE 17.5. Intralobular Lines in Idiopathic Pulmonary Fibrosis (IPF). A targeted thin-section CT through the right lower lobe in a patient with IPF shows thickening of intralobular (*red arrows*) and interlobular (*blue arrowheads*) lines associated with ground glass opacity.

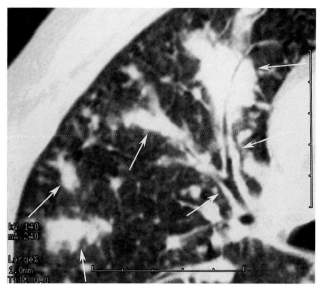

FIGURE 17.6. Thickened Bronchovascular Structures in Lymphangitic Carcinomatosis. In a patient with lymphangitic carcinomatosis, a thin-section CT shows both smooth and nodular thickening of the bronchovascular structures (*arrows*) that represents lymphatic tumor surrounding the axial interstitium.

Honeycomb cysts are small (6 to 10 mm) cystic spaces with thick (1 to 3 mm) walls, most often in the posterior subpleural regions of the lower lobes and result from end-stage pulmonary fibrosis from a variety of etiologies. Pathologically, the cysts are lined by bronchiolar epithelium and are the result of bronchiolectasis. Most patients show additional signs of interstitial disease, including thickened interlobular and intralobular lines, parenchymal bands, irregularity of lung interfaces, and areas of ground glass opacity. Honeycombing is frequently seen in

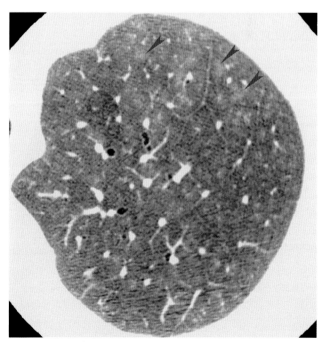

FIGURE 17.7. Centrilobular Ground Glass Nodules in Subacute Hypersensitivity Pneumonitis. Thin-section CT shows the typical poorly defined centrilobular nodules (*arrowheads*) of subacute hypersensitivity pneumonitis.

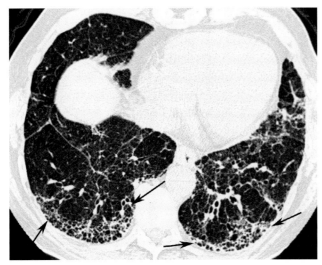

FIGURE 17.8. Honeycomb Lung in Idiopathic Pulmonary Fibrosis (IPF). Thin-section CT in a patient with IPF shows peripheral honeycombing (*arrows*) resulting from end-stage pulmonary fibrosis.

UIP (Fig. 17.8) and chronic hypersensitivity pneumonitis and occasionally in sarcoidosis.

Thin-walled cysts are a common manifestation of late stages of Langerhans' cell histiocytosis of lung (LCH), also referred to as eosinophilic granulomatosis, and lymphangioleiomyomatosis (LAM). These cysts are slightly larger in diameter (10 mm) and have thinner walls than honeycomb cysts. Honeycomb cysts usually have shared walls, whereas the cysts of LCH and LAM do not. The cysts of LCH and LAM are usually evenly distributed from central to peripheral portions of the upper lobes (Fig. 17.9), with or without lower lobe involvement, whereas honeycombing tends to occur in the subpleural regions of the lower lobes. Normal lung may be found in the intervening spaces between the cysts of LCH and LAM. Honeycombing uniformly destroys lung and produces distortion of lung interfaces and traction bronchiectasis, features not typically found in either LCH or LAM.

Irregularity of Lung Interfaces. A common thin-section CT sign of interstitial disease, irregularity of the normally smooth interface between the bronchovascular bundles and the surrounding lung, reflects edema or fibrosis or infiltration of the axial interstitium by granulomas (Fig. 17.5) or tumor. Similarly, irregularity of the interface between fissures or pleural surfaces and adjacent lung indicates peripheral interstitial disease. UIP and sarcoidosis are the most common causes of irregular lung interfaces.

Micronodules. These 1- to 3-mm, sharply marginated, round opacities seen on thin-section CT represent conglomerates of granulomas or tumor cells within the interstitium. These are most often seen in sarcoidosis, LCH, silicosis (Fig. 17.10), miliary tuberculosis (TB) or histoplasmosis, metastatic adenocarcinoma, and lymphangitic carcinomatosis. They may be seen along the central bronchovascular structures (sarcoidosis, LCH), within interlobular septa or subpleural interstitium (sarcoidosis, lymphangitic carcinomatosis, silicosis), or within the substance of the pulmonary lobules (metastatic adenocarcinoma, miliary granulomatous infection). Nodules predominating in the peribronchovascular, interlobular, and subpleural regions—those portions of the interstitium where the lymphatics lie—are said to have a "perilymphatic" distribution.

Ground Glass Opacity. Ground glass opacity is defined as an area of increased attenuation (on thin-section CT) within which the normal parenchymal structures are visible. Multifocal areas of ground glass opacity can sometimes be identified in patients with diffuse interstitial lung disease. These regions often respect lobular borders and do not demonstrate air-bronchograms. They result from abnormalities below the resolution of the CT scan and are most often produced by thickening of the alveolar septa, with or without the lining of the alveolar spaces, by inflammatory exudate or fluid. Diseases commonly associated with this appearance include desquamative interstitial pneumonia (DIP), *Pneumocystis jiroveci* (formerly *P carinii*) pneumonia, acute hypersensitivity pneumonitis (Fig. 17.11), nonspecific interstitial pneumonia (NSIP), and interstitial pulmonary edema. The ground glass densities are occasionally confined to the immediate centrilobular regions of the pulmonary lobules, where they appear as fuzzy nodular densities that outline the normally invisible centrilobular bronchiole (Fig. 17.7). This reflects involvement of the peribronchovascular interstitium and surrounding

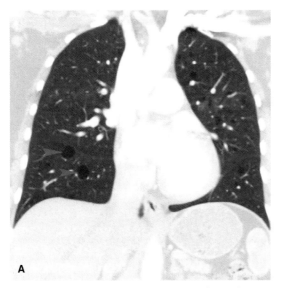
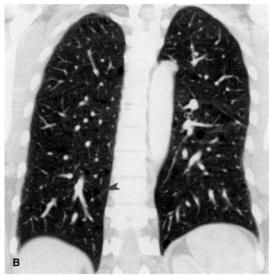

FIGURE 17.9. Thin-Walled Cysts in Lymphangioleiomyomatosis (LAM). A and **B.** Coronal reconstructions of a thin-section CT of a patient with LAM show multiple, thin-walled cysts (*arrowheads*). Although variably sized, the cysts are fairly uniform in shape.

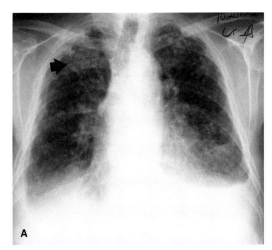
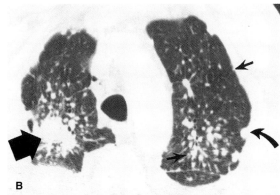

FIGURE 17.10. **Nodules and a Conglomerate Mass in Silicosis. A.** Posteroanterior radiograph of a 79-year-old patient with silicosis shows diffuse nodules as well as a conglomerate mass in the right upper lobe (*arrow*). **B.** Thin-section CT scan through the upper lobes shows peribronchovascular and subpleural micronodules (*small arrows*), larger nodules (*curved arrow*), and a conglomerate mass representing progressive massive fibrosis in the right upper lobe (*large arrow*). The pleural effusions are caused by concomitant congestive heart failure.

alveoli by an inflammatory process and is seen in hypersensitivity pneumonitis, COP, and panbronchiolitis. The presence of ground glass opacities is important because it often implies an active inflammatory process or edema that is reversible and warrants aggressive treatment. Ground glass abnormality associated with a predominant pattern of honeycombing indicates microscopic pulmonary fibrosis, however.

Architectural Distortion and Traction Bronchiectasis. Processes that result in extensive parenchymal fibrosis can distort the normal architecture of the lung, creating irregularities of the lung–mediastinal, lung–pleural, and lung–vascular interfaces. Parenchymal distortion is often better appreciated on thin-section CT than on plain radiographs. Sarcoidosis and UIP (Fig. 17.12) are the diseases most commonly associated with architectural distortion.

A finding commonly associated with architectural distortion is *traction bronchiectasis,* in which fibrosis causes traction on the walls of bronchi, resulting in irregular dilatation. While this usually involves segmental and subsegmental bronchi, it also can be seen at the intralobular level, where traction bronchiolectasis contributes to honeycombing. Traction bronchiectasis is most commonly seen in UIP

(Fig. 17.12), but is also common in fibrotic sarcoidosis and radiation fibrosis.

Conglomerate Masses. In some patients with extensive pulmonary fibrosis, masses of fibrotic tissue develop in the parahilar regions of the upper lobes, often associated with peripheral bullae. On CT, these masses are seen to contain crowded vessels and dilated bronchi. They are most often seen in patients with end-stage sarcoidosis but can occur in complicated silicosis with progressive massive fibrosis (PMF) (Fig. 17.10) or radiation fibrosis following treatment of Hodgkin lymphoma or lung cancer. A similar finding is seen rarely in IV drug users when a granulomatous fibrosis results as a response to IV talc or starch mixed with narcotics.

Consolidation refers to increased lung density that obscures underlying blood vessels; air bronchograms are commonly present. This finding can be seen with any airspace-filling process (Fig. 17.13) but occasionally occurs in interstitial diseases such as UIP and sarcoidosis.

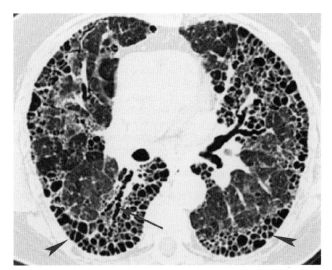

FIGURE 17.11. **Ground Glass Opacity in Acute Hypersensitivity Pneumonitis.** A thin-section CT through the upper lobes shows widespread ground glass opacity in a patient with hypersensitivity pneumonitis. Note that the pulmonary vessels are still visible within the areas of abnormality.

FIGURE 17.12. **Architectural Distortion and Traction Bronchiectasis in Idiopathic Pulmonary Fibrosis.** Thin-section CT through the lower lobes shows extensive peripheral honeycombing (*blue arrowheads*), traction bronchiectasis (*red arrow*), and architectural distortion.

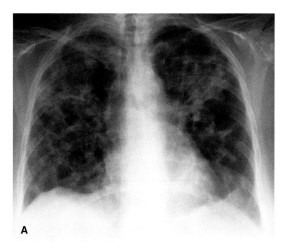
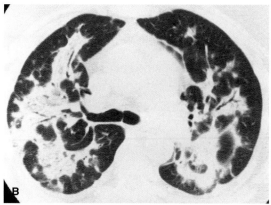

FIGURE 17.13. Consolidation in Cryptogenic Organizing Pneumonia (COP). A. Posteroanterior radiograph in a 53-year-old patient with fever, dyspnea, and a dry cough shows patchy consolidation and diminished lung volumes. **B.** Thin-section CT scan shows multifocal areas of consolidation in a peribronchial distribution. Note air bronchograms with mild bronchial dilatation (*arrows*) within the consolidated areas. An open lung biopsy showed COP.

CHRONIC INTERSTITIAL LUNG DISEASE

Chronic interstitial lung disease usually results from diffuse inflammatory processes that primarily affect the axial and parenchymal interstitium of the lung. A wide variety of disease processes can result in diffuse damage to the pulmonary interstitium (2). Careful evaluation of all available radiologic studies and correlation with clinical findings and laboratory data are essential to the accurate diagnosis of chronic interstitial lung disease (Table 17.4). However, the majority of patients with interstitial lung disease will require histologic examination of lung tissue for definitive diagnosis.

Chronic Interstitial Pulmonary Edema

Chronic elevation of pulmonary venous pressure may lead to increased interstitial markings on plain radiographs. The interstitial thickening is caused by distention of pulmonary lymphatics and chronic interstitial edema and is seen most commonly in patients with long-standing mitral stenosis or LV failure. Radiographically, peribronchial cuffing, tram tracking, poor definition of vascular markings, and linear or reticular opacities may be seen. Redistribution of blood flow to the upper lobes, a manifestation of pulmonary venous hypertension, and prominence of the fissures caused by subpleural edema and fibrosis are concomitant findings. Honeycombing is not a feature of chronic pulmonary venous hypertension; its presence in a patient with cardiac disease should suggest another cause of pulmonary fibrosis (e.g., amiodarone lung toxicity).

Connective Tissue Disease

These disorders are associated with immunologically mediated inflammation and damage to connective tissues throughout the body. The most common thoracic manifestations of this group of heterogeneous disorders are vasculitis and interstitial fibrosis, although the pleura, chest wall, diaphragm, and heart may also be affected (3).

Rheumatoid Lung Disease (Table 17.5). Rheumatoid arthritis produces a chronic arthritis of peripheral joints. Extra-articular manifestations are seen in up to 75% of patients. In contrast to the disease as a whole, which is more common in women, pulmonary involvement is more common in men. The pleuropulmonary manifestations of rheumatoid disease typically follow the onset of joint disease and tend to be seen in patients with high serum rheumatoid factor titers and eosinophilia, but in up to 15% of patients, pleuropulmonary involvement precedes the joint disease.

The most common radiographic manifestation of parenchymal lung involvement is an interstitial pneumonitis and fibrosis, which histologically is a form of UIP. This begins as an alveolitis (inflammation of the alveolar interstitium) that is seen radiographically as fine reticular or ground glass opacities with a lower zone predominance. There is gradual progression to end-stage pulmonary fibrosis with the development of a bibasilar medium or coarse reticular or reticulonodular pattern (honeycombing) (Fig. 17.14). Thin-section CT is more sensitive in detecting the earliest parenchymal changes than conventional radiographs and is also more sensitive in depicting the development of interstitial fibrosis (Fig. 17.15). Predominant upper lobe fibrosis, cavitation, and bulla formation are rare. This less common pattern of lung involvement is indistinguishable from that seen with ankylosing spondylitis and must be distinguished from postprimary fibrocavitary TB by acid-fast staining of sputum.

Less common parenchymal manifestations of rheumatoid disease are lung nodules (Fig. 17.15) and changes attributable to COP. Necrobiotic (rheumatoid) nodules in the lung can produce peripheral well-defined nodular opacities on chest radiographs that are histologically indistinguishable from the subcutaneous rheumatoid nodules seen on the extensor surfaces of the elbows and knees in these patients. The lung nodules commonly evolve into thick-walled cavities, which tend to wax and wane in parallel with the flares of arthritis. Similar nodules may develop in the lungs of coal miners and silica or asbestos workers with rheumatoid arthritis as a hypersensitivity response to inhaled dust particles (Caplan syndrome). Caplan syndrome is usually indistinguishable radiographically from the necrobiotic nodules of simple rheumatoid disease, although the presence of the associated characteristic small nodular or irregular parenchymal opacities of simple pneumoconiosis helps make this distinction. COP and bronchiolitis obliterans (constrictive bronchiolitis) are also associated with rheumatoid disease. The clinical, functional, and radiographic findings are similar to those of COP or bronchiolitis obliterans associated with systemic lupus erythematosus (SLE), drugs, or viral infection.

Pleuritis is the most common thoracic manifestation of rheumatoid disease and is found in 20% of patients. As with

TABLE 17.4

DIFFERENTIAL DIAGNOSTIC FEATURES IN CHRONIC INTERSTITIAL LUNG DISEASE

■ FINDING	■ DIFFERENTIAL DIAGNOSIS	■ FINDING	■ DIFFERENTIAL DIAGNOSIS

Upper zone distribution	Tuberculosis (postprimary)
	 Chronic fungal infection
	   Histoplasmosis
	     Coccidioidomycosis
	 Sarcoidosis
	 Eosinophilic granuloma
	 Silicosis
	 Ankylosing spondylitis
	 Hypersensitivity pneumonitis
	   (chronic)
	 Radiation fibrosis from treatment
	   of head and neck malignancy
		Hilar/mediastinal lymph node enlargement	Sarcoidosis
			 Lymphangitic carcinomatosis
			 Lymphoma
			 Hematogenous metastases
			 Tuberculosis
			 Fungal infection
			 Silicosis

Lower zone distribution	Idiopathic pulmonary fibrosis
	 Asbestosis
	 Rheumatoid lung
	 Scleroderma
	 Neurofibromatosis
	 Dermatomyositis/polymyositis
	 Chronic aspiration
		Pleural disease	Asbestosis (plaques)
			 Lymphangitic carcinomatosis
			   (effusion)
			 Rheumatoid lung disease (effusion/
			   thickening)
			 Lymphangioleiomyomatosis
			   (chylous effusion)

Normal or increased lung volumes	Sarcoidosis
	 Eosinophilic granuloma
	 Lymphangioleiomyomatosis
	 Tuberous sclerosis
	 Interstitial disease superimposed
	   on emphysema
		Abnormalities of soft tissues and bony thorax	Skin nodules
			   Neurofibromatosis
			 Subcutaneous calcifications
			   Dermatomyositis
			   Scleroderma
			 Erosion of distal clavicles
			   Rheumatoid lung
			   Scleroderma
			 Rib lesions
			 Ribbon ribs/erosion of inferior
			   rib margins
			   Neurofibromatosis
			 Erosion of superior margins
			   Rheumatoid lung
			   Scleroderma
			 Kyphoscoliosis
			   Neurofibromatosis
			 Lytic bone lesions
			   Metastases
			   Eosinophilic granuloma

Honeycombing	Idiopathic pulmonary fibrosis Sarcoidosis Eosinophilic granuloma Rheumatoid lung Scleroderma Pneumoconiosis Hypersensitivity pneumonitis Chronic aspiration Radiation fibrosis		

Miliary nodules	Tuberculosis
	 Fungi
	   Histoplasmosis
	   Coccidioidomycosis
	   Cryptococcosis
	 Silicosis
	 Metastases
	   Thyroid carcinoma
	   Renal cell carcinoma
	   Bronchogenic carcinoma
	   Melanoma
	   Choriocarcinoma
	 Sarcoidosis
	 Eosinophilic granuloma		

pulmonary involvement, there is a male predilection for pleural disease. Pleural effusions are exudative and have a characteristically low glucose concentration.

Enlargement of the central pulmonary arteries and right heart dilatation may be seen on chest radiographs in patients with pulmonary arterial hypertension. This is an uncommon manifestation of rheumatoid disease that usually develops secondary to diffuse interstitial fibrosis. Rarely, the pulmonary arteries are involved as a part of the systemic vasculitis seen in extra-articular rheumatoid disease. There are no parenchymal abnormalities associated with rheumatoid pulmonary arteritis.

Abnormalities that may be seen in the chest wall of individuals with rheumatoid arthritis include tapered erosion of the distal clavicles, rotator cuff atrophy with a high-riding humeral head, bilateral symmetric glenohumeral joint space narrowing with or without superimposed degenerative joint disease, and superior rib notching or erosion.

Systemic Lupus Erythematosus (SLE). This disease of young and middle-aged women typically involves inflammation of multiple organs mediated by auto-antibodies and circulating immune complexes. The thorax is commonly affected and may be the initial site of involvement. The thoracic disease is often limited to the pleura and pericardium, although the lung, heart,

TABLE 17.5

MANIFESTATIONS OF RHEUMATOID LUNG DISEASE

■ MANIFESTATION	■ RADIOGRAPHIC FINDINGS
Serositis	
Pleuritis	Pleural effusion, thickening
Pericarditis	Pericardial effusion
Interstitial pneumonitis	Pulmonary fibrosis (basilar predominance)
Necrobiotic nodules	Multiple peripheral cavitating nodules
Caplan syndrome	Multiple peripheral cavitating nodules
Bronchiolitis obliterans	Hyperinflation
Pulmonary arteritis	Pulmonary arterial hypertension and right heart enlargement Pulmonary hemorrhage

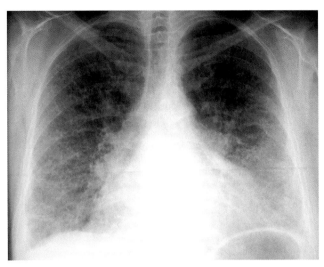

FIGURE 17.14. **Honeycombing in Rheumatoid Lung.** Posteroanterior radiograph in a patient with end-stage rheumatoid lung disease demonstrates medium reticular opacities caused by honeycomb cysts. Note the predominant peripheral distribution of disease. Bilateral pleural effusions and cardiac enlargement caused by pericardial effusion are also evident.

diaphragm, and intercostal muscles are involved in as many as one-third of patients. In the pleura and pericardium, a fibrinous serositis produces painful exudative pleural and pericardial effusions (see Fig. 19.5). Radiographically, the pleural effusions are small or moderate in size and can be unilateral or bilateral. The effusions usually resolve with corticosteroid therapy. Pleural fibrosis results in diffuse pleural thickening and is present in the majority of patients with long-standing disease.

Pulmonary involvement may take the form of acute lupus pneumonitis or chronic interstitial disease. Acute lupus pneumonitis is characterized by rapid onset of fever, dyspnea, and hypoxemia and may require mechanical ventilation. These patients have pathologic changes that are indistinguishable from those seen in ARDS, with diffuse alveolar damage producing an exudative intra-alveolar edema with hyaline membrane formation. Radiographically, rapidly coalescent bilateral airspace opacities are seen, whereas the typical thin-section CT finding is one of ground glass opacity (Fig. 17.16). These findings are difficult to distinguish from those seen in diffuse alveolar hemorrhage associated with pulmonary vascu-

litis, severe pneumonia related to immunosuppressive therapy, or pulmonary edema secondary to renal failure. The diagnosis of acute lupus pneumonitis is made by excluding pneumonia and pulmonary edema and by noting an improvement following the initiation of immunosuppressive therapy.

Radiographic evidence of UIP is distinctly uncommon in SLE, but fibrosis is said to be present pathologically in one-third of patients. When seen radiographically, the pattern is one of bibasilar reticular opacities that are indistinguishable from those seen in rheumatoid lung disease or scleroderma. Therefore, the presence of severe interstitial fibrosis in a patient with clinical features of SLE should prompt consideration of the diagnosis of an overlap syndrome (mixed connective tissue disease). As with rheumatoid lung disease and scleroderma, thin-section CT is the most sensitive technique for demonstrating early interstitial disease.

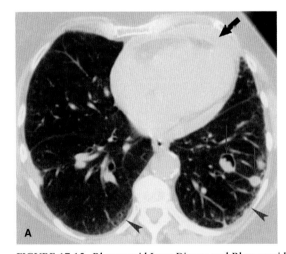
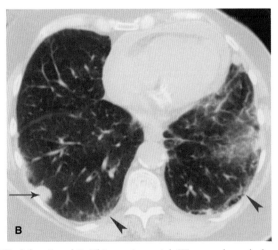

FIGURE 17.15. **Rheumatoid Lung Disease and Rheumatoid Nodules. A** and **B.** Thin-section axial CT scans through the lung bases in a patient with rheumatoid arthritis show asymmetric subpleural reticulation (*blue arrowheads*) reflecting interstitial pneumonitis. Note cavitating and solid bilateral rheumatoid nodules (*red arrows*) and pericardial effusion (*black arrow*), additional findings seen in patients with rheumatoid chest disease.

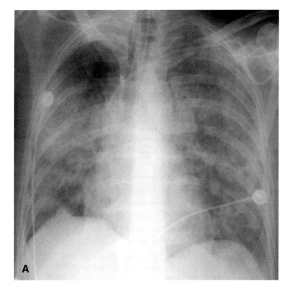

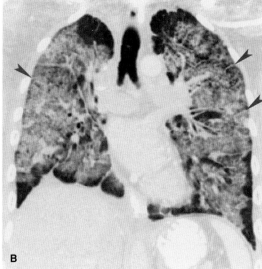

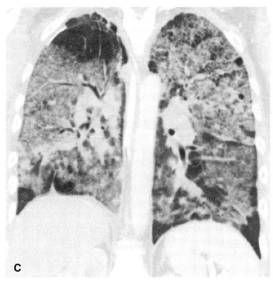

FIGURE 17.16. **Acute Lupus Pneumonitis. A.** Frontal chest radiograph in a 45-year-old woman with lupus and acute respiratory failure shows diffuse bilateral airspace and ground glass opacities. CT with coronal reformations through the mid- **(B)** and posterior **(C)** thorax shows bilateral ground glass opacities with foci of consolidation and associated interlobular septal thickening (*arrowheads*), findings seen in diffuse alveolar damage.

Additional chest radiographic findings in SLE include elevation of the hemidiaphragms with decreased lung volumes and resultant bibasilar areas of linear atelectasis. Diaphragmatic elevation is present in as many as 20% of patients and is the result of diaphragmatic weakness from a primary myopathy unrelated to corticosteroid therapy. Rarely, the central pulmonary arteries are enlarged from pulmonary arterial hypertension secondary to pulmonary vasculitis. Pulmonary embolism with or without infarction may produce peripheral parenchymal opacities and results from deep venous thrombosis that develops in the presence of a circulating lupus anticoagulant. COP has been described in patients with SLE but is indistinguishable clinically and radiographically from lupus pneumonitis, because both conditions produce parenchymal opacities that are responsive to steroids. Superior rib erosions may be present and are indistinguishable from similar findings in rheumatoid arthritis or scleroderma.

Scleroderma (progressive systemic sclerosis) produces inflammation and fibrosis of the skin, esophagus, musculoskeletal system, heart, lungs, and kidneys in young and middle-aged women. The etiology and pathogenesis are unknown. The lungs are involved pathologically in nearly 90% of patients, although only 25% of patients have respiratory symptoms or radiographic evidence of pulmonary involvement. Pulmonary

function testing is more sensitive than conventional radiography in the diagnosis of lung disease and shows the typical diminished lung volumes, preserved flow rates, and low diffusing capacity of interstitial pulmonary fibrosis. Pathologically, the parenchymal changes are those of interstitial fibrosis with a pattern of nonspecific interstitial pneumonia (NSIP). Severe pulmonary involvement is reflected radiographically as a coarse reticular or reticulonodular pattern involving the subpleural regions of the lower lobes. The most common thin-section CT findings are ground glass opacities, reticulation and eventually traction bronchiectasis in a lower zone, subpleural distribution (Fig. 17.17). Thin-section CT is more sensitive than the chest radiograph in detecting and evaluating interstitial disease. Progressive loss of lung volume is seen with advancing pulmonary fibrosis. The development of large (1 to 5 cm) subpleural lower lobe cysts may lead to spontaneous pneumothorax.

Pulmonary arterial hypertension with enlarged central pulmonary arteries and RV dilatation is seen in up to 50% of patients with scleroderma and may be seen in the absence of interstitial fibrosis. In these patients, thickening and obliteration of small muscular pulmonary arteries and arterioles are responsible for the development of pulmonary arterial hypertension. Pleural effusions are significantly less common in scleroderma than in rheumatoid disease or SLE and may be a

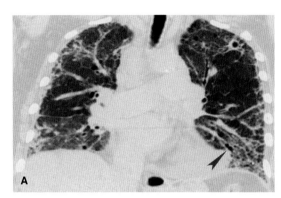
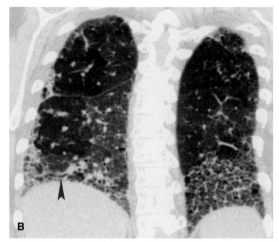

FIGURE 17.17. **Scleroderma With Fibrotic Nonspecific Interstitial Pneumonitis (NSIP).** CT with coronal reformations through the mid- (**A**) and posterior (**B**) thorax in a patient with biopsy-proven NSIP complicating scleroderma shows bilateral lower lobe predominant peripheral reticulation and ground glass opacities, with traction bronchiectasis (*arrowheads*) and minimal honeycomb cyst formation.

helpful distinguishing feature. Pleural thickening is more often attributable to extension of pulmonary interstitial fibrosis into the interstitial layer of the pleura than to pleuritis.

Several additional chest radiographic findings may be seen in patients with scleroderma. Eggshell calcification of mediastinal lymph nodes has been reported, although it is more common in silicosis and sarcoidosis. A dilated air-filled esophagus may be identified on the upright chest radiograph and is a manifestation of esophageal dysmotility from smooth muscle atrophy and fibrosis. An air–fluid level within a dilated esophagus suggests secondary distal esophageal stricture formation from chronic reflux esophagitis. Functional or anatomic esophageal obstruction may result in aspiration with the development of lower lobe pneumonia. Because patients with scleroderma are at a greater risk for developing lung cancer, particularly bronchioloalveolar cell carcinoma, the appearance of a mass or persistent airspace opacity should raise this possibility. Patients with the CREST syndrome (subcutaneous calcification, Raynaud phenomenon, esophageal dysmotility, sclerodactyly, and telangiectasia), a variant of scleroderma, may have radiographically visible calcifications within the subcutaneous tissues of the chest wall. Superior rib notching or erosion may also be seen.

Dermatomyositis and polymyositis involve autoimmune inflammation and destruction of skeletal muscle, producing proximal muscle pain and weakness (polymyositis) and occasionally associated with a skin rash (dermatomyositis). The thoracic manifestations of these diseases include respiratory and pharyngeal muscle weakness. Interstitial pneumonitis is seen in 5% to 10% of patients and is indistinguishable from that associated with rheumatoid lung disease, SLE, scleroderma, or IPF. A fine reticular interstitial pattern in acute disease leads to a chronic, coarse reticular or reticulonodular process that is predominantly basilar in distribution. Most patients with polymyositis and interstitial lung disease have clinical manifestations of rheumatoid arthritis or scleroderma, and these patients tend to respond favorably to corticosteroids. As with scleroderma, the early parenchymal changes may be subradiographic but can be demonstrated on thin-section CT studies through the lower lobes. Airspace consolidation and ground glass opacity representing organizing pneumonia and diffuse alveolar damage, respectively (Fig. 17.18). Additional chest radiographic findings in polymyositis reflect the involvement of skeletal muscle. Small lung volumes with diaphragmatic elevation and basilar linear atelectasis are secondary to diaphragmatic and intercostal muscle involvement. Pharyngeal

and upper esophageal muscle weakness predispose to aspiration pneumonia. The chest radiograph should be examined carefully for lung masses because bronchogenic carcinoma accounts for a significant percentage of the malignancies seen with a higher-than-normal frequency in patients with dermatomyositis or polymyositis.

Sjögren Syndrome. This autoimmune disorder of middle-aged women is characterized by the sicca syndrome (dry eyes [keratoconjunctivitis sicca], dry mouth [xerostomia], and dry nose [xerorhinia]), which results from lymphocytic infiltration of the lacrimal, salivary, and mucous glands, respectively. Most patients with the sicca syndrome have associated manifestations of other collagen vascular diseases, such as rheumatoid arthritis, scleroderma, or SLE.

The chest is involved in approximately one-third of patients with Sjögren syndrome with or without associated collagen vascular disease. The most common manifestation is interstitial fibrosis, which is indistinguishable from that seen with other collagen vascular disorders. Involvement of tracheobronchial mucous glands leads to thickened sputum with mucus plugging and recurrent bronchitis, bronchiectasis, atelectasis, and

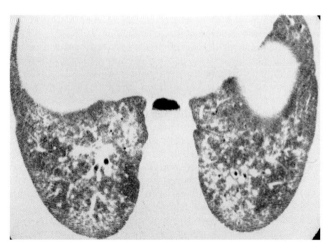

FIGURE 17.18. **Polymyositis.** Thin-section CT through the lung bases shows reticulation and ill-defined centrilobular nodules, likely reflecting interstitial pneumonitis and organizing pneumonia, respectively, in a patient with polymyositis.

pneumonia. Thin-section CT demonstrates both interstitial opacities and the presence of small airways involvement with bronchiolectasis and a "tree-in-bud" appearance. Pleuritis and pleural effusion are less common.

Patients with Sjögren syndrome are at increased risk for developing lymphocytic interstitial pneumonitis (LIP) and non-Hodgkin pulmonary lymphoma. The radiographic appearance of LIP is lower lobe coarse reticular or reticulonodular opacities that are indistinguishable from interstitial fibrosis. Thin-section CT shows ground glass opacity with scattered, thin-walled cysts. The development of lymphoma in these patients should be suspected when nodular or alveolar opacities develop in the lung in association with mediastinal lymph node enlargement.

Ankylosing Spondylitis. Approximately 1% to 2% of individuals with ankylosing spondylitis develop pulmonary disease in the form of upper lobe pulmonary fibrosis. The fibrotic changes are commonly associated with the development of bullae and cavities, which are prone to mycetoma formation with *Aspergillus.* The diagnosis should be suspected in a young to middle-aged man with characteristic spine changes (kyphosis and spinal ankylosis) who has abnormally increased lung volumes and upper lobe fibrobullous disease, the latter of which simulates postprimary fibrocavitary TB.

Overlap Syndromes and Mixed Connective Tissue Disease. Some patients with collagen vascular disease have features of more than one of the recognized syndromes discussed above. These patients are classified as having an overlap syndrome with thoracic manifestations characteristic of the other disorders. Patients with a distinct form of overlap syndrome, called *mixed connective tissue disease,* have clinical features of SLE, scleroderma, and polymyositis and have serum antibodies to extractable nuclear antigen. The thoracic manifestations of mixed connective tissue disease include UIP, pulmonary arterial hypertension caused by plexogenic pulmonary arteriopathy, and pleural effusion and thickening from a fibrinous pleuritis like that found inpatients with SLE.

Idiopathic Chronic Interstitial Pneumonias

The idiopathic interstitial pneumonias are characterized by an inflammatory process in the lung that can result in pulmonary fibrosis. These disorders are most accurately characterized by their histologic appearance and include UIP, acute interstitial pneumonia (AIP), COP, respiratory bronchiolitis-associated interstitial lung disease (RB-ILD), DIP, and NSIP (2). Unfortunately, confusion arises when clinical terms are used interchangeably with the aforementioned histologic terms in describing these disorders. When possible (when the histology is known), it is most accurate to use the histologic term to describe a particular disorder, whereas reserving clinical terms such as *IPF* or *rheumatoid lung* for interstitial disease associated with specific clinical diseases for which histology is unavailable.

Usual Interstitial Pneumonia. UIP is the most common of the idiopathic interstitial pneumonias. It is likely the result of repetitive injury to the lung. The initial response in the lung is inflammation, which is followed by repair and eventually fibrosis. The pathologic abnormalities seen in UIP represent a spectrum of findings, characterized in the early stage of disease by marked proliferation of macrophages in the alveolar airspaces associated with a mild and uniform thickening of the interstitium by mononuclear cells. Late in the course of disease, the pathologic findings are characterized by thickening of the alveolar interstitium by mononuclear inflammatory cells and fibrous tissue. A distinguishing histologic feature of UIP is that different stages of the disease are seen simultaneously within different portions of the lung (temporal heterogeneity).

Patients with UIP typically present in the fifth to seventh decades, with a slight male preponderance. Presenting symptoms include progressive dyspnea or a nonproductive cough. Pulmonary function tests show restrictive disease and a decreased diffusing capacity for carbon monoxide (DLCO). Most cases of UIP are idiopathic, but up to 30% of patients with UIP have an associated collagen vascular or immunologic disorder. This is most often rheumatoid arthritis, but it can also be SLE, scleroderma, or dermatomyositis/polymyositis.

The radiographic manifestations of UIP parallel the pathologic changes. In the early phase of disease, the chest radiograph may appear normal despite the presence of clinical symptoms and abnormalities on pulmonary function testing. The earliest radiographic changes are bibasilar fine to medium reticular opacities or ground glass density (Fig. 17.19A). As the disease progresses, a coarse reticular or reticulonodular pattern is seen, which almost invariably leads to the formation of honeycomb cysts (3 to 10 mm in diameter) and progressive loss of lung volume. Extensive pulmonary fibrosis may be associated with findings of pulmonary arterial hypertension.

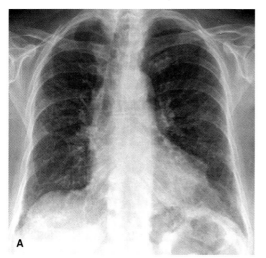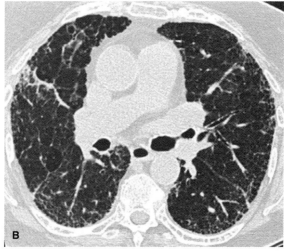

FIGURE 17.19. Usual Interstitial Pneumonia (UIP). A. Posteroanterior radiograph in a patient with UIP demonstrates bilateral coarse reticular opacities. **B.** A thin-section CT through the mid-lungs shows peripheral reticulation and ground glass opacities.

Upper lobe bullae may be seen and predispose to the development of spontaneous pneumothorax. Hilar lymph node enlargement and pleural effusions have been described but are rare and should suggest an alternative diagnosis.

Thin-section CT findings in UIP differ with the stage of the disease and vary from one lung region to another. Patients with active inflammatory areas of disease, as demonstrated histologically by interstitial and intra-alveolar inflammatory changes, show areas of ground glass density on thin-section CT. As fibrosis develops, findings include irregular septal or subpleural thickening (in contrast to the smooth septal thickening seen with edema or lymphangitic spread of carcinoma), intralobular lines, irregular interfaces, honeycombing, and traction bronchiectasis [Figs. 17.12, 17.19B]). The changes are typically most severe in the peripheral and basal portions of the lungs, which can be helpful in differential diagnosis. Mildly enlarged mediastinal lymph nodes are often seen.

In most patients, the disease progresses inexorably, with an overall mean survival of less than 5 years. Patients with early, active disease (positive gallium scan, ground glass, or airspace opacities radiographically) may benefit from immunosuppressive therapy with corticosteroids or cyclophosphamide, whereas those with end-stage fibrosis (honeycombing) will not. Most patients succumb to respiratory failure, often precipitated by infection or cardiac disease. There is an increased incidence of bronchogenic carcinoma, with adenocarcinoma the most common histologic subtype.

Acute Interstitial Pneumonia. Also known as the Hamman-Rich syndrome, acute interstitial pneumonia is an acute, aggressive form of idiopathic interstitial pneumonitis and fibrosis. Patients with acute interstitial pneumonia typically present with a brief history of cough, fever, and dyspnea that progress rapidly to severe hypoxemia and respiratory failure requiring mechanical ventilation. The pathologic manifestations of acute interstitial pneumonia are those of ARDS, and the disease has been termed *idiopathic ARDS.* The histologic findings are those of diffuse alveolar damage with minimal mature collagen deposition. A characteristic of the process is that it is diffuse and temporally homogeneous.

Chest radiographs and thin-section CT scans show findings of ARDS, with diffuse ground glass opacity and consolidation with air bronchograms (Fig. 17.20) (4). On CT, there is often a gradient of increasing density from anterior to posterior lung. Linear opacities, honeycombing, and traction bronchiectasis are uncommon. As in other forms of ARDS, the mortality rate ranges from 60% to 90%. Fibrosis can develop but tends to stabilize and does not progress beyond the recovery phase.

Cryptogenic Organizing Pneumonia and Bronchiolitis Obliterans With Organizing Pneumonia. The terms cryptogenic organizing pneumonia (COP) and bronchiolitis obliterans with organizing pneumonia (BOOP), refer to a disorder characterized by the widespread deposition of granulation tissue (fibroblasts, collagen, and capillaries) within peribronchiolar airspaces and bronchioles. Most cases of are idiopathic and properly referred to as COP. A number of conditions have been associated with this disorder in which case it is usually referred to as BOOP. These include viral infection (influenza, adenovirus, and measles); toxic fume inhalation (sulfur

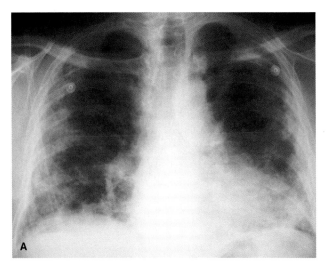

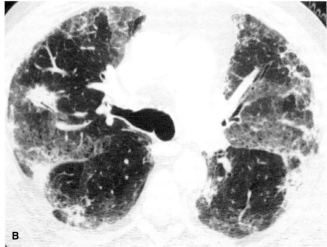

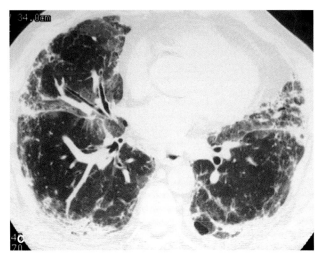

FIGURE 17.20. **Acute Interstitial Pneumonia (Hamman-Rich Syndrome).** Frontal radiograph (**A**) in a patient with biopsy-proven acute interstitial pneumonia demonstrates peripheral airspace and ground glass opacity. CT scans through the upper lobe bronchus (**B**) and lower lungs (**C**) show predominantly peripheral ground glass and reticular opacities with scattered airspace opacities.

dioxide and chlorine); collagen vascular disease (rheumatoid arthritis and SLE); organ transplantation (bone marrow, lung, and heart–lung); drug reactions; and chronic aspiration. Although the terms are similar, BOOP is a different disease than bronchiolitis obliterans (obliterative bronchiolitis). For the purposes of this discussion, the COP will be used to refer to both COP and BOOP.

Patients with COP often have a subacute illness, with several months' history of nonproductive cough and dyspnea. The physical examination may reveal rales or wheezes. Pulmonary function tests usually show a restrictive pattern of disease with diminished lung volumes and normal to increased flow rates. The DLCO is significantly decreased. Pathologically, a mononuclear cell exudate in the bronchioles and surrounding alveoli organizes to form intrabronchiolar and intra-alveolar granulation tissue. A characteristic of this disease is the uniformity of the histologic changes and the absence of parenchymal distortion and fibrosis; these features help distinguish COP from UIP, which can have similar clinical, functional, and radiographic features.

Radiographs in patients with COP reveal patchy bilateral airspace or ground glass opacities (Fig. 17.13A), with scattered nodular opacities in some patients. The most common thin-section CT findings are patchy consolidation or ground glass opacity with either a subpleural or peribronchial pattern of distribution (Fig. 17.13B). More recently, a thin-section CT finding of patchy ground glass opacities surrounded by crescentic regions of more dense consolidation, termed the so-called "reversed halo" sign, has been described in patients with COP, which while not specific should suggest the diagnosis (Fig. 17.21). Small ill-defined peribronchial nodules are seen less commonly. Bronchiectasis and bronchial wall thickening are commonly seen in the involved areas of lung.

The diagnosis of COP can only be made by recognizing the characteristic histologic changes on open lung biopsy. The distinction of COP from UIP may be difficult but is important because COP has a more favorable prognosis and usually responds rapidly to corticosteroid therapy. COP complicating heart–lung transplantation generally has a worse prognosis but may respond favorably to immunosuppressive therapy.

Respiratory Bronchiolitis-Associated Interstitial Lung Disease. RB-ILD is a disorder seen only in cigarette smokers and is characterized by inflammation within and around the respiratory bronchioles. The histology of RB-ILD overlaps with that of DIP, and some authors have suggested that RB-ILD is an early form of DIP. Patients with RB-ILD are typically young, heavy smokers with mild cough and dyspnea. Pulmonary function tests show restrictive or mixed restrictive–obstructive patterns. Symptoms respond to smoking cessation or steroid therapy, and there is no progression to end-stage fibrosis.

The chest radiograph is normal in up to 21% of cases of RB-ILD, but diffuse linear and nodular opacities and bibasilar atelectasis are often seen. The most common thin-section CT findings are scattered ground glass opacities and small centrilobular nodules, often with an upper lobe–predominant distribution (Fig. 17.22). Linear opacities are rare and honeycombing is not seen. Emphysema is often a concomitant finding.

Desquamative Interstitial Pneumonia. DIP is a disorder characterized by the accumulation of macrophages within alveolar spaces. Ninety percent of patients with DIP are cigarette smokers. While focal areas of macrophage accumulation can be seen as a component of UIP, in DIP it is diffuse and temporally homogeneous. There are also distinguishing clinical features that support the concept of two distinct entities. DIP affects younger individuals, with a mean age at diagnosis of 40 to 45 years, and is almost invariably associated with heavy cigarette smoking. Most importantly, DIP is more steroid-responsive than UIP and therefore carries a more favorable prognosis; the median survival for patients with DIP is 12 years, compared with 4 years for those with UIP.

DIP cannot be reliably distinguished from UIP radiographically. The typical radiographic findings in DIP are bibasilar reticular opacities with normal or minimally diminished lung volumes. Ground glass opacities are seen in only 33% of cases, whereas honeycombing is rare. Up to 22% of patients have a normal chest radiograph. Thin-section CT shows ground glass opacities, most often within the peripheral aspects of the bases (Fig. 17.23). Irregular linear opacities, honeycombing, and traction bronchiectasis can be seen but are much less common than in UIP. Ground glass abnormalities often improve or completely resolve with corticosteroid therapy.

Nonspecific Interstitial Pneumonitis. NSIP is a recently introduced term used to describe interstitial pneumonias that cannot be otherwise classified as UIP, AIP, COP, RB-ILD, or DIP. Many cases of NSIP are seen in association with collagen

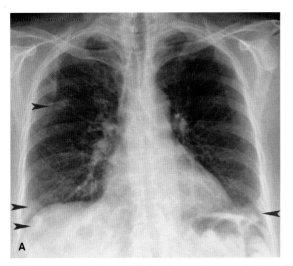 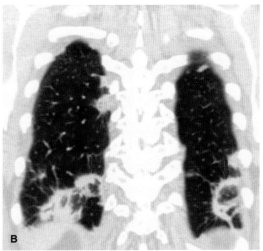

FIGURE 17.21. "Reversed Halo" Sign in Cryptogenic Organizing Pneumonia. A. Frontal chest radiograph in a 53-year-old woman with dry cough and shortness of breath shows ill-defined densities in the peripheral right lung and both lung bases (*arrowheads*). **B.** CT with coronal reformation shows bilateral, lower zone predominant peripheral mass-like opacities, several of which demonstrate dense peripheral consolidation or a reversed halo sign (*arrows*). Diagnosis was by open lung biopsy.

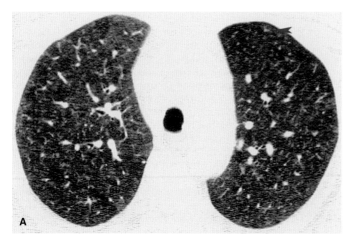
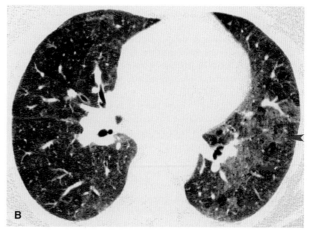

FIGURE 17.22. Respiratory Bronchiolitis-Associated Interstitial Lung Disease (RB-ILD). Thin-section CT scans through the upper lobes (**A**) and lower lobes (**B**) in a patient with biopsy-proven RB-ILD demonstrate bilateral centrilobular (*arrowheads*) and geographic regions of ground glass opacity.

vascular disease or as drug reactions. The pathologic changes are temporally homogeneous, as compared to UIP, which is typically heterogeneous. Pathologists generally divide NSIP into cellular and fibrotic forms of disease, with correlative findings on thin-section CT. Those with cellular NSIP show areas of ground glass and consolidation on thin-section CT in a peripheral and lower zone distribution (Fig. 17.24). Bronchial dilatation and linear opacities are more typical of the fibrotic form of NSIP (Fig. 17.17), but in distinction to UIP, honeycombing is rare. While cellular NSIP is usually responsive to steroids, fibrotic NSIP has a poor prognosis, similar to that of UIP.

Other Chronic Interstitial Lung Diseases

Neurofibromatosis (NF) is an autosomal dominant neurocutaneous syndrome, which is divided into two types: type 1, or von Recklinghausen disease, and type 2. The classic manifesta-

tions of NF 1 are cutaneous café-au-lait spots and neurofibromas of cutaneous and subcutaneous peripheral nerves and nerve roots. In addition, there is often involvement of the skeletal, vascular, and pulmonary systems. The condition is also associated with a variety of neoplasms, including meningiomas, optic gliomas, neurofibrosarcomas, and pheochromocytomas.

There are several thoracic manifestations of NF 1. Cutaneous and subcutaneous neurofibromas may be seen along the chest wall or projecting over the lungs. The spine may show a kyphoscoliosis, with scalloping of the posterior aspect of the vertebral bodies caused by dural ectasia. "Ribbon rib" deformities and rib notching may be seen. Mediastinal masses in patients with NF 1 include neurofibromas, lateral thoracic meningoceles, and extra-adrenal pheochromocytomas.

Parenchymal lung disease is seen in approximately 20% of patients with NF 1. The findings include diffuse interstitial fibrosis and bulla formation. The interstitial fibrosis is predominantly lower zonal and bilaterally symmetric. Bullae usually develop

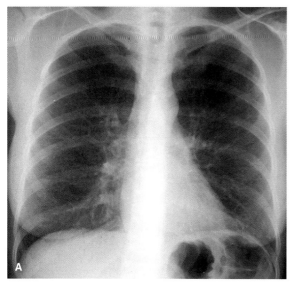
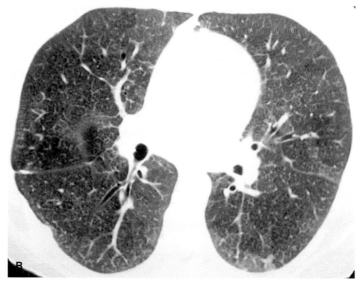

FIGURE 17.23. Desquamative Interstitial Pneumonia (DIP). Chest radiograph (**A**) and thin-section CT (**B**) show fine reticular or ground glass opacities in a smoker with DIP.

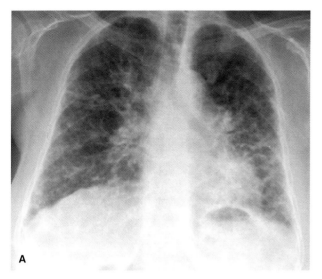

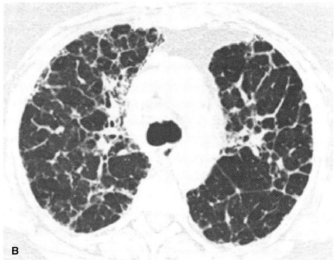

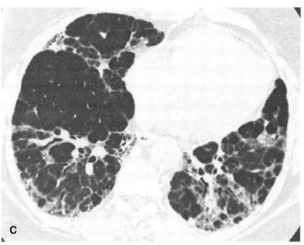

FIGURE 17.24. **Nonspecific Interstitial Pneumonia (NSIP). A.** Frontal chest radiograph demonstrates coarse interstitial markings throughout both lungs. **B.** Thin-section CT scan at the level of the carina demonstrates thickened interlobular septa with medial upper lobe traction bronchiectasis. **C.** Thin-section CT through the lung bases shows traction bronchiectasis, minimal honeycombing, and ground glass opacities. Open lung biopsy demonstrated NSIP.

in the upper zones, with asymmetric involvement of the lungs. Pulmonary symptoms are usually minimal or absent, with pulmonary function tests showing a mixed obstructive/restrictive pattern. A small number of patients will develop respiratory failure caused by pulmonary fibrosis, with secondary development of pulmonary arterial hypertension and cor pulmonale.

Tuberous Sclerosis (TS) is an autosomal dominant neurocutaneous syndrome with variable expression. The classical clinical triad of TS is seizures, mental retardation, and adenoma sebaceum. Additional manifestations include intracranial calcifications, cerebral cortical and periventricular hamartomas, renal angiomyolipomas, cardiac rhabdomyomas, retinal phakomas, and sclerotic bone lesions.

Pulmonary involvement in TS is rare and is seen in approximately 1% of cases. Patients with pulmonary TS tend to be older and have a lower incidence of seizures and mental retardation. The pulmonary involvement is indistinguishable clinically, pathologically, and radiographically from that seen in LAM. Pathologically, there is smooth muscle proliferation in the peribronchovascular and parenchymal interstitium of the lung. Small adenomatoid nodules measuring several millimeters in diameter may be seen scattered throughout the lungs.

Radiographically, there are symmetric bilateral reticular or reticulonodular opacities. In the later stages of disease, a pattern of coarse reticular or small cystic opacities may be seen. The cysts are uniform in size and smaller than 1 cm in diameter. Thin-section CT is best at depicting the presence of thin-walled pulmonary cysts and can help detect associated extrapulmo-

nary abnormalities, including renal angiomyolipomas and periventricular tubera. A helpful feature in distinguishing TS from other chronic interstitial lung diseases is the normal to increased lung volumes in patients with TS caused by small airways obstruction and expiratory air trapping. In distinction to EG of lung and sarcoidosis, which have a predominant upper zone distribution of disease, pulmonary TS tends to affect the entire lung uniformly. Pneumothorax is common and results from the rupture of a subpleural cyst. Pleural effusions are uncommon. The pulmonary involvement often leads to pulmonary arterial hypertension and cor pulmonale, which are associated with a high mortality.

Lymphangioleiomyomatosis (LAM) is an uncommon condition that is seen exclusively in women. The average age at diagnosis is 43 years. Although LAM shares many features with pulmonary TS, it is not an inherited condition and lacks the extrapulmonary features of TS.

On gross pathologic examination, patients with advanced LAM show replacement of the normal lung architecture by cysts. These cysts, which range from 0.2 to 2.0 cm in diameter, are separated by thickened interstitium containing numerous interlacing bundles of smooth muscle. Smooth muscle proliferation is also seen within the walls of pulmonary veins, bronchioles, and lymphatics. The smooth muscle proliferation within lymphatic channels causes lymphatic obstruction and dilatation that may lead to the development of chylothorax, chyloperitoneum, or chylopericardium. Similarly, smooth muscle proliferation within mediastinal and retroperitoneal lymph

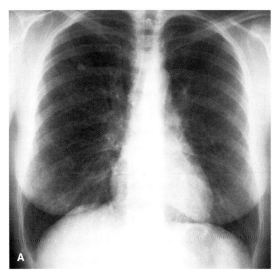
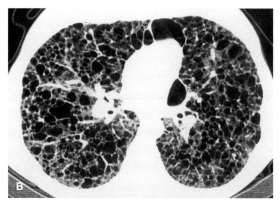

FIGURE 17.25. **Lymphangioleiomyomatosis (LAM). A.** Posteroanterior radiograph in a 36-year-old patient with LAM shows diffuse coarse reticular opacities with normal lung volumes. **B.** Thin-section CT in another patient with LAM shows almost complete replacement of the parenchyma by thin-walled cysts.

nodes may result in nodal enlargement. The perilymphatic smooth muscle proliferation and nodal enlargement help distinguish LAM pathologically from the pulmonary involvement of TS.

The patient with LAM is typically a woman of childbearing age who presents with progressive dyspnea or a spontaneous pneumothorax. Hemoptysis may be seen in some patients, presumably related to pulmonary venous obstruction by the smooth muscle proliferation.

The chest radiograph may be normal early in the disease. Eventually, symmetric bilateral fine reticular or reticulonodular opacities are seen. The late radiographic pattern is one of cysts and honeycombing; the cysts tend to have thinner walls than those seen with IPF or NF (Fig. 17.25A). As in TS, the lung volumes are typically normal or increased. Large, recurrent chylous pleural effusions may be unilateral or bilateral. Spontaneous pneumothorax is also a common finding and may be bilateral.

Thin-section CT demonstrates thin-walled cysts distributed throughout the lungs (Fig. 17.25B). In less severely involved areas, the intervening lung is normal. Interlobular septal thickening is generally mild or absent. Although thin-walled cysts are seen in a variety of other diseases, the thin-section CT findings, in a patient with a characteristic history (a woman with dyspnea, spontaneous pneumothorax, and chylous pleural effusions) are diagnostic (5).

The prognosis of patients with symptomatic LAM is poor, with approximately 70% of patients dying within 5 years. In some patients, the administration of antiprogesterone agents such as tamoxifen may slow the progression of disease.

Alveolar Septal Amyloidosis. Amyloidosis encompasses a group of diseases characterized by the extracellular deposition of insoluble fibrillary proteins termed *amyloid.* Amyloid represents a number of proteins that are distinctive biochemically but similar physically in that their polypeptide chains form beta-pleated sheets. Amyloidosis has traditionally been classified into four forms: (*1*) primary, in which there is no associated chronic disease or in which there is an underlying plasma cell disorder; (*2*) secondary, in which an underlying chronic abnormality such as TB is present; (*3*) familial, which is very uncommon and usually localized to nervous tissue; and (*4*) senile, which affects many organs in patients older than 70

years. More recently, a classification scheme has been developed that is based on the specific protein comprising amyloid. In this scheme, the most important forms are amyloid L (AL), usually seen with plasma cell dyscrasias and associated with the deposition of immunoglobulin light chains, and amyloid A (AA), which occurs in patients with chronic inflammatory diseases such as familial Mediterranean fever and certain neoplasms, including Hodgkin disease.

There are three major patterns of amyloid deposition within the lungs and airways: tracheobronchial, nodular parenchymal, and diffuse parenchymal (alveolar septal). In most cases these patterns occur independently, but can overlap.

In alveolar septal amyloidosis, the amyloid is deposited in the parenchymal interstitium and within the media of small blood vessels. Within the alveolar septa, amyloid deposits are located between the endothelial cells lining the septal capillaries and the alveolar epithelium; inflammatory cells are typically absent.

This process is usually seen in older patients who have symptoms of chronic progressive dyspnea. Recurrent hemoptysis may also be seen as a result of medial dissection of the involved pulmonary arteries. Radiographically, patients with parenchymal alveolar septal disease show evidence of interstitial disease, with fine reticular or reticulonodular opacities that may become more coarse and confluent over time. Thin-section CT demonstrates interlobular septal thickening, reticulation, and micronodules. Fibrosis and lymph node enlargement are uncommon (4). The radiographic appearance simulates that seen in silicosis or sarcoidosis.

The diagnosis is made on lung biopsy by the identification of amorphous eosinophilic material thickening the alveolar septa that appears apple green in color when stained with Congo red and viewed under polarized light. There is no effective treatment.

Chronic Aspiration Pneumonia. Patients who repeatedly aspirate may develop chronic interstitial abnormalities on chest radiographs. With repeated episodes of aspiration over months to years, a residuum of irregular reticular interstitial opacities may persist, probably representing peribronchial scarring. A reticulonodular pattern may be seen as the result of granulomas forming around food particles. These chronic interstitial abnormalities can be observed between episodes of acute aspiration pneumonitis.

INHALATIONAL DISEASE

Pneumoconiosis

The term *pneumoconiosis* is used to describe the nonneoplastic reaction of the lungs to inhaled inorganic dust particles (6). The inorganic dust pneumoconioses result from the inhalation and retention of asbestos, silica, or coal particles within the lung. With time, the accumulation of these particles leads to two types of pathologic reaction that may be seen alone or in combination: fibrosis, which may be focal and nodular or diffuse and reticular; and the aggregation of particle-laden macrophages. Organic dust inhalational syndromes, which are discussed at the end of this section, are not associated with the retention and accumulation of particles within the lungs. Instead, the organic dusts induce a hypersensitivity reaction known as hypersensitivity pneumonitis or extrinsic allergic alveolitis.

Asbestosis. Asbestos is the generic term for a group of fibrous silicates that are resistant to heat and various chemical insults. Asbestos is divided into two major subgroups: the serpentines and the amphiboles. The serpentines are curly, flexible, and smooth; the only commercially important serpentine is chrysotile. The amphiboles have straight, needlelike fibers; this subgroup includes crocidolite and amosite. The different types of asbestos fibers vary in their potential to cause disease, with the amphiboles having a greater fibrogenic and carcinogenic potential than the serpentines. At present, more than 90% of the asbestos used in the United States is chrysotile.

Asbestos inhalation may cause disease of the pleura, parenchyma, airways, and lymph nodes. Pleural disease is the most common of these and usually manifests as parietal pleural plaques. Other pleural manifestations include pleural effusion, localized visceral pleural fibrosis, diffuse pleural fibrosis, and mesothelioma. The pleural manifestations of asbestos exposure are discussed in more detail in Chapter 19. The pulmonary parenchymal manifestations of asbestos inhalation include interstitial fibrosis (asbestosis), rounded atelectasis, and bronchogenic carcinoma.

Asbestosis is defined as a diffuse parenchymal interstitial fibrosis caused by the inhalation of asbestos fibers. The development of asbestosis depends on both the length and severity of exposure, and clinical manifestations are usually not apparent for 20 to 40 years following initial exposure. Pathologically, a large number of "asbestos bodies" will be seen in lung tissue. This characteristic structure consists of a core transparent asbestos fiber surrounded by a coat of iron and protein. Asbestos bodies are usually found within interstitial fibrous tissue or airspaces and only rarely in pleural plaques. The number of asbestos bodies and fibers per gram of digested lung tissue is roughly proportional to the degree of occupational exposure and the severity of interstitial fibrosis. On gross examination of affected lungs, fibrosis is most prominent in the subpleural regions of the lower lobes. Microscopically, the appearance varies from a slight increase in interstitial collagen to complete obliteration of normal architecture and formation of thick fibrous parenchymal bands and cystic spaces (honeycombing).

The majority of patients with asbestos-related pleuropulmonary disease are asymptomatic. Patients beyond the early stages of interstitial fibrosis will often experience shortness of breath and a restrictive pattern on pulmonary function tests. These patients are also at risk of developing asbestos-associated neoplasia, particularly bronchogenic carcinoma and pleural mesothelioma, and require close clinical follow-up.

The radiographic findings in asbestosis occur in two forms: small and large opacities. Small opacities may be reticular, nodular, or a combination of the two. The changes produced on chest radiographs are divided into three stages. The earliest finding is a fine reticulation, predominantly in the lower lung zones, which is a manifestation of early interstitial pneumonitis and fibrosis. With time, the small irregular opacities become more prominent, creating a coarse reticular pattern of disease. In later stages, the reticular opacities may extend into the mid-lung and upper lung zones, with progressive obscuration of the cardiac and diaphragmatic margins and progressive diminution of lung volumes. Large opacities, that is, those measuring greater than 1 cm in diameter, are invariably associated with widespread interstitial fibrosis and pleural plaques. These large opacities show lower zone predominance and may be well-defined or ill-defined and multiple.

Thin-section CT is a sensitive means of detecting both the pleural and parenchymal changes associated with clinical asbestosis. Interlobular septal thickening is the most common thin-section CT finding in asbestos-exposed individuals. Intralobular septal thickening and small centrilobular "dot-like" opacities, the latter caused by peribronchiolar fibrosis, are also common. Many cases will progress to honeycombing. The thin-section CT findings are similar to those of IPF (Figs. 17.12, 17.19), but patients with asbestosis may also have pleural disease, which may help to distinguish between these two entities (Fig. 17.26). Additionally, ground glass opacity is relatively uncommon in asbestosis compared with IPF and other forms of UIP.

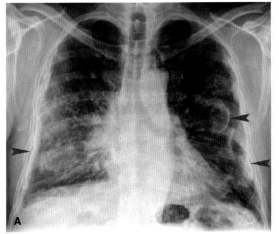
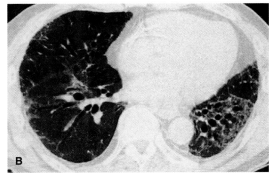

FIGURE 17.26. Asbestosis. A. Frontal chest radiograph shows course bibasilar interstitial markings and calcified pleural plaques (*arrowheads*) **B.** Thin-section CT through the lung bases shows left lower lobe honeycombing, peripheral ground glass opacities, and traction bronchiectasis bilaterally.

Identification of intrafissural plaques, especially if they contain calcification, is also possible with thin-section CT. Characteristic CT features of focal lung masses in asbestos-exposed individuals may allow for conservative management of these lesions. For example, a wedge-shaped or round mass adjacent to focal pleural thickening, with evidence of lobar volume loss and a "comet tail" bronchovascular bundle coursing into it, can be confidently diagnosed as rounded atelectasis by thin-section CT, obviating biopsy.

Silicosis. Silica is an abundant mineral composed of regularly arranged molecules of silicon dioxide. It is ubiquitous in the earth's crust and exposure to a high concentration may lead to pathologic and radiologic changes. Occupations associated with such levels of exposure include mining, quarrying, foundry work, ceramic work, and sandblasting. Two distinct histopathologic reactions to inhaled silica are *silicotic nodules* and *silicoproteinosis.*

Silicotic nodules measure from 1 to 10 mm in diameter and are made up of dense concentric lamellae of collagen. They are typically most numerous in the upper lobes and parahilar regions of lung; calcification or ossification of the nodules is common. Coalescence of these nodules produces areas of progressive massive fibrosis (PMF). PMF may occupy an entire lobe, with areas of emphysema often present adjacent to these masses. Focal necrosis is common within the central portions of these large conglomerate lesions and is often the result of ischemia or superinfection by TB or anaerobic bacteria. Exposure of 10 to 20 years is usually required for the radiographic changes of fibrotic silicosis to develop. The classic radiographic appearance is multiple well-defined nodules ranging from 1 to 10 mm in diameter. These tend to be diffuse with an upper zone predominance nodules and calcify in approximately 20% of cases. A reticular pattern of disease may be seen preceding or associated with the nodular pattern and is sometimes the earliest radiographic finding. This pattern of reticulonodular opacities is often referred to as "simple" silicosis, in contrast to the large conglomerate opacities that characterize "complicated" silicosis (Fig. 17.10). These conglomerate opacities represent areas of PMF and most commonly develop in the peripheral portions of the upper and mid-lung zones. The opacities tend to migrate toward the hila, leaving areas of emphysema between the pleural surface and the areas of progressive fibrosis. These conglomerate areas may cavitate, often in association with superimposed tuberculous infection. Hilar lymph node enlargement may be seen at any stage, and these hilar nodes often demonstrate peripheral "eggshell" calcification. Clinically, the diagnosis of fibrotic silicosis is based on identification of a diffuse reticular, nodular, or reticulonodular pattern on the chest radiograph in a patient with an appropriate exposure history. Patients may be asymptomatic for many years, but may worsen functionally in conjunction with progression of the radiographic changes. The pulmonary fibrosis and associated restrictive functional impairment of silicosis may progress even after the individual is removed from the offending environment.

Silicoproteinosis usually occurs in individuals exposed to very high concentrations of silica. It is characterized by filling of alveolar spaces with lipoproteinaceous material similar to that seen in idiopathic alveolar proteinosis. There is little collagen deposition associated with this reaction and the well-defined collagenous nodule is not typically seen. Acute silicoproteinosis presents radiographically with diffuse airspace disease and is indistinguishable in appearance from idiopathic alveolar proteinosis. As do patients with fibrotic silicosis, those with acute silicoproteinosis have an increased susceptibility to TB. They are also predisposed to superinfection with *Nocardia*, which may produce mass-like consolidation and chest wall involvement.

Coal Worker's Pneumoconiosis. The inhalation of large amounts of carbon-containing inorganic material may lead to significant pulmonary disease. The exposure levels required to cause this disease occur almost exclusively in the workplace. Since the most common occupation producing this entity is coal mining, the resultant disease is termed coal worker's pneumoconiosis (CWP).

CWP has two characteristic pathologic findings: the coal dust macule and PMF. The coal dust macule results from the deposit of carbonaceous material within the lung. Coal dust macules are round or stellate nodules ranging in size from 1 to 5 mm. They are composed of pigment-laden macrophages with minimal or absent collagen formation. They are found within the interstitium adjacent to respiratory bronchioles and are scattered throughout the lungs with a predilection for the apices. The coal dust macule or nodule is the hallmark of simple CWP and is generally not associated with functional impairment. In fact, radiographic abnormalities may be absent in simple CWP. Complicated CWP is characterized by the presence of PMF. PMF is defined as nodular or mass-like lesions exceeding 2 to 3 cm in diameter that are composed of irregular fibrosis and pigment. PMF is most common in the posterior segments of the upper lobes and superior segments of the lower lobes. The conglomerate masses may cross interlobar fissures. Central cavitation is common and is most often a result of infarction from obliteration of pulmonary vessels by the fibrotic masses. Occasionally, superinfection of the masses by TB or fungus accounts for central necrosis and cavitation. The mass lesions of complicated CWP are similar to those seen in complicated silicosis. It should be noted that despite their name, the lesions of PMF may not progress with time and are not necessarily massive in size.

Patients with CWP usually present with respiratory difficulties only when PMF has developed, as those with simple pneumoconiosis are generally asymptomatic. In complicated CWP, there is progressive dyspnea, which may lead to cor pulmonale. Because many coal workers also smoke cigarettes, the development of centrilobular emphysema and chronic bronchitis may complicate the clinical picture.

Radiographically, "simple" CWP presents typically as upper zone reticulonodular or small nodular opacities (6). A purely reticular pattern may also be seen, especially in the early stages of the process. The nodules range from 1 to 5 mm in diameter and correspond to conglomerates of coal dust macules seen pathologically. The lesions are indistinguishable radiographically from the nodules of simple silicosis. In as many as 10% of coal miners, some of these nodules will calcify centrally. This is in distinction to the diffuse calcification of silicotic nodules. The nodular opacities of simple CWP do not progress after coal dust exposure has ceased. The lesions of complicated pneumoconiosis (PMF) range in size from 2 cm to an entire lobe and are seen in the upper portion of the lungs. PMF usually begins peripherally as a mass with a smooth, well-defined lateral border and an ill-defined medial border. PMF gradually "migrates" toward the hilum, creating a zone of emphysema between the opacities and the chest wall. These lesions may mimic primary carcinoma, particularly if a background of nodular opacities is not appreciated. The PMF seen with CWP may develop years after exposure to coal dust has ceased and may progress in the absence of further exposure.

Certain complicating factors may alter the radiographic appearance of CWP. TB is relatively common in patients with CWP and may produce central cavitation in some patients with PMF. Caplan syndrome or "rheumatoid pneumoconiosis," seen in coal workers with rheumatoid arthritis, is characterized radiographically by nodular opacities 0.5 to 5 cm in diameter that develop rapidly and tend to appear in crops. The nodules are more sharply defined and seen more peripherally than the masses of PMF. These lesions are not specific for CWP and may be seen in patients with silicosis or asbestosis.

Miscellaneous Pneumoconioses. A variety of inorganic dusts other than asbestos, silica, and coal dust can cause pleuropulmonary disease but are far less common. Chronic berylliosis produces a reaction that mimics sarcoidosis and is discussed in the section "Granulomatous Diseases." Aluminum workers may develop disabling pulmonary fibrosis after years of exposure to aluminum dust, usually from bauxite mining. Radiographic changes include fine to coarse reticular or reticulonodular opacities distributed throughout the lungs, along with greatly diminished lung volumes and marked pleural thickening. Apical bullae may be seen, which produce spontaneous pneumothoraces. Hard metal pneumoconiosis, formerly called giant cell interstitial pneumonitis, may result from exposure to cobalt and tungsten alloys and can cause interstitial pneumonitis with varying degrees of fibrosis. The chest radiograph demonstrates a reticulonodular pattern that may be very coarse and, if advanced, may be associated with small cystic shadows. Lymph node enlargement may be seen.

Hypersensitivity Pneumonitis

Hypersensitivity pneumonitis or *extrinsic allergic alveolitis* is an immunologic pulmonary disorder associated with the inhalation of one of the antigenic organic dusts. These dusts must be of small particle size to penetrate into the alveolar spaces and incite a host inflammatory response. A wide variety of etiologic agents have been implicated, including many thermophilic bacteria, true fungi, and various animal proteins. Some of the more common disease entities include farmer's lung (exposure to moldy hay), humidifier lung (exposure to water reservoirs contaminated by thermophilic bacteria), and bird-fancier's lung (exposure to avian proteins in feathers and excreta).

The development of hypersensitivity pneumonitis depends upon the size, number, and immunogenicity of the inhaled organic particles as well as the immune response of the host. Two forms of the disease are distinguished by their clinical presentation and immunopathogenesis. Acute disease develops 4 to 6 hours following exposure to the inciting antigen and is mediated by a type 3 (immune complex) reaction. Typical symptoms include cough, dyspnea, and fever. Chronic disease is often insidious and commonly results in interstitial pulmonary fibrosis. Patients with chronic disease often have malaise, chronic cough, and progressive dyspnea. This form of disease appears to be mediated by a type 4 (cell-mediated) immune reaction.

The histopathologic features of the different types of hypersensitivity pneumonitis are usually indistinguishable, except in rare situations where antigenic material can be identified in the pathologic preparations. The pathologic features are dependent on the intensity of exposure to the allergen and on the stage of disease when tissue biopsy is obtained. Early findings include capillary congestion and inflammation within alveolar septae. In later stages of acute disease, bronchiolitis and alveolitis with granuloma formation are present. With repeated antigenic exposure, there is a progressive increase in interstitial fibrosis, which is initially patchy in distribution but may progress to diffuse interstitial fibrosis.

The radiographic changes of hypersensitivity pneumonitis parallel the pathologic findings. The chest radiograph may be normal early in the acute stage of disease. Within hours, fine nodular or ground glass opacities develop, most often in the lower lobes; progressive airspace opacification may simulate pulmonary edema. Within hours to days, the opacities resolve and the chest radiograph becomes normal. With continued or repeated exposures, the chest radiograph will remain abnormal between acute episodes. The chronic changes appear as diffuse coarse reticular or reticulonodular opacities in the mid-lung and upper lung zones; a honeycomb pattern with loss of lung volume may be seen. The diagnosis of hypersensitivity pneumonitis should be considered when repeated episodes of rapidly changing ground glass or airspace opacification are seen in a patient with underlying coarse interstitial lung disease. Hilar or mediastinal lymph node enlargement and pleural effusion are uncommon findings in patients with hypersensitivity pneumonitis.

Thin-section CT may be very helpful in the diagnosis of hypersensitivity pneumonitis, particularly in the subacute phase, when chest radiographs may be normal or quite nonspecific. The most common findings in the acute phase of disease are airspace opacities. The subacute phase is characterized by patchy areas of ground glass opacity and poorly defined ("fuzzy") centrilobular nodules (Figs. 17.7, 17.11) (7). These findings may be superimposed on one another and both show a predilection in the mid- and lower lung zones. In the chronic phase of the disease, findings are those of fibrosis: interlobular and intralobular interstitial thickening, honeycombing, and traction bronchiectasis (Fig. 17.27). Distribution of disease is varied, but sometimes there is relative sparing of the costophrenic angles, which may help to distinguish hypersensitivity pneumonitis from UIP.

The diagnosis of hypersensitivity pneumonitis is made by eliciting a history that suggests a temporal relationship between the patient's symptoms and certain exposures. The intermittent exposure of susceptible persons to high concentrations of antigen leads to recurrent episodes that typically begin 4 to 6 hours following exposure. The symptoms usually persist for 12 hours and then resolve spontaneously if the exposure has been terminated. Repeated exposure to the inciting antigen will result in acute exacerbations, with typical symptoms and radiographic findings. Chronic disease is more difficult to diagnose and develops when there is a continuous low level of exposure to the antigen. The prognosis for patients whose disease is recognized at an early stage is good if the offending agent can be removed from the patient's environment. In the more insidious chronic form of disease, the diagnosis is often delayed and considerable interstitial fibrosis may be present at the time of diagnosis. These patients generally suffer from chronic respiratory insufficiency.

GRANULOMATOUS DISEASES

Sarcoidosis

Sarcoidosis is a multisystem granulomatous disease of unknown etiology characterized histologically by noncaseating granulomas that may progress to fibrosis. The disease is seen more commonly in blacks than whites and is rare in Asians. Black women are at particular risk for this disease. Most patients are 20 to 40 years of age at the time of diagnosis; however, because patients with this disease are often asymptomatic, many cases are never identified.

The etiology of sarcoidosis is unknown, although an inhaled infectious agent such as *Mycobacterium, Yersinia,* or a virus has been suggested. Whatever the etiologic agent, the underlying pathogenesis involves activation of pulmonary macrophages, which, in turn, recruit mononuclear cells to the pulmonary interstitium, leading to the formation of granulomas. The activated macrophages also stimulate proliferation of T-helper lymphocytes in the lung, which induces an overactivity of B lymphocytes, resulting in the hypergammaglobulinemia characteristically seen in this disease. The excess number of T-helper lymphocytes in the lung may be detected in bronchoalveolar lavage (BAL) fluid of patients with sarcoidosis and is helpful in the differential diagnosis of this condition.

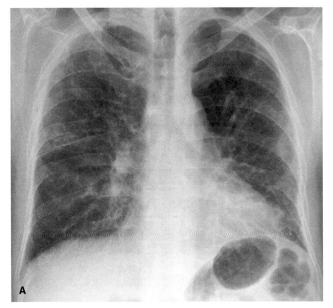

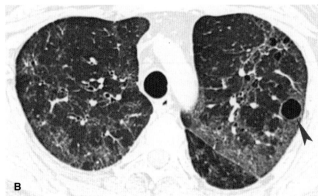

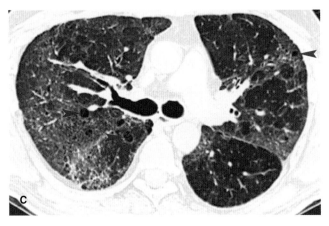

FIGURE 17.27. **Chronic Hypersensitivity Pneumonitis. A.** Chest radiograph in a farmer with chronic progressive dyspnea shows bilateral reticular opacities without zonal predilection. Axial CT scans through the upper (**B**) and mid-lungs (**C**) shows bilateral areas of reticulation and ground glass opacity. Note the presence of cysts (*arrowheads*), which have been described in hypersensitivity pneumonitis and likely reflect overdistending regions of lung distal to small airway involvement.

The pathologic changes of sarcoidosis follow a fairly predictable pattern. The earliest changes involve the pulmonary interstitium, with the development of a nonspecific lymphocytic and histiocytic infiltrate. This progresses to the formation of microscopic granulomas. The granulomas contain palisading epithelioid histiocytes with intermixed multinucleated giant cells and, in contrast to tuberculous granulomas, are typically noncaseating. The giant cells in the granulomas may contain dark-staining lamellated structures within their cytoplasm called Schaumann bodies, which are characteristic of sarcoidosis. The granulomas are found most commonly within the axial (peribronchovascular) and peripheral or subpleural interstitium of the lung, but may involve the parenchymal (alveolar) interstitium and airway mucosa; the airway lesions may be visualized bronchoscopically. Involvement of the axial interstitium of the lung accounts for the high (approximately 90%) diagnostic yield of blind transbronchial biopsy in sarcoidosis, since this technique usually provides samples of the bronchial wall, the surrounding axial interstitium, and adjacent airspaces. The small granulomas usually resolve after months or years. In some patients, the microscopic granulomas coalesce to form larger nodules. Rarely, these nodules grow to form large, well-defined masses or poorly marginated opacities that contain air bronchograms and simulate an airspace-filling process. In this "alveolar" form of sarcoidosis, the airspaces are not filled with material but are compressed and obliterated by the exuberant granuloma formation within the surrounding interstitium.

In 20% of patients, fibrous tissue is deposited at the periphery of the granulomas and eventually grows inward to replace the granulomas, resulting in interstitial fibrosis. The fibrosis tends to progress over time, with the development of broad bands of fibrous tissue extending from the hilar regions toward the lung apices, producing hilar elevation and distortion of the hilar vessels and upper mediastinum. Masses of fibrous tissue may develop in the parahilar regions of the upper lobes, with peripheral areas of emphysema or cyst formation. These cysts predispose a patient to spontaneous pneumothoraces and provide a site for mycetoma formation.

Lymph node involvement in sarcoidosis is characterized by replacement of the normal nodal architecture with granulomas that are indistinguishable from those found in the pulmonary parenchyma. As with parenchymal involvement, these may regress, coalesce, or undergo fibrosis.

The clinical presentation of sarcoidosis may be dominated by pulmonary or extrapulmonary manifestations of the disease, but a considerable percentage of patients are asymptomatic and are identified by incidental findings on chest radiographs. Pulmonary symptoms are present in 25% of patients and include dyspnea and a nonproductive cough. Common extrapulmonary findings include fever, malaise, uveitis, and erythema nodosum. In a minority of patients, involvement of the liver, heart, kidneys, or CNS may dominate the clinical picture.

Common laboratory findings in sarcoidosis include hypercalcemia, hypergammaglobulinemia, and elevated serum

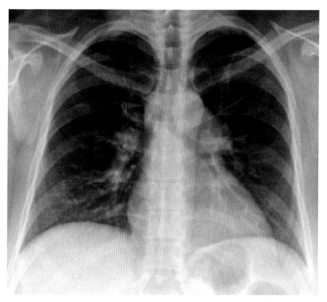

FIGURE 17.28. Sarcoidosis. Posteroanterior radiograph in an asymptomatic 26-year-old shows enlargement of right paratracheal (*blue arrowhead*), bilateral hilar (*red arrowheads*), and aortopulmonary window (*red arrow*) lymph nodes, characteristic of sarcoidosis.

angiotensin-converting enzyme levels. Cutaneous anergy to purified protein derivative tuberculin skin test (PPD) reflects an abnormality of delayed hypersensitivity found in these patients. Pulmonary function tests vary from normal in those with minimal or no parenchymal disease to a severe restrictive pattern with low diffusing capacity in patients with end-stage pulmonary fibrosis.

Lymph Node Enlargement. Enlargement of mediastinal and hilar lymph nodes is found in 80% of patients with sarcoidosis and is associated with radiographically normal lungs in slightly more than half of these patients (8). The classic appearance on chest radiographs is the combination of right paratracheal and bilateral symmetric hilar lymph node enlargement (Fig. 17.28). The symmetric enlargement is a key feature that allows distinction from malignancy and TB, conditions that usually produce unilateral or asymmetric lymph node enlargement. Left paratracheal lymph node enlargement is common, as determined by CT, although enlargement of these nodes is usually not appreciated on radiographs because the region is obscured by the aorta and great vessels on frontal radiographs. The enlarged nodes tend to have a lobulated contour because the individual nodes remain discrete. Mediastinal (paratracheal) lymph node enlargement without concomitant hilar enlargement is uncommon and should suggest lymphoma or metastatic disease. Similarly, unilateral hilar nodal enlargement is unusual, seen in only 5% of individuals. CT has shown that involvement of anterior mediastinal, posterior mediastinal, subcarinal, and aortopulmonary lymph nodes occurs with greater frequency than was previously thought based on the radiographic appearance.

The enlarged lymph nodes regress within 2 years in 75% of affected patients. A small percentage of patients will have persistent lymph node enlargement for years. The development of parenchymal opacities concomitant with the resolution of lymph node enlargement is a helpful feature in differentiating sarcoidosis from lymphoma, in which enlarged lymph nodes do not regress when parenchymal abnormalities develop. Calcification of involved lymph nodes is seen in up to 20% of patients and may involve only the periphery of the node ("eggshell" calcification).

Lung Disease. The lung is involved radiographically in only 40% to 50% of patients with sarcoidosis, despite the nearly 90% yield from transbronchial biopsy of the lung. The most common parenchymal abnormality is bilateral symmetric reticulonodular opacities show a predilection for the mid- and upper lung zones (Fig. 17.29). The reticulonodular opacities represent the combination of granulomas and fibrosis. CT shows that most nodules lie predominantly in a peribronchovascular and subpleural location (Fig. 17.30A). The appearance of reticulonodular opacities never precedes the enlargement of hilar and mediastinal lymph nodes. The earliest parenchymal finding is a diffuse micronodular pattern, identical in appearance to miliary TB, which represents the superimposition of microscopic granulomas (Fig. 17.30B). This pattern, which is rarely identified radiographically, may precede the development of hilar lymph node enlargement.

In approximately 10% of patients, the coalescence of granulomas produces one of two unusual radiographic manifestations of parenchymal sarcoidosis. Exuberant interstitial granulomas can obliterate adjacent airspaces, producing poorly defined airspace opacities that may contain air bronchograms. In some cases, intra-alveolar inflammation and granulomas contribute to the alveolar pattern of disease. These airspace opacities are primarily seen in the peripheral portions of the mid-lung zone, thereby simulating eosinophilic pneumonia and cryptogenic organizing radiographically. The presence of reticulonodular opacities elsewhere in the lung or concomitant symmetric hilar and mediastinal lymph node enlargement, best seen on CT and thin-section CT, provide important clues to the diagnosis.

Nodular or mass-like sarcoidosis develops in a manner similar to alveolar disease. These masses can be quite large and typically have a sharp margin. Air bronchograms are often demonstrated on CT and thin-section CT (Fig. 17.30C); cavitation is extremely rare.

Pulmonary fibrosis develops in 20% of patients with longstanding parenchymal involvement. The chest radiograph shows coarse linear opacities extending obliquely from the hila toward the upper and mid-lung zones. There is considerable distortion and elevation of the hila, with scalloping of the lung–mediastinal interface. Occasionally, conglomerate masses of fibrosis form in the upper perihilar regions that simulate the PMF of complicated silicosis. On CT, these masses contain air bronchograms with traction bronchiectasis. Distortion and obstruction of the airways from fibrosis can lead to secondary air trapping, with resultant alveolar septal disruption and paracicatricial emphysema or bullae formation (Fig. 17.31). An increase in radiographic lung volumes may accompany these cystic changes, a finding that is characteristic of bullous sarcoidosis. Mycetomas can develop within the cysts and lead to massive hemoptysis from erosion into bronchial arteries. Cysts may also rupture into the pleural space and produce spontaneous pneumothoraces.

Pleural Changes. Pleural thickening or effusion occurs in approximately 7% of patients with sarcoidosis and is the result of granulomatous inflammation of the visceral and parietal pleura. Aggregation of nodules along the pleural surface can cause pleural pseudoplaques.

Miscellaneous Findings. Endobronchial granulomas can result in fibrosis of the bronchial wall and bronchial stenosis. Pulmonary arterial hypertension is an uncommon finding and is usually secondary to long-standing pulmonary fibrosis.

Thin-section CT Findings. Thin-section CT is clearly more sensitive than chest radiographs in detecting the parenchymal abnormalities of sarcoidosis. A variety of thin-section CT findings have been described in this disease, which represent both the granulomatous and fibrotic response seen histologically (Figs. 17.29B, 17.30). The most frequent finding is the

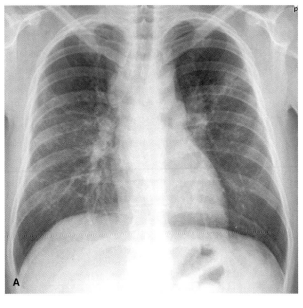

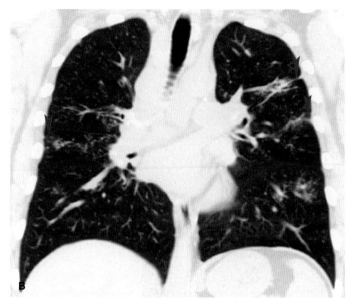

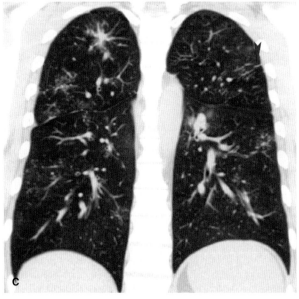

FIGURE 17.29. Sarcoidosis With Reticulonodular Opacities. A. Frontal radiograph in a patient with sarcoidosis shows bilateral predominantly midzone reticulonodular opacities in association with bilateral hilar and paratracheal lymph node enlargement. CT scans with coronal reformations through the mid- (**B**) and posterior (**C**) lungs shows patchy areas of clustered micronodules with some admixed reticulation (*arrowheads*) in the upper and mid-lungs.

presence of interstitial nodules, 3 to 10 mm in diameter, seen as nodular thickening of the peribronchoarterial (axial) interstitium and interlobular septa or as subpleural nodules. The nodules correlate closely with the coalescing noncaseating granulomas seen microscopically on tissue specimens. Septal thickening, thickening of bronchovascular bundles, architectural distortion, lung cysts, honeycombing, and central conglomerate masses with crowded, ectatic bronchi are findings indicative of fibrosis from long-standing disease. Segmental or mass-like airspace opacities, termed "alveolar" sarcoid, usually indicate the presence of active disease and resolve with corticosteroid therapy. Likewise, the finding of patchy areas of ground glass density has been shown to correlate with increased uptake on gallium scans and may be indicative of an active alveolitis. Several recent papers have showed good correlation between conventional CT and thin-section CT findings and pulmonary function tests.

Radiographic Staging of Sarcoidosis. The chest radiographic manifestations of sarcoidosis have been divided into five stages (Table 17.6). These stages generally parallel the

course of disease and are useful for prognostic purposes. Stage 1 disease is associated with a 75% rate of resolution, whereas only 30% of patients with stage 2 and 10% of patients with stage 3 disease resolve.

The diagnosis of sarcoidosis is usually based on the histologic demonstration of noncaseating granulomas involving multiple organs. Tissue is most often obtained by bronchoscopically guided transbronchial biopsy, which provides a diagnosis in up to 90% of patients. Biopsy of organs likely to be involved in this disease, such as the liver and scalene lymph nodes, will provide a diagnosis in a majority of patients. Percutaneous needle biopsy can provide diagnostic tissue specimens in those with mass-like pulmonary lesions. In certain situations, the diagnosis of sarcoidosis is made on a constellation of chest radiographic findings and characteristic eye or skin changes. In such patients, gallium scintigraphy showing a pattern of increased uptake in the hilar lymph nodes, lung, and salivary glands may be used as a confirmatory test. Gallium scanning has also been used to assess the degree of disease activity.

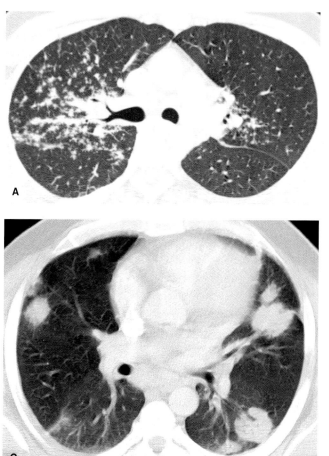

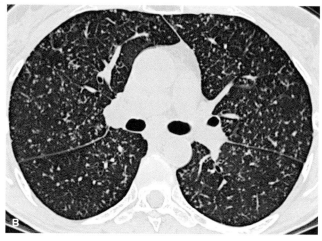

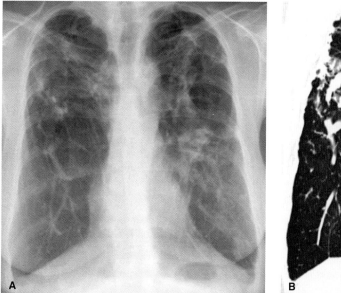

FIGURE 17.30. CT Appearances of Pulmonary Sarcoidosis. Sarcoidosis in three different patients showing (A) typical perilymphatic nodules, (B) miliary nodules, and (C) mass-like opacities. The latter two appearances are uncommon.

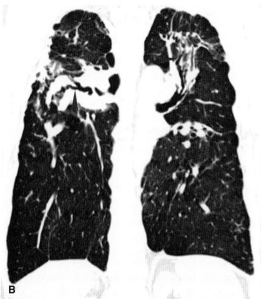

FIGURE 17.31. Stage IV (Fibrotic) Sarcoidosis. A. In a 65-year-old woman with a 25-year history of sarcoidosis, frontal chest radiograph shows coarse reticular opacities with marked elevation and distortion of the hila and mediastinal reflections. B. CT scan with coronal reformation shows perihilar fibrosis with traction bronchiectasis (*arrowheads*). Note the relative absence of nodules in this stage of disease.

TABLE 17.6

RADIOGRAPHIC STAGING OF SARCOIDOSIS

■ STAGE	■ RADIOGRAPHIC FINDINGS
0	Normal chest radiograph
1	Bilateral hilar lymph node enlargement
2	Bilateral hilar lymph node enlargement and parenchymal disease
3	Parenchymal disease only
4	Pulmonary fibrosis

Berylliosis

Although berylliosis is actually an inhalational lung disease, it is discussed here because of the clinical, pathologic, and radiographic similarities to sarcoidosis. This uncommon disease produces noncaseating granulomas in multiple organs, with primary lung involvement. The radiographic features of berylliosis are indistinguishable from those of sarcoidosis. Hilar and mediastinal lymph node enlargement and bilateral reticulonodular opacities are the most common findings. Progression to end-stage interstitial fibrosis with honeycombing or upper lobe bullous disease may occur, with the latter predisposing the patient to aspergilloma formation and spontaneous pneumothoraces.

Langerhans Cell Histiocytosis of Lung

The entity of LCH includes several disorders with similar pathologic features that differ in age at the time of diagnosis, mode of presentation, specific organs involved, and prognosis. The form of this disease affecting adults, also called eosinophilic granuloma (EG), presents with predominant involvement of lung and bones. The disease most commonly affects young adults and has no sex predilection. There is a very high association between pulmonary involvement and cigarette smoking.

Pathologically, LCH of lung demonstrates multiple small nodules, which are found predominantly in the axial interstitial tissues of the upper and mid-lung zones around small bronchioles. The nodules are granulomas composed predominantly of cells with eosinophilic cytoplasm, previously called histiocytosis X cells, and now known as Langerhans cells. They are normally found in the skin, where they act as antigen-processing cells, and appear to proliferate in the lung and other organs in response to an unidentified antigenic stimulus. In some patients, the nodular phase of disease may be preceded by an exudative phase, with filling of the alveolar spaces with a cellular exudate containing the Langerhans cells. The small peribronchiolar nodules may coalesce to form larger nodules, which may cavitate, or they may extend to infiltrate the alveolar septa and induce an interstitial inflammatory reaction. The nodules may resolve completely, but in most patients, the central portions of the nodules undergo fibrosis, producing a stellate nodular lesion that is characteristic of pulmonary LCH histologically. In the late stages, characteristic findings include fibrosis and the development of small, uniform, thin-walled cysts. Larger peripheral cysts or bullae may develop in the apical regions, presumably as a result of bronchiolar obstruction by fibrosis, with distal air trapping.

Pulmonary symptoms are present in two-thirds of patients with LCH of lung at presentation. Cough and the gradual

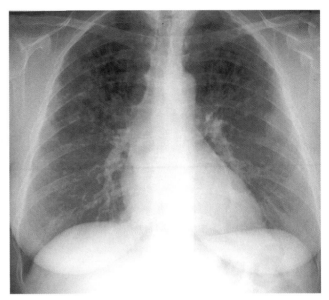

FIGURE 17.32. Langerhans Cell Histiocytosis (LCH) of Lung. Posteroanterior radiograph in a 52-year-old woman with LCH shows a nodular pattern with a middle and upper zone predominance.

onset of dyspnea are the most common complaints. Pleuritic chest pain may indicate the development of a spontaneous pneumothorax from rupture of a subpleural cyst. Pulmonary function tests reflect the fibrosis and cystic changes seen in this disorder, with characteristic restrictive and obstructive patterns of disease and a diminished diffusing capacity.

The radiographic findings in LCH of the lung usually follow a predictable pattern (9). Although the earliest changes in LCH of the lung are associated with filling of alveoli, the radiographic demonstration of airspace opacities is uncommon. The earliest findings are small to medium nodular opacities that tend to have an upper and mid-lung zone distribution (Fig. 17.32). In some cases the nodules coalesce to form larger nodules or masses, which rarely cavitate. The nodular pattern may resolve completely or be replaced by a predominantly reticulonodular or reticular pattern that represents the fibrotic phase of the disease. Late stages of the disease are characterized by a coarse reticular pattern with intermixed thin-walled cysts. These cysts account for the relative preservation or increase in lung volumes typical of LCH, which is a distinguishing feature of this disease. Hilar or mediastinal lymph node enlargement is distinctly uncommon, a feature that helps distinguish LCH from sarcoidosis. Pneumothorax from rupture of a cyst or bulla is the presenting finding or develops during the course of disease in up to 25% of patients. Pleural effusion in the absence of a pneumothorax is rare. Extrapulmonary manifestations include well-defined lytic rib or vertebral lesions.

The parenchymal changes of LCH of the lung are best demonstrated on thin-section CT. Thin-section CT in patients with a relatively short duration of symptoms (<6 months) shows well-defined interstitial nodules of varying size, sometimes with cavitation, and cyst formation in the upper lungs. More long-standing disease is characterized by larger cysts (Fig. 17.33) and honeycombing. Nodules and thick-walled cysts can transform into thin-walled cysts, suggesting that the sequence of evolution of LCH lesions is as follows: nodule right arrow cavitated nodule right arrow thick-walled cyst right arrow thin-walled cyst.

Features that help distinguish LCH of lung from emphysema are the presence of nodules (with or without cavitation) and thin-walled cysts in LCH that lack a constant relationship to the centrilobular core structures. The thin-section CT distinction of LCH from LAM in a woman is more difficult; an

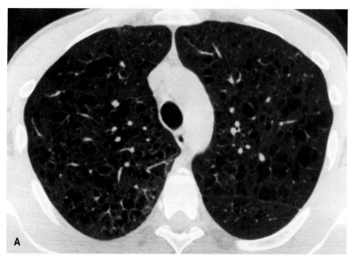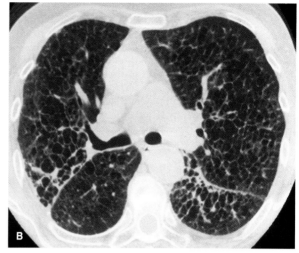

FIGURE 17.33. **Langerhans Cell Histiocytosis on Thin-Section CT. A.** Thin-section CT in a 39-year-old smoker with eosinophilic granuloma (EG) shows multiple cysts with thin but well-defined walls. **B.** In another patient with EG, the cysts are more extensive, with little normal intervening parenchyma. Note the irregular shape of many of these cysts.

upper zone distribution and the presence of nodules favor LCH. Nodules in LAM also tend to be more uniform in shape, whereas nodules in LCH can be bizarre appearing.

The diagnosis of LCH of lung is made by noting the characteristic stellate nodular lesions with Langerhans cells on open lung biopsy specimens. The treatment for symptomatic patients is corticosteroid therapy, although more than half of the patients with lung disease stabilize or improve spontaneously.

Wegener Granulomatosis

Wegener granulomatosis is a systemic autoimmune disorder characterized pathologically by a necrotizing granulomatous vasculitis involving the upper and lower respiratory tracts and kidneys. The characteristic lesions in the lungs are discrete nodules or masses of granulomatous inflammation with central necrosis and cavitation. The lesions involve pulmonary vessels, accounting for the high incidence of central necrosis and for

the occasional presentation with pulmonary hemorrhage. Mucosal and submucosal lesions may be present in the tracheobronchial tree and are seen almost exclusively in women.

Most patients with Wegener granulomatosis are middle-aged, with a slight male predominance. The respiratory tract is affected in 100% of patients, with symptoms usually dominated by sinus and nasal mucosal involvement. Pulmonary involvement may be asymptomatic or manifested by cough, dyspnea, or chest pain. Presentation with pulmonary hemorrhage and hemoptysis may mimic other pulmonary-renal syndromes such as Goodpasture syndrome and idiopathic pulmonary hemorrhage. Renal involvement usually follows involvement of the respiratory tract and is seen in almost 90% of patients.

The characteristic chest radiographic features of lung involvement in Wegener granulomatosis are multiple sharply marginated nodules or masses (Fig. 17.34); solitary lesions are seen in up to one-third of patients. Irregular, thick-walled cavitary lesions are seen in 50% of patients during the course of disease (10). Localized or diffuse areas of airspace opacification can represent hemorrhage or pneumonia, the latter often

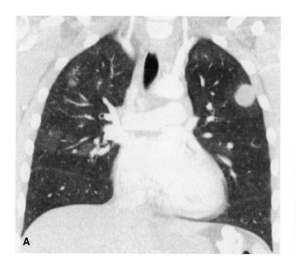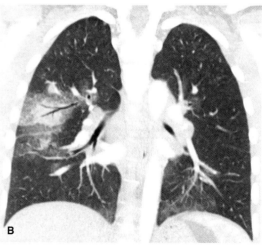

FIGURE 17.34. **Wegener Granulomatosis. A and B.** Coronal reconstructions of a CT scan in a patient with Wegener granulomatosis show a large mass with indistinct margins in the right upper lobe, a large area of ground glass opacity in the right upper lobe, and diffuse centrilobular ground glass nodules.

a result of complicating *Staphylococcus aureus* infection. Tracheal or bronchial lesions may be present and are usually best appreciated on CT, where they appear as calcified mucosal or submucosal deposits, which produce irregular narrowing of the airway lumen. The airway lesions are usually not associated with parenchymal disease, but endobronchial lesions may produce distal atelectasis. Pleural effusion from pleural involvement is not uncommon. Pneumothorax may result from rupture of a cavitary lesion into the pleural space. Lymph node enlargement is not seen in this disease.

The diagnosis of Wegener granulomatosis is be made by biopsy of involved tissues, usually nasal mucosa or lung, showing granulomatous inflammation and vasculitis that are characteristic of this disease. The pathologic changes in the kidneys are often nonspecific and therefore renal biopsy is often nondiagnostic. This disease usually responds dramatically to cyclophosphamide (Cytoxan) therapy. Some patients with disease limited to the chest respond to oral co-trimoxazole (Bactrim). Untreated patients invariably die of renal failure or, less commonly, progressive respiratory disease. High serologic titers for the presence of antineutrophil cytoplasmic antibody are specific for the diagnosis of Wegener granulomatosis, although a negative test does not exclude the diagnosis, particularly in patients with limited or inactive disease.

EOSINOPHILIC LUNG DISEASE

This term refers to a heterogeneous group of allergic diseases characterized by excess eosinophils in the lung and occasionally blood. Fraser and Pare have classified these diseases into three groups: idiopathic, those of known etiology, and those associated with autoimmune or collagen vascular disorders (Table 17.7).

TABLE 17.7

EOSINOPHILIC LUNG DISEASE

Idiopathic	Simple pulmonary eosinophilia (Löffler syndrome)
	Chronic eosinophilic pneumonia
	Hypereosinophilic syndrome
Known etiology	Drugs
	Antibiotics
	Penicillins
	Nitrofurantoin
	Nonsteroidal anti-inflammatory agents
	Aspirin
	Chemotherapeutic agents
	Bleomycin
	Methotrexate
	Parasites
	Filaria
	Strongyloides
	Ascaris
	Hookworm
Autoimmune disease	Wegener granulomatosis
	Sarcoidosis
	Rheumatoid lung disease
	Polyarteritis nodosa
	Allergic angiitis and granulomatosis (Churg-Strauss syndrome)

Müller NL, Colman N, Pare PD, Fraser RS. Fraser and Pare's Diagnosis of Diseases of the Chest (4 volume set). 4th ed. Philadelphia, PA: W.B. Saunders, 1999.

Idiopathic Eosinophilic Lung Disease

The idiopathic disorders associated with eosinophilic lung disease include simple pulmonary eosinophilia, chronic eosinophilic pneumonia, and hypereosinophilic syndrome (11).

Simple pulmonary eosinophilia, also known as Löffler syndrome, is a transient pulmonary process characterized pathologically by pulmonary infiltration with an eosinophilic exudate. Most patients have a history of allergy, most commonly asthma. The characteristic radiographic findings are peripheral, homogeneous, ill-defined areas of airspace opacities that may parallel the chest wall (Fig. 17.35); this latter feature is best appreciated on CT. The opacities in Löffler syndrome have been described as fleeting because there is a tendency for rapid clearing in one area with new involvement in other areas. A dry cough, dyspnea, and peripheral blood eosinophilia are common but are not invariably present. The diagnosis is based on the combination of pulmonary symptoms, blood eosinophilia, and characteristic radiographic findings. Most patients have a self-limiting illness that resolves spontaneously within 4 weeks.

Chronic Eosinophilic Pneumonia. Patients with symptoms and radiographic abnormalities that last longer than 1 month are considered to have chronic eosinophilic pneumonia. The clinical and radiographic features are similar to those of Löffler syndrome, although there is a distinct predilection for women. Patients are usually symptomatic with fever, malaise, and dyspnea. The pulmonary symptoms and radiographic opacities respond dramatically to corticosteroid therapy and improve within 4 to 7 days, although relapse upon discontinuation of treatment is common.

Hypereosinophilic syndrome is a systemic disorder with a male predominance that is characterized by multiple organ damage from eosinophilic infiltration of tissues. Blood eosinophilia is prolonged and marked in this condition. The major chest radiographic findings are associated with cardiac involvement causing congestive heart failure: cardiomegaly, pulmonary edema, and pleural effusions. Pulmonary parenchymal infiltration with eosinophils may produce interstitial or airspace opacities.

Eosinophilic Lung Disease of Identifiable Etiology

Pulmonary eosinophilia of known etiology includes drug and parasite-induced eosinophilic lung disease. Drugs associated with pulmonary eosinophilia include nitrofurantoin and penicillin. The parasitic infections most commonly responsible are filaria and the roundworms *Ascaris lumbricoides* and *Strongyloides stercoralis.* These parasites may produce pulmonary eosinophilia as they migrate through the alveolar capillaries and into the alveoli during their tour of the body. These disorders are usually indistinguishable clinically and radiographically from Löffler syndrome.

Eosinophilic Lung Disease Associated With Autoimmune Diseases

A number of autoimmune disorders are associated with eosinophilic pulmonary infiltrates. These include Wegener granulomatosis, sarcoidosis, rheumatoid lung disease, polyarteritis nodosa, and allergic angiitis and granulomatosis. The first three disorders have a variety of thoracic manifestations and are discussed elsewhere. The predominant chest radiographic finding in polyarteritis nodosa is hemorrhage caused by a vasculitis involving the bronchial arterial circulation. This

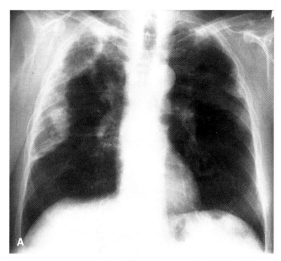
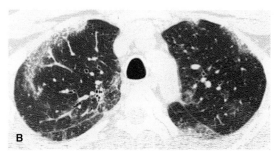

FIGURE 17.35. Eosinophilic Pneumonia. **A.** In a 38-year-old man with asthma, shortness of breath, and peripheral eosinophilia, a frontal chest film demonstrates bilateral peripheral airspace opacities. The patient's symptoms and the radiographic findings improved rapidly following initiation of corticosteroid therapy. **B.** CT scan in a different patient with eosinophilic pneumonia shows peripheral ground glass opacity with reticulation in the upper lungs.

condition is discussed in Chapter 14. Allergic angiitis and granulomatosis (Churg-Strauss syndrome) is a multisystem disorder in which asthma, blood eosinophilia, necrotizing vasculitis, and extravascular granulomas are invariable features. Pulmonary involvement, as seen radiographically or pathologically, is indistinguishable from chronic eosinophilic pneumonia.

DRUG-INDUCED LUNG DISEASE

Drugs can induce a variety of adverse effects in the chest (13). The majority of cases of drug-induced chest disease are iatrogenic, although accidental or intentional drug overdoses may also result in severe pulmonary disease. The clinical and imaging findings are often difficult to distinguish from infection, pulmonary edema, or a pulmonary manifestation of the disease being treated. The major histologic principal patterns of drug-induced lung damage are diffuse alveolar damage, UIP, NSIP, BOOP, eosinophilic lung disease, and pulmonary hem-

orrhage (Table 17.8). DAD, eosinophilic lung disease, and pulmonary hemorrhage are usually the result of an acute lung insult. UIP, NSIP, and BOOP are more commonly due to chronic toxicity.

Patterns of Drug-Induced Lung Disease

Diffuse alveolar damage most commonly results from an acute insult to the lungs resulting in damage to type II pneumocytes and the alveolar endothelium. The initial manifestation is pulmonary edema, frequently in a geographic or nondependent distribution without much associated pleural fluid or interlobular septal thickening. After discontinuation of the offending drug, it may resolve, stabilize or progress to fibrosis, frequently in an UIP pattern (Fig. 17.36). Drugs that commonly cause diffuse alveolar damage include chemotherapeutic agents (busulphan, bleomycin, BCNU, and cyclophosphamide), gold salts, mitomycin, and melphalan. Opiates can also cause acute pulmonary edema.

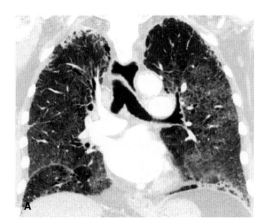
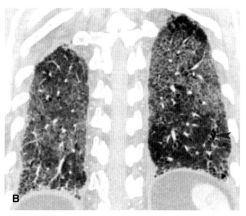

FIGURE 17.36. **Cytoxan-Induced Diffuse Alveolar Damage.** CT scans with coronal reformations through the mid- (**A**) and posterior (**B**) lungs in a patient with biopsy proven mixed proliferative and organizing diffuse alveolar damage from Cytoxan shows bilateral ground glass and reticular opacities, with foci of traction bronchiectasis (*arrowheads*).

TABLE 17.8

HISTOLOGIC PATTERNS IN DRUG-INDUCED LUNG TOXICITY

■ HISTOLOGY	■ COMMON CAUSES
DAD	Cyclophosphamide Bleomycin Carmustine (BCNU, bis-chloronitrosurea) Gold salts Mitomycin Melphalan
UIP	Cyclophosphamide Bleomycin Methotrexate
NSIP	Carmustine Amiodarone Methotrexate Gold salts Chlorambucil
Eosinophilic pneumonia	Penicillamine Sulfasalazine Nitrofurantoin NSAIDs Para-amino salicylic acid
BOOP	Bleomycin Gold salts Cyclophosphamide Methotrexate Amiodarone Nitrofurantoin Penicillamine Sulfasalazine
Hemorrhage	Anticoagulants Amphotericin B Cyclophosphamide Mitomycin Cytarabine (Ara-C, arabinofuranosyl cytidine) Penicillamine

DAD, diffuse alveolar damage; BCNU, bis-chloronitrosurea; UIP, usual interstitial pneumonitis; NSIP, nonspecific interstitial pneumonia; NSAIDs, nonsteroidal anti-inflammatory drugs; BOOP, bronchiolitis obliterans with organizing pneumonia.

UIP can be the result of diffuse alveolar damage or occur as a result of chronic drug toxicity. The drugs most commonly implicated in this form of lung disease are amiodarone, nitrofurantoin, and the chemotherapeutic agents cyclophosphamide, bleomycin, and methotrexate. Radiographically, patients present with bilateral, predominantly lower lobe, coarse reticular and linear opacities with diminished lung volumes. In patients undergoing chemotherapy for malignancy, the findings are difficult to distinguish from those of lymphangitic carcinomatosis, pulmonary hemorrhage, or opportunistic pneumonia. Pulmonary edema is the major differential diagnosis in patients on amiodarone therapy. The diagnosis can usually be made by excluding one of these other processes or thin-section CT.

NSIP (also referred to as chronic interstitial pneumonia when known to result from drug toxicity) is most commonly encountered with amiodarone, methotrexate, and BCNU therapy. Gold salts and chlorambucil are less common causes.

BOOP is a relatively common result of pulmonary drug toxicity and usually responds well to cessation of therapy and steroids. A large number of drugs have been reported to cause BOOP, most commonly bleomycin, cyclophosphamide, methotrexate and gold salts, and less commonly amiodarone, nitrofurantoin, penicillamine, and sulfasalazine. Biological agents including the TNF-alpha monoclonal antibody rituximab, used in non-Hodgkin lymphoma and rheumatoid arthritis, has been shown to rarely produce organizing pneumonia with associated interstitial pneumonitis (Fig. 17.37).

Eosinophilic pneumonia results from a hypersensitivity response to a metabolite of the drug combined with an endogenous protein. Antibody production directed against this hapten–protein complex leads to antibody-mediated immediate or immune complex hypersensitivity reactions. It is usually associated with fever, skin rash, and blood eosinophilia. Radiographically, fleeting peripheral patchy airspace opacities develop hours to days after the initiation of drug therapy. The opacities often respond to corticosteroid therapy. Penicillin and sulfonamide antibiotics are the drugs most often associated with hypersensitivity reactions.

Pulmonary hemorrhage may be caused by drug-induced pulmonary vasculitis, complicate anticoagulation therapy or result from drug-induced thrombocytopenia. Penicillamine therapy has been associated with pulmonary hemorrhage in patients with rheumatoid arthritis, but the mechanism is unknown. Affected individuals typically have hemoptysis and a falling hematocrit associated with the rapid development of diffuse bilateral airspace opacities. The diagnosis of hemorrhage is usually confirmed by bloody fluid return on bronchoalveolar lavage. Lavage also shows an increased percentage of alveolar macrophages containing hemosiderin. The opacities of diffuse pulmonary hemorrhage resolve completely without residual scarring unless accompanied by pulmonary infarction, which may leave pleural and parenchymal scars.

Other Manifestations. Pulmonary nodules are an uncommon manifestation of chronic lung injury from bleomycin or Cytoxan, and in this situation, they are radiographically indistinguishable from pulmonary metastases.

A number of drugs, most commonly procainamide, hydralazine, and isoniazid, have been associated with a lupus-like syndrome that is often indistinguishable from SLE. Pleural and pericardial effusions are common. Basilar interstitial disease has been described but is uncommon.

Obliterative bronchiolitis is a small airways inflammatory process that results in granulation tissue within bronchioles causing air-trapping, which can be severe enough to result in respiratory insufficiency. It can result from a variety of insults including aspiration, organ transplantation, viral infection, collagen vascular disease, and drugs, especially penicillamine, and is described in more detail in Chapter 18.

A chronic granulomatous vasculitis may develop as a response to particulate substances such as talc or starch mixed with illicit IV drugs. This can lead to obliteration of the pulmonary vasculature, producing pulmonary hypertension and RV failure. Radiographically, the lungs may show an interstitial pattern of disease, with enlargement of the central pulmonary arteries and right heart (12). The radiographs may rarely show central conglomerate masses that are indistinguishable from PMF of silicosis or end-stage sarcoidosis.

Enlargement of the hilar and mediastinal lymph nodes on chest radiographs is an uncommon manifestation of drug toxicity. Dilantin and methotrexate are the main drugs associated with this rare complication. The lymphadenopathy is usually part of a systemic hypersensitivity reaction and regresses with removal of the offending agent.

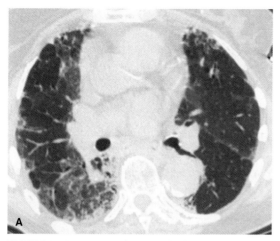
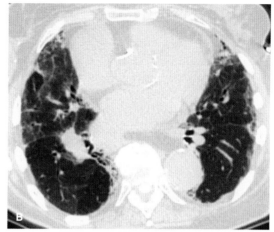

FIGURE 17.37. **Rituximab-Induced Diffuse Lung Disease. A.** Chest radiograph in a patient receiving rituximab to prevent renal transplant rejection shows a diffuse bilateral pattern of ground glass and basilar airspace opacification. **B.** CT with coronal reformation shows a mixed pattern of ground glass opacity and patchy air space opacities (*arrowheads*) and minimal reticulation. Open lung biopsy showed a mixed pattern of organizing pneumonia and interstitial pneumonitis. The patient responded to discontinuation of the rituximab and corticosteroid administration.

Common Drugs Exhibiting Pulmonary Toxicity (Table 17.9)

Nitrofurantoin is an oral antibiotic used widely in the treatment of urinary tract infections. There are two distinct patterns of nitrofurantoin-associated pulmonary reaction: acute and chronic. The acute form, seen in approximately 90% of cases, most likely represents a hypersensitivity reaction. The chest radiograph demonstrates interstitial or mixed alveolar/interstitial infiltrates with a basal predominance, often accompanied by small pleural effusions. The chronic form occurs after weeks to years of continuous therapy and is probably caused by direct toxic damage. Interstitial pneumonitis and fibrosis indistinguishable from IPF are seen pathologically (13) (Fig. 17.38).

Bleomycin is a cytotoxic antibiotic used in the treatment of lymphoma, squamous cell carcinoma, and testicular cancer. Bleomycin-induced lung disease is related to the cumulative dosage of the drug. Free oxygen radicals within the lung are felt to play a major role in the lung injury and account for the deleterious effects of supplemental oxygen administration in patients with bleomycin toxicity. The typical radiographic pattern is that of bilateral lower lobe reticular opacities. A minority of patients will demonstrate acute patchy or confluent airspace opacities as a result of a hypersensitivity reaction to the drug or DAD. The reticular or airspace opacities tend to have a basal predominance. Solitary or multiple pulmonary nodules constitute an unusual radiographic appearance of bleomycin lung toxicity that is indistinguishable radiographically from pulmonary metastases, but the lesions generally disappear following cessation of the drug.

Alkylating Agents. Drugs such as busulfan, which is used in the treatment of myeloproliferative disorders, and cyclophosphamide (Cytoxan), used widely in the treatment of malignancies and autoimmune disease, cause clinically recognizable pulmonary toxicity in 1% to 4% of patients. Pathologic findings include organizing intra-alveolar exudate, fibrosis, and the presence of large atypical type 2 pneumocytes. Radiographically, a diffuse reticular pattern with basal predominance is seen; airspace opacities may be present and are more common with busulfan than cyclophosphamide.

TABLE 17.9

SPECIFIC DRUG TOXICITIES

■ DRUG	■ PRIMARY PATHOLOGY	■ TREATMENT	■ INCIDENCE	■ PROGNOSIS
Cyclophosphamide	Diffuse alveolar damage, NSIP, BOOP	Discontinue drug	Common	Good
Carmustine	Diffuse alveolar damage, NSIP	Discontinue drug	20%–50%	Good
Bleomycin	Diffuse alveolar damage, NSIP, BOOP	Discontinue drug	3%–5%	Poor
Amiodarone	NSIP, BOOP, pleural effusions	Discontinue drug	5%–10%	Good
Gold salts	Diffuse alveolar damage, NSIP, BOOP	Discontinue drug	1%	Good
Methotrexate	NSIP, HSP, BOOP	None	5%–10%	Good
Nitrofurantoin	NSIP	Discontinue drug		Good

NSIP, nonspecific interstitial pneumonia; BOOP, bronchiolitis obliterans with organizing pneumonia; HSP, hypersensitivity pneumonitis.

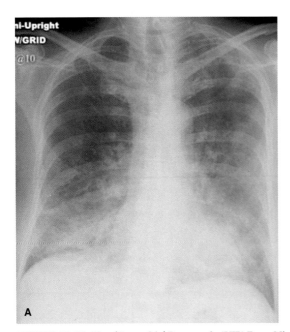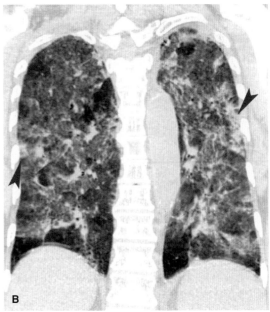

FIGURE 17.38. Usual Interstitial Pneumonia (UIP) From Nitrofurantoin Administration. Axial CT scans through the mid (**A**) and lower (**B**) lungs in an elderly woman receiving nitrofurantoin prophylaxis for recurrent urinary tract infections shows bilateral subpleural reticulation with traction bronchiectasis (*arrowheads*) consistent with UIP.

Cytosine arabinoside (Ara-C) is an antimetabolic agent generally used to treat acute leukemia. Pulmonary toxicity develops in 15% to 30% of treated patients within 30 days of administration and is manifested as pulmonary edema resulting from increased capillary permeability.

Methotrexate is an antimetabolite used for the treatment of malignancies and autoimmune diseases such as rheumatoid arthritis and psoriasis. In contrast to bleomycin and the alkylating agents, methotrexate usually causes reversible pulmonary disease caused by a hypersensitivity reaction rather than direct toxic damage to the lung. Diffuse alveolar damage leading to restrictive lung disease is seen in approximately 10% of cases, however, and appears radiographically as a diffuse reticular pattern.

Amiodarone, an antiarrhythmic agent, is an important cause of drug-induced pulmonary damage, affecting approximately 5% of individuals on chronic therapy. Amiodarone is concentrated in the lung and has a long tissue half-life. The exact mechanism of lung damage is unknown but relates to the accumulation of phospholipids, which disturb metabolic functions in the lung. Pathologically, there is inflammation and fibrosis of the alveolar septae, with an accumulation of lipid-laden alveolar macrophages and hyperplasia of type 2 pneumocytes.

Pulmonary toxicity begins months to years after the initiation of therapy. Patients typically present with dyspnea or a nonproductive cough, which may be difficult to distinguish from congestive heart failure or pneumonia. The chest film typically shows airspace and reticular opacities. CT findings show significant overlap with findings of pulmonary edema—which is common in these patients—with reticulation and ground glass and airspace opacities. Findings of fibrosis and high attenuation within parenchymal abnormalities should strongly suggest amiodarone toxicity (Fig. 17.39). Amiodarone should be withdrawn or the dose diminished at the earliest sign of toxicity because the drug has an extraordinarily long half-life (approximately 90 days). The cessation of amiodarone at an early stage of toxicity, with occasional use of corticosteroids, usually provides relief.

MISCELLANEOUS DISORDERS

Pulmonary alveolar proteinosis (PAP) is a rare disease in which the lipoproteinaceous material surfactant deposits in abnormal amounts within the airspaces of the lung. Idiopathic PAP has a predilection for 20- to 40-year-old men, although the disease has been reported in children. In adults, PAP has been seen in patients with acute silicoproteinosis and immunocompromised patients with lymphoma, leukemia, or AIDS. These conditions are associated with an acquired defect of alveolar macrophages that causes them to fail to phagocytize surfactant, resulting in the accumulation of surfactant within the alveolar spaces. Pathologically, the alveoli are filled with a lipoproteinaceous material that stains deep pink with periodic acid-Schiff. The interstitium is usually not involved, but some patients may have chronic interstitial inflammation and fibrosis.

Patients with PAP are often asymptomatic, although some complain of progressive dyspnea and a nonproductive cough. The absence of orthopnea is an important clinical feature distinguishing PAP from pulmonary edema secondary to congestive heart failure.

The typical radiographic finding in alveolar proteinosis is bilateral symmetric perihilar airspace opacification, which is indistinguishable in appearance from pulmonary edema (Fig. 17.33). Airspace nodules are commonly seen at the periphery of the confluent opacities. Cardiomegaly, pleural effusions, and evidence of pulmonary venous hypertension are notably absent. Thin-section CT scans typically show geographic ground glass opacities superimposed upon thickened interlobular and intralobular septa, a pattern that has been described as "crazy paving." While crazy paving in the proper clinical setting is characteristic of this disease, a number of other conditions can produce this pattern on thin-section CT, most commonly pulmonary edema (particularly permeability edema), atypical pneumonia and pulmonary hemorrhage, and rarely, bronchoalveolar cell carcinoma (14).

Patients with PAP are particularly prone to superinfection of the lung with *Nocardia, Aspergillus, Cryptococcus,* and atypical mycobacteria. The factors responsible for this may

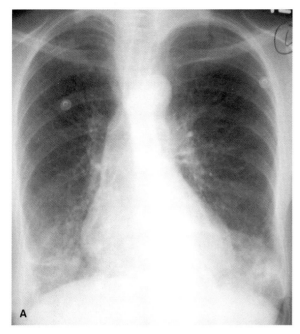

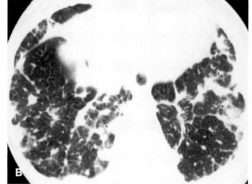

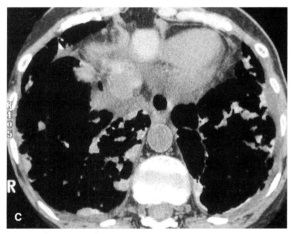

FIGURE 17.39. Amiodarone Lung Toxicity. A. Frontal chest radiograph in a 64-year-old patient who experienced progressive shortness of breath while receiving amiodarone for ventricular tachycardia shows cardiomegaly, bibasilar coarse interstitial opacities, and small pleural effusions. Thin-section unenhanced CT scan through the lung bases at lung windows (**B**) shows coarse reticular and nodular opacities, which were high attenuation at mediastinal windows (**C**), consistent with amiodarone lung toxicity.

include macrophage dysfunction and the favorable culture medium of intra-alveolar lipoproteinaceous material. Infection by one of these organisms should be suspected in any patient with PAP who develops symptoms of pneumonia or radiographic findings of focal parenchymal opacification or cavitation and pleural effusion. CT helps in the early detection of opportunistic infection because pneumonia or abscess formation may be obscured by the underlying process on conventional radiographs (Fig. 17.40).

Prior to the advent of BAL, one-third of patients died from respiratory failure or opportunistic infections, whereas the remaining two-thirds either stabilized or resolved spontaneously. Repeated BAL with saline has significantly reduced the mortality from this disease. The duration of treatment with BAL varies; some patients require repetitive long-term therapy, whereas others resolve after a single treatment. Recently, the recognition that patients with PAP have deficient levels of granulocyte macrophage–colony-stimulating factor (GM-CSF) in alveolar macrophages has led to therapy with GM-CSF, which is an alternative to lung lavage for treatment of this disease.

Alveolar microlithiasis is a rare disorder characterized by the deposition of minute calculi within the alveolar spaces. While alveolar microlithiasis can affect individuals of any age without sex predilection, there is a very high incidence of this disease in siblings. The underlying abnormality responsible for the formation of these calculi, known as calcospherites, is unknown. These are small calculi, measuring less than 1 mm in diameter, which are composed of calcium phosphate. Pathologically these calculi are found within normal alveoli; interstitial fibrosis may develop in long-standing disease. The radiographic findings are specific: confluent bilateral dense micronodular opacities that, because of their high intrinsic density, produce the so-called "black pleura sign" at their interface with the chest wall. Apical bullous disease is common and may lead to spontaneous pneumothorax. The diagnosis is made by a history of alveolar microlithiasis in a sibling of an affected individual in combination with typical radiographic findings. Biopsy is usually unnecessary. The majority of patients are asymptomatic at presentation despite the marked radiographic abnormalities, a feature that is characteristic of this disorder. Most patients develop progressive respiratory insufficiency, although some remain stable for years. There is no effective treatment.

Diffuse pulmonary ossification is an uncommon condition characterized by the formation of bone within the lung parenchyma. The nodular form of this disease is seen in mitral stenosis, whereas more irregular ossification is seen in chronic inflammatory conditions such as amyloidosis and UIP. The condition is appreciated as nodular or linear areas of high attenuation on thin-section CT. Other conditions that can produce

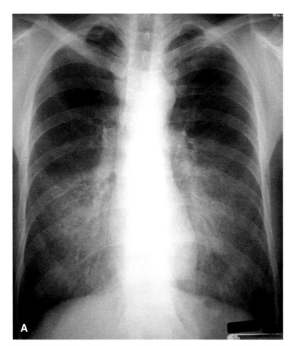 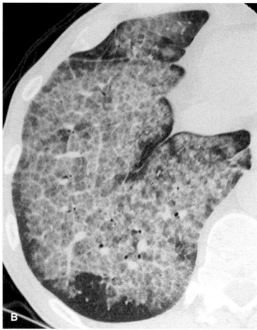

FIGURE 17.40. **Pulmonary Alveolar Proteinosis (PAP). A.** Frontal chest radiograph in a 34-year-old man with PAP demonstrates subtle bilateral ground glass opacities. **B.** A CT scan viewed at the lung windows shows a mixed pattern of ground glass attenuation superimposed on thickened interlobular and intralobular lines, which has been termed "crazy paving" and is characteristic of this disorder.

high-attenuation material in the lung parenchyma include pulmonary calcification in secondary hyperparathyroidism, in which there is an upper lobe predilection, and amiodarone lung toxicity, in which the deposition of an iodinated metabolite of amiodarone accumulates in the lung, liver, and thyroid.

References

1. Kazerooni EA. High-resolution CT of the lungs. AJR Am J Roentgenol 2001;177:501–519.
2. Pandit-Bhalla M, Diethelm L, Ovella T, et al. Idiopathic interstitial pneumonias: an update. J Thorac Imaging 2003;18:1–13.
3. Kim EA, Lee KS, Johkoh T, et al. Interstitial lung diseases associated with collagen vascular diseases: radiologic and histopathologic findings. Radiographics 2002;22:S151–S165.
4. Aylwin ACB, Gishen P, Copley SJ. Imaging appearance of thoracic amyloidosis. J Thorac Imaging 2005;20:41–46.
5. Pallisa E, Sanz P, Roman A, et al. Lymphangiomyomatosis: pulmonary and abdominal findings with pathologic correlation. Radiographics 2002;22:S185–S198.
6. Kim KI, Kim CW, Lee MK, et al. Imaging of occupational lung disease. Radiographics 2001;21:1371–1391.
7. Lynch DA, Rose CS, Way D, King TE. Hypersensitivity pneumonitis: sensitivity of high-resolution CT in a population-based study. AJR Am J Roentgenol 1992;159:469–472.
8. Koyama T, Ueda H, Togashi K, et al. Radiologic manifestations of sarcoidosis in various organs. Radiographics 2004;24:87–104.
9. Sundar KM, Gosselin MV, Chung H, Cahill BC. Pulmonary Langerhans cell histiocytosis: emerging concepts on pathobiology, radiology, and clinical evolution of disease. Chest 2003;123:1673–1683.
10. Mayberry JP, Primack SL, Muller NL. Thoracic manifestations of systemic autoimmune diseases: radiographic and high-resolution CT findings. Radiographics 2000;20:1623–1635.
11. Johkoh T, Muller NL, Akira M, et al. Eosinophilic lung diseases: diagnostic accuracy of thin-section CT in 111 patients. Radiographics 2000;216:773–780.
12. Ng CS, Wells AU, Padley SPG. A CT sign of chronic pulmonary arterial hypertension: the ratio of main pulmonary artery to aortic diameter. J Thor Imaging 1999;14:270–278.
13. Rossi SE, Erasmus JJ, McAdams HP. Pulmonary drug toxicity: radiologic and pathologic manifestations. Radiographics 2000;20:1245–1259.
14. Holbert JM, Costello P, Li W, et al. CT features of pulmonary alveolar proteinosis. AJR Am J Roentgenol 2001;176:1287–1294.

CHAPTER 18 ■ AIRWAYS DISEASE

JEFFREY S. KLEIN

Trachea and Central Bronchi Congenital Tracheal Anomalies Focal Tracheal Disease Diffuse Tracheal Disease Tracheal and Bronchial Injury Broncholithiasis	**Chronic Obstructive Pulmonary Disease** Asthma and Chronic Bronchitis Bronchiectasis Emphysema **Bullous Lung Disease** **Small Airways Disease**

TRACHEA AND CENTRAL BRONCHI

Congenital Tracheal Anomalies

Tracheal agenesis, cartilaginous abnormalities of the trachea, tracheal webs and stenosis, tracheoesophageal fistulas, and vascular rings and slings present as breathing and feeding difficulties in the neonatal and infancy period. These are uncommon congenital lesions that are discussed in Chapter 50.

Tracheoceles, also known as paratracheal air cysts, are true diverticula that represent herniation of the tracheal air column through a weakened posterior tracheal membrane. These lesions occur almost exclusively in the cervical trachea because the pressure gradient from the extrathoracic trachea to the atmosphere with the Valsalva maneuver favors their formation in this region. Tracheoceles are usually asymptomatic and are easily recognized on CT as circular lucencies along the right posterolateral trachea at the thoracic inlet.

Tracheal bronchus or bronchus suis, so called because it is the normal pattern of tracheal branching in pigs, consists of an accessory bronchus to all or a portion of the right upper lobe that arises from the right lateral tracheal wall within 2 cm of the tracheal carina (Fig. 18.1). However, it most often supplies the apical segment of the right upper lobe. While it is usually an incidental finding on chest CT in 0.5% to 1.0% of the population, there is an association with congenital tracheal stenosis and an aberrant left PA. Most patients are asymptomatic.

Focal Tracheal Disease

Focal disorders of the trachea may produce narrowing or dilatation of the tracheal lumen (Table 18.1) (1). Focal narrowing may be produced by extrinsic or intrinsic mass lesions, retraction, or inflammatory disorders of the tracheal wall.

Extrinsic Mass Effect. The most common cause of extrinsic mass effect on the trachea is a tortuous or dilated aortic arch or brachiocephalic artery, typically seen in older individuals as a rightward deviation of the distal trachea. An intrathoracic goiter or a large paratracheal lymph node mass is an additional cause of extrinsic tracheal mass effect. Extrinsic mass effect can also be seen with congenital vascular anomalies, such as an aberrant left pulmonary artery and aortic ring, or with a large mediastinal bronchogenic cyst. Because the tracheal cartilage provides resiliency, extrinsic masses tend to displace the trachea without narrowing its lumen. Traction deformity of the trachea is generally seen in cicatrizing processes that asymmetrically affect the lung apices, most commonly postprimary tuberculosis (TB), histoplasmosis, and radiation fibrosis. Occasionally the distal trachea is narrowed in patients with sclerosing mediastinitis, although this disorder normally affects the central bronchi.

Focal Tracheal Stenosis. Focal tracheal or central (main and proximal lobar) bronchial narrowing may result from inflammatory disorders that affect the tracheal or central bronchial walls. Cartilaginous damage or the development of granulation tissue and fibrosis from a tracheostomy or at the site of a previously inflated endotracheal tube balloon cuff can lead to focal tracheal narrowing (Fig. 18.2). The tracheal stenosis has a typical hourglass deformity on frontal radiographs. Those patients with tracheomalacia from cartilage damage may manifest narrowing only during phases of the respiratory cycle when extratracheal pressure exceeds intratracheal pressure. Therefore, patients with extrathoracic tracheomalacia, most often at the site of a prior tracheostomy, demonstrate tracheal narrowing on inspiration, whereas patients with intrathoracic tracheomalacia, usually from prior endotracheal intubation, have tracheal narrowing on expiration. Postintubation stenosis is rare with the low-pressure, high-volume endotracheal tube cuffs in current use. Wegener's granulomatosis can produce a necrotizing granulomatous inflammation of the trachea and central bronchi, leading to focal cervical tracheal narrowing or, in advanced disease, narrowing of the entire length of the trachea. The diagnosis of tracheal involvement by Wegener granulomatosis is made by the radiographic demonstration of tracheal narrowing in association with upper airway and renal involvement and characteristic findings on biopsy. Cyclophosphamide therapy administered early in the course of the disease may reduce inflammation and improve tracheal narrowing. Sarcoidosis involving the central airways may rarely cause focal tracheal or bronchial stenosis.

A number of infectious processes may result in tracheal or bronchial inflammation and stenosis. Endotracheal and endobronchial TB is usually associated with cavitary TB, where the production of large volumes of infected sputum predisposes

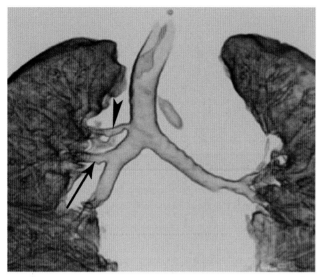

FIGURE 18.1. Tracheal Bronchus. Shaded surface rendering of a helical CT data set reveals an anomalous bronchus (*arrowhead*) supplying a portion of the right upper lobe arising from the right lateral tracheal wall above the tracheal carina. Note the right upper lobe bronchus (*arrow*).

to tracheal and central bronchial infection. Upper tracheal inflammation and stenosis may result from histoplasmosis and coccidioidomycosis. Invasive tracheobronchitis from aspergillosis, candidiasis, and mucormycosis has been described in immunocompromised patients. Tracheal scleroma is a chronic granulomatous disorder caused by infection with *Klebsiella rhinoscleromatis*. This disease is uncommon in the United States and is seen most commonly in people of lower socioeconomic standing in Central and South America and Eastern Europe. The infection begins as an inflammation of the nasal mucosa and paranasal sinuses, extending inferiorly to involve the larynx, pharynx, and trachea in a minority of patients. In its chronic phase, intense granulation tissue and fibrosis lead to stenosis of the nasal cavity, pharynx, larynx, and upper trachea; the latter is seen in fewer than 10% of patients. Radiographically, the upper trachea shows irregular nodular narrowing, which may extend to involve the length of the trachea. The diagnosis is made on biopsy, which reveals granulation tissue containing large foamy histiocytes filled with the causative organism (Mikulicz cells). Antibiotic treatment is effective if administered in the early phases of infection before extensive fibrosis has developed.

Tracheal and bronchial masses are mostly neoplasms and are discussed in Chapter 15.

Focal tracheal dilatation is caused by congenital or acquired abnormalities of the elastic membrane or cartilaginous rings of the trachea. Localized tracheal dilatation may be seen with tracheoceles, with acquired tracheomalacia related to prolonged endotracheal intubation, or as a result of tracheal traction from severe unilateral upper lobe parenchymal scarring.

Diffuse Tracheal Disease

Diffuse disorders of the trachea manifest as either narrowing or dilatation of the tracheal lumen. Diffuse tracheal narrowing may be seen with saber-sheath trachea, amyloidosis, tracheobronchopathia osteochondroplastica, relapsing polychondritis, Wegener's granulomatosis, or tracheal scleroma (Table 18.2) (2). The latter two conditions may cause diffuse tracheal narrowing, but more

TABLE 18.1

CAUSES OF FOCAL TRACHEAL DISEASE

Narrowing	Extrinsic	
		Thyroid goiter
		Paratracheal lymph node mass
		Asymmetric or unilateral upper lobe fibrosis
		Tuberculosis
		Histoplasmosis
	Intrinsic	
		Tracheomalacia
		Endotracheal tube cuff
		Tracheostomy site
	Wegener granulomatosis	
	Sarcoidosis	
	Infection	
		Tuberculosis
		Fungus
		Histoplasmosis
		Coccidioidomycosis
		Aspergillosis
		Scleroma
Masses	Neoplasm	
	Malignant	
	Primary	
		Squamous cell carcinoma
		Adenoid cystic carcinoma (cylindroma)
	Metastatic	
		Direct invasion
		Laryngeal carcinoma
		Thyroid carcinoma
		Esophageal carcinoma
		Bronchogenic carcinoma
		Hematogenous (endobronchial)
		Breast carcinoma
		Renal cell carcinoma
		Colon carcinoma
		Melanoma
	Benign	
		Chondroma
		Fibroma
		Squamous cell papilloma
		Hemangioma
		Granular cell myoblastoma
	Nonneoplastic	
		Ectopic thyroid or thymus
		Mucus
Dilatation	Tracheoceles	
	Tracheomalacia	
	Upper lobe fibrosis	

commonly the involvement is limited to the cervical trachea. These conditions are discussed in the section on focal tracheal narrowing.

Diffuse Tracheal Narrowing. Congenital tracheal stenosis is a rare condition in which there is incomplete septation of the cartilage rings, producing a long segment tracheal narrowing or "napkin ring" trachea. This anomaly is often associated with other congenital cardiovascular anomalies, in particular anomalous origin of the left PA from the right PA ("PA sling") and anomalous origin of the right upper lobe bronchus from the trachea ("tracheal bronchus" or "bronchus suis").

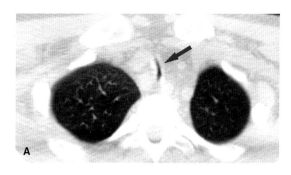

FIGURE 18.2. Tracheal Stenosis From Prior Intubation. Axial CT scan at lung windows through the upper trachea (**A**) and shaded surface rendering from helical CT scan (**B**) show marked narrowing (*arrows*) of the trachea in the coronal plane because of prior intubation with resultant stenosis.

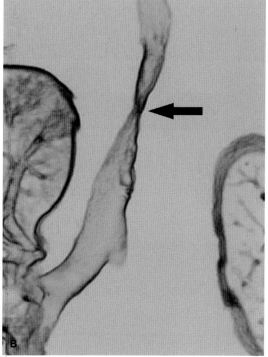

Saber-sheath trachea is a fixed deformity of the intrathoracic trachea in which the coronal diameter is diminished to less than two-thirds of the sagittal diameter. The tracheal wall is uniformly thickened, and calcification of the cartilaginous rings is present in most cases. This entity exclusively affects older men with functional evidence of chronic obstructive pulmonary disease. The tracheal narrowing likely reflects the chronic transmission of increased intrapleural pressure seen in obstructive lung disease and tracheal injury from chronic cough. The characteristic findings are apparent on frontal radiographs and CT (Fig. 18.3).

Amyloidosis is characterized by the deposition of a fibrillar protein–polysaccharide complex in various organs. It may involve the airways as part of localized or systemic disease. Submucosal deposits in the tracheobronchial tree are more commonly a manifestation of localized disease and may be associated with nodular or alveolar septal deposits in the lungs. Mass-like circumferential deposits that irregularly narrow the tracheal lumen are best demonstrated on CT and can

result in recurrent atelectasis and pneumonia. Calcification of these deposits occurs in only 10% of cases. The diagnosis is made by the presence of typical protein–polysaccharide deposits demonstrated following Congo red staining of tracheal or bronchial wall biopsy specimens. This typically demonstrates apple-green birefringence when viewed under polarized light (Fig. 18.4).

Tracheobronchopathia osteochondroplastica is a rare disorder characterized by the presence of multiple submucosal osseous and cartilaginous deposits within the trachea and central bronchi of elderly men. The lesions arise as enchondromas from the tracheal and bronchial cartilage, and then project internally to produce nodular submucosal deposits that irregularly narrow the tracheal lumen and have a characteristic

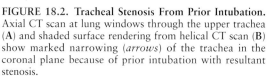

TABLE 18.2

CAUSES OF DIFFUSE TRACHEAL DISEASE

Tracheal narrowing	Congenital tracheal stenosis (complete cartilage rings)
	Saber-sheath trachea
	Amyloidosis
	Tracheobronchopathia osteochondroplastica
	Relapsing polychondritis
	Wegener granulomatosis
	Tracheal scleroma
Tracheal dilatation	Tracheobronchomegaly (Mounier–Kuhn syndrome)
	Tracheomalacia
	Pulmonary fibrosis

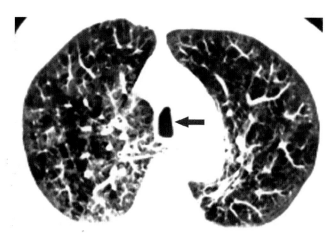

FIGURE 18.3. Saber-Sheath Trachea in Chronic Obstructive Pulmonary Disease (COPD). HRCT scan just above the tracheal carina in a 65-year-old man with COPD reveals coronal narrowing of the trachea (*arrow*), representing a saber-sheath tracheal deformity. Note the additional findings associated with cigarette smoking: centrilobular emphysema and bronchial wall thickening, the latter reflecting chronic bronchitis.

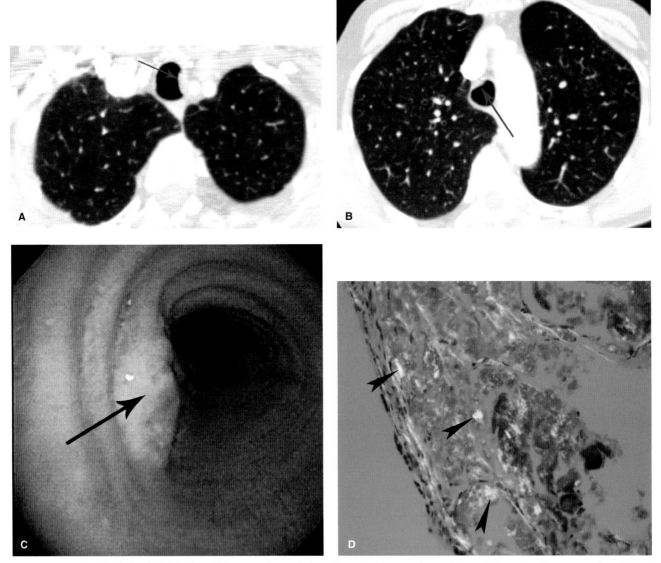

FIGURE 18.4. Amyloidosis of the Trachea. CT scans at lung windows through the upper (**A**) and lower (**B**) trachea demonstrate broad-based nodular lesions (*arrows*) along the tracheal wall. **C.** Image from fiberoptic bronchoscopy shows a raised yellowish lesion (*arrow*) along the left lateral proximal tracheal wall. **D.** Photomicrograph obtained under polarized light following Congo red staining of the endobronchial biopsy specimen shows typical apple-green birefringent crystals (*arrowheads*) characteristic of amyloid deposits.

appearance and feel on bronchoscopy. The diagnosis is generally made on bronchoscopy and CT, where calcified plaques can be seen involving the anterior and lateral walls of the trachea. Sparing of the membranous posterior wall of the trachea, which lacks cartilage, is a helpful feature that distinguishes this entity from tracheobronchial amyloid (Fig. 18.5). While usually asymptomatic, patients may have recurrent infection related to bronchial obstruction by the masses.

Relapsing polychondritis is a systemic autoimmune disorder that commonly affects the cartilage of the earlobes, nose, larynx, tracheobronchial tree, joints, and large elastic arteries. Early in the disease, tracheal wall inflammation associated with cartilage destruction leads to an abnormally compliant and dilated trachea. Later in the disease, fibrosis leads to diffuse fixed narrowing of the tracheal lumen. Respiratory complications secondary to involvement of the upper airway cartilage accounts for nearly 50% of all deaths from this condition. The diagnosis is made by noting recurrent inflammation at two or more cartilaginous sites, most commonly the pinnae of the ear (producing cauliflower ears) and the bridge of the nose (producing a saddlenose

deformity). Radiographs and CT show diffuse smooth thickening of the wall of the trachea and central bronchi with narrowing of the lumen.

Diffuse Tracheal Dilatation. *Tracheobronchomegaly* (Mounier–Kuhn syndrome) is a congenital disorder of the elastic and smooth muscle components of the tracheal wall. An association with Ehlers–Danlos syndrome, a congenital defect in collagen synthesis, and cutis laxa, a congenital defect in elastic tissue, has been reported. The disease is found almost exclusively in men under the age of 50. Abnormal compliance of the trachea and central bronchi leads to central bronchial collapse during coughing. The airways obstruction impairs mucociliary clearance, predisposing the patient to recurrent episodes of pneumonia and bronchiectasis. Symptoms are indistinguishable from those associated with chronic bronchitis and bronchiectasis. On frontal radiographs, the trachea and central bronchi measure greater than 3.0 cm and 2.5 cm, respectively, in coronal diameter. The trachea has a corrugated appearance caused by the herniation of tracheal mucosa and

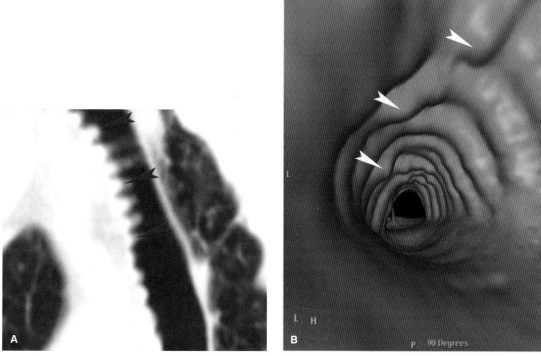

FIGURE 18.5. Tracheobronchopathia Osteochondroplastica. Sagittal CT scan at lung windows (**A**) and endoluminal rendering of helical CT scan (**B**) demonstrate nodular protrusions (*arrowheads*) extending from the cartilaginous rings of the tracheal wall.

submucosa between the tracheal cartilages (Fig. 18.6). The lungs are typically hyperinflated and may demonstrate bullae.

Tracheobronchomalacia (TBM) with diffuse tracheal and central bronchial dilatation may result from a congenital or acquired defect of tracheal cartilage (3). Congenital disorders most often associated with TBM include relapsing polychondritis, Ehlers–Danlos syndrome, and mucopolysaccharidosis. Acquired TBM is more common than the congenital form and is most often the result of prolonged intubation, prior tracheostomy, and extrinsic tracheal compression by mediastinal masses and vascular anomalies. Symptoms and radiographic findings are similar to those of tracheobronchomegaly-cough, dyspnea, wheezing, and recurrent respiratory infection. The imaging hallmark of tracheomalacia is excessive airway collapse on expiration, seen best on CT performed at total lung capacity (i.e., inspiration) in comparison to dynamic expiratory CT with a low-dose CT acquisition performed during a forced expiratory maneuver. A reduction in the cross-sectional area of the trachea exceeding 50% on the expiratory CT, particularly if there is a crescentic "frown-like" configuration to the trachea in cross section, is strongly suggestive of the diagnosis (Fig. 18.7).

In some patients with long-standing interstitial pulmonary fibrosis, diffuse tracheal dilatation may be seen. The etiology of the tracheal dilatation may relate to long-standing elevation in transpulmonary pressures caused by diminished lung compliance or to chronic coughing.

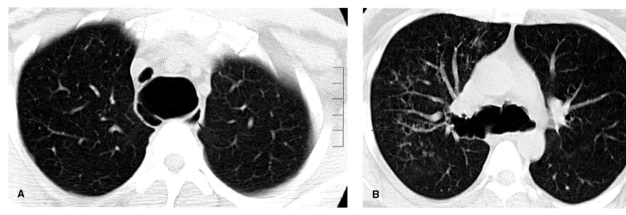

FIGURE 18.6. Tracheobronchomegaly (Mounier–Kuhn Syndrome). CT scans at lung windows at the level of the trachea (**A**) and carina (**B**) show marked tracheal and main bronchial dilatation in a patient with Mounier–Kuhn syndrome. Note the presence of characteristic diverticula along the central airways (*arrows*) and concomitant varicose bronchiectasis within the right upper lobe (*arrowheads*). (Case courtesy of Matthew Brewer, M.D., Milwaukee, WI.)

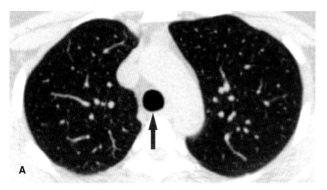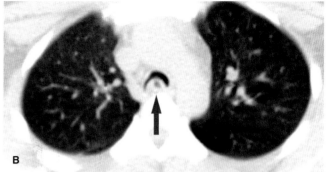

FIGURE 18.7. Tracheobronchomalacia in Ehlers–Danlos Syndrome. Paired inspiratory (**A**) and low-dose expiratory (**B**) CT scans through the mid trachea (*arrows*) at lung windows show a normal rounded configuration of the trachea on inspiration with marked collapse during dynamic expiratory CT with a "frown-like" configuration with buckling of the posterior tracheal membrane.

Tracheal and Bronchial Injury

Injury to the trachea or main bronchi is most often seen with blunt chest trauma from a deceleration-type injury. Concomitant aortic laceration, great vessel injury, or rib (particularly an upper anterior rib), sternum, scapula, or vertebral fracture is the rule and may dominate the clinical picture. The mechanism of injury is forceful compression of the central tracheobronchial tree against the thoracic spine during impact. The fractures generally involve the proximal main bronchi (80%) or distal trachea (15%) within 2 cm of the tracheal carina; the peripheral bronchi are involved in 5% of cases. Horizontal laceration or transection parallel to the tracheobronchial cartilage is the most common form of injury.

The diagnosis of tracheobronchial injury is often first suggested on early post-trauma chest radiographs by the presence of pneumothorax and pneumomediastinum, particularly in a patient not receiving mechanical ventilation (Fig. 18.8A). Typically, the pneumothorax fails to respond to chest tube drainage owing to a large air leak at the site of airway interruption. The subtended lung remains collapsed against the lateral chest wall ("fallen lung" sign) (Fig. 18.8B). An aberrant endotracheal tube or an overdistended balloon cuff is a further clue to the presence

of an unsuspected tracheobronchial disruption. As many as one third of tracheobronchial injuries have a delayed diagnosis; these patients may present with a collapsed lung or pneumonia secondary to bronchial stenosis. Definitive diagnosis is by bronchoscopy. MDCT with three-dimensional reconstruction with shaded surface display may be useful in patients who develop bronchial occlusion or stenosis because of a delay in diagnosis.

Penetrating tracheal injuries usually involve the cervical trachea and result from gunshot or stab wounds to the neck. Injury to the intrathoracic trachea is usually associated with fatal penetrating cardiovascular injury.

Broncholithiasis

Broncholithiasis, the presence of calcified material within the tracheobronchial tree, develops from erosion of a calcified peribronchial lymph node into the bronchial lumen (Fig. 18.9). Most calcified lymph nodes result from granulomatous lymph node inflammation caused by histoplasmosis or TB. Broncholiths may occlude the airway and lead to bronchiectasis, obstructive atelectasis, or pneumonia. Patients are often asymptomatic but

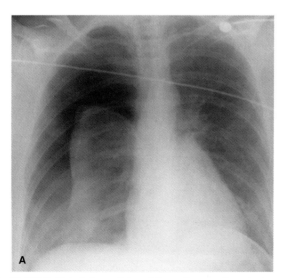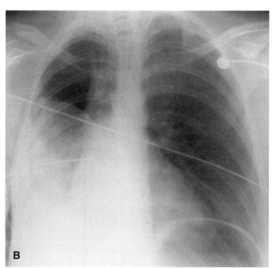

FIGURE 18.8. Injury of the Right Main Bronchus. A. An upright chest film shows a broken right clavicle with a large right pneumothorax and pneumomediastinum in a 24-year-old woman struck by a car. **B.** A film obtained following chest tube placement shows a persistent pneumothorax. A large air leak was noted from the tube. Bronchoscopy revealed complete disruption of the right main bronchus, which was confirmed at thoracotomy.

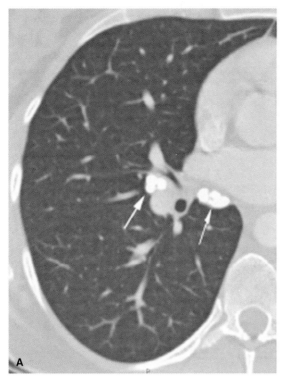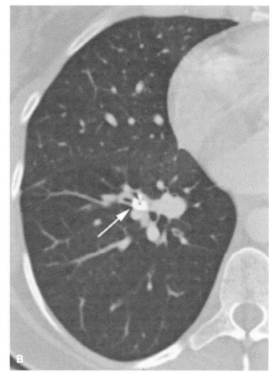

FIGURE 18.9. **Broncholithiasis.** Targeted reconstruction of the right lung from a CT in a 33-year-old woman with hemoptysis at the level of the middle lobe bronchus (**A**) and proximal basal segmental right lower lobe bronchi (**B**) show calcified lymph nodes (*arrows*) in the right hilum and azygoesophageal recess (*arrows* in **A**) with a calcified node within the anterior basal segmental bronchus (*arrow* in **B**).

may have cough productive of stones or calcified material (lithoptysis). Hemoptysis may develop from erosion of the broncholith into a bronchial vessel.

CHRONIC OBSTRUCTIVE PULMONARY DISEASE

The diseases known collectively as chronic obstructive pulmonary disease (COPD) include asthma, chronic bronchitis, bronchiectasis, and emphysema (4). The common pathophysiology in this group of diseases is obstruction to expiratory airflow.

Asthma and Chronic Bronchitis

Asthma is an airways disorder characterized by the rapid onset of bronchial narrowing with spontaneous resolution or improvement as a result of therapy. A wide variety of inciting factors and agents have been identified. Many patients have an allergic history and develop episodic bronchial constriction from excessive production of immunoglobulin E following exposure to antigenic stimuli. This results in bronchial smooth muscle contraction, bronchial wall inflammation, and excessive mucus production. These responses narrow the bronchial lumen and produce symptoms of coughing, wheezing, and dyspnea.

The radiographic findings in uncomplicated asthma are primarily the result of diffuse airways narrowing. Hyperinflation producing increased lung volume, flattening or inversion of the diaphragm, attenuation of the peripheral vascular markings, and prominence of the retrosternal airspace is the result of expiratory air trapping. Bronchial wall inflammation and thickening appear radiographically as peribronchial cuffing

and "tram tracking." In some patients, the hila are prominent from transient pulmonary arterial hypertension caused by hypoxic vasoconstriction.

There are several reasons to obtain a chest radiograph in patients with asthma. Tracheal and central bronchial narrowing from extrinsic or intrinsic lesions may produce dyspnea and wheezing and be mistaken for asthma. Bacterial pneumonia may induce airway hyperreactivity and present as an acute asthmatic attack. Complications of asthma may be detected on chest radiographs obtained during and following the asthmatic episode. Mucus plugs can cause bronchial obstruction and resorptive atelectasis; pneumonia can develop in these collapsed regions. Expiratory airflow obstruction with resultant alveolar rupture and dissection of air medially may produce pneumomediastinum (Fig. 18.10). If the extra-alveolar air dissects peripherally to the subpleural space to form subpleural blebs, pneumothorax may result. Both pneumomediastinum and pneumothorax may be exacerbated in ventilated patients receiving high-positive-pressure ventilation.

Chronic bronchitis is a clinical and not a radiographic diagnosis. It is defined as the excess production and expectoration of sputum that occurs on most days for at least 3 consecutive months in at least 2 consecutive years. The majority of individuals with chronic bronchitis are cigarette smokers. Morphologically, the lower lobe bronchi are most often affected, with thickening of their walls from mucous gland hyperplasia. The ratio of mucous gland thickness to bronchial wall thickness is known as the Reid index; an abnormally high index (>50%) correlates strongly with symptoms of excess mucus production. Fifty percent of patients with a history of chronic bronchitis have normal chest films. Some patients show peribronchial cuffing or tram tracks when the thick-walled and mildly dilated bronchi are viewed end on or in length, respectively. Other patients have a "dirty chest," in which the peripheral

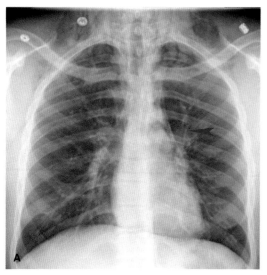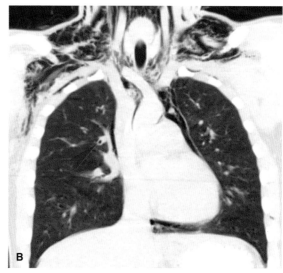

FIGURE 18.10. **Asthma Complicated by Pneumomediastinum. A.** Frontal chest radiograph in a patient with an acute asthma exacerbation shows perihilar bronchial cuffing (*arrowhead*) and pneumomediastinum extending into the neck producing subcutaneous emphysema. **B.** Coronal reformatted CT scan at the level of the ascending aorta displayed at lung windows shows airways thickening (*arrowhead*) and confirms pneumomediastinum extending into the neck.

lung markings are accentuated. This radiographic appearance lacks a definite pathologic correlate but may represent thickened airway walls, smoking-related small airways disease (i.e., respiratory bronchiolitis), or prominent PAs from pulmonary arterial hypertension complicating associated centrilobular emphysema. CT in patients with chronic bronchitis may show bronchial wall thickening and mucus plugging (Fig. 18.11).

Bronchiectasis

Bronchiectasis is defined as an abnormal permanent dilatation of bronchi. This is distinguished from transient bronchial dila-

tation that can be seen within areas of airspace consolidation in patients with pneumonia. Morphologically, bronchiectasis is divided into three groups: cylindric, varicose, and saccular (cystic). Cylindric bronchiectasis is characterized by mild diffuse dilatation of the bronchi. Varicose bronchiectasis is cystic bronchial dilatation interrupted by focal areas of narrowing, an appearance that has been likened to a string of pearls. Cystic bronchiectasis is seen as clusters of bronchi with marked localized saccular dilatation. Bronchiectasis may be localized or generalized. Localized bronchiectasis is most commonly a result of prior TB, whereas generalized bronchiectasis is seen in patients with cystic fibrosis. Patients usually have a history of chronic sputum production and recurrent lower

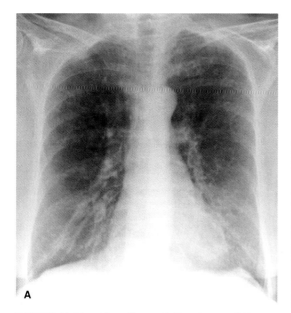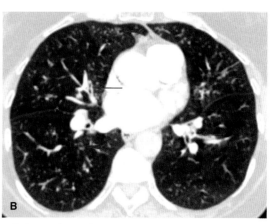

FIGURE 18.11. **"Dirty Chest" of Chronic Bronchitis. A.** Frontal chest radiograph in a patient with a history of chronic bronchitis and chronic obstructive pulmonary disease shows hyperinflation with increased parenchymal markings. **B.** CT scan at the level of the mid lungs at lung windows demonstrates bronchial thickening (*arrows*), centrilobular tree-in-bud opacities (*arrowheads*) and mosaic attenuation, the latter likely due to airways disease.

respiratory infections. Hemoptysis associated with enlargement of bronchial arteries is common and may be massive and life-threatening.

The chest radiographic findings of bronchiectasis are typically nonspecific. Scarring, volume loss, and loss of the sharp definition of the normal bronchovascular markings are present in the affected regions. Parallel linear shadows representing the walls of cylindrically dilated bronchi seen in length may be visualized. Cystic bronchiectasis has a characteristic appearance of multiple peripheral thin-walled cysts, with or without air-fluid levels, that tend to cluster together in the distribution of a bronchovascular bundle. The findings tend to be peripheral in most cases of localized bronchiectasis; central bronchiectasis is seen only in allergic bronchopulmonary aspergillosis, cystic fibrosis, bronchial atresia, or acquired central bronchial obstruction.

CT has all but eliminated the need for contrast bronchography in the evaluation of bronchiectasis. As compared to bronchography, thin-section CT scans obtained at regular intervals have an accuracy exceeding 95% in the diagnosis of bronchiectasis (5). The CT appearance of bronchiectasis depends on the site of involvement and the type of bronchiectasis. In the upper and lower lobes, all bronchi are imaged in cross section, and their luminal diameter can be directly compared to that of the accompanying PAs. Cylindric bronchiectasis in these regions appears as multiple dilated thick-walled circular lucencies, with the adjoining smaller artery giving each dilated bronchus the appearance of a "signet ring" (Fig. 18.12). In the

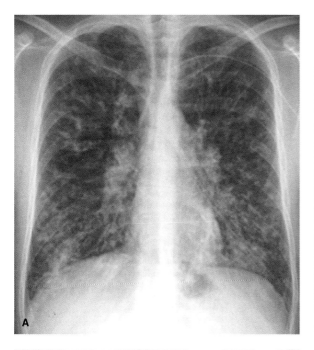

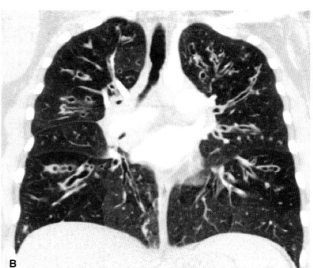

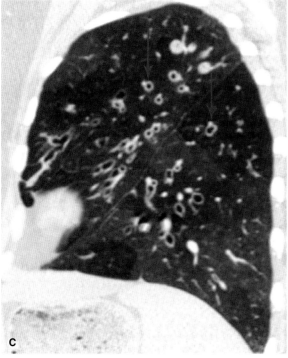

FIGURE 18.12. Bronchiectasis in Cystic Fibrosis. A. Chest radiograph in a patient with cystic fibrosis. The lungs are hyperinflated with multiple linear and tubular branching opacities. Note the bilateral hilar enlargement as a result of pulmonary arterial hypertension and reactive lymph node enlargement. B. Coronal reformatted CT scan through the trachea shows bilateral cylindrical bronchiectasis (arrows) and mosaic attenuation due to airways disease. C. Sagittal reformation through the left lung shows the left lung cylindrical bronchiectasis in cross section as "signet rings" (arrows).

TABLE 18.3

SPECIFIC CAUSES OF BRONCHIECTASIS

Localized	Tuberculous scarring, upper lobes (postprimary disease)
	Bronchial disease
	Extrinsic compression
	Enlarged hilar nodes
	Bronchial stenosis/occlusion
	Bronchial atresia
	Tuberculosis
	Sarcoidosis
	Prior bronchial injury
	Endobronchial mass
	Carcinoid tumor
	Bronchogenic carcinoma
	Foreign body
Diffuse	Cystic fibrosis
	Dysmotile cilia syndrome
	Congenital immunodeficiency
	Postinfectious
	Adenovirus (Swyer–James syndrome)
	Measles
	Pertussis
	Chronic aspiration
	Allergic bronchopulmonary aspergillosis
	Pulmonary fibrosis (traction bronchiectasis)
	α-1-antitrypsin deficiency

mid-lung, where the bronchi course horizontally, the appearance is that of parallel linear opacities (tram tracks). Mucoid impaction within dilated upper or lower lobe bronchi may be mistaken for lung nodules unless one observes the vertical nature of the opacity on sequential axial images. In the mid-lung regions, impacted bronchi sectioned in length are recognized as branching, fingerlike opacities. Cystic bronchiectasis in any region is easily recognized as clusters of rounded lucencies, often containing air-fluid levels; this appearance has been likened to a cluster of grapes. Varicose bronchiectasis cannot be differentiated from cylindric bronchiectasis unless sectioned longitudinally in the mid-lung regions, where the pattern of dilatation simulates the contour of a caterpillar. The detection of varicose bronchiectasis in an asthmatic patient should suggest the diagnosis of allergic bronchopulmonary aspergillosis.

CT has replaced bronchography for the diagnosis of bronchiectasis because it is noninvasive and highly accurate. High-resolution or volumetric CT can be used to detect the presence and extent of disease.

Bronchiectasis is caused by a variety of disorders, all of which predispose the bronchi to chronic inflammation, with resultant cartilage damage and dilatation (Table 18.3).

Cystic fibrosis is a hereditary disease in young Caucasians characterized in the lung by the production of abnormally thick, tenacious mucus. The thick mucus plugs the small airways and leads to bronchial obstruction and infection. A vicious cycle of recurrent infection, most often with *Pseudomonas aeruginosa* or *Staphylococcus aureus*, eventually causes severe bronchiectasis. The bronchiectasis is associated with functional airways obstruction and dyspnea. Hemoptysis, sometimes massive, may complicate the bronchiectasis and may require treatment by transcatheter bronchial artery embolization. Chest radiographs in affected patients show hyperinflation with predominantly upper lobe bronchiectasis with mucus plugging. Thin-section CT delineates the severity and extent

of bronchiectasis and shows associated small airways disease seen as tree-in-bud opacities and mosaic attenuation due to air trapping (Fig. 18.12). Distal atelectasis and obstructive pneumonitis are common findings. The pulmonary hila may be prominent from enlarged lymph nodes caused by chronic infection or from vascular dilatation associated with pulmonary arterial hypertension. The diagnosis rests on a positive family history and a sweat test showing an abnormally high concentration of chloride. Improvements in antibiotic therapy and pulmonary physiotherapy have increased long-term survival, but the overall prognosis remains poor, with most patients succumbing to respiratory insufficiency in young adulthood. Recently, the use of inhaled recombinant DNAase to reduce the viscosity of tracheobronchial secretions has brought symptomatic and functional improvement to a number of patients. Lung or heart/lung transplantation is an option in selected individuals.

Dysmotile cilia syndrome is a disorder in which the epithelial cilial motion is abnormal and ineffective. A variety of structural cilial abnormalities may be found, the most common of which is an absence of the outer dynein arms of the peripheral microtubules of the cilia. The abnormality may result in rhinitis, sinusitis, bronchiectasis, dysmotile spermatozoa and sterility, situs inversus, and dextrocardia. The triad of sinusitis, situs inversus, and bronchiectasis is known as Kartagener syndrome. Chest radiographs show diffuse bronchiectasis and hyperinflation; situs inversus is seen in approximately 50% of patients. The diagnosis is made on the basis of the clinical and radiographic findings along with studies of cilial anatomy and motion on samples obtained from nasal biopsy.

Postinfectious Bronchiectasis. Severe childhood pneumonia, usually a sequela of infection with adenovirus, measles, or pertussis (the latter two are seen not uncommonly in nonimmunized Asian immigrants), may cause severe bronchial damage and recurrent infection with resultant bronchiectasis (Fig. 18.13). In some patients, childhood bronchitis and bronchiolitis are associated with obstructive airways disease and an underdeveloped lung, the latter known as Swyer–James syndrome (see "Small Airways Disease" section).

Allergic bronchopulmonary aspergillosis represents a hypersensitivity reaction to *Aspergillus* and is characterized clinically by asthma, blood eosinophilia, bronchiectasis with mucus plugging, and circulating antibodies to *Aspergillus* antigen. An immediate (type 1) hypersensitivity reaction to *Aspergillus* antigen accounts for acute episodes of wheezing and dyspnea, while an immune complex-mediated (type 3) hypersensitivity within the lobar bronchi leads to bronchial wall inflammation and proximal bronchiectasis. Affected patients invariably have an allergic history, and it is often associated with known asthma or cystic fibrosis. Patients with this disorder have recurrent episodes of cough, wheezing, and expectoration of mucus plugs. The chest radiograph is diagnostic and shows proximal, predominantly upper lobe bronchiectasis; consolidation due to associated eosinophilic pneumonia is seen in the majority of patients during the acute phase of the disease. The dilated bronchi may be seen as dilated air-filled tubules or as broadly branching opacities characteristic of mucoid impaction within the dilated bronchi. CT is helpful in characterizing the opacities as dilated bronchi (Fig. 18.14). The detection of varicose bronchiectasis in a susceptible patient should suggest the diagnosis. Corticosteroids are the treatment of choice.

Bronchial Obstruction. Bronchiectasis can develop distal to an endobronchial obstruction caused by neoplasm, atresia, or stenosis. Slow-growing central bronchogenic neoplasms that have a large endoluminal component (e.g., carcinoid tumor) may obstruct the distal bronchi and produce bronchiectasis with mucus plugging (mucoceles). Similarly, bronchial atresia or bronchostenosis from trauma or

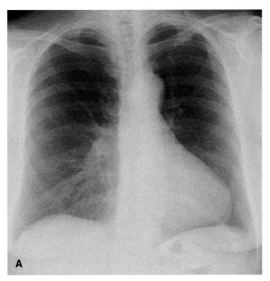
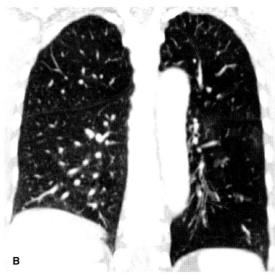

FIGURE 18.13. **Unilateral Hyperlucent Lung (Swyer–James) Syndrome. A.** Chest radiograph shows subtle decrease in left lung volume with a small left hilum and attenuated vascularity. **B.** Coronal reformatted CT scan through the level of the descending aorta at lung windows shows left lung hyperlucency with mild central bronchial dilatation and thickening (*arrowhead*).

chronic bronchial infection (e.g., endobronchial TB) can lead to distal bronchial dilatation. The plain radiographic recognition of mucocele formation in patients with endobronchial obstruction is dependent on adequate collateral ventilation to the lung supplied by the obstructed airway. Unfortunately, in most patients, collapse of lung around the dilated mucus-filled bronchus precludes diagnosis on plain radiographs. CT will show the central airway obstruction and dilated mucus bronchograms and can help guide bronchoscopic examination and biopsy.

FIGURE 18.14. **Allergic Bronchopulmonary Aspergillosis (ABPA).** Coronal reformatted CT scan through the posterior chest at lung windows in a patient with ABPA shows bilateral lower lobe mucoid impaction (*arrows*) and patchy upper lobe ground-glass opacities (*arrowheads*).

Peribronchial Fibrosis. Traction bronchiectasis is a term used to describe the effect of severe pulmonary fibrosis on the peripheral airways. Airways that traverse regions of parenchymal fibrosis and honeycombing often become irregularly dilated as their walls are retracted by the fibrotic process. This occurs most commonly in the upper lobes in patients with long-standing TB and in the subpleural regions of the lower lobes in patients with end-stage idiopathic pulmonary fibrosis. Because the accompanying fibrosis precludes visualization of the dilated bronchi radiographically, traction bronchiectasis is best appreciated on HRCT studies of the lung.

Emphysema

Definition and Subtypes. Emphysema is a pathologic diagnosis that is defined as an abnormal, permanent enlargement of the airspaces distal to the terminal bronchiole, accompanied by destruction of alveolar walls, and without obvious fibrosis. The pathologic classification of emphysema is based on the portion of the secondary pulmonary lobule affected. *Centrilobular emphysema* is the most common and is characterized by airspace distention in the central portion of the lobule, with sparing of the more distal portions of the lobule. This form of emphysema affects the upper lobes to a greater extent than the lower lobes (Fig. 18.15). *Panlobular emphysema* results in uniform distention of the airspaces throughout the substance of the lobule, from the central respiratory bronchioles to the peripheral alveolar sacs and alveoli. In contrast to centrilobular emphysema, this form has a predilection for the lower lobes (Fig. 18.16). *Paraseptal emphysema* is seen as selective distention of peripheral airspaces adjacent to interlobular septa, with sparing of the centrilobular region. This form of emphysema is most often seen in the immediate subpleural regions of the upper lobes (Fig. 18.15). Paraseptal emphysema may coalesce to form apical bullae; rupture of these bullae into the pleural space may give rise to spontaneous pneumothoraces. *Paracicatricial* or *irregular emphysema* refers to destruction of lung tissue associated with fibrosis that bears no consistent relationship to a given portion of the lobule. It is most

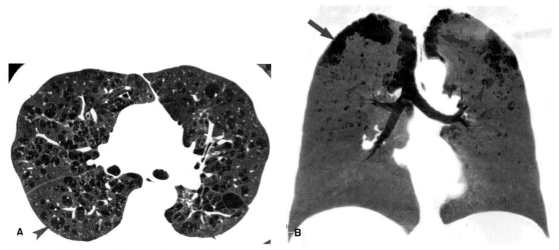

FIGURE 18.15. Centrilobular and Paraseptal Emphysema on CT. A. CT scan through the mid lungs in a patient with centrilobular emphysema shows discrete lucencies (*arrowheads*) lacking perceptible walls and containing centrilobular artery branches. **B.** In another patient with both centrilobular and paraseptal emphysema, a coronal minimum intensity reconstruction shows subpleural lucencies, reflecting paraseptal emphysema (*arrows*) with associated centrilobular emphysema (*arrowheads*).

often seen in association with old granulomatous inflammation (Fig. 18.17).

Etiology and Pathogenesis. The most common etiologic factor for the development of emphysema is cigarette smoking. This is associated predominantly with centrilobular emphysema but may be a contributing factor in the development of panlobular emphysema. The pathogenesis of centrilobular emphysema is complex and has not been completely elucidated. Cigarette smoke leads to excess neutrophil deposition in the lung. This results in the release of proteases (e.g., elastase) and antiprotease inhibitors, which in turn leads to destruction of alveolar septa. Inflammation and obstruction of small airways likely contributes to distal airspace distention and alveolar septal disruption. The association between deficiency of the serum protein α-1-antitrypsin (α-1-protease inhibitor) and the development of panlobular emphysema is well established. This disease is inherited as an autosomal recessive trait. Individuals who are homozygous for both recessive genes (ZZ phenotype) develop panlobular emphysema by middle age. Heterozygotes (MZ phenotype) have only a slightly increased incidence of emphysema.

Cigarette smoking, by producing excess antiprotease inhibitors, can accelerate the development of emphysema in patients with the ZZ and MZ phenotypes.

Clinical Findings and Functional Abnormalities. Because a definitive diagnosis of emphysema requires tissue, the diagnosis during life is based on a combination of clinical, functional, and radiographic findings. The vast majority of patients with emphysema are long-term cigarette smokers. Symptoms associated with emphysema include dyspnea and a productive cough; the latter is attributed to chronic bronchitis, which often accompanies centrilobular emphysema. The functional hallmarks of emphysema are decreased airflow and diffusing capacity. Expiratory airflow obstruction is expressed as a decrease in the volume of air expired in the first second of a forced expiratory maneuver from total lung capacity (FEV_1) and a decrease in the ratio of FEV_1 to the total volume of air expired during a forced expiratory maneuver (FEV_1/FVC). Airflow obstruction is secondary to increased airways resistance and decreased driving pressure (i.e., elastic recoil). In patients with moderate to severe emphysema, the predominant factor limiting expiratory airflow is the

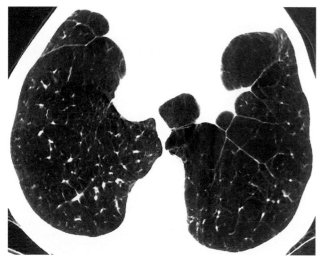

FIGURE 18.16. Panlobular Emphysema. HRCT scan through the lower lobes shows uniform destruction of secondary pulmonary lobules.

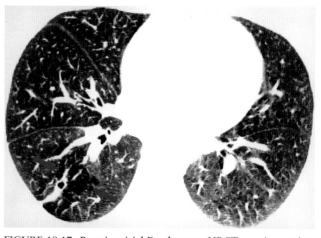

FIGURE 18.17. Paracicatricial Emphysema. HRCT scan in a patient with focal right lower lobe postinflammatory scarring and bronchiectasis shows focal hyperlucency (*arrows*) representing paracicatricial emphysema.

TABLE 18.4

RADIOGRAPHIC FINDINGS IN PULMONARY EMPHYSEMA

■ FINDING	■ EXPLANATION
Diffuse hyperlucency (panlobular)	Destruction of pulmonary capillary bed and alveolar septa
Flattening and depression of the hemidiaphragms; increased retrosternal airspace (panlobular > centrilobular)	Hyperinflation caused by loss of elastic recoil of lung
Bulla	Thin-walled region of confluent (panlobular > centrilobular) emphysematous destruction
Enlarged central PAs; right heart enlargement (centrilobular)	Loss of pulmonary capillary bed; associated chronic hypoxemia causes increased pulmonary vascular resistance
Increased peripheral vascular markings (centrilobular)	Small airways disease Increased pulmonary vascularity

decreased elastic recoil that results from parenchymal destruction. Airflow obstruction, however, is not invariably present in patients with mild emphysema. Diffusing capacity, measured by the diffusion of carbon monoxide from the alveoli into the bloodstream during a single breath hold ($DL_{CO}SB$), assesses the integrity and surface area of the alveolocapillary membrane. The diffusing capacity in emphysema is decreased because the volume of pulmonary parenchyma available for gas exchange is diminished. The severity of the emphysema correlates well with the $DL_{CO}SB$. Although an abnormal diffusing capacity is more sensitive than abnormal spirometry in diagnosing emphysema, it is nonspecific. Since $DL_{CO}SB$ depends on both the surface area available for gas diffusion and the number and hemoglobin content of red blood cells within the pulmonary capillaries, any process affecting these factors can alter the measurement of $DL_{CO}SB$. For example, a decreased $DL_{CO}SB$ can be seen in any disease that diminishes the volume of pulmonary capillaries available for gas diffusion (e.g., pulmonary embolism); interferes with gas exchange across the alveolocapillary membrane (e.g., interstitial pulmonary fibrosis), or produces airway obstruction, thereby diminishing the gas-exchanging airspaces (i.e., cystic fibrosis). Furthermore, some patients with mild to moderate morphologic emphysema can have a normal $DL_{CO}SB$.

Radiologic Evaluation. Frontal and lateral chest radiographs are the initial radiographic examinations obtained in patients with suspected emphysema. The plain radiographic findings of emphysema are listed in Table 18.4 (6). Hyperinflation is the most important plain radiographic finding and reflects the loss of lung elastic recoil. It is the radiographic equivalent of an abnormally increased total lung capacity. The abnormal increase in lung volumes is best detected by noting inferior displacement and flattening of the normally convex superior hemidiaphragms, right or obtuse angles to the normally acute-angled costophrenic sulci, and an increase

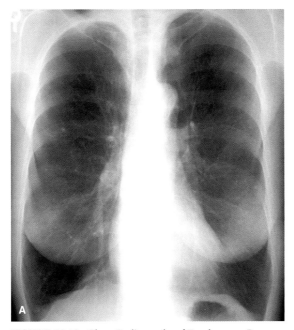
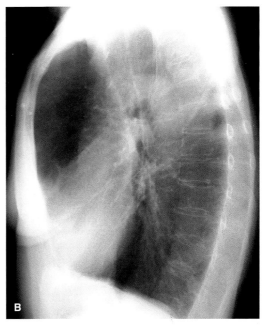

FIGURE 18.18. Chest Radiographs of Emphysema. Posteroanterior (**A**) and lateral (**B**) chest radiographs in a 62-year-old woman with emphysema show hyperinflation with hyperlucency, upper lobe vascular attenuation, flattening of the diaphragms, and an increased retrosternal airspace, reflecting severe emphysema.

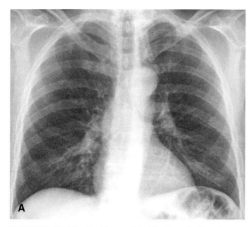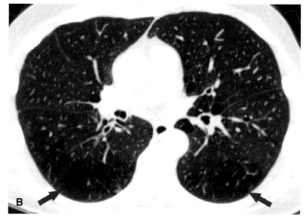

FIGURE 18.19. **Radiographically Occult Emphysema. A.** Chest radiograph in a patient with chronic obstructive pulmonary disease is normal, without signs of emphysema. **B.** Axial CT scan through the mid lungs at lung windows shows minimal left upper lobe (*arrowheads*) and confluent superior segment lower lobe (*arrows*) emphysema.

in anteroposterior chest diameter (best appreciated by noting an increase in the depth of the retrosternal clear space) (Fig. 18.18). Absent or attenuated peripheral vascular markings are caused by parenchymal destruction and obliteration of peripheral pulmonary arteries traversing emphysematous areas. When the characteristic thin walls of bullae are seen marginating the peripheral avascular regions, emphysema can be diagnosed with certainty. Increased radiolucency of the lungs on radiographs resulting from pulmonary hyperinflation and attenuation of peripheral vascular markings is difficult to detect because it is subject to various patient and technical factors and therefore is an inaccurate indicator of the presence of emphysema. It is well recognized that many patients with severe centrilobular emphysema have minimal or no hyperinflation on chest radiographs, and they tend to show increased lung markings rather than peripheral vascular attenuation. In such patients, the increased markings may reflect the presence of smoking-related small airways disease (e.g., respiratory bronchiolitis-associated interstitial lung disease [RB-ILD]). The effects of emphysema and chronic hypoxemia on the right side of the heart may be appreciated as enlargement of the central pulmonary arteries and right ventricle in those with complicating pulmonary arterial hypertension and cor pulmonale.

The use of the term *chronic obstructive pulmonary disease* to describe patients with the plain radiographic findings of emphysema is inaccurate and should be discouraged. COPD is a functional diagnosis, whereas the chest radiograph depicts anatomy only. In fact, patients with radiographic findings of hyperinflation and vascular attenuation, while they invariably have emphysema morphologically, may rarely lack functional evidence of airflow obstruction and therefore do not have COPD.

Widespread, extensive emphysema may be accurately diagnosed on chest radiographs, but mild disease is often not evident radiographically (Fig. 18.19). The use of chest CT has allowed for the diagnosis of emphysema in the absence of chest radiographic findings of hyperinflation or parenchymal abnormalities. CT is ideally suited to the diagnosis of emphysema because of its cross-sectional nature and high contrast resolution. Early reports on the use of CT to diagnose emphysema depended on recognition of either large avascular areas or regions with abnormally low Hounsfield attenuation numbers. Thin-section CT provides better characterization of centrilobular emphysema than standard scans of 5 to 10 mm collimation. MDCT with the use of coronal and sagittal reconstructions is useful for assessing the distribution of emphysema, particularly in patients considered for lung volume reduction surgery (LVRS).

Centrilobular emphysema on thin-section CT scan is seen as discrete, well-defined areas of abnormally low attenuation that lack definable walls and is situated centrally within the secondary pulmonary lobule adjacent to the bronchovascular bundle (Fig. 18.15). MDCT or high-resolution CT, with its thin-collimation technique and high spatial resolution, can detect mild centrilobular emphysema that may be imperceptible on chest radiography (Fig. 18.19) and missed on 5- to 10-mm collimated scans because of partial volume averaging of small emphysematous areas within the thickness of the scan section.

Treatment of Emphysema. Advances in operative techniques now provide two surgical options and an endobronchial intervention for the treatment of emphysema. Recently, a surgical technique first developed in the 1950s—lung volume reduction surgery (LVRS)—has been reintroduced as a method of relieving patient dyspnea by resecting severely emphysematous regions of lung and improving respiratory mechanics. This technique, which was evaluated in the National Emphysema Treatment Trial, was shown to benefit only a select group of patients with emphysema, specifically those with mostly upper lobe emphysema and low exercise capacity prior to surgery. An alternative surgical technique available to treat patients with emphysema, particularly younger patients with α-1-antitrypsin deficiency, is single or double lung transplantation. Several centers now administer intravenously pooled α-1-antitrypsin to patients with associated emphysema to prevent further damage to the lungs. Most recently, the bronchoscopic placement of one-way endobronchial valves that prevent air entry but allow air egress from emphysematous lung has shown modest improvement in lung function and dyspnea in select patients with emphysema.

BULLOUS LUNG DISEASE

Bullae are thin-walled cystic spaces that exceed 1 cm in diameter and are found within the lung parenchyma (Fig. 18.19). Three morphologic types have been described: type 1 bullae, which are apical, subpleural rounded gas collections without septations containing a narrow neck; type 2 bullae, which are also subpleural in location but have wide necks and contain strands of residual tissue; and type 3 bullae, which are morphologically similar to type 2 bullae but are located deep within the lung substance. Bullae most often represent confluent areas of emphysematous lung and may be seen as part of generalized emphysema. However, in a minority of patients, bullae are not associated with emphysema. For example, the increased lung weight and chronically elevated transpleural pressure in patients with lower lobe interstitial pulmonary fibrosis predispose to bullae formation. Bullae may also be seen in diseases that cause chronic upper lobe fibrosis, such as

TABLE 18.5

CAUSES OF PRIMARY BULLOUS LUNG DISEASE

Familial

Vanishing lung disease

Marfan syndrome

Ehlers–Danlos syndrome

IV drug use

HIV infection

Birt–Hogg–Dube syndrome

sarcoidosis, pulmonary Langerhans cell histiocytosis, and ankylosing spondylitis. In these diseases, chronic bronchiolar obstruction leads to distal airspace distention, alveolar septal disruption, and the development of bullae. A rare cause of lung cysts or bullae is Birt–Hogg–Dube syndrome, which is an autosomal dominant disorder characterized by skin fibrofolliculomas, malignant renal tumors, and thin-walled lung cysts, the latter predisposing to spontaneous pneumothorax.

Primary bullous disease (Table 18.5) is a group of disorders in which bullae are isolated lesions without intervening areas of emphysema or interstitial lung disease. Primary bullous lung disease may be familial and has been found in association with Marfan or Ehlers–Danlos syndrome, IV drug use, HIV infection, and vanishing lung syndrome, which is an accelerated form of paraseptal emphysema seen in young adult men (Fig. 18.20). Most patients are asymptomatic unless large bullae compress normal parenchyma and cause compressive atelectasis and dyspnea. Radiographically, isolated bullae have an upper lobe distribution and appear as rounded, thin-walled lucencies of varying size. These lesions can become huge as a result of air trapping and cause depression of the ipsilateral lung and hemidiaphragm and may even produce contralateral mediastinal shift. CT is useful in evaluating the extent of bullous disease and the amount of compressed pulmonary tissue.

Spontaneous pneumothorax occurs when a subpleural bulla ruptures into the pleural space. These patients may be difficult to manage; persistent air leaks lead to prolonged and often unsuccessful closed tube drainage of the pleural space and reexpansion of the lung. When a bulla becomes secondarily infected, chest

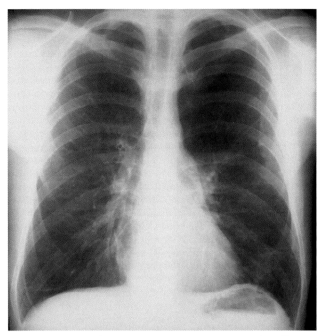

FIGURE 18.20. Bullous Lung Disease. Posteroanterior chest film in a 27-year-old man shows left lung and right upper lobe bullae, representing vanishing lung disease.

radiographs or CT will demonstrate an air-fluid level within the bulla that resolves over several weeks with the administration of antibiotics. A cancer may rarely develop within the wall of a bulla. Symptomatic patients and those with enlarging bullae should be considered for bullectomy. Radioisotopic lung perfusion studies may be performed preoperatively to assess the amount of perfused and potentially functional lung parenchyma compressed by the bullae.

SMALL AIRWAYS DISEASE

Bronchiolitis refers to an inflammation of the small noncartilaginous airways (7) (Table 18.6). *Infectious bronchiolitis* is often a disease of young children caused by respiratory syncytial

TABLE 18.6

CLINICAL AND IMAGING FEATURES OF SMALL AIRWAYS DISEASE

■ ENTITY	■ ASSOCIATED CONDITIONS	■ CT FINDINGS
Infectious bronchiolitis	Viral/atypical/mycobacterial infection	Tree-in-bud opacities
Diffuse panbronchiolitis	None	Tree-in-bud opacities, bronchial dilatation/thickening
Respiratory bronchiolitis-associated interstitial lung disease	Cigarette smoking	Centrilobular and geographic ground-glass opacities
Hypersensitivity pneumonitis (subacute)	Inhaled organic antigen	Centrilobular ground-glass nodules, air trapping on expiratory scans
Follicular bronchiolitis	Rheumatoid arthritis, Sjögren syndrome	Centrilobular ground-glass nodules
Constrictive bronchiolitis	Transplant patients, drug reactions, inhalation injury, postinfectious	Mosaic attenuation with air trapping on expiratory scans, bronchial dilatation (late)
Diffuse idiopathic pulmonary neuroendocrine cell hyperplasia (DIPNECH)	Carcinoid tumor	Mosaic attenuation with air trapping on expiratory scans, bronchial thickening, nodule(s)

virus or adenovirus and produces respiratory distress and radiographic hyperinflation that are indistinguishable from asthma. However, there is an increasing recognition of infectious bronchiolitis in adults caused by a variety of microorganisms. A specific but uncommon cause of bronchiolitis is *diffuse* or *Asian panbronchiolitis,* which is associated with sinus disease and results in progressive pulmonary symptoms of airways disease, including cough and sputum production. Bronchiolar and peribronchial inflammation is commonly a result of heavy cigarette smoking. This latter disease is termed *respiratory bronchiolitis-associated interstitial lung disease* (RB-ILD), and it presents with signs and symptoms of interstitial lung disease. RB-ILD is reviewed in Chapter 17. Bronchiolitis is also a prominent feature of patients with subacute hypersensitivity pneumonitis, which is also reviewed in Chapter 17. *Follicular bronchiolitis* reflects a form of diffuse lymphoid hyperplasia of peribronchiolar lymphoid follicles of unclear clinical significance seen in patients with rheumatoid arthritis or Sjögren syndrome. Thin-section CT shows ill-defined centrilobular ground-glass nodules and occasional bronchial dilatation.

Constrictive bronchiolitis, also known as *bronchiolitis obliterans,* is a subacute disease characterized pathologically by a mononuclear cell inflammatory process within the walls of respiratory bronchioles that leads to the formation of granulation tissue, which plugs small airways. This results in dyspnea and functional airways obstruction. This disorder may be idiopathic or secondary to viral infection, toxic fume inhalation (e.g., silo filler's disease), drug reaction (e.g., penicillamine), collagen vascular disorders (e.g., rheumatoid arthritis), organ transplantation, or chronic aspiration. Lung, heart–lung, and bone marrow transplant patients (Fig. 18.21) are particularly prone to constrictive bronchiolitis. Constrictive bronchiolitis in the adult also may be the result of an early childhood lower respiratory infection with adenovirus, measles, or mycoplasma, in which case it is known as unilateral hyperlucent lung or Swyer–James syndrome. In Swyer–James syndrome, the bronchiolitis causes diffuse small airways obliteration, air trapping, and destruction of alveolar walls and emphysema owing to overdistention of peripheral airspaces. Because postinfectious bronchiolitis obliterans affects the lungs asymmetrically and

usually occurs during a period of lung growth and development, the affected lung is typically small and hyperlucent and the ipsilateral PA is hypoplastic. Most patients with the Swyer–James syndrome are asymptomatic, whereas some patients complain of dyspnea or recurrent lower respiratory tract infections. A rare form of constrictive bronchiolitis termed diffuse idiopathic pulmonary neuroendocrine cell hyperplasia (DIPNECH) is seen in middle-aged woman who demonstrate severe airflow limitation and thin-section CT findings of air trapping with bronchial thickening and dilatation in association with one or multiple small nodules representing neuroendocrine cell tumorlets.

The chest radiograph in patients with pure constrictive bronchiolitis may be normal despite the presence of severe dyspnea and functional evidence of airflow obstruction. The most common radiographic abnormality in this disorder is diffuse reticulonodular opacities with associated hyperinflation. Central bronchiectasis has been described particularly in those with constrictive bronchiolitis that developed as a complication of heart–lung transplantation. In patients with Swyer–James syndrome, the affected lung is normal or small in volume, and marked unilateral air trapping is seen on fluoroscopy or expiratory films. The air trapping is caused by bronchiolar obstruction with collateral air drift to the distal airspaces on inspiration that cannot escape on expiration. The ipsilateral hilum is small and the pulmonary vasculature is reduced, accounting for the hyperlucency seen radiographically and on CT (Fig. 18.13). Perfusion lung scanning shows decreased perfusion of the affected lung, while the ventilation study shows decreased ventilation with markedly delayed radioisotope washout. This latter finding helps distinguish the Swyer–James syndrome from primary central PA occlusion or hypoplastic lung, conditions in which ventilation is maintained.

HRCT in Small Airways Disease. HRCT is a sensitive indicator of the presence of small airways disease (7). Both

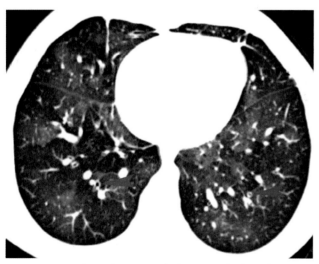

FIGURE 18.21. Constrictive Bronchiolitis (Bronchiolitis Obliterans). Thin-section CT scan in a 53-year-old male with prior bone marrow transplantation for myelodysplasia and biopsy-proven constrictive bronchiolitis shows mosaic attenuation with attenuation of vessels with lucent regions (*asterisks*) and mild central bronchial wall thickening and dilatation (*arrowheads*).

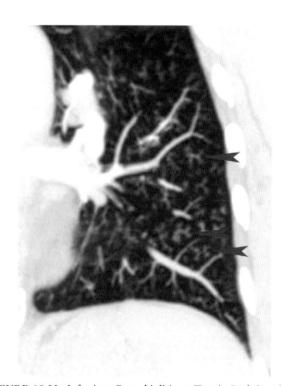

FIGURE 18.22. Infectious Bronchiolitis as Tree-in-Bud Opacities. Coned-down coronal maximum intensity projection (MIP) CT image through the left lower lobe in a patient with mycoplasma pneumonia shows centrilobular tree-in-bud opacities (*arrowheads*).

direct and indirect findings may be evident on HRCT that allow detection of this process. The direct sign of small airways disease is centrilobular nodular and tree-in-bud opacities which represent diseased preterminal bronchioles. This is seen on HRCT as sharply defined or ground-glass nodules with or without Y- or V-shaped tubular branching opacities centrally situated within the secondary pulmonary lobule within 5 mm of the pleural surface (Fig. 18.22). Pathologically, the opacities reflect dilatation and mucus plugging of small bronchioles or peribronchiolar inflammation and fibrosis.

The indirect signs of small airways disease result from expiratory air trapping and are most easily seen on HRCT. Those portions of lung most severely affected by small airways disease are poorly ventilated and perfused and appear relatively hyperlucent adjacent to areas of normal lung. This results in an appearance on HRCT, termed "mosaic attenuation," that is virtually indistinguishable from the changes seen in primary pulmonary arterial occlusive disease. Furthermore, infiltrative processes such as *Pneumocystis jiroveci* pneumonia and desquamative interstitial pneumonitis, which produce patchy ground-glass opacification, also result in a mosaic attenuation appearance on HRCT. The use of both inspiratory and expiratory HRCT scans helps distinguish between these various disorders. In a patient with mosaic attenuation, attenuated vessels within the lucent regions of lung indicate that the lucent regions are abnormal because of decreased perfusion. This finding allows distinction from ground-glass opacification, where the caliber of vessels in normal and abnormal lung are comparable. The presence of small airways disease is confirmed on expiratory HRCT by noting air trapping within the hyperlucent regions.

References

1. Marom EM, Goodman PC, McAdams HP. Focal abnormalities of the trachea and main bronchi. AJR Am J Roentgenol 2001;176:707–711.
2. Marom EM, Goodman PC, McAdams HP. Diffuse abnormalities of the trachea and main bronchi. AJR Am J Roentgenol 2001;176:713–717.
3. Carden KA, Boiselle PM, Waltz DA, Ernst A. Tracheomalacia and tracheobronchomalacia in children and adults: an in-depth review. Chest 2005;127:984–1005.
4. Washko GR. Diagnostic imaging in COPD. Semin Respir Crit Care Med 2010;31:276–285.
5. Hansell DM. Bronchiectasis. Radiol Clin North Am 1998;36:107–128.
6. Foster WL, Gimenez EI, Roubidoux MA, et al. The emphysemas: radiologic-pathologic correlation. Radiographics 1993;13:311–328.
7. Lynch DA. Imaging of small airways disease and chronic obstructive lung disease. Clin Chest Med 2008;29:165–179.

CHAPTER 19 ■ PLEURA, CHEST WALL, DIAPHRAGM, AND MISCELLANEOUS CHEST DISORDERS

JEFFREY S. KLEIN AND JIMMY S. GHOSTINE

PLEURA

Anatomy, Physiology, and Pathophysiology

The pleura is a serous membrane subdivided into visceral pleura, which covers the lung and forms the interlobar fissures, and parietal pleura, which lines the mediastinum, diaphragm, and thoracic cage. Both the visceral and parietal pleurae consist of a single layer of mesothelial cells and their basement membrane, and a dense sheet of irregular connective with varying ratios of collagen to elastin (1). The potential space between the visceral and parietal pleura is the pleural space. The parietal and visceral pleurae meet at the hila and form a thin double-layered fold at the medial lung base inferior to the inferior pulmonary veins termed the pulmonary ligament (see Fig. 12.8). A small amount of fluid totaling 2 to 5 mL is normally present in the pleural space to serve as a lubricant that allows smooth gliding of the visceral pleura along the parietal pleura during breathing. The volume of fluid within the pleural space is the result of a dynamic equilibrium between formation and resorption (2). The formation of pleural fluid follows Starling's law and depends upon hydrostatic and oncotic forces in both the systemic capillaries of the parietal pleura and the pleural space (1). Under normal conditions, pleural fluid is formed by filtration from systemic capillaries in the parietal pleura and resorbed via the parietal pleural lymphatics. (Fig. 19.1).

The radiologically detectable manifestations of pleural diseases are limited and include effusion, thickening, and calcification (3).

Pleural Effusion

Pleural effusions form when an imbalance occurs between formation and reabsorption (Table 19.1). Pleural effusions may be classified by their gross appearance (bloody, chylous, purulent, serous), the underlying disease process (Table 19.2), or by the pathophysiology of abnormal pleural fluid formation (i.e., transudative versus exudative) (Tables 19.1 and 19.3). This latter differentiation is made by measuring the protein, lactic acid dehydrogenase (LDH), and glucose concentration of the pleural fluid obtained by thoracentesis (Table 19.3).

Specific Causes of Pleural Effusion. *Congestive heart failure* is the most common condition to produce a transudative pleural effusion. The effusions are typically bilateral and larger on the right (4). An isolated right effusion is twice as common as an isolated left effusion.

Parapneumonic Effusion and Empyema. A parapneumonic effusion is defined as an effusion associated with pneumonia. Peripheral parenchymal infection produces an exudative pleural effusion by causing visceral pleural inflammation that increases pleural capillary permeability. Inflammatory thickening of the pleural membranes with lymphatic obstruction may also be a contributing factor. Empyema results when the parenchymal infection extends into the pleural space. Parenchymal infections that typically result in empyema formation are bacterial pneumonia, septic emboli, and lung abscess, whereas fungal, viral, and parasitic infections are uncommon causes. Less commonly, infection may extend into the pleural space from the spine, mediastinum, and chest wall.

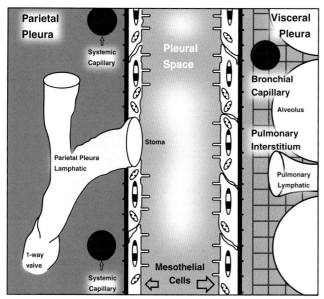

FIGURE 19.1. Normal Pleural Physiology. (Modified from Miserocchi G. Physiology and pathophysiology of pleural fluid turnover. Eur Respir J 1997;10:219–225.)

Forty percent of bacterial pneumonias have an associated pleural effusion. *Staphylococcus aureus* and gram-negative pneumonias are the most common cause of parapneumonic effusion and empyema. The natural history of parapneumonic effusions may be divided into three stages (5–7). Stage 1 is an exudative stage; visceral pleural inflammation causes increased capillary permeability and pleural fluid accumulation. Most of these sterile exudative effusions resolve with appropriate antibiotic therapy. A stage 2 parapneumonic effusion is a fibrinopurulent pleural fluid collection containing bacteria and neutrophils. Fibrin deposition on the visceral and parietal pleura impairs fluid resorption and produces loculations. If the infection is not treated, the loculations will impair attempts at closed pleural fluid drainage. A stage 3 parapneumonic effusion develops 2 to 3 weeks after initial pleural fluid formation and is characterized by the ingrowth of fibroblasts over the pleura, which produces pleural fibrosis and entraps the lung. Dystrophic calcification

TABLE 19.1

MECHANISMS OF ABNORMAL PLEURAL FLUID FORMATION

Increased interstitial fluid production
  CHF, parapneumonic effusions, ARDS, and lung
    transplantation

Increased hydrostatic pressure
  LV or RV failure, SVC syndrome, pericardial tamponade

Increased capillary permeability
  ↑Cytokine levels producing increased permeability

Decreased oncotic pressure gradient
  Hypoproteinemic states

Impaired reabsorption
  Obstruction of lymphatics

Elevation of systemic venous pressure

CHF, congestive heart failure; ARDS, acute respiratory distress syndrome; SVC, superior vena cava.

TABLE 19.2

ETIOLOGY OF PLEURAL EFFUSIONS

Infectious	Bacterial/mycobacterial
	Viral
	Fungal
	Parasitic
Cardiovascular	Heart failure
	Pericarditis
	Superior vena cava obstruction
	Postcardiac surgery
	Myocardial infarction
	Pulmonary embolism
Neoplastic	Bronchogenic carcinoma
	Metastases
	Lymphoma
	Pleural or chest wall neoplasms (mesothelioma)
Immunologic	Systemic lupus erythematosus
	Rheumatoid arthritis
	Sarcoidosis (rare)
	Wegener granulomatosis
Inhalational	Asbestos
Trauma	Blunt or penetrating chest trauma
Abdominal disease	Cirrhosis (hepatic hydrothorax)
	Pancreatitis
	Subphrenic abscess
	Acute pyelonephritis
	Ascites (from any cause)
	Splenic vein thrombosis
Miscellaneous	Drugs
	Myxedema
	Ovarian tumor

of the pleura may develop following resolution of the pleural infection. Tuberculous pleural effusion or empyema resulting from the rupture of subpleural caseating granulomas may complicate pulmonary infection or occur as the primary manifestation of disease. Effusions in tuberculosis (TB) are more common in young adults with pulmonary disease and in HIV-positive individuals with severe immunodeficiency. The pleural fluid is characteristically straw colored, with greater than 70% lymphocytes and a low glucose concentration.

TABLE 19.3

CHARACTERIZATION OF PLEURAL EFFUSIONS

Transudate	Exudate
$TP_{fluid}/TP_{serum} < 0.5$	$TP_{fluid}/TP_{serum} > 0.5$
$LDH_{fluid}/LDH_{serum} < 0.6$	$LDH_{fluid}/LDH_{serum} > 0.6$
$LDH_{fluid} < 200$ IU/L	$LDH_{fluid} > 200$ IU/L
Specific gravity < 1.016	Specific gravity > 1.016
Diff Dx:	**Diff Dx:**
Cardiogenic	Infection
Hypoproteinemic	Infarction
Myxedematous	Neoplasm
Cirrhotic (hepatic hydrothorax)	Inflammation (serositis)
Nephrotic syndrome	

LDH, lactic acid dehydrogenase.

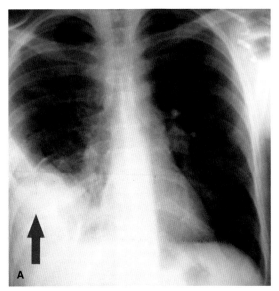
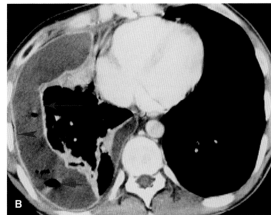

FIGURE 19.2. **Empyema on Chest Radiograph and CT. A.** Posteroanterior chest film in a patient with a recent right lower pneumonia demonstrates an oval opacity in the right lateral costophrenic sulcus containing gas (*arrow*). **B.** An enhanced CT scan shows a circumferential pleural fluid collection with enhancing visceral (*long red arrow*) and parietal (*red arrowhead*) pleural layers representing an empyema. Note the contained gas pockets (*short blue arrow*), indicating loculations within the collection itself.

Radiographically, empyema most often appears as a loculated pleural fluid collection. On CT, it is elliptic in shape and is seen most often within the posterior (costal pleura) and inferior (subpulmonic) pleural space. The collection conforms to and maintains a broad area of contact with the chest wall (Fig. 19.2). The distinction of empyema from peripheral lung abscess has important therapeutic implications; empyemas require external drainage, whereas lung abscesses usually respond to postural drainage and antibiotic therapy. Contrast-enhanced chest CT is most useful in making this distinction (Table 19.4) (8). Detection of an empyema may be difficult when there is extensive parenchymal consolidation. In these cases, CT and US are useful in detecting parapneumonic fluid collections and guiding diagnostic thoracentesis and pleural drainage. Findings on CT that are fairly specific for the presence of an exudative pleural effusion include thickening and enhancement of the parietal pleura, the presence of loculations, and the detection of discrete soft tissue lesions along the parietal pleura outlined by low-attenuation pleural fluid. Hemorrhagic effusions can occasionally be recognized on CT by their intrinsic high attenuation or the presence of a fluid–fluid level caused by dependent cellular blood elements.

Neoplasms. Pleural effusion may be seen with benign or malignant intrathoracic tumors. The tumors most commonly associated with pleural effusion are, in order of frequency, lung carcinoma, breast carcinoma, pelvic tumors, gastric carcinoma, and lymphoma. Pleural fluid may result from pleural involvement by tumor or from lymphatic obstruction anywhere from the parietal pleura to the mediastinal nodes. The effusions are exudative and may be bloody. Demonstration of malignant cells on cytologic examination of pleural fluid obtained at thoracentesis is necessary for the diagnosis of a malignant effusion. Image-guided closed or thoracoscopic biopsy is reserved for patients with negative cytologic examination. Clues to the presence of a malignant pleural effusion include smooth or nodular pleural thickening, mediastinal or hilar lymph node enlargement or mass, and solitary or multiple parenchymal nodules. CT is useful in demonstrating pleural masses or underlying parenchymal lesions in those with large effusions (Fig. 19.3).

Trauma. Blunt or penetrating trauma to the chest, including iatrogenic trauma from thoracotomy, thoracostomy, or placement of central venous catheters, may result in a hemothorax. Hemothorax results from laceration of vessels within the lung, mediastinum, chest wall, or diaphragm. Intrapleural blood coagulates rapidly, and septations form early. In some individuals, pleural motion causes defibrination, which lyses the clotted blood. In the acute setting, pleural fluid of high

TABLE 19.4

EMPYEMA VERSUS LUNG ABSCESS ON CT

■ FEATURE	■ EMPYEMA	■ ABSCESS
Shape	Oval, oriented longitudinally	Round
Margin	Thin, smooth ("split pleura" sign)	Thick, irregular
Angle with chest wall	Obtuse	Acute
Effect on lung	Compression	Consumption
Treatment	External drainage	Antibiotics, postural drainage

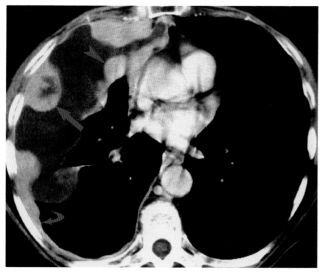

FIGURE 19.3. Malignant Pleural Disease: CT Diagnosis. CT in a patient with lung cancer shows discrete nodules on the parietal pleura (*straight arrow*), the visceral pleura (*arrowhead*), and the nodular thickening (*curved arrow*) of the parietal pleura, all representing manifestation of pleural metastases. The diagnosis of bronchogenic carcinoma metastatic to the pleura was confirmed by US-guided biopsy.

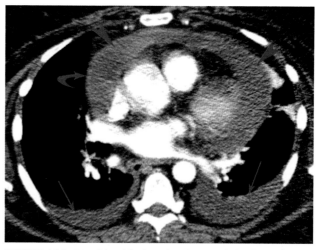

FIGURE 19.5. Serositis with Pleural and Pericardial Effusions. Axial CT scan in a 54-year-old patient with lupus erythematosus shows bilateral pleural (*arrows*) and a pericardial (*arrowheads*) effusion. Note subtle thickening and enhancement of the pericardium (*curved arrow*) indicating the presence of pericarditis.

CT attenuation (>80 H) may be seen (Fig. 19.4); associated rib fractures or subcutaneous emphysema should suggest the diagnosis. An acute hemothorax is treated with thoracostomy tube drainage, whereas thoracotomy is generally reserved for persistent bleeding or hypotension.

Esophageal perforation from prolonged vomiting (Boerhaave syndrome) or as a complication of esophageal dilatation may produce a pleural effusion, most commonly on the left side.

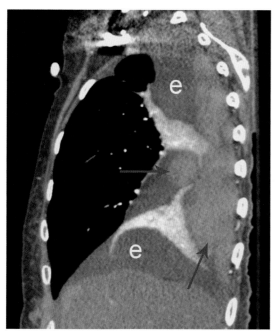

FIGURE 19.4. Hemothorax. Sagittal CT-reconstruction through the right hemithorax in a patient who has sustained blunt chest trauma with a right rib fracture shows a pleural effusion (*e*) containing dependent high-attenuation material (*arrows*) representing clotted blood in a traumatic hemothorax.

Extravascular placement of a central line can result in a hydrothorax when intravenous solution is inadvertently infused into the pleural or extrapleural space.

Collagen Vascular and Autoimmune Disease. Systemic lupus erythematosus has a reported incidence of pleural effusions ranging from 33% to 74% (Fig. 19.5). These exudative effusions are a result of pleural inflammation; patients often present with pleuritic chest pain. In some cases, the nephrotic syndrome associated with systemic lupus erythematosus may produce transudative effusions. Cardiomegaly is a common associated radiographic finding and may be caused by pericardial effusion, hypertension, renal failure, or lupus-associated endocarditis or myocarditis. Pleural effusion is the most common intrathoracic manifestation of rheumatoid arthritis and is most frequently seen in male patients following the onset of joint disease. The effusions occur independent of pulmonary parenchymal involvement, but may develop following intrapleural rupture of peripheral rheumatoid nodules. The effusions of rheumatoid arthritis are exudative, with lymphocytosis, low glucose concentration, and low pH (<7.2). Rheumatoid effusions may persist unchanged for years. Autoimmune syndromes producing pleural and pericardial effusions have been described following myocardial infarction (Dressler syndrome) or cardiac surgery (postpericardiotomy syndrome). Both are characterized by fever, pleuritis, pneumonitis, and pericarditis developing within days to weeks of the precipitating event. The radiographic findings include enlargement of the cardiac silhouette, pleural effusions, and parenchymal airspace opacities. A serosanguineous exudative pleural effusion is seen in over 80% of patients. Treatment with nonsteroidal anti-inflammatory drugs usually results in symptomatic and radiographic improvement.

Abdominal Disease. Radioisotope studies have demonstrated that peritoneal fluid may enter the pleural space via transdiaphragmatic lymphatic channels or through defects in the diaphragm. The lymphatic channels are larger on the right side, accounting for the higher incidence of right-sided effusions associated with ascites or liver failure (hepatic hydrothorax).

Pancreatitis. Acute or chronic pancreatitis can cause pleural effusions that are most often left-sided because of the proximity of the pancreatic tail to the left hemidiaphragm. The effusion associated with acute pancreatitis is typically exudative and may be bloody. Pleural effusion from chronic pancreatitis

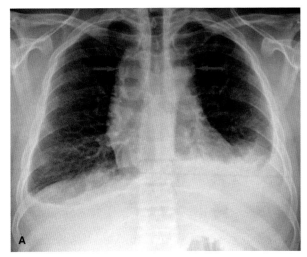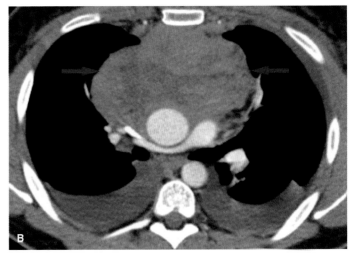

FIGURE 19.6. Chylous Pleural Effusions Caused by Hodgkin Lymphoma. **A.** Chest radiograph in a 26-year-old man with nodular sclerosing Hodgkin lymphoma shows an anterior mediastinal mass (*arrows*) with bilateral pleural effusions. **B.** Contrast-enhanced axial CT scan shows a large heterogeneous anterior mediastinal mass (*arrows*) associated with bilateral pleural effusions. Chylous fluid was obtained at left-sided thoracentesis.

may cause pleuritic chest pain and shortness of breath. Rupture of the pancreatic duct can lead to a pancreaticopleural fistula. A high amylase concentration in the pleural fluid should suggest the pancreas as the etiology of the effusion, although elevated amylase may be seen in pleural effusions caused by malignancy or esophageal perforation.

Subphrenic abscess complicating abdominal surgery or perforation of a hollow viscus can cause diaphragmatic paresis, basilar atelectasis, and pleural effusion. Patients with a pleural effusion associated with upper abdominal pain, fever, and leukocytosis should have CT or US examination and when applicable, percutaneous catheter drainage of the abscess.

Pelvic Tumors. An association between benign pleural effusions and pelvic tumors has long been recognized. First described with ovarian fibroma (Meigs syndrome), a number of pelvic and abdominal tumors, including pancreatic and ovarian malignancy, lymphoma, and uterine leiomyomas, have been found to cause pleural effusion. The effusions in Meigs syndrome are usually transudative and resolve after removal of the pelvic tumor.

Chylothorax is a pleural collection containing triglycerides in the form of chylomicrons resulting from extravasation of thoracic duct contents secondary to malignancy, iatrogenic trauma, or TB (Fig. 19.6). The thoracic duct originates from the cisterna chyli at the level of the first lumbar vertebra and ascends along the right paravertebral space, entering the thorax via the aortic hiatus. The duct crosses from right to left at the level of the sixth thoracic vertebra to lie alongside the upper esophagus. A knowledge of this anatomy is useful, as disruption of the upper duct caused by direct trauma or obstruction with rupture produces a left chylothorax, whereas injury to the lower intrathoracic duct produces a right chylothorax. At the level of the left subclavian artery, the duct arches anteriorly to empty into the confluence of the left internal jugular and subclavian veins. The radiographic appearance is indistinguishable on plain radiographs and CT from other causes of free-flowing effusions. The diagnosis is confirmed by triglyceride levels exceeding 110 mg/dL in the pleural fluid.

Pulmonary Embolism. Infarction complicating pulmonary embolism is a well-recognized cause of pleural effusion. The effusion may be associated with elevation of the ipsilateral diaphragm and peripheral wedge-shaped opacities (Hampton hump). The pleural effusion is typically a small, unilateral, serosanguineous exudate.

Drugs may cause pleural effusions as a result of pleural inflammation (methysergide) or by producing a lupus-like syndrome (phenytoin, isoniazid, hydralazine, procainamide). Nitrofurantoin has been associated with an immunologic reaction that causes pleuropulmonary disease with eosinophilia.

Management of Pleural Effusion. Transudative pleural effusions are managed by treatment of the underlying disorder because the pleura is intrinsically normal in these diseases. Management of parapneumonic effusions is best guided by evaluation of the likelihood that the effusion, if not drained, would result in prolonged hospitalization, pleural fibrosis with resultant respiratory impairment, local spread of infection, or death. This likelihood is based on the anatomy, bacteriology, and chemistry (i.e., ABCs) of the fluid collection. In general, larger, loculated collections with positive gram stains or cultures and pH less than 7.20 are associated with a moderate to high risk for poor outcome as detailed above and should be drained if possible (5). The choice of drainage procedure depends on various factors, including patient age and underlying condition, length of illness, and access to image-guided therapy and thoracoscopy. Although intrapleural fibrinolytic therapy with tissue plasminogen activator will help a certain subset of patients with complex parapneumonic effusions (Fig. 19.7), some will require open pleural drainage by video-assisted thoracoscopic surgery (VATS) or thoracotomy with decortication. In contrast, malignant pleural effusions most often require closed drainage and pleural sclerosis, with talc being the current agent of choice. Trials of other pleurodesis agents have not shown superiority while being marred by higher cost. It is notable that talc pleurodesis can cause FDG-18 PET positive nodularity, which is a source of false-negative PET evaluations. Some patients may benefit from VATS drainage and sclerosis. Select patients can be managed as outpatients with indwelling silastic catheters (e.g., PleurX™catheter, CareFusion Corp, San Diego, CA), which allow intermittent patient-directed drainage of fluid. Patients with chylothorax secondary to lymphoma or TB require therapy directed at this underlying, whereas patients with traumatic disruption of the thoracic duct often require surgical ligation of the duct.

Patients with pleural effusions from trauma, pulmonary embolism, autoimmune disorders, and drug reactions often require no specific therapy. Exceptions include the postpericardi-

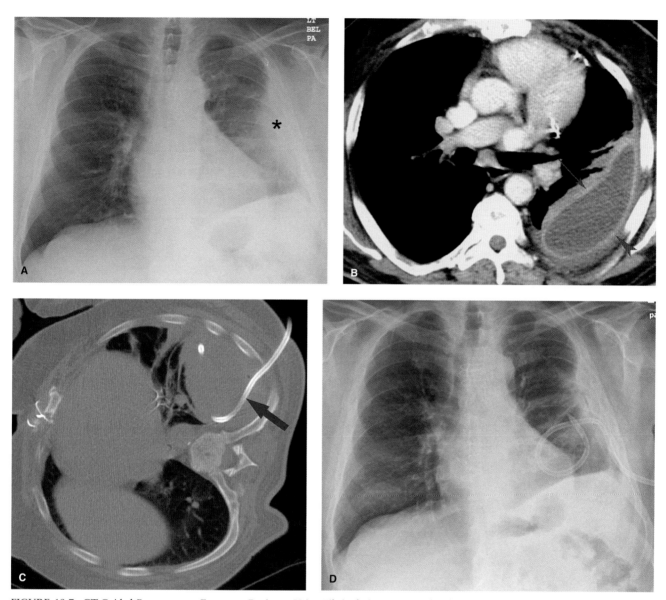

FIGURE 19.7. CT-Guided Percutaneous Empyema Drainage Using Fibrinolytics. A. Frontal radiograph in a 58-year-old man with fever and dyspnea shows a left lateral pleural opacity (*asterisk*). B. Contrast-enhanced axial CT confirms a loculated left posterolateral effusion with enhancing visceral (*arrow*) and parietal (*arrowhead*) pleurae indicative of an empyema (the "split pleura" sign). C. CT scan during image-guided catheter drainage with the patient in the right lateral decubitus position shows a drainage catheter (*arrow*) curled within the collection. Repeat chest radiograph (D) following daily intrapleural fibrinolytic therapy shows significant improvement in the left-sided collection.

otomy or post-MI patients (Dressler syndrome), who are treated with nonsteroidal anti-inflammatory agents, and patients with large hemothoraces requiring large bore tube drainage to prevent pleural fibrosis and lung entrapment.

Bronchopleural Fistula

A bronchopleural fistula is a communication between the lung and the pleural space that often originates from a peripheral airway. A bronchopleural fistula from a bronchus typically results in an empyema, whereas an air leak from peripheral airspaces may cause an intractable pneumothorax without associated infection. Bronchopleural fistulas often develop from dehiscence of a bronchial stump following lobectomy or pneumonectomy, or as the result of a necrotizing pulmonary infection. Presenting symptoms include fever, cough, and dys-

pnea; large air leaks may be noted in patients with pleural drains. Radiographically, a bronchopleural fistula presents as a loculated intrapleural air and fluid collection. An air–fluid level in the postpneumonectomy space should suggest the diagnosis. CT is useful in evaluating patients with suspected bronchopleural fistula and empyema (Fig. 19.8) (6). It can distinguish a hydropneumothorax from a peripheral lung abscess and occasionally demonstrates the actual fistulous communication.

Following pneumonectomy, the residual space gradually fills with fluid and appears radiographically as an opaque hemithorax with ipsilateral mediastinal shift. The radiographic findings suggesting bronchopleural fistula formation complicating pneumonectomy are described in the previous section. CT and MR are useful in evaluating the postpneumonectomy space for evidence of tumor recurrence, and may help in the diagnosis of postoperative bronchopleural fistula and empyema.

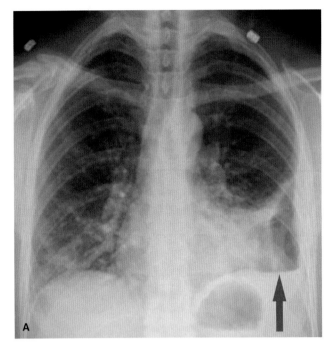

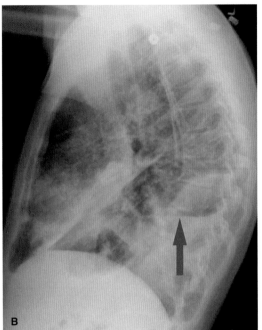

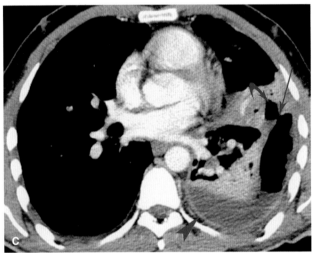

FIGURE 19.8. **Bronchopleural Fistula and Empyema Complicating Pneumonia.** Frontal (**A**) and lateral (**B**) radiographs demonstrate bilateral lower lobe and lingular consolidation, with a left lower loculated hydropneumothorax (*arrows*). **C.** Axial contrast-enhanced CT shows lingular and left lower lobe consolidation with a cavitation in the lingula (*curved arrow*) associated with a bronchopleural fistula (*long arrow*). A loculated pleural air and fluid collection is present with enhancement of the parietal pleura (*arrowhead*).

Pneumothorax

Pneumothorax results from air entering the pleural space and may be traumatic or spontaneous (Table 19.5). Spontaneous pneumothorax is further subdivided into a primary form, which has no identifiable etiology, and a secondary form, which is associated with underlying parenchymal lung disease (7). Patients with a pneumothorax typically present with the sudden onset of dyspnea and pleuritic chest pain.

Radiographically, pneumothorax on upright radiography is recognized by nondependent lucency that parallels the chest wall and displaces the visceral pleural line medially. In a supine patient, such as in the ER or ICU setting, a pneumothorax can be undetectable as air in the pleural space rises nondependently and creates indiscernible increased lucency over the lower thorax and upper abdomen. Signs of pneumothorax on supine radiography include a hyperlucent upper abdomen (particularly on the right over the normally dense liver), the "deep sulcus" sign (Fig. 19.9), the "double diaphragm" sign, the epicardial fat pad sign (for left pneumothorax), and an unusually sharp heart border. In patients with preexisting pleural adhesions, a pneumothorax can present as a loculated lucency within the pleural space including the interlobar fissures.

On CT, pneumothorax is identified by nondependent lucency over the lower anterior thorax. It is not uncommon in trauma patients to detect a small basilar pneumothorax overlying the lower chest that is not evident radiographically.

Traumatic Pneumothorax. Trauma is the most common cause of pneumothorax. Penetrating injuries can produce pneumothorax by introducing air from the atmosphere into the pleural space or by laceration of the visceral pleura, resulting in an air leak from the lung. Gunshot and knife wounds to the chest and upper abdomen, central line placement, thoracentesis, transbronchial biopsy, and percutaneous needle biopsy are common penetrating injuries that cause traumatic pneumothorax. Blunt chest trauma may cause pneumothorax by two different mechanisms: (1) An acute increase in intrathoracic pressure results in extra-alveolar interstitial air because of alveolar disruption, which tracks peripherally and ruptures into the pleural space. (2) Laceration of the tracheobronchial tree can produce a pneumothorax with a large bronchopleural fistula. In patients with rib fractures, the free edge of the fractured ribs can project inward to lacerate the lung and cause pneumothorax.

TABLE 19.5

ETIOLOGY OF PNEUMOTHORAX

Trauma	Iatrogenic
	Thoracic/abdominal surgery
	Percutaneous interventional procedures
	Lung/pleural biopsy
	Thoracentesis
	Central line placement
	Aberrant feeding tube placement
	Mechanical ventilation
	Esophagoscopic biopsy/dilatation
	Bronchoscopic biopsy
	Not iatrogenic
	Penetrating injury
	Stab wound
	Gunshot wound
	Blunt injury
	Tracheobronchial disruption
	Esophageal rupture
	Rib fractures
Spontaneous	Primary (idiopathic)
	Secondary
	Obstructive airways disease
	Asthma
	Emphysema
	Infection
	Cavitating pneumonia
	Lung abscess
	Septic emboli
	Pneumatoceles
	Pulmonary infarction (rare)
	Neoplasm
	Bronchogenic carcinoma
	Pleural or chest wall neoplasm
	Metastases (sarcomas, squamous cell)
	Cystic lung disease
	Sarcoidosis
	Langerhans cell histiocytosis
	Cystic fibrosis
	Tuberous sclerosis
	Lymphangioleiomyomatosis
	Birt-Hogg Dube syndrome
	Catamenial pneumothorax (pleural endometriosis)
	Connective tissue disorders
	Marfan syndrome
	Ehlers-Danlos syndrome
	Cutis laxa

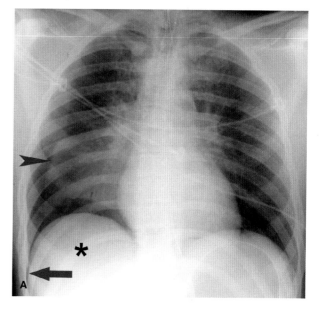

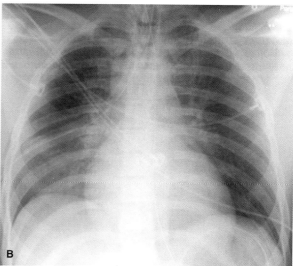

FIGURE 19.9. Pneumothorax on Supine Radiograph. A. Supine portable chest radiograph in a 17-year-old patient who sustained severe blunt head and chest trauma shows abnormal lucency over the upper right abdomen (*asterisk*) and a deep right lateral costophrenic sulcus (*arrow*). Air in the pleural space is visible laterally outlining a consolidated middle lobe due to contusion (*arrowhead*). **B.** Repeat radiograph following right chest tube placement shows resolution of the pneumothorax.

Primary spontaneous pneumothorax most often occurs in young or middle-aged men. A familial incidence and a propensity for tall, thin individuals has been noted. Affected patients may have blebs or bullae in the lung apices that are responsible for the development of recurrent pneumothoraces. Treatment of the initial episode is with closed tube drainage, with thoracoscopic bullectomy reserved for recurrent episodes or persistent air leak.

Secondary Spontaneous Pneumothorax. Multiple entities have been associated with secondary spontaneous pneumothorax, although in some patients the lungs are intrinsically normal. In the majority of the latter, there is usually a history of sudden increases in intrathoracic pressure. Chronic obstructive pulmonary disease is the most common predisposing condition. Acute obstruction to expiration from bronchoconstriction (asthma) or the performance of the Valsalva maneuver (crack

cocaine or marijuana smoking, transvaginal childbirth) may cause spontaneous pneumothorax. Pneumothorax may complicate cystic lung changes in sarcoidosis, Langerhans cell histiocytosis of lung, and lymphangioleiomyomatosis. Necrotizing pneumonia or lung abscess caused by gram-negative or anaerobic bacteria, TB, or *Pneumocystis jiroveci* pneumonia can lead to pneumothorax, particularly in the mechanically ventilated patient. Metastases to the lung are an infrequent cause of pneumothorax and rarely are a presenting feature of disease. In these cases, pneumothorax develops when necrotic subpleural metastases rupture into the pleural space (Fig. 19.10).

Sarcomas, particularly osteogenic sarcoma, lymphoma, and germ cell malignancies, are the most common primary malignancies to produce spontaneous pneumothorax. Marfan syndrome is the most common connective tissue disease producing pneumothorax; it usually results from the rupture of

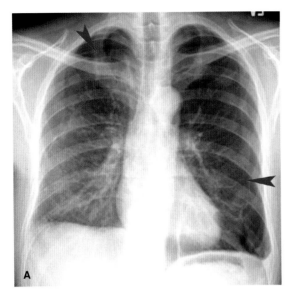

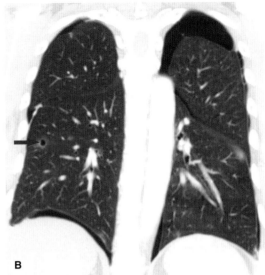

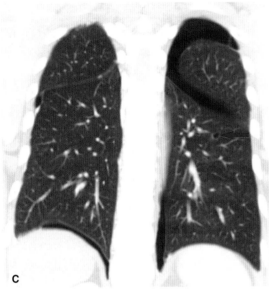

FIGURE 19.10. Spontaneous Pneumothorax from Cavitary Metastases. A. Chest radiograph in a patient with a history of a lower extremity sarcoma demonstrates bilateral spontaneous pneumothoraces (*arrowheads*). Coronal-reformatted chest CT at the level of the descending aorta (**B**) and thoracic spine (**C**) confirms the pneumothoraces and shows thin-walled cavitary nodules (*arrows*) reflecting metastases.

apical bullae. Other connective tissue diseases that can produce pneumothorax are Ehlers-Danlos syndrome and cutis laxa.

Mechanically ventilated patients are particularly at risk for pneumothorax because of the administration of positive pressure, emphysema, underlying or complicating necrotizing pneumonia, and frequent line placements and other invasive procedures. Not uncommonly, patients with ARDS develop small peripheral cystic airspaces, which can rupture into the pleural space. When these are seen to develop on serial chest radiographs, impending pneumothorax can be suggested.

A particularly rare type of recurrent pneumothorax that occurs with menstruation is catamenial pneumothorax. This condition affects women in their fourth decade and is most likely caused by the cyclical necrosis of pleural endometrial implants, which creates an air leak between the lung and pleura. Rarely, air entering the peritoneal cavity during menstruation gains access to the pleural cavity via diaphragmatic defects. The predilection for right-sided pneumothoraces in this disorder indicates a key role for right-sided diaphragmatic defects. The pneumothoraces tend to be small and resolve spontaneously. Catamenial pneumothorax is managed by preventing menstruation with the administration of oral contraceptives.

Tension pneumothorax is a critical condition that most often results from iatrogenic trauma in mechanically ventilated patients. Tension pneumothorax results from a check-valve pleural defect that allows air to enter but not exit the pleural space. This leads to a pleural air collection that has a pressure exceeding atmospheric pressure during at least a portion of the respiratory cycle, causing complete collapse of the underlying lung and impairing venous return to the heart. Clinically, patients present with tachypnea, tachycardia, cyanosis, and hypotension. Radiographically, the involved hemithorax is expanded and hyperlucent, with a medially retracted lung, ipsilateral diaphragmatic depression or inversion, and contralateral mediastinal shift (Fig. 19.11). It is important to remember that contralateral mediastinal shift from pneumothorax does not invariably indicate tension, since a relative inequality in the degree of negative intrapleural pressure can produce shift in the absence of tension. Therefore, tension pneumothorax remains a clinical diagnosis. Immediate evacuation of the pleural space should be performed with a needle, catheter, or large-bore thoracostomy tube.

Focal Pleural Disease

Focal pleural disease may be divided into localized pleural thickening, pleural calcification, or pleural mass (Table 19.6) (8).

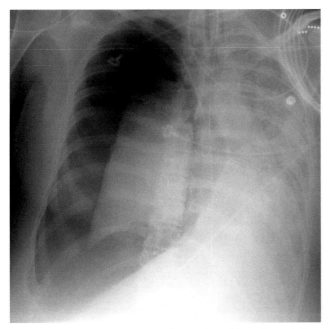

FIGURE 19.11. Tension Pneumothorax. Portable radiograph in a 27-year-old woman with acute respiratory distress syndrome (ARDS) complicating pneumonia demonstrates a large right pneumothorax with enlargement of the right hemithorax, marked diaphragmatic depression, and contralateral mediastinal shift.

Localized pleural thickening from fibrosis is usually the end result of peripheral parenchymal and pleural inflammatory disease, with pneumonia the most common cause. Additional causes include pulmonary embolism with infarction, asbestos exposure, trauma, prior chemical pleurodesis, and drug-related pleural disease.

TABLE 19.6

FOCAL PLEURAL DISEASE

Opacities that mimic focal pleural thickening	Apical cap
	Companion shadows of first and second ribs
	Subpleural deposits of fat
Thickening	Pneumonia
	Pulmonary infarct
	Trauma
	Asbestos exposure (bilateral)
Calcification	Visceral pleura
	Hemothorax
	Empyema (tuberculosis)
	Parietal pleura
	Asbestos exposure (bilateral)
Pleural/extrapleural mass	Neoplasm
	Benign
	Localized fibrous tumor
	Lipoma
	Neurofibroma
	Malignant
	Metastases (usually multiple)
	Mesothelioma (usually diffuse pleural thickening)
	Loculated pleural effusion/empyema
	Hematoma

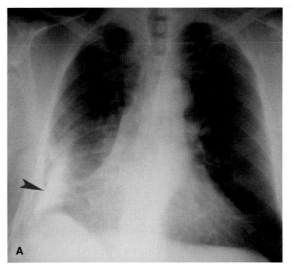

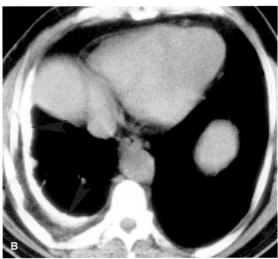

FIGURE 19.12. Pleural Calcification Caused by Tuberculosis. **A.** Posteroanterior chest radiograph in a 61-year-old man with prior TB demonstrates a small right hemithorax and a dense opacity inferolaterally. **B.** A CT scan through the lung bases shows a thick rind of pleural calcification (*arrowheads*) surrounding a contracted lung.

Pleural calcification is most often unilateral and involves the visceral pleura. It is usually the result of prior hemothorax or empyema (e.g., TB), although pleural thickening from any cause may calcify. Asbestos exposure can cause bilateral multifocal calcified parietal pleural plaques. Visceral pleural calcifications from pleural hemorrhage or infection are indistinguishable radiographically. Initially, the calcification is punctate, but it often progresses to become sheetlike. CT is particularly useful in characterizing pleural calcification (Fig. 19.12). The presence of fluid within calcified pleural layers seen on CT suggests an active empyema and is most often seen in patients with prior TB. The use of CT and HRCT in the evaluation of asbestos-related focal pleural disease and calcification is discussed in a subsequent section.

Pleural Mass. Focal pleural masses are usually benign neoplasms such as lipomas; loculated pleural fluid can mimic a pleural mass radiographically. Thoracic lipomas may arise in the chest wall or subpleural fat. Subpleural lipomas produce a pleural mass and can change shape during respiration or with changes in patient positioning because of their pliable nature. Homogeneous fat attenuation on CT scan (−30 to −100 H) is diagnostic (Fig. 19.13).

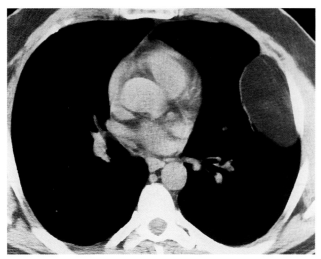

FIGURE 19.13. **Pleural Lipoma.** CT scan in a patient with an asymptomatic mass discovered as an incidental chest radiographic finding shows a left anterolateral pleura-based mass with homogeneous fatty attenuation representing a lipoma.

TABLE 19.7

DIFFUSE PLEURAL DISEASE

Smooth thickening	Pleural fibrosis
	Hemothorax
	Prior empyema or exudative effusion (including asbestos exposure)
	Interstitial pulmonary fibrosis
	Pleural effusion (particularly on supine radiographs)
Lobulated/nodular	Primary
	Mesothelioma
	Metastatic
	Adenocarcinoma of lung, breast, ovary, kidney, GI tract
	Invasive thymoma
	Lymphoma (subpleural deposits)
	Multiloculated pleural effusion/empyema

Localized fibrous tumors of pleura (LFTP) are uncommon pleural tumors (8). While most often benign, approximately 15% will recur locally after resection. These lesions appear as well-defined, spherical or oblong masses that arise from subpleural mesenchymal cells and are benign in approximately 80% of cases. These tumors are occasionally attached to the pleura by a narrow pedicle, a finding that is virtually pathognomonic and accounts for changes in intrapleural location seen with changes in patient positioning in some individuals (Fig. 19.14). CT usually shows a smoothly marginated, pleura-based soft tissue mass with either uniform soft tissue attenuation or inhomogeneous enhancement caused by areas of necrosis. An association between LFTP and hypertrophic pulmonary osteoarthropathy and hypoglycemia is recognized. Unlike malignant mesothelioma, there is no association between LFTP and asbestos exposure.

Diffuse Pleural Disease

Diffuse pleural disease represents diffuse pleural fibrosis (fibrothorax), pleural malignancy, or multiloculated pleural effusion (Table 19.7) (9).

Fibrothorax (diffuse pleural fibrosis) is defined as pleural thickening extending over more than one-fourth of the costal pleural surface (Fig. 19.15). Fibrothorax most commonly results from the resolution of an exudative pleural effusion (including asbestos-related effusions), empyema, or hemothorax. It may also be seen as a subpleural extension of diffuse interstitial fibrosis. The fibrothorax can encompass the entire lung and produce entrapment. When this causes a restrictive ventilatory defect, pleurectomy (decortication) may be necessary to restore function to the underlying lung.

Pleural Malignancy. Metastatic disease to the pleura commonly causes irregular or nodular pleural thickening, usually in association with a pleural effusion. The malignant tumors

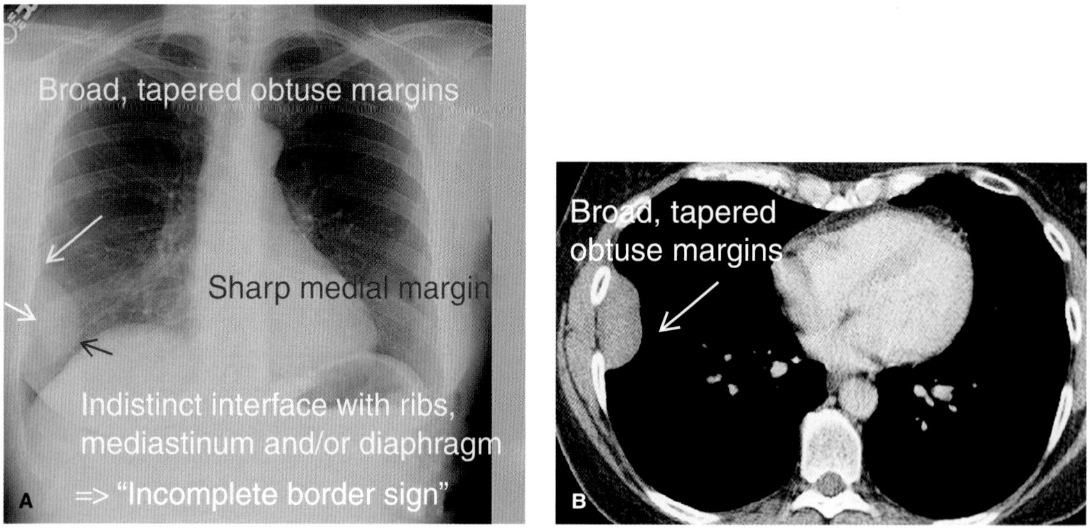

Broad, tapered obtuse margins

Sharp medial margin

Indistinct interface with ribs, mediastinum and/or diaphragm
=> "Incomplete border sign"

Broad, tapered obtuse margins

FIGURE 19.14. **Localized Fibrous Tumor of Pleura. A.** Chest radiograph in a 47-year-old woman shows a smooth intrathoracic mass (*arrows*) in the lower right lateral chest with obtuse superior and inferior margins. **B.** Axial CT scan shows a sharply defined soft tissue mass with tapered obtuse margins, typical of a pleural mass. Note the absence of chest wall involvement. Biopsy confirmed a localized fibrous tumor of pleura.

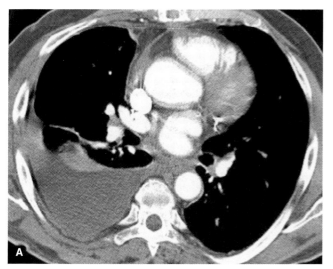 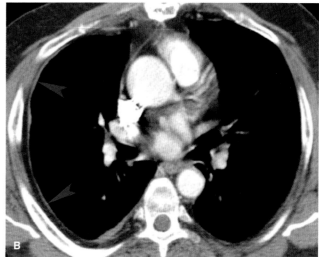

FIGURE 19.15. **Diffuse Pleural Fibrosis. A.** Axial CT scan shows a right pleural effusion. **B.** Repeat CT years later obtained for evaluation of shortness of breath with restrictive disease on pulmonary function tests shows thickening along the right costal pleural surface (*arrowheads*) with hypertrophy of the extrapleural fat and volume loss in the right hemithorax. Note sparing of the mediastinal pleural surface, typical of benign pleural disease.

with a propensity to metastasize to the pleura include adenocarcinomas of the lung, breast, ovary, kidney, and GI tract. Malignant mesothelioma is seen almost exclusively in asbestos-exposed individuals.

Malignant pleural disease is most often caused by one of four conditions: metastatic adenocarcinoma (see Fig. 15.15), invasive thymoma or thymic carcinoma, mesothelioma, and rarely lymphoma. Pleural malignancy presents radiographically as multiple discrete pleural masses or nodular pleural thickening. The pleural lesions are often obscured by an associated malignant pleural effusion. Contrast-enhanced CT can distinguish solid pleural masses from loculated pleural fluid and can show discrete pleural masses or thickening in patients with large effusions. In contrast to benign pleural thickening, malignant pleural disease is more likely when the pleural thickening on CT is circumferential and nodular, greater than 1 cm in thickness, and/or involves the mediastinal pleura (9). Mesothelioma is radiographically indistinguishable from metastatic pleural disease and will be discussed in the next section. Chest wall invasion by pleural tumor, seen as rib destruction or soft tissue infiltration of the subcutaneous fat and musculature, is better appreciated on CT or MR than on plain films. The diagnosis of malignant pleural disease is made by cytologic examination of fluid obtained at thoracentesis, closed or thoracoscopically guided pleural biopsy, or by thoracotomy.

Asbestos-Related Pleural Disease

Prolonged exposure to the inorganic silicate mineral fibers generically known as asbestos can result in a variety of pleural and pulmonary disorders. Benign pleural disease is the most common thoracic manifestation of asbestos inhalation and includes pleural plaques, pleural effusions, and diffuse pleural fibrosis. Rounded atelectasis is reviewed in Chapter 12. Malignant asbestos-related pleural disease manifests as malignant mesothelioma.

Benign Asbestos-Related Pleural Disease. *Pleural plaques* are the most common benign manifestation of asbestos inhalation. These plaques develop 20 to 30 years after the initial asbestos exposure and are more frequent with increasing length and severity of exposure. Asbestos plaques are found on the parietal pleura, most commonly over the diaphragm and lower posterolateral chest wall. The mediastinal pleural surface and costophrenic sulci are characteristically spared. The plaques are discrete, bilateral, slightly raised (2 to 10 mm thick) foci of pleural thickening that are pearly white and shiny in gross appearance. Histologically, the plaques are composed of dense bands of collagen. Punctate or linear calcification within the plaques is common and is more frequent as the plaques enlarge. Asbestos bodies (short, straight asbestos fibers coated with iron and protein that microscopically look like small dumbbells) are not seen within the plaques. Visceral pleural plaques, seen as discrete flat regions of pleural thickening within the major fissures on HRCT, are most commonly associated with interstitial fibrosis. Most patients with isolated asbestos-related pleural plaques are asymptomatic.

Detection of pleural plaques on conventional radiographs is best performed with 45° oblique views that profile the anterolateral and posterolateral plaques. When viewed en face, the calcified plaques appear as geographic areas of opacity that have been likened to a holly leaf (Fig 19.16). CT and HRCT studies are extremely sensitive in detecting calcified and noncalcified pleural plaques in asbestos-exposed individuals and can distinguish pleural plaques and diffuse pleural fibrosis from subpleural fat deposits that may mimic pleural disease on conventional radiographs. Although plaques are invariably bilateral on gross examination of the pleural space in affected individuals, it is not unusual to see unilateral plaques (most often left-sided) on conventional radiographs or HRCT.

Pleural effusion occurs 10 to 20 years after the initial exposure and is the earliest manifestation of asbestos-related pleural disease. The development of asbestos-related effusions appears to be dose related. The effusions are usually small, unilateral or bilateral, and exudative and may be bloody. The diagnosis of a benign asbestos-related pleural effusion is one of exclusion and, in addition to a history of exposure, requires the exclusion of TB or pleural malignancy (i.e., mesothelioma or metastatic adenocarcinoma). A long latency period between the initial exposure and the development of pleural effusion (>20 years) should prompt a diagnostic evaluation for malignant mesothelioma. While most asbestos-related pleural effusions

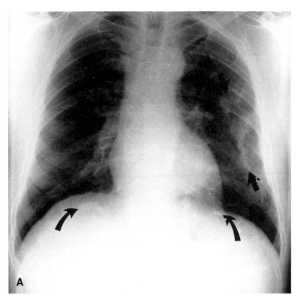
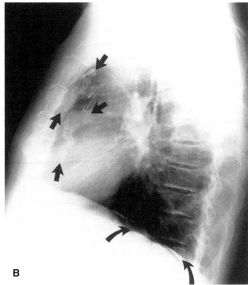

FIGURE 19.16. Calcified Pleural Plaques. Posteroanterior (**A**) and lateral (**B**) chest films in a 64-year-old man show bilateral diaphragmatic (*curved arrows*) and anterolateral (*straight arrows*) pleural plaques, reflecting prior asbestos exposure.

resolve spontaneously, up to one-third recur and some patients develop diffuse pleural fibrosis.

Diffuse pleural thickening or fibrosis may follow asbestos-related pleural effusion or result from the confluence of pleural plaques. Diffuse asbestos pleural thickening is defined as smooth, flat pleural thickening extending over one-fourth of the costal pleural surface. In distinction to pleural plaques, which affect the parietal pleura alone, diffuse pleural fibrosis involves both the parietal and visceral pleura. Radiographically, diffuse pleural thickening is seen as a smooth thickening of the pleura involving the lower thorax with blunting of the costophrenic sulci (Fig. 19.17). CT and HRCT are useful to determine the extent of pleural thickening, involvement of the interlobar fissures, and to detect underlying fibrotic or emphysematous lung disease. Diffuse pleural fibrosis can result in symptomatic restrictive lung disease.

Malignant Asbestos-Related Pleural Disease. *Malignant mesothelioma* is a rare malignant pleural neoplasm associated with asbestos exposure. Unlike other pleural and parenchymal manifestations of asbestos, it does not appear to be dose related. Mesothelioma most often occurs 30 to 40 years after the initial exposure. Although the incidence increases with heavy exposure, malignant mesothelioma may also develop after minimal exposure and contrasts with the linear relationship between the development of benign asbestos pleural disease and the dose of asbestos exposure. Crocidolite is the fiber type most often implicated in the development of malignant mesothelioma, although chrysotile likely accounts for the majority of asbestos-related mesotheliomas because it is the most widely used form of asbestos. Pathologically, mesothelioma is divided into epithelial, sarcomatous, and mixed types, with the epithelial form the most

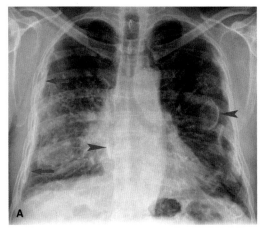
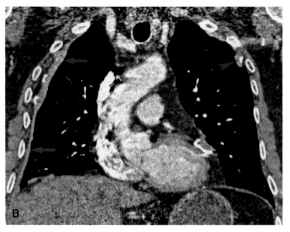

FIGURE 19.17. Diffuse Pleural Fibrosis from Asbestos. A. Frontal chest radiograph shows bilateral calcified plaques (*arrowheads*) and more diffuse thickening along the right lateral pleural surface (*arrows*). **B.** Coronal-reformatted CT at the level of the ascending aorta confirms the presence of bilateral pleural plaques (*arrowhead*) and also shows thickening along the right lateral pleural surface (*arrows*). Note the subtle decrease in volume of the right hemithorax, best evidenced by narrowing of the intercostal spaces. The absence of mediastinal pleural involvement is typical for benign pleural processes.

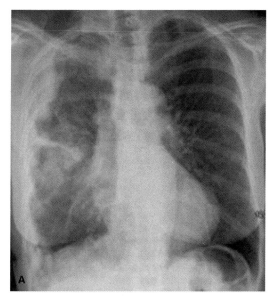
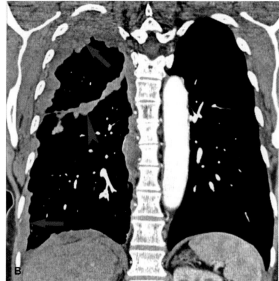

FIGURE 19.18. Mesothelioma. A. Chest radiograph shows marked nodular right pleural thickening. **B.** Coronal-reformatted contrast-enhanced CT at the level of the descending aorta shows circumferential nodular right pleural thickening with extension into the right oblique fissure (*arrowheads*). CT-guided biopsy confirmed an epithelial subtype of mesothelioma.

common and associated with a better prognosis than the sarcomatous and mixed subtypes.

Mesothelioma typically grows by contiguous spread from the pleural space into the lung, chest wall, mediastinum, and diaphragm; distant metastases are not uncommon. It most often appears radiographically as thick (>1 cm) and nodular diffuse pleural thickening (10). Calcification or, rarely, ossification is seen in 20% of tumors, although calcified pleural plaques may be seen in uninvolved areas of the pleura. A pleural effusion is often present, which, if large, may obscure the pleural tumor. Malignant involvement of the mediastinal pleural surface may prevent contralateral mediastinal shift despite extensive pleural tumor volume and effusion, a finding that may help distinguish mesothelioma from metastatic disease. CT is the imaging modality of choice in the evaluation of malignant mesothelioma and depicts the extent of pleural involvement and invasion of the chest wall and mediastinum (Fig. 19.18). Diaphragmatic invasion by tumor, best assessed by coronal MR or reformatted multidetector CT (MDCT) scans, is important only in those patients who are considered for resection. Adenopathy is seen in the ipsilateral hilum and mediastinum in approximately 50% of patients. While the radiologic findings may be highly suggestive of mesothelioma, metastatic pleural malignancy can have a similar appearance, so histologic confirmation is necessary.

The diagnosis of malignant mesothelioma is made histologically and often requires the use of special stains. The epithelial type of malignant mesothelioma may be indistinguishable from adenocarcinoma on light microscopy. While surgical resection by pleurectomy or extrapleural pneumonectomy may benefit selected patients with limited disease and good pulmonary reserve, the median survival from the time of diagnosis is only 6 to 12 months.

CHEST WALL

Disorders of the soft tissues or bony structures of the chest wall may come to attention because of local symptoms or physical findings, during evaluation of pulmonary or pleural disease, or as an incidental finding on radiographic studies (Table 19.8).

Soft Tissues

Congenital absence of the pectoralis muscle results in hyperlucency of the affected hemithorax on frontal radiographs. *Poland syndrome* is an autosomal recessive disorder characterized by unilateral absence of the sternocostal head of the pectoralis major, ipsilateral syndactyly, and rib anomalies. There may be associated aplasia of the ipsilateral breast. Patients who have had a mastectomy will also show unilateral

TABLE 19.8

CHEST WALL LESIONS

Tumors	Benign
	Mole
	Nevus
	Wart
	Neurofibroma
	Lipoma
	Hemangioma
	Desmoid
	Malignant
	Fibrosarcoma
	Liposarcoma
	Metastases
	Melanoma
	Bronchogenic carcinoma
	Askin tumor (primitive neuro-ectodermal tumor)
Infection (abscess)	*Staphylococcus*
	Tuberculosis
Trauma	Hematoma

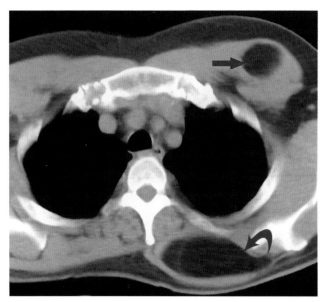

FIGURE 19.19. Chest Wall Lipomas. Unenhanced CT scan shows sharply circumscribed homogeneous fatty masses in the left pectoral (*straight arrow*) and rhomboid major (*curved arrow*) muscles.

hyperlucency. In those who have undergone a modified radical mastectomy, the horizontally oriented inferior edge of the hypertrophied pectoralis minor muscle may be identified on frontal radiographs.

A variety of skin lesions such as moles, nevi, warts, neurofibromas, and accessory nipples may produce a nodular opacity on frontal radiographs that mimics a solitary pulmonary nodule. Examination of the skin surface should be performed in any patient with a new nodular opacity seen on chest radiographs, and repeat radiographs obtained with a radiopaque marker over the skin lesion will confirm the nature of the opacity and avoid unnecessary follow-up radiographs and chest CT. Chest wall abscesses may present as localized, painful, fluctuant subcutaneous masses. *Staphylococcus* and *Mycobacterium*

tuberculosis are the most common organisms responsible. The diagnosis is usually obvious clinically. Chest radiographs demonstrate a poorly defined opacity on the frontal radiograph when the abscess involves the anterior or posterior chest wall. CT shows a localized fluid collection with an enhancing wall and is used to determine the location and extent of the collection prior to open drainage.

Soft tissue neoplasms of the chest wall are rare (11). They are most often detected clinically as a mass protruding from the chest wall and appear as nonspecific extrathoracic soft tissue masses on chest radiographs. The most common benign neoplasm of the chest wall is a lipoma. Lipomas may be intrathoracic or extrathoracic, or they may project partially within and outside the thorax (dumbbell lipoma). CT shows a sharply circumscribed mass of fatty density (Fig. 19.19), whereas MR shows characteristic high and intermediate signal intensity on T1WIs and T2WIs, respectively. A desmoid tumor is a rare fibroblastic tumor arising within striated muscle that is histologically benign but has a tendency for local invasion. Desmoids are most common in the abdominal wall musculature of multiparous women but may arise in the chest wall musculature following local trauma. Hemangiomas are uncommon chest wall tumors. While they are often indistinguishable from other soft tissue tumors radiographically, the recognition of phleboliths, hypertrophy of involved bones, or the identification of vascular channels on contrast-enhanced CT or MR studies should suggest the diagnosis.

Fibrosarcomas and liposarcomas are the most common malignant soft tissue neoplasms of the chest wall in adults. Malignant tumors often present with symptoms of localized chest wall pain and a visible, palpable mass. Patients who have received chest wall radiation are at particular risk for developing sarcomas. Radiographically, these soft tissue masses are often associated with bony destruction. CT best depicts the bone destruction and intrathoracic component of tumor, whereas MR shows the extent of tumor and delineates tumor from surrounding muscle and subcutaneous fat (8). A rare malignant neoplasm arising from the chest wall of children and young adults is an Askin tumor, which arises from primitive neuroectodermal rests in the chest wall (Fig. 19.20). These lesions are very aggressive and associated with a high mortality rate.

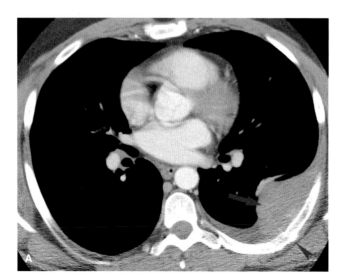
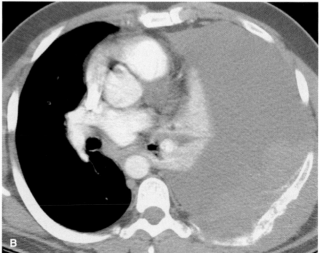

FIGURE 19.20. Askin Tumor (Primitive Neuroectodermal Tumor) of Chest Wall. A. Contrast-enhanced CT in a 32-year-old man demonstrates a left pleural mass (*arrow*) with adjacent involvement of the rib (*arrowhead*) and associated pleural effusion. B. Repeat CT obtained 1 month later shows enlargement of the mass with progressive rib involvement and a large pleural effusion with contralateral mediastinal shift. Surgical resection revealed an Askin tumor.

TABLE 19.9

RIB LESIONS

Congenital	Fusion anomalies
	Cervical rib
	Ribbon ribs
	Rib notching
	Inferior
	Coarctation of the aorta
	Tetralogy of Fallot
	Superior vena cava obstruction
	Blalock-Taussig shunt
	(unilateral right)
	Neurofibromatosis
	Superior
	Paralysis
	Collagen vascular disease
	Rheumatoid arthritis
	Systemic lupus erythematosus
Trauma	Healing rib fracture
Nonneoplastic tumors	Fibrous dysplasia
	Eosinophilic granuloma
	Brown tumor
Neoplasms	Benign
	Osteochondroma
	Enchondroma
	Osteoblastoma
	Malignant
	Primary
	Chondrosarcoma
	Osteogenic sarcoma
	Fibrosarcoma
	Metastatic
	Multiple myeloma
	Metastases
	Breast carcinoma
	Bronchogenic carcinoma
	Renal cell carcinoma
	Prostate carcinoma
Osteomyelitis	*Staphylococcus aureus*
	Tuberculosis
	Actinomycosis
	Nocardiosis

The Bony Thorax

Congenital Anomalies (Table 19.9) (12). The most common congenital anomalies of the ribs are bony fusion and bifid ribs, neither of which have clinical significance. Intrathoracic ribs are extremely rare congenital anomalies where an accessory rib arises from a vertebral body or the posterior surface of a rib and extends inferolaterally into the thorax, usually on the right side. Osteogenesis imperfecta and neurofibromatosis may be associated with thin, wavy, "ribbon" ribs. A relatively common congenital anomaly is the cervical rib, which arises from the seventh cervical vertebral body. Cervical ribs are usually asymptomatic, although in a minority of individuals with the thoracic outlet syndrome, the rib or associated fibrous bands can compress the subclavian artery, producing second weakness, and swelling of the upper extremity. Surgical resection of the cervical rib can relieve the symptoms in selected patients.

Rib notching is seen in a variety of pathologic conditions. Inferior rib notching is much more common than superior rib notching and is caused by enlargement of one or more of the structures that lie in the subcostal grooves (intercostal nerve, artery, or vein). The notching predominantly affects the posterior aspects of the ribs bilaterally and may be narrow, wide, deep, or shallow.

The most common cause of bilateral inferior rib notching is coarctation of the aorta distal to the origin of the left subclavian artery. In this condition, blood circumvents the aortic obstruction and reaches the descending aorta via the subclavian, internal mammary, and intercostal arteries. The increased blood flow in the intercostal arteries produces tortuosity and dilatation of these vessels, which erodes the inferior margins of the adjacent ribs. Other causes of aortic obstruction that can lead to inferior rib notching include aortic thrombosis and Takayasu aortitis. Congenital heart diseases associated with decreased pulmonary blood flow may be associated with rib notching as the intercostal arteries enlarge in an attempt to supply collateral blood flow to the oligemic lungs. Superior vena cava obstruction can cause increased flow through intercostal veins and produce rib notching.

Patients with aortic coarctation develop rib notching gradually; it is most common in adolescents and is rare in children younger than 7 years. The first two ribs are uninvolved because the first and second intercostal arteries arise from the superior intercostal branch of the costocervical trunk of the subclavian artery and therefore do not communicate with the descending thoracic aorta. Coarctation may produce unilateral left rib notching when the aortic narrowing occurs proximal to an aberrant right subclavian artery. Unilateral right-sided notching occurs when the coarctation is proximal to the left subclavian artery. Additional causes of unilateral inferior rib notching include subclavian artery obstruction and surgical anastomosis of the proximal subclavian artery to the ipsilateral pulmonary artery (Blalock-Taussig procedure).

Multiple intercostal neurofibromas in neurofibromatosis type 1 are the most common nonvascular cause of inferior rib notching. The neurofibromas appear kyphoscoliosis, and scalloping of the posterior aspect of the vertebral bodies caused by dural ectasia.

Superior rib notching is much less common than inferior rib notching. The pathogenesis of superior rib notching is unknown, although a disturbance of osteoblastic and osteoclastic activity and the stress effect of the intercostal muscles are proposed mechanisms. Paralysis is the most common condition associated with superior rib notching. Other etiologies include rheumatoid arthritis, systemic lupus erythematosus, and rarely, marked tortuosity of the intercostal arteries from severe, long-standing aortic obstruction.

Trauma. Rib and costal cartilage fractures may result from blunt or penetrating trauma to a normal ribcage or from minimal trauma to abnormal ribs, such as those affected by metastases. An acute rib fracture is seen as a thin vertical lucency; malalignment of the superior and inferior cortices of the rib may occasionally be the only radiographic finding. The tendency to affect the posterolateral aspects of the ribs explains the utility of obtaining ipsilateral posterior oblique radiographs for suspected fracture because this projection best displays the fracture line. In any patient with an acute rib fracture, a careful search should be made for associated pneumothorax, hemothorax, and pulmonary contusion or laceration. Since the first three ribs are well protected by the clavicles, scapulae, and shoulder girdles, fracture of these ribs indicates severe trauma and should prompt a careful evaluation for associated great vessel and visceral injuries. Fracture of the tenth, eleventh, or twelfth ribs may be associated with injury to the liver or spleen. Severe blunt trauma to the ribcage, in which multiple contiguous ribs are fractured in more

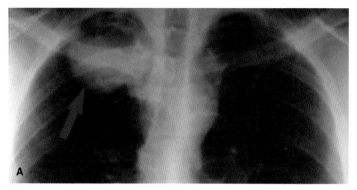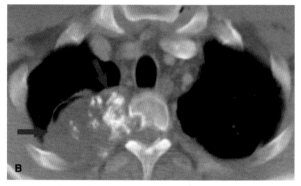

FIGURE 19.21. Chondrosarcoma of Rib. A. Cone-down view of a posteroanterior chest radiograph in a 37-year-old man with a 3-month history of right shoulder pain demonstrates a right apical extrapulmonary mass (*arrow*). **B.** A CT scan reveals a bone-forming mass (*arrows*) arising from the right third costotransverse junction, with erosion of the adjacent vertebral body. This chondrosarcoma was successfully resected by a combined thoracic and neurosurgical approach.

than one place, is termed a "flail chest." This results in a free segment of the chest wall that moves paradoxically inward on inspiration and outward on expiration. Healing rib fractures will demonstrate callus formation, which may be exuberant in patients receiving corticosteroids. Multiple contiguous healed rib fractures, particularly if bilateral, should suggest chronic alcoholism or a prior motor vehicle accident.

Nonneoplastic Lesions. The ribs are the most common site of involvement by monostotic fibrous dysplasia. The typical appearance is an expansile lesion in the posterior aspect of the rib with a lucent or ground glass density; rarely, the lesion is sclerotic. Multiple rib involvement from polyostotic fibrous dysplasia can result in severe restrictive pulmonary disease. Eosinophilic granuloma can cause lytic lesions in patients younger than 30 years. These are usually solitary lytic lesions, which can be expansile but do not have sclerotic margins; this latter feature helps distinguish these lesions from fibrous dysplasia. Brown tumors from hyperparathyroidism can also produce lytic rib lesions.

Neoplasms. Primary osteochondral neoplasms or metastatic disease can involve the ribs. Osteochondromas are the most common benign neoplasm of the ribs in adults. Chondrosarcoma is the most common primary rib malignancy, with osteogenic sarcoma and fibrosarcoma less common (Fig. 19.21). Rib involvement from multiple myeloma or metastatic carcinoma can produce solitary or multiple lytic lesions and is much more common than primary tumors. Myeloma can also cause permeative bone destruction that is indistinguishable from severe osteoporosis. The diagnosis of myeloma is made by identification of a monoclonal spike on serum protein electrophoresis and typical findings of abnormal aggregates of plasma cells on bone marrow biopsy. The most common metastatic lesions to ribs are from bronchogenic and breast carcinoma, which produce multiple lytic lesions when dissemination is hematogenous or localized rib destruction when invasion is by direct contiguous spread. Expansile lytic rib metastases are seen most commonly from renal cell and thyroid carcinoma. Sclerotic rib metastases are most commonly seen in breast and prostate carcinoma, although lung cancer can produce blastic metastases (Fig. 19.22).

Infection. Chest wall infection and osteomyelitis of the ribs usually develop from contiguous spread from the lung, pleural space, and vertebral column. Less commonly, infection complicates penetrating chest trauma or spreads to the ribs hematogenously. Pleuropulmonary infections that may traverse the pleural space and produce a chest wall infection include TB, fungus, actinomycosis, and nocardiosis. Radiographs may demonstrate bone destruction, periostitis, and sub-

cutaneous emphysema; bone scans can detect subradiographic bone involvement. CT can demonstrate bone destruction, soft tissue swelling, and abscesses within the chest wall. Additionally, CT may show involvement of the adjacent pleural space, lung, sternum, or vertebral column.

Costal Cartilages. Ossification of the costal cartilages is a normal finding on frontal chest radiographs in adults. Female costal cartilage ossification involves the central portion of the cartilage, extending from the rib toward the sternum in the shape of a solitary finger, whereas male costal cartilage ossification involves the peripheral portion of the cartilage and has the appearance of two fingers ("peace" sign). These typical patterns of male and female costal cartilage ossification are seen in 70% of patients (Fig. 19.23) and do not apply to the first rib.

Scapula. Scapular abnormalities that are visible on frontal radiographs include congenital, posttraumatic, and neoplastic lesions. *Sprengel deformity* is a congenital anomaly in which the scapula is hypoplastic and elevated. The association of Sprengel deformity with an omovertebral bone, fused cervical vertebrae, hemivertebrae, kyphoscoliosis, and rib anomalies is termed the *Klippel-Feil syndrome.* Scapular fractures may result from direct trauma to the upper back and shoulder or from impaction of the humeral head into the glenoid. A winged scapula is identified when the scapula is superiorly displaced from its normal position and the inferior portion is posteriorly displaced from the chest wall, thereby foreshortening its appearance on the frontal radiograph. This deformity results from disruption in the innervation of the serratus anterior muscle that maintains the scapula against the chest wall. Metastatic disease to the scapula is recognized by the presence of lytic destructive lesions; bronchogenic and breast carcinomas are the most common primary malignancies.

Clavicle. A variety of diseases can affect the clavicle. The clavicle is involved in cleidocranial dysostosis, in which there is partial or complete aplasia of the clavicle. The distal third of the clavicle is commonly fractured in blunt trauma. Rheumatoid arthritis and hyperparathyroidism are associated with erosion of the distal clavicles. The distal clavicle is sharply defined in rheumatoid arthritis and tapers to a point, whereas in hyperparathyroidism it is often widened and irregular. Additional findings in rheumatoid arthritis include narrowing of the glenohumeral joint and a high riding humeral head caused by rotator cuff atrophy. Primary malignant neoplasms of the clavicle include Ewing or osteogenic sarcoma. Metastases to the clavicle are usually associated with lesions in other portions of the bony thorax. Osteomyelitis of the clavicle is uncommon and is most often seen in intravenous drug users.

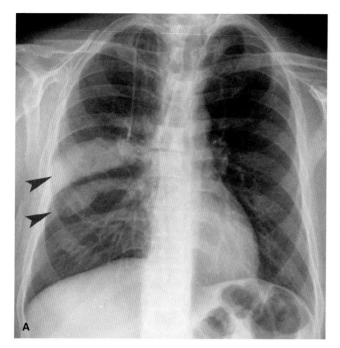

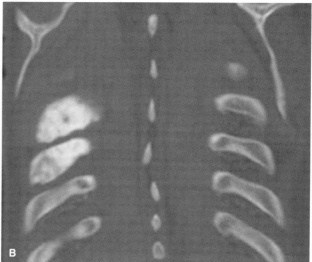

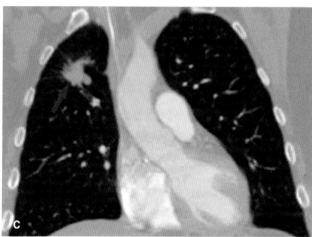

FIGURE 19.22. Blastic Bone Metastases from Lung Cancer. A. Chest radiograph shows sclerotic, expansile changes in two contiguous right posterior ribs (*arrowheads*) and the midthoracic spine. **B.** Coronal-reformatted CT through the posterior chest wall shows blastic changes in the two contiguous ribs. **C.** Coronal-reformatted CT through the ascending aorta shows a spiculated right upper lobe nodule (*arrow*) reflecting the patient's primary non–small-cell lung cancer.

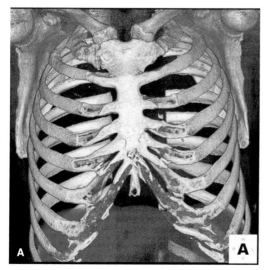

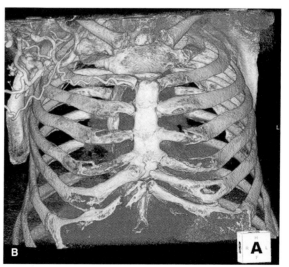

FIGURE 19.23. Normal Ossification Patterns in Men and Women. Shaded-surface three-dimensional reconstructions of the anterior chest wall show typical ossification patterns of costal cartilages in a woman (**A**) and a man (**B**).

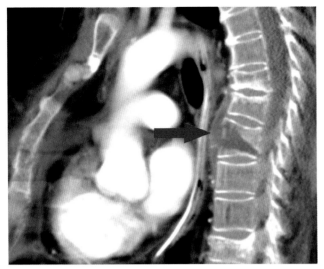

FIGURE 19.24. Vertebral Osteomyelitis. Sagittal maximum intensity projection reconstruction in a 72-year-old woman with back pain and staphylococcal sepsis shows an expansile lesion (*arrow*) of a midthoracic vertebral body with prevertebral soft tissue mass. CT-guided aspiration of the paravertebral mass revealed *Staphylococcus*.

Paget disease can involve the clavicle, but there is often concomitant pelvic bone and calvarial involvement.

Thoracic Spine. Numerous thoracic spine abnormalities are visible on chest radiographs. Congenital anomalies, including hemivertebrae, butterfly vertebra, spina bifida, and scoliosis, can be seen on well-penetrated frontal radiographs. Vertebral compression fractures caused by trauma, osteoporosis, or metastases are best seen on lateral radiographs and may produce an exaggerated kyphosis. Large bridging osteophytes may mimic a paraspinal mass on frontal radiographs or a pulmonary nodule on lateral films. Vertebral osteomyelitis is seen as destruction of vertebral bodies and intervertebral discs, often associated with a paraspinal abscess (Fig. 19.24). Chronic anemia in patients with thalassemia major or sickle cell disease may result in prevertebral or paravertebral masses of extramedullary hematopoiesis, which represent herniated hyperplastic bone marrow. Sickle cell anemia produces a characteristic appearance of H-shaped or "Lincoln log" vertebrae on lateral chest radiographs, which is pathognomonic of this disease. Similarly, a "rugger jersey" appearance to the thoracic spine on lateral chest films suggests renal osteosclerosis.

Sternum. Developmental sternal deformities include pectus excavatum (funnel chest), pectus carinatum (pigeon breast), and abnormal segmentation. In pectus excavatum, the sternum is inwardly depressed and the ribs protrude anterior to the sternum. It often has an autosomal dominant pattern of inheritance but may occur sporadically.

Pectus excavatum is commonly associated with congenital connective tissue disorders, such as Marfan syndrome, Poland syndrome, osteogenesis imperfecta, and congenital scoliosis. Most patients are asymptomatic. A clinically insignificant systolic murmur can result from compression of the right ventricular outflow tract, although some patients with pectus deformities and systolic murmurs have mitral valve prolapse. Pectus excavatum has a characteristic appearance on frontal chest radiograph. The heart is displaced to the left, and the combination of the depressed soft tissues of the anterior chest wall and the vertically oriented anterior ribs results in loss of the right heart border. The findings on frontal radiographs may be mistakenly attributed to middle lobe opacification from pneumonia or atelectasis. The typical inward depression of the midsternum and lower sternum is seen on lateral chest radiographs (Fig. 19.25). CT helps define the deformity and its effect upon the heart and mediastinal structures.

Pectus carinatum is an outward bowing of the sternum that may be congenital or acquired. The congenital form is seen more commonly in boys and in families with a history of chest wall deformities or scoliosis. Congenital atrial or ventricular septal defects and severe childhood asthma account for the majority of the acquired cases of pectus carinatum. Affected

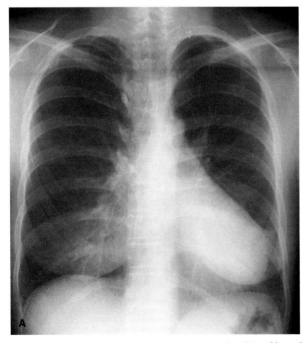
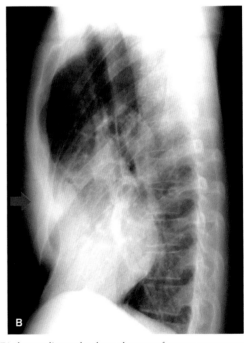

FIGURE 19.25. Pectus Excavatum. Posteroanterior (**A**) and lateral (**B**) chest radiographs show changes of pectus excavatum (*arrow*). Note the apparent middle lobe opacity that is typical of this condition.

patients are asymptomatic. The characteristic outward bowing of the sternum with deepening of the retrosternal airspace is seen on lateral radiographs.

Severe blunt trauma to the chest, most often associated with deceleration injury from a motor vehicle accident, can result in fracture or dislocation of the sternum. Sternal body fracture and sternomanubrial dislocation are associated with a 25% to 45% mortality rate from concomitant injuries to the aorta, diaphragm, heart, tracheobronchial tree, and lung. Sternal films or lateral radiographs will show the fracture and often demonstrate a retrosternal hematoma; CT may be useful in those patients with normal plain films and a high suspicion of sternal injury. A prior median sternotomy is the most common sternal abnormality seen on conventional radiographs and chest CT. Circular wires encompassing the sternum are seen spaced along its length within the interspaces between costal cartilages. The vertical lucency representing the sternotomy may heal, but in many patients bony union does not occur. In the early postoperative period, a retrosternal hematoma may be seen, which normally resolves within the first several weeks. The radiologist plays a key role in the evaluation of possible sternal wound infection. Plain film evidence of bony destruction and air in the sternal incision appearing days to weeks after sternotomy are specific but insensitive findings for osteomyelitis. Bone scans are not particularly useful, as there will be increased radionuclide uptake for months following sternotomy. CT is the modality of choice in the evaluation of sternal wound infection. The CT findings of sternal osteomyelitis include bone destruction, peristernal soft tissue mass, enhancing fluid collection, and gas. The extent of infection, specifically associated mediastinitis, can also be determined.

DIAPHRAGM

Unilateral Diaphragmatic Elevation. The differential diagnosis of unilateral diaphragmatic elevation is listed in Table 19.10. Eventration of the diaphragm is a result of congenital absence

TABLE 19.10

UNILATERAL DIAPHRAGMATIC ELEVATION

Eventration	
Diminished lung volume	Congenital
	Hypoplastic lung
	Acquired
	Lobar/lung atelectasis
	Pulmonary resection
Paralysis	Idiopathic
	Iatrogenic phrenic nerve injury
	Phrenic crush (tuberculosis)
	Intraoperative
	Malignant invasion of phrenic nerve
	Bronchogenic carcinoma
	Inflammation of diaphragmatic muscle
	Pleuritis
	Lower lobe pneumonia
	Subphrenic abscess
Upper abdominal mass	Hepatomegaly or liver mass
	Splenomegaly
	Gastric/colonic distention
	Ascites (usually bilateral)
	Diaphragmatic hernia[a]
	Subpulmonic pleural effusion[a]

[a]Apparent diaphragmatic elevation.

or underdevelopment of diaphragmatic musculature. This produces a localized elevation of the anteromedial portion of the hemidiaphragm on frontal radiographs in older individuals (Fig. 19.26), which is indistinguishable on the right from the rare foramen of Morgagni hernia. Complete diaphragmatic

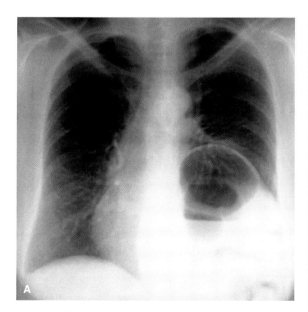
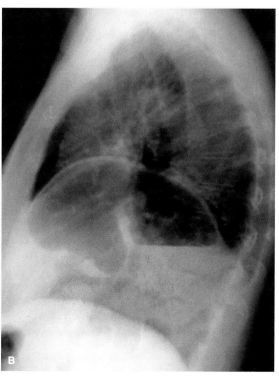

FIGURE 19.26. **Eventration of the Diaphragm.** Posteroanterior (**A**) and lateral (**B**) chest radiographs in an asymptomatic 61-year-old woman reveal marked elevation of the left hemidiaphragm representing diaphragmatic eventration.

eventration is usually left sided and is indistinguishable radiographically from diaphragmatic paralysis.

Unilateral diaphragmatic paralysis is usually caused by surgical injury or neoplastic involvement of the phrenic nerve, which affects the right and left hemidiaphragms with equal frequency. Idiopathic phrenic nerve dysfunction resulting from a viral neuritis is a common cause of diaphragmatic paralysis in male patients and is usually right sided. A positive fluoroscopic or ultrasonographic sniff test (paradoxical superior movement of the diaphragm with sniffing, a result of the effects of negative intrathoracic pressure on a flaccid diaphragm during inspiration) is diagnostic. Chronic loss of lung volume, particularly from collapse or resection of the lower lobe, results in diaphragmatic elevation. This is also a common sequela of chronic cicatrizing atelectasis of the upper lobe from TB.

An enlarged liver or hepatic mass can produce right hemidiaphragmatic elevation by direct pressure on the undersurface of the hemidiaphragm. Similarly, an enlarged spleen, gas-distended stomach, or enlarged splenic flexure can produce an elevated left hemidiaphragm. Irritation of the superior surface of the hemidiaphragm by a pleural or pleura-based parenchymal process (e.g., infarct, pneumonia) or of the undersurface of the diaphragm by a subphrenic abscess, hepatitis, or cholecystitis may cause the diaphragm to become flaccid, leading to elevation. A subpulmonic effusion may simulate an elevated hemidiaphragm.

Bilateral diaphragmatic elevation that is not effort related may be caused by a neuromuscular disturbance or intrathoracic or intra-abdominal disease. Radiographically, the diaphragms are elevated on both frontal and lateral views. Bibasilar linear atelectasis or passive lobar or segmental lower lobe atelectasis may be seen. Bilateral phrenic nerve disruption or intrinsic diaphragmatic muscular disease will produce bilateral diaphragmatic paralysis and elevation. Common disorders include cervical cord injury, multiple sclerosis, and the myopathy associated with systemic lupus erythematosus. In these patients, fluoroscopic or real-time US imaging of the diaphragms demonstrates a positive sniff test.

Lung restriction caused by interstitial fibrosis, bilateral pleural fibrosis, or chest wall disease (most commonly from obesity) can produce bilateral diaphragmatic elevation. An increase in intra-abdominal volume, most often from ascites, hepatosplenomegaly, or pregnancy, can restrict diaphragmatic motion. These conditions may be distinguished from bilateral paralysis by observation of normal but diminished inferior excursion of the diaphragms on fluoroscopy, US, or inspiratory/expiratory radiographs.

Diaphragmatic Depression. Depression and flattening of one hemidiaphragm is seen with unilateral overinflation of a lung, usually as a compensatory mechanism when the contralateral lung is small or as a result of a large ipsilateral pneumothorax. Distinction between these two entities is usually possible by the clinical history and by characteristic findings in those with pneumothorax. A tension pneumothorax may cause inversion of the hemidiaphragm. Bilateral diaphragmatic depression is either a permanent finding—a result of abnormally increased lung compliance in patients with emphysema—or a transient finding in those with asthma and expiratory air trapping.

Diaphragmatic Hernias. There are three types of nontraumatic diaphragmatic hernias. The most common is the *esophageal hiatal hernia*, which represents herniation of a portion of the stomach through the esophageal hiatus. These are usually seen as incidental asymptomatic masses on chest radiographs, although some patients may have symptoms of gastroesophageal reflux or, rarely, severe pain from strangulation of the herniated stomach. Hiatal hernias are seen projecting behind the heart on frontal chest radiographs in the immediate supradiaphragmatic region of the posterior mediastinum. An air–fluid level may be seen in the hernia. An esophagram is confirmatory. CT shows widening of the esophageal hiatus and depicts the contents of the hernia sac, which often include stomach, omental fat, and, rarely, ascitic fluid (Fig. 19.27).

Bochdalek Hernia. The foramen of Bochdalek is a defect in the hemidiaphragm at the site of the embryonic pleuroperitoneal canal. Large hernias through the Bochdalek foramen present in the neonatal period with hypoplasia of the ipsilateral lung and respiratory distress. In adults, small hernias through this foramen are common and are predominantly seen on the left side, presumably because of the protective effect of the liver, which prevents herniation of right infradiaphragmatic fat through the right foramen of Bochdalek. The hernia typically appears as a posterolateral mass above the left hemidiaphragm, although it can occur anywhere along the posterior diaphragmatic surface (Fig. 19.28). CT shows the diaphragmatic defect with herniation of retroperitoneal fat, omentum, spleen, or kidney.

Morgagni Hernia. A defect in the parasternal portion of the diaphragm, the foramen of Morgagni, is the least common type of diaphragmatic hernia. A Morgagni hernia is

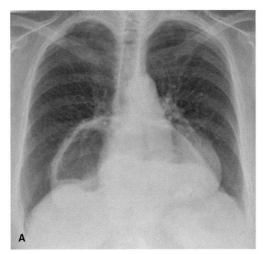
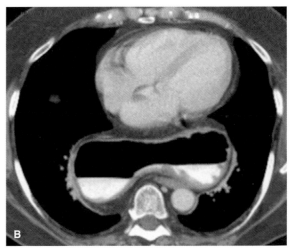

FIGURE 19.27. Hiatal Hernia. Chest radiograph (**A**) and CT scan with coronal reconstruction (**B**) in a 73-year-old man shows a sliding hiatal hernia in the posterior mediastinum.

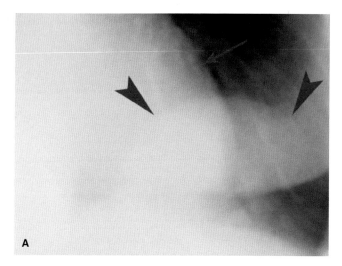

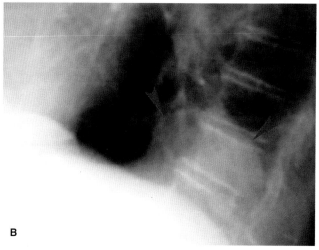

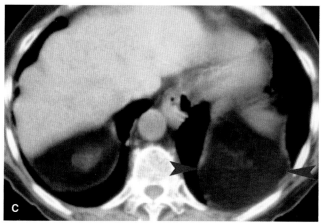

FIGURE 19.28. Foramen of Bochdalek Hernia. A. Cone-down view of the left lung base from a posteroanterior chest radiograph in an asymptomatic 82-year-old man shows a mass (*arrowheads*) arising from the posterolateral aspect of the left hemidiaphragm. *Arrow* indicates the left heart border. **B.** Cone-down view of the posterior left lung base from a lateral chest radiograph shows the same well-marginated mass (*arrowheads*). **C.** CT scan through the diaphragm shows fat herniating through the Bochdalek hernia (*arrowheads*).

invariably right sided and appears as an asymptomatic cardiophrenic angle mass (Fig. 19.29). The diagnosis is made by noting herniation of omental fat, liver, or transverse colon through the paracardiac portion of the right hemidiaphragm on CT scans through the lung bases. The presence of omental vessels within a fatty paracardiac mass is diagnostic (Fig. 19.29C). Coronal CT can demonstrate the diaphragmatic defect, distinguishing this entity from partial eventration of the hemidiaphragm.

Traumatic Hernia. Traumatic herniation of abdominal contents through a tear or rupture of the central or posterior aspect of the hemidiaphragm may follow blunt thoracoabdominal trauma or penetrating injury (13). The left side is affected in more than 90% of cases because the liver dissipates the traumatic forces and protects the right hemidiaphragm from injury. Radiographically, the diagnosis should be suspected when the left hemidiaphragmatic contour is indistinct or elevated or when gas-filled loops of bowel or stomach are seen in the left lower thorax following severe trauma. Early diagnosis is often difficult because associated thoracic and abdominal injuries may obscure the clinical and radiographic findings. The diagnosis is often made after the traumatic episode, with symptoms caused by intestinal obstruction with strangulation (pain, vomiting, fever), compression of the left lung (cough, dyspnea, chest pain), or as an incidental finding, particularly if only fat and no viscus has herniated through the defect (Fig. 19.30). In addition to the stomach, the small intestine, colon, omentum, spleen, kidney, fat, and the left lobe of the liver can also herniate through the defect. The diagnosis is usually made by upper or lower GI contrast studies demonstrating bowel herniating into the thorax through a

constricting diaphragmatic defect. The resultant narrowing or "waist" of the herniated intestine as it traverses the diaphragmatic defect differentiates a hernia from simple diaphragmatic elevation. Large diaphragmatic defects may be demonstrated on MDCT scans with coronal and sagittal reconstructions, which also characterize the herniated tissues and detect associated visceral injuries (Fig. 19.31). In addition to the detection of intrathoracic herniation of abdominal contents, MDCT can directly depict the diaphragmatic defect, even in the absence of visceral herniation. Other CT findings suggestive of traumatic diaphragmatic injury include thickening or retraction of the diaphragm away from the traumatic injury, a narrowing or waist of the diaphragm on the herniated viscus ("collar" or "waist" sign) (Fig. 19.31C), and contact between the posterior ribs and the liver (right-sided injury) or stomach (left-sided injury), termed the "dependent viscera" sign. US or MR are difficult to obtain in the acute trauma setting but are occasionally useful (12).

Diaphragmatic Tumors. Primary diaphragmatic tumors are rare, with an equal incidence of benign and malignant lesions. Benign lesions include lipomas, fibromas, schwannomas, neurofibromas, and leiomyomas. Echinococcal cysts and extralobar sequestrations may be found within the diaphragm. Fibrosarcomas are the most common primary malignant diaphragmatic lesion. Radiographically, they appear as focal extrapulmonary masses obscuring all or part of the hemidiaphragm and are indistinguishable from masses arising within the diaphragmatic pleura. CT may show the origin of the mass, although the relationship of the mass to the diaphragm is best appreciated on coronal MR images or transabdominal US. Direct invasion of the diaphragm by lower lobe bronchogenic

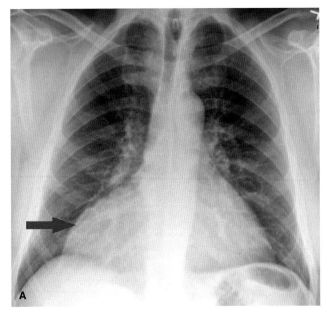
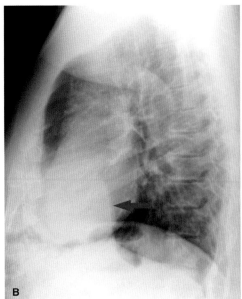
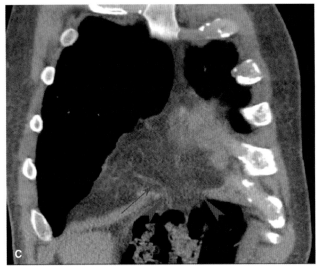

FIGURE 19.29. Foramen of Morgagni Hernia. Frontal (**A**) and lateral (**B**) chest radiographs in a 60-year-old woman reveal a large mass in the right cardiophrenic angle (*arrows*). **C.** Coronal-reformatted CT scan at the level of the anterior diaphragm shows a fatty precardiac mass containing omental vessels (*arrow*). The defect in the medial diaphragm is visible (*arrowheads*).

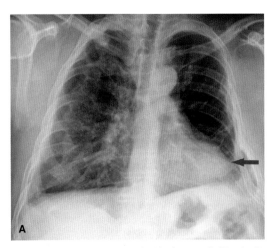
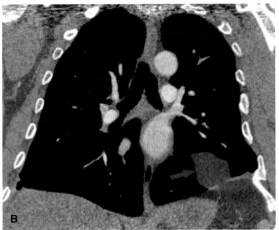

FIGURE 19.30. Posttraumatic Diaphragmatic Hernia Containing Fat. A. Frontal chest radiograph in a patient with a history or prior motor vehicle accident shows multiple healed bilateral rib fractures. There is a vague left retrocardiac opacity (*arrow*). **B.** Coronal-reformatted CT through the midthorax shows a fatty hernia (*arrow*) extending into the thorax via a central left diaphragmatic defect (*curved arrow*).

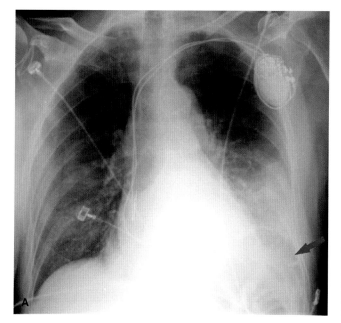

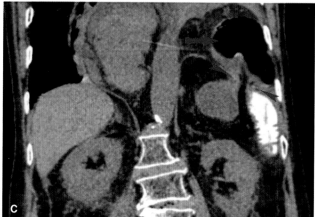

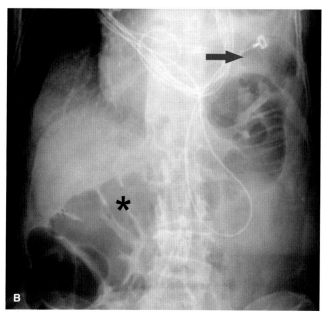

FIGURE 19.31. Traumatic Diaphragmatic Hernia with Incarcerated Colon. A. Portable chest radiograph in a trauma patient shows left lower lobe opacity. Note some dilated bowel (*arrow*) projecting over the left lower chest. B. An abdominal radiograph confirms a superiorly displaced splenic flexure of colon (*arrow*), with dilatation of the transverse colon (*asterisk*). C. Coronal-reformatted unenhanced CT shows a loop of colon (*arrow*) extending through a narrow diaphragmatic defect that produces a waist on the herniated bowel (*arrowheads*).

carcinoma, mesothelioma, or a subphrenic neoplasm is much more common than primary diaphragmatic malignancy.

CONGENITAL LUNG DISEASE

Bronchogenic cysts represent anomalous outpouchings of the primitive foregut that no longer communicate with the tracheobronchial tree. They are commonly present as asymptomatic mediastinal masses and are discussed in detail in Chapter 13.

Congenital cystic adenomatoid malformation (CCAM) is a lesion usually seen in newborn infants, although it occasionally presents in childhood or early adulthood. Three pathologic subtypes of CAM have been described. The most common subtype is composed of one or several large cysts that are lined by respiratory epithelium with scattered mucous glands, smooth muscle, and elastic tissue in their walls. Multiple smaller cystic structures are present in the intervening lung

between the larger cysts. Radiographically, these lesions often appear as round, air-filled masses, which exert mass effect on the adjacent lung and mediastinum (Fig. 19.32). A CAM in the left lower lobe may be difficult to distinguish from a congenital diaphragmatic hernia. Delayed clearance of fetal fluid in the newborn may give the radiographic appearance of an intrapulmonary soft tissue mass. These lesions may be identified on prenatal US examination.

Bronchial atresia, a developmental stenosis or atresia of a lobar or segmental bronchus, produces bronchial obstruction with resultant distal bronchiectasis. Most patients are asymptomatic and are first recognized by typical findings on frontal chest radiographs, namely a rounded, oval, or branching central lung opacity representing the obstructed, mucus-filled, dilated bronchus (mucocele) with hyperlucency in that portion of lung supplied by the atretic bronchus. The overinflated lobe or segment results from air trapping in the obstructed lung as air enters by collateral air drift on inspiration but cannot empty through the proximal tracheobronchial tree on expiration. The

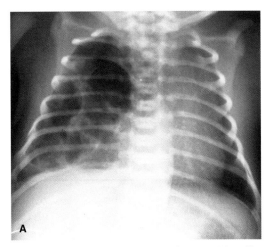
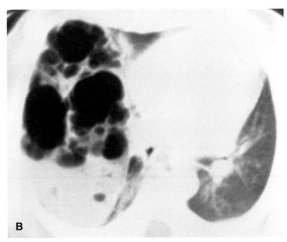

FIGURE 19.32. Congenital Cystic Adenomatoid Malformation (CCAM). A. Frontal chest radiograph in a newborn shows a multicystic mass in the right midlung and lower lung. **B.** CT scan demonstrates a complex mass occupying the middle and right lower lobes with air-filled cysts and a solid component posteriorly. Surgery revealed a CCAM of the middle lobe.

most common site of involvement is the apicoposterior segment of the left upper lobe, followed by the segmental bronchi of the right upper and middle lobes. The combination of a central mucocele with peripheral hyperlucency in a young, asymptomatic patient is virtually diagnostic of this disorder (Fig. 19.33) (14).

Neonatal lobar hyperinflation (congenital lobar emphysema) may develop from a variety of disorders that produce a check-valve bronchial obstruction. These include extrinsic compression by mediastinal bronchogenic cysts, anomalous left pulmonary artery, congenital deficiency of bronchial cartilage, and congenital or acquired bronchial stenosis. The bronchial obstruction leads to air trapping on expiration, with resultant overinflation of the distal lung. In order of decreasing frequency, the left upper lobe, right middle lobe, and right upper lobe are the most common sites of involvement. Respiratory difficulties are usually evident within the first month of life,

with a minority presenting later. Radiographically, hyperlucency of the affected lobe is seen with compression of adjacent lung, diaphragmatic depression, and contralateral mediastinal shift (Fig. 19.34). These findings are accentuated on expiratory films or on decubitus films obtained with the affected side down. CT, particularly when performed in expiration or with the affected side down, shows a hyperlucent, overexpanded lobe with attenuated blood vessels. Because many of these cases are not truly congenital but rather arise in the neonatal period from acquired abnormalities and because overinflation of normal alveoli without destruction of alveolar walls is seen pathologically, the term *neonatal lobar hyperinflation* has been used to more appropriately describe this syndrome. Treatment is surgical for symptomatic patients, whereas relatively asymptomatic patients are observed for spontaneous resolution. The findings in bronchial atresia and congenital lobar emphysema are reviewed in Table 19.9.

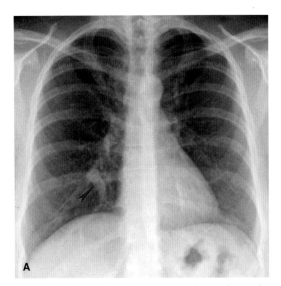
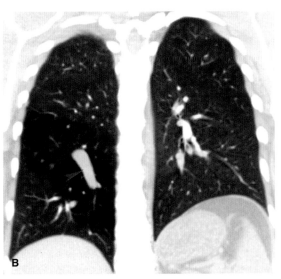

FIGURE 19.33. Bronchial Atresia. A. Chest radiograph in a 43-year-old woman with a history of asthma shows a curvilinear opacity (*arrowhead*) in the lower right lung. **B.** Coronal-reformatted CT through the posterior thorax at lung windows shows a hyperlucent portion of the right lower lobe, within which there is a broad tubular opacity (*arrowhead*) reflecting a bronchocele in a patient with bronchial atresia.

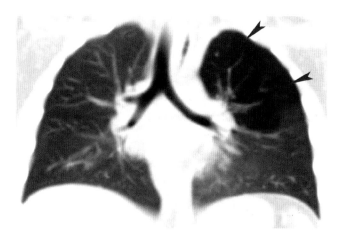

FIGURE 19.34. Neonatal Lobar Hyperinflation (Congenital Lobar Emphysema). Coronal-reformatted CT through the central airways in a neonate with respiratory distress shows a hyperlucent left upper lobe (*arrowheads*) with attenuated vascular markings indicative of congenital lobar emphysema.

Bronchopulmonary sequestration is a congenital abnormality resulting from the independent development of a portion of the tracheobronchial tree that is isolated from the normal lung and maintains its fetal systemic arterial supply. Grossly, the sequestered lung is cystic and bronchiectatic. These patients most often present with recurrent pneumonia from recurrent infection in the sequestered lung, although some (mostly extralobar sequestrations) are discovered as asymptomatic posterior mediastinal masses on routine radiographs.

Pulmonary sequestration is divided into intralobar and extralobar forms (Table 19.11). *Intralobar sequestration* is contained within the visceral pleura of the normal lung. *Extralobar sequestration* is enclosed by its own visceral pleural envelope and may be found adjacent to the normal lung or within or below the diaphragm. Most patients with intralobar sequestration present with pneumonia. Extralobar sequestration is usually asymptomatic and is seen as an incidental finding in a neonate with other severe congenital anomalies. Intralobar sequestration is more common than the extralobar type, by a ratio of 3 to 1. Both forms are found in the lower lobes, but extralobar sequestration is predominantly left sided (90%), whereas one-third of intralobar sequestrations are right sided. A major differentiating feature between the two types is the arterial supply to and venous drainage from the sequestered lung. An intralo-

bar sequestration is supplied by a single large artery that arises from the infradiaphragmatic aorta and enters the sequestered lung via the pulmonary ligament. The venous drainage is typically via the pulmonary veins, although systemic venous drainage can occur. In contrast, an extralobar sequestration receives several small branches from systemic and occasionally pulmonary arteries, with venous drainage into the systemic venous system (inferior vena cava, azygos, or hemiazygos veins). Sequestration appears as a solid posterior mediastinal mass or as a solitary or multicystic air collection (14). Air–fluid levels are seen when infection has produced communication of the sequestered lung with the normal tracheobronchial tree. The definitive diagnosis is made by the demonstration of abnormal systemic arterial supply to the abnormal lung, which is usually accomplished by thoracic aortography, contrast-enhanced MDCT (Fig. 19.35), US, or coronal MR and MR angiography. Arteriography is usually reserved for preoperative patients in whom precise demonstration of the origin and number of the systemic feeders is necessary.

Hypoplastic lung is a developmental anomaly resulting in a small lung. It occurs secondary to congenital pulmonary arterial deficiency or following compression of the developing lung in utero from a variety of causes. Grossly, the lung is small, with a decrease in the number and size of airways, alveoli, and pulmonary arteries. Radiographically, the small lung and hemithorax are associated with ipsilateral diaphragmatic elevation and mediastinal shift, with herniation of the hyperinflated contralateral lung anteriorly toward the affected side. Hypoplastic lung can simulate total lung collapse radiographically but can usually be distinguished on clinical grounds and review of prior radiographic studies that show a small lung without evidence of pleural or parenchymal scarring.

Hypogenetic lung-scimitar syndrome, a variant of the hypoplastic lung, is characterized by an underdeveloped right lung with abnormal venous drainage of the lung to the inferior vena cava just above or below the right hemidiaphragm. The systemic venous drainage of the lung produces an extracardiac left-to-right shunt. The anomalous vein, which drains all or most of the right lung, may be seen as a vertically oriented curvilinear density shaped like a scimitar in the medial right lower lung, thereby giving this syndrome its common name of scimitar syndrome. The anomalies of venous drainage and lobar bronchial anatomy (usually bilateral left-sided [hyparterial] bronchial branching) have given rise to the term *congenital pulmonary venolobar syndrome.* The right pulmonary artery is invariably hypoplastic, with supply to all or part of the lung (usually the lower lobe) from the systemic circulation. Associated anomalies include eventration of the right hemidiaphragm, horseshoe

---

TABLE 19.11

BRONCHIAL ATRESIA VERSUS NEONATAL LOBAR HYPERINFLATION

■ DIAGNOSTIC VARIABLE	■ BRONCHIAL ATRESIA	■ NEONATAL LOBAR HYPERINFLATION
Age at presentation	Teens/young adults	Neonatal period
Symptoms	Asymptomatic	Respiratory distress
Location	LUL > RUL > RML	LUL > RML > RUL
Radiographic/CT findings	Hyperlucent segment with mucocele	Hyperlucent lobe Diaphragmatic depression Mediastinal displacement
Treatment	None	Resection

LUL, left upper lobe; RUL, right upper lobe; RML, right middle lobe.

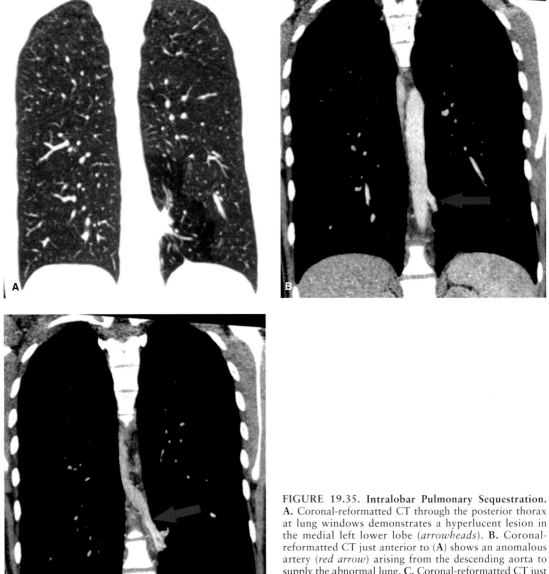

FIGURE 19.35. Intralobar Pulmonary Sequestration. A. Coronal-reformatted CT through the posterior thorax at lung windows demonstrates a hyperlucent lesion in the medial left lower lobe (*arrowheads*). B. Coronal-reformatted CT just anterior to (A) shows an anomalous artery (*red arrow*) arising from the descending aorta to supply the abnormal lung. C. Coronal-reformatted CT just posterior to (B) shows venous drainage (*blue arrow*) into the azygos vein, somewhat atypical for intralobar sequestration.

lung (congenital fusion of the right and left lungs posteroinferiorly), and cardiac anomalies such as atrial septal defect (most common), coarctation of the aorta, patent ductus arteriosus, and tetralogy of Fallot. The frontal chest radiographic findings are diagnostic and include a small right hemithorax with diaphragmatic elevation or eventration, dextroposition of the heart, and herniation of left lung anteriorly into the right hemithorax (Fig. 19.36). The classic appearance of a solitary scimitar vein is seen in only one-third of cases, with the remainder having multiple small draining veins. Although plain film findings are usually diagnostic, CT or MR shows the abnormal draining vein and associated abnormalities. Most patients are asymptomatic, but some may present with recurrent infection or symptoms related to a left-to-right shunt or the associated cardiac anomalies.

Arteriovenous malformations (AVMs) are abnormal vascular masses in which a focal collection of congenitally weakened capillaries dilates to become a tortuous complex of vessels fed by a single pulmonary artery and drained by a single pulmonary vein. Most pulmonary AVMs do not come to attention until early adulthood. They are detected either incidentally, as part of a screening evaluation in patients with hereditary hemorrhagic telangiectasia (a condition present in approximately 80% of all patients with pulmonary AVMs), or because of a variety of symptoms. The most common pulmonary symptoms are hemoptysis and dyspnea, the latter attributable to hypoxia caused by the intrapulmonary right-to-left shunt. Nonpulmonary symptoms most often relate to CNS disease. Stroke may occur from paradoxical right-to-left cerebral emboli or from thrombosis resulting from secondary polycythemia caused by chronic hypoxemia. Brain abscess may develop from paradoxical septic emboli.

The chest radiograph of a pulmonary AVM usually shows a solitary pulmonary nodule, most often located in the subpleural portions of the lower lobes. Approximately one third of patients have multiple lesions. The lesion is often lobulated and has feeding and draining vessels emanating from the mass and extending toward the hilum. The morphology of the lesions is best demonstrated on MDCT with reconstructions. The feeding and

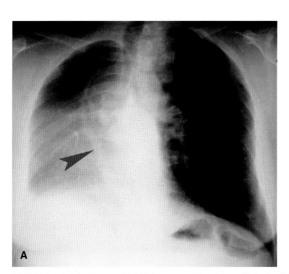
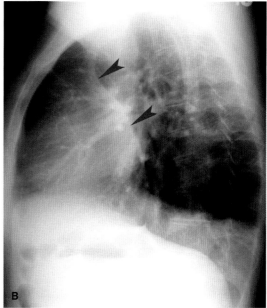

FIGURE 19.36. **Congenital Pulmonary Venolobar (Scimitar) Syndrome.** Frontal (**A**) and lateral (**B**) chest radiographs in a patient with Scimitar syndrome show a small right lung with rightward cardiomediastinal shift and a characteristic draining vein (*blue arrowhead*). The lateral film shows the interface of the hypoplastic right lung with the anteriorly situated heart and mediastinal fat (*red arrowheads*) that have shifted as a result of the hypoplasia.

draining vessels can be demonstrated by CT or MR. Angiography is reserved for preoperative evaluation and for patients undergoing therapeutic transcatheter embolization with spring coils or detachable occlusion balloons, which is the treatment of choice for patients with multiple AVMs.

TRAUMATIC LUNG DISEASE

Pulmonary contusion usually follows blunt chest trauma and typically develops adjacent to the site of impact. Blood and edema fluid fill the alveoli of the lung within the first 12 hours after trauma, producing scattered areas of airspace opacification that may rapidly become confluent and may be difficult to distinguish from aspiration pneumonia (Fig. 19.37). Patients may have shortness of breath and hemoptysis; blood can usually be suctioned from the endotracheal tube. The typical radiographic course is stabilization of opacities by 24 hours and improvement within 2 to 7 days. Progressive opacities seen more than 48 hours after trauma should raise the suspicion of aspiration pneumonia or developing ARDS.

Pulmonary Laceration, Traumatic Lung Cyst, and Pulmonary Hematoma. Pulmonary laceration is a common sequela of penetrating or blunt chest trauma. In the latter situation, it

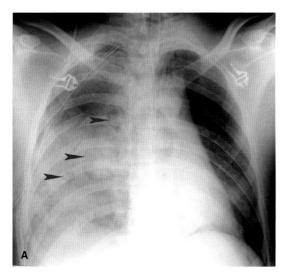
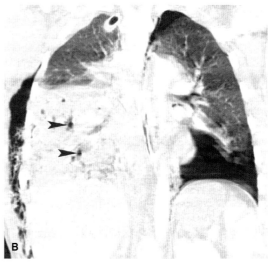

FIGURE 19.37. **Pulmonary Contusions. A.** Portable chest radiograph in a trauma patient shows extensive right lung and left lower lobe retrocardiac air space opacification. Subtle lucencies are visible within the consolidated areas (*arrowheads*). **B.** Coronal-reformatted CT through the posterior thorax shows dense right lower lobe consolidation reflecting lung contusion, with scattered lucencies representing traumatic lung cysts (*arrowheads*). Note the presence of multiple right rib fractures and a left pneumothorax. The patient also sustained a traumatic aortic laceration (not shown).

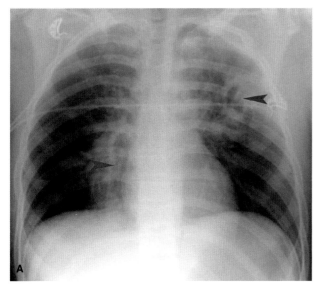

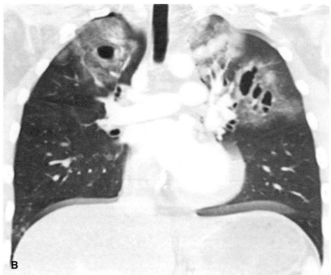

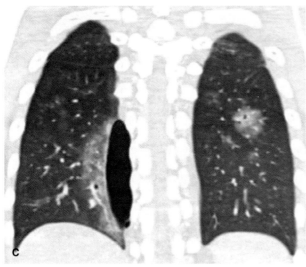

FIGURE 19.38. Traumatic Lung Cysts. A. Portable chest radiograph in a 23-year-old man involved in a motor vehicle accident shows right lower and left upper lobe consolidation. Lucencies (*arrows*) within the affected regions are discernible. Coronal-reformatted CT scan at lung windows through the posterior thorax (**B**) and trachea (**C**) show multifocal ground glass opacities containing thin-walled cysts. There is a small right apical pneumothorax.

represents a shearing injury to the substance of the lung. The elastic properties of the lung quickly transform the linear laceration into a rounded air cyst. These cysts may be filled with varied amounts of blood as a result of laceration of pulmonary capillaries; those that are completely filled with blood are more appropriately termed *pulmonary hematomas*. On radiographs and CT, these cysts appear as rounded lucencies that may contain air or an air–fluid level (Fig. 19.38) (15). Initially, these cysts are often obscured by the adjacent contused lung, only to be recognized after resorption of the blood. The cysts tend to shrink gradually over a period of weeks to months. The term *traumatic air cysts* rather than *pneumatoceles* should be used for these lesions; the latter term is reserved for air cysts that result from a check-valve overdistention of the distal lung, as seen in staphylococcal pneumonia.

ASPIRATION

Aspiration pneumonia and *pneumonitis* are terms used to describe the different pulmonary inflammatory responses to aspirated material. As was discussed in the chapter on infection, aspiration pneumonia describes a mixed anaerobic infection resulting from the aspiration of infected oropharyngeal contents. The aspiration of oropharyngeal or gastric secretions

may also occur in a "pure" form uncomplicated by anaerobic infection, producing aspiration pneumonitis.

Aspiration of oropharyngeal or gastric secretions, with or without food particles, is not an uncommon event. It is seen in debilitated patients with chronic diseases, in patients with tracheal or gastric tubes, in unconscious patients, and in those who have suffered strokes, seizures, or trauma. More chronic and less easily recognizable forms of aspiration may occur in patients with anatomic abnormalities of the upper GI tract (Zenker diverticulum, esophageal stricture) or functional disorders (gastroesophageal reflux, neuromuscular dysfunction).

Gastric fluid is highly irritating to the lungs and often stimulates explosive coughing and associated deep inspirations, leading to widespread distribution of the fluid throughout both lungs and into the peripheral airspaces. The hydrochloric acid contained in gastric fluid causes direct damage to both the bronchiolar lining and the alveolar wall. The severity of the resultant pneumonitis depends upon several factors: it is increased with a pH of the aspirated fluid less than 2.5, large volume of aspirated fluid, large particulate matter in the aspirated fluid, and young age. The massive aspiration of gastric contents is known as Mendelson syndrome. When the aspirate includes particulate material, the particles are distributed by gravity and may incite a granulomatous foreign body–type reaction. Three basic radiographic patterns of aspiration

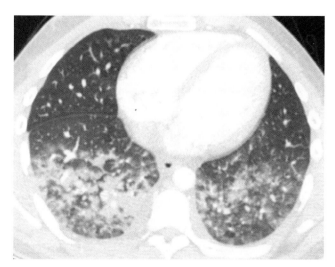

FIGURE 19.39. Aspiration Bronchiolitis/Pneumonitis. Axial CT scan at lung windows through the lower thorax shows a dependent bilateral lower lobe process characterized by ground glass, tree-in-bud opacities and air-space consolidation reflecting aspiration bronchiolitis and bronchopneumonia.

pneumonitis have been observed: (*1*) extensive bilateral airspace opacification, (*2*) diffuse but discrete airspace nodular opacities, and (*3*) irregular parenchymal opacities that are not obviously airspace filling in nature (16). Parenchymal involvement is most often bilateral, with a predilection for the basal and perihilar regions (Fig. 19.39). When a significant amount of admixed food is present, the opacities are usually posterior and segmental. Atelectasis is often present, presumably caused by airways obstruction by food particles. The radiographic appearance may worsen over the first few days but then demonstrates rapid improvement. A worsening of the radiographic appearance at this stage suggests development of a complicating infection, ARDS, or pulmonary embolism.

Chronic Aspiration Pneumonitis. Patients who repeatedly aspirate may develop chronic interstitial abnormalities on chest radiographs. With repeated episodes of aspiration over

months to years, irregular reticular interstitial opacities may persist, probably representing peribronchial scarring. A reticulonodular pattern may be seen, caused by granulomas forming around food particles. These chronic interstitial abnormalities can be observed in between episodes of acute aspiration pneumonitis.

Exogenous Lipoid Pneumonia. Multifocal areas of consolidation or masses can result from the aspiration of lipid material and are classically seen in older patients with swallowing disorders or gastroesophageal reflux who ingest mineral oil as a laxative or inhale oily nose drops. When solitary, lesions can mimic lung cancer. CT findings of fat attenuation with a compatible clinical history are diagnostic of this entity (Fig. 19.40).

RADIATION-INDUCED LUNG DISEASE

The pulmonary effects of external irradiation, most commonly administered for palliation of unresectable bronchogenic carcinoma or metastatic disease to the chest or treatment of mediastinal Hodgkin lymphoma, depend upon several variables. The volume of lung treated will affect the incidence of radiation injury; the greater the volume irradiated, the more likely that radiation injury will occur. Most radiation treatment is limited to less than one-third to one-half of the lung, as an equivalent dose administered to an entire lung or both lungs would cause serious lung injury. The total dose and the method of fractionation will affect the incidence of radiation injury. Doses under 20 Gy rarely produce lung injury, whereas doses exceeding 30 Gy, particularly if administered to a significant portion of the lungs, have a significant incidence of radiation pneumonitis. Administration of a single large dose is more deleterious than fractionation of a similar total dose over the course of several weeks. There is variation in the susceptibility to radiation among individuals; a given dose may cause pneumonitis in one patient, whereas another remains unaffected. The concomitant use of chemotherapeutic agents (particularly bleomycin) or the withdrawal of corticosteroid therapy may accentuate the deleterious effects of radiation. The mechanism of radiation-induced lung injury is not completely understood,

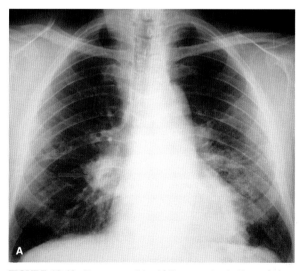

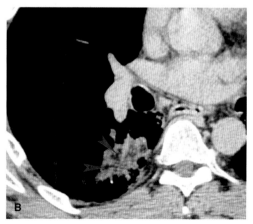

FIGURE 19.40. Exogenous Lipoid Pneumonia. A. Frontal chest radiograph in a 77-year-old man who used mineral oil as a laxative shows a superior segment right lower lobe mass (*arrow*) with associated lower lung interstitial changes present for 3 years. **B.** Thin-section CT at mediastinal windows shows fat attenuation (*arrowheads*) within the mass, which is indicative of lipoid pneumonia.

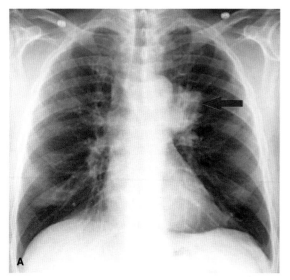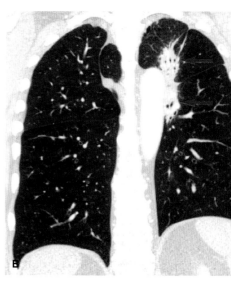

FIGURE 19.41. Radiation Fibrosis. A. Chest radiograph in a patient previously irradiated for unresectable non–small-cell carcinoma shows a left perihilar opacity (*arrow*). **B.** Coronal-reformatted CT through the posterior thorax shows dense juxta-aortic consolidation containing air bronchograms representing radiation fibrosis (*arrows*). Note the elevation of the left oblique fissure and left diaphragm resulting from cicatricial atelectasis of the irradiated lung.

but the acute effects involve injury to capillary endothelial and pulmonary epithelial cells that line the alveoli. This diffuse alveolar damage produces a cellular, proteinaceous intra-alveolar exudate and hyaline membranes that is indistinguishable histologically from ARDS. These changes develop 4 to 12 weeks following the completion of therapy. Although most patients with acute radiation pneumonitis are asymptomatic, dyspnea and a nonproductive cough may be present.

Radiographically, a sharply marginated, localized area of airspace opacification is seen that does not conform to lobar or segmental anatomic boundaries and directly corresponds to the radiation port (17). Adhesive atelectasis of the involved portion of lung is common because the radiation produces a loss of surfactant by damaging type 2 pneumocytes. The pneumonitis may resolve completely with or without the administration of corticosteroids, or it may progress to pulmonary fibrosis. Pulmonary fibrosis corresponds histologically to a reparative phase, with regeneration of type 2 pneumocytes, reorganization of the parenchyma, ingrowth of granulation tissue, and eventually interstitial fibrosis. Fibrosis appears as coarse linear opacities or occasionally as a homogeneous parenchymal opacity with severe cicatrizing atelectasis of the involved portion of the lung. The sharp margination of the parenchymal fibrotic changes may be difficult to appreciate on plain radiographs, but is usually obvious on cross-sectional CT or MR studies. Fibrotic tissue is characteristically low signal on T2W MR sequences, a finding that is helpful in distinguishing fibrosis from recurrent tumor, which typically produces high signal on T2WIs. The parenchymal changes are usually stable by 1 year following radiation therapy. Pleural thickening caused by fibrosis is a common finding. Small pleural and pericardial effusions are also common.

The diagnosis of radiation pneumonitis is usually made by excluding infection or malignancy as a cause of the patient's symptoms and by the presence of typical radiographic findings following a course of radiation therapy to the chest. This distinction may require bronchoalveolar lavage and transbronchial biopsy. An increased number of lymphocytes in the bronchoalveolar lavage fluid and an absence of malignant cells confirm the diagnosis. The demonstration of airspace opacifi-cation on CT that conforms to a known portal of radiation is usually sufficient for the diagnosis (Fig. 19.41). Treatment is generally supportive, with severe cases requiring corticosteroid therapy.

References

1. Light RW. Physiology: changes with pleural effusion and pneumothorax. In: Light RW, Lee G. Textbook of Pleural Diseases. 2nd ed. London: Hodder Arnold, 2008:43–58.
2. Miserocchi G. Physiology and pathophysiology of pleural fluid turnover. Eur Respir J 1997;10:219–225.
3. Leung AN, Muller NL, Miller RR. CT in differential diagnosis of diffuse pleural disease. AJR Am J Roentgenol 1990;154:487–492.
4. Peterman TA, Brothers SK. Pleural effusions in congestive heart failure and in pericardial disease. N Engl J Med 1983;309:313.
5. Colice GL, Curtis A, Deslauriers J, et al. Medical and surgical treatment of parapneumonic effusions. An evidence-based guideline. Chest 2000;18: 1158–1171.
6. Stern EJ, Sun H, Haramati LB. Peripheral bronchopleural fistulas: CT imaging features. AJR Am J Roentgenol 1996;167:117–120.
7. Baumann MH, Strange C, Heffner JE, et al. Management of spontaneous pneumothorax. An American College of Chest Physicians Delphi Consensus Statement. Chest 2001;119:590–602.
8. Muller NL. Imaging of the pleura. Radiology 1993;186:297–309.
9. Leung AN, Muller NL, Miller RR. CT in the differential diagnosis of diffuse pleural disease. AJR Am J Roentgenol 1990;154:487–492.
10. Wang ZJ, Reddy GP, Gotway MB, et al. Malignant pleural mesothelioma: evaluation with CT, MR imaging, and PET. Radiographics 2004;24: 105–119.
11. Jeung M-Y, Gangi A, Gasser B, et al. Imaging of chest wall disorders. Radiographics 1999;19:617–637.
12. Guttentag AR, Salwen JK. Keep Your Eyes on the Ribs: The Spectrum of Normal Variants and Diseases That Involve the Ribs. Radiographics 1999;19:1125–1142.
13. Iochum S, Ludig T, Walter F, et al. Imaging of diaphragmatic injury: a diagnostic challenge. Radiographics 2002;22:S103–S116.
14. Zylak CJ, Eyler WR, Spizarny DL, Stone CH. Developmental lung anomalies in the adult: radiologic-pathologic correlation. Radiographics 2002;22:S25–S43.
15. Wagner RB, Crawford WO Jr, Schimpf PP. Classification of parenchymal injuries of the lung. Radiology 1988;167:77–82.
16. Landay MJ, Christensen EE, Bynum LJ. Pulmonary manifestations of acute aspiration of gastric contents. AJR Am J Roentgenol 1978;131:587–592.
17. Choi YW, Munden RF, Erasmus JJ, et al. Effects of radiation therapy on the lung: radiologic appearances and differential diagnosis. Radiographics 2004;24:985–997.

SECTION EDITOR: Karen K. Lindfors

CHAPTER 20 ■ BREAST IMAGING

KAREN K. LINDFORS AND HUONG T. LE-PETROSS

Breast imaging has two purposes. The first purpose is to screen asymptomatic women for early breast cancer. The second purpose is to evaluate breast abnormalities in symptomatic patients or patients with indeterminate screening mammograms. Screening is accomplished with standard two-view mammography, but diagnostic evaluation often requires the additional use of special mammographic views, breast US, MR, and interventional procedures.

SCREENING FOR BREAST CANCER

Breast cancer survival is influenced by the size of the tumor and the lymph node status at the time of diagnosis. Small tumors with negative axillary lymph nodes have survival rates well above 90%. Such cancers are detected far more often with screening mammography than with physical examination. It follows that screening mammography should lower mortality from breast cancer. Several randomized controlled trials have proven the efficacy of this technique.

In 1963 the Health Insurance Plan of New York (HIP) invited 31,000 women aged 40 to 64 years to participate in four annual screenings for breast cancer by mammography and physical examination. This study group was compared with a control group of women who received routine medical care. Nine years after beginning the study there was a 29% reduction in breast cancer mortality in the group receiving annual screening (1).

Other trials of mammographic screening were begun in the late 1970s and early 1980s. Four of these were carried out in Sweden and were similar in design. They were population based, meaning that all women living within a spe-

cific geographical area who were within the age range under study were included in the trial. Breast cancer mortality was compared between women invited to screening and those not invited (controls). When the data from all centers were combined, the reduction in breast cancer mortality among women aged 40 to 74 years was 24% in the group invited to mammographic screening (2).

The actual benefit of screening mammography for women of all ages is likely to exceed that which has been demonstrated by the randomized clinical trials. Breast cancer mortality data on all women invited for screening, regardless of whether they actually underwent mammography, were used in calculating the reduction of mortality attributable to screening. Compliance rates for obtaining mammography among trial invitees ranged from 61% to 89%. The technology used for mammography has improved greatly since the time that the trials began, resulting in earlier detection of breast cancer (3). Recent evaluations of the impact of mammographic screening in the community setting (service screening) have shown breast cancer mortality reductions of up to 50% among screened women; however, it is difficult to determine the contribution of screening relative to that of improvements in therapy in lowering the death rate from breast cancer (4,5).

Screening Guidelines

Data from the randomized, controlled trials of mammographic screening as well as information from large community-based screening programs were used to formulate the American Cancer Society (ACS) guidelines for breast cancer screening in average risk women, which are shown in Table 20.1 (6). Both

TABLE 20.1

AMERICAN CANCER SOCIETY GUIDELINES FOR BREAST CANCER SCREENING
IN AVERAGE-RISK WOMEN

■ AGE	■ CLINICAL EXAMINATION	■ MAMMOGRAPHY
20–39 years	Every 3 years	Not recommended
40 years and older	Annually	Annually

clinical examination and mammography are essential components of a screening program because all cancers are not seen mammographically. False-negative mammograms occur in 9% to 16% of palpable breast cancers.

There is controversy over the age at which mammographic screening should begin and also the frequency of such screening. In late 2009, the U.S. Preventive Services Task Force (USPSTF) withdrew its support for mammographic screening for women in their forties and recommended that women ages 50 to 74 years be screened biennially (7). The USPSTF concluded that the benefit gained from screening was not high enough to offset the downsides of screening (false-positive results, anxiety, and possible overdiagnosis and overtreatment). They chose to use a 15% reduction in mortality in their meta-analysis even though mortality reductions of up to 44% have been reported with screening in this age group. The National Cancer Institute advises that women at average risk for breast cancer and age 40 years and older should undergo screening mammography every 1 to 2 years (8). Observational studies have shown that women aged 40 to 49 years were more likely to have late-stage cancers diagnosed if they were screened at 2-year intervals when compared with a 1-year screening interval (9). Other studies of cancers that occur between screens have shown that a greater proportion of breast cancers grow faster in younger women than in older women (10–12). It is for this reason that the ACS has recommended *annual* mammographic screening for women at age 40 and older, yet the chance of being diagnosed with breast cancer between the ages of 40 and 49 is 1 in 66 women or 2%, and the chance of dying from breast cancer is 0.3%. Although it is clear both that mammographic screening can reduce breast cancer mortality for women in their forties and that annual mammographic screening is more effective in reducing breast cancer deaths for women in this age group; economic considerations may favor modifications in screening strategies.

For postmenopausal women, there is some question regarding the additional benefit gained by annual screening since studies have shown that there is no increase in late-stage cancers diagnosed if screening is done every 2 years instead of annually (9). The incidence of breast cancer does increase with age. The age at which mammographic screening should cease is not specified in the ACS or NCI guidelines. There are no data on breast cancer mortality reduction for women who are screened beyond age 74. For elderly women, general health status and quality of life should be considered when deciding whether to undergo mammography. Experts suggest that mammographic screening should stop when life expectancy is less than 5 to 7 years or when abnormal results of screening would not be acted on because of age or comorbid conditions (13).

Women potentially at high risk for development of breast cancer should seek expert advice regarding the age at which screening should begin, the periodicity of mammography, and the possible addition of other screening modalities. A risk assessment should be performed. Factors known to increase a woman's risk include the following: (1) A personal history of breast or ovarian cancer. (2) Laboratory evidence that the woman is a carrier of the BRCA1 or BRCA2 genetic mutation. These mutations confer an estimated risk of up to 80% for development of breast cancer by age 70. (3) Having a mother, sister, or daughter with breast cancer. (4) Atypical ductal hyperplasia (ADH) or lobular neoplasia diagnosed on a previous breast biopsy. (5) A history of chest irradiation received between the ages of 10 and 30 years. Women who are at high risk (lifetime risk for breast cancer of greater than 20%) should undergo annual screening MR in addition to mammographic screening (14). Screening with US can be considered in high-risk women who cannot undergo MR screening.

When adopting a screening policy, the physician must remember that all women are at risk for developing breast cancer. The ACS estimates that one woman in every eight will develop the disease during her lifetime. The majority of women who contract breast cancer will not have histories that place them at higher risk.

Screening Outcomes

What are the expected outcomes in a group of 1000 asymptomatic women undergoing bilateral screening mammography for the first time? Approximately 80 of these women will be recalled for additional studies. These may include magnification or other special mammographic views and US. Biopsy will be recommended in about 16 of these women, and cancer will be found in about 6 of them. With subsequent screenings of the same women, the numbers of cancers found will decrease and the positive predictive value, or percentage of women undergoing biopsy who actually have cancer, should increase.

The goal of screening asymptomatic women is to find breast cancer in its earliest stages when survival is greatest. In a well-established screening program, over 50% of cancers will be minimal; minimal cancers are defined as those that are noninvasive or invasive, but less than 1 cm in size with negative nodes. Over 80% of breast cancer discovered by screening mammography should be node negative (15,16).

Optimal effectiveness of a breast cancer screening program requires the use of physical examination in addition to mammographic screening. About 9% to 16% of cancers are not visualized mammographically; such cancers are discovered on physical examination. The minimum size of breast cancers that can be felt on physical examination averages between 1.5 and 2 cm.

False-negative mammograms can occur for a variety of reasons. The palpable abnormality may not be included on a film. Dense breast parenchyma may obscure visualization of a mass. The imaging technique may be suboptimal for visualization of an abnormality. The particular tumor type may not be visible mammographically or there may be observer error in the interpretation of the mammogram. It must be emphasized that a negative mammogram should not deter further diagnostic evaluation of a clinically palpable mass.

Some breast cancers will arise in the interval between screening examinations. The number of such cancers will depend on the frequency of screening. Interval cancers tend to be more advanced at diagnosis when compared with those diagnosed at screening (11); they may be biologically more aggressive. Additionally, a previous negative mammogram or the knowledge that screening will be performed regularly may be a disincentive for patients to seek immediate medical care for a breast mass found in the interval between screens. Physicians must stress that any breast mass requires immediate attention, regardless of whether the patient has had a recent negative mammogram.

Radiation Risk

An increased susceptibility to breast cancer has been documented among women exposed to high doses of radiation (1 to 20 Gy). The survivors of the atomic bomb explosions in Japan, patients undergoing radiation therapy, and sanatoria patients undergoing multiple chest fluoroscopies for monitoring of tuberculosis therapy are all groups having an increased incidence of breast cancer. Such data raised questions about the risk incurred from the low doses of radiation received during screening mammography (approximately 2 mGy per view).

A controlled study of the effects of low doses of radiation such as those received during mammography would require large numbers of women in both the study and control groups. Close to 100 million patients in each group would be required in order to provide statistically significant data. Clearly, this would not be practical or possible. As such, estimates or risk have been hypothesized by extrapolation from data obtained at higher doses using a linear dose-response model.

Follow-up data from the Japanese atomic bomb survivors have shown progressively decreasing radiation risk with increased age at exposure. Women exposed in their youth and teens suffered the highest increase in risk. No increased risk was demonstrable for women aged 40 years or older at exposure. Studies of the other populations sustaining significant breast radiation exposure have also supported a diminished risk with advancing age at exposure. Estimated lifetime risk of breast cancer death from a single mammogram in the age group from 40 to 49 years is approximately 2 in 1 million. In women aged 50 to 59 years, this risk is reduced to less than 1 in 1 million; progressive reductions in risk are seen at older ages (17).

These theoretical risks should be weighed against the risk of dying from spontaneous breast cancer, which would be approximately 700 per million in women aged 40 to 49 years and 1000 per million in women aged 50 to 59 years. This risk increases steadily with advancing age.

The Use of Other Imaging Modalities for Breast Cancer Screening

Mammography is the only imaging modality that has been proven to reduce breast cancer mortality when used to screen asymptomatic women. MR is being used for breast cancer screening in conjunction with mammography in high-risk women. Other modalities are under investigation for their potential use in screening.

Although the impact of screening with MR on breast cancer mortality remains unknown, prospective studies in high-risk women have shown significantly higher sensitivities for MR screening in addition to mammography (86% to 100%) compared to mammography alone (25% to 60%) (18). MR does, however, have a much higher false-positive rate than mammography and leads to more negative biopsies. It is important to emphasize that MR cannot replace mammography as a screening modality; it must be used as a supplemental method of screening in high-risk women. The addition of MR adds considerable cost to a breast cancer screening program.

Several single institution studies have shown that whole breast screening US can detect small nonpalpable invasive cancers not seen mammographically. Prevalence rates for cancers seen only on sonography are approximately 3/1000, but positive predictive values for biopsies based on US alone are approximately half of those for biopsies of lesions discovered on mammography (19). A multi-institution trial of screening breast US as an adjunct to mammography in high-risk women reported an incremental cancer detection rate of 4.2/1000 women screened with both modalities as compared to mammography alone; however, false positives were also increased substantially when US was used (20).

Studies comparing mammography, breast US, and breast MR for screening in high-risk women have shown that supplemental screening with US adds no benefit to screening with mammography and breast MR. US screening may, however, be useful in high-risk women in whom MR is contraindicated or cannot be tolerated. In addition to high false-positive rates, there are challenges to the incorporation of US as a screening modality. US is highly dependent on the operator and on the equipment and technique used for scanning. It is also a time consuming, labor intensive examination, which should be performed by a radiologist trained in the technique. Automated scanners are under investigation to address these issues, but at present there are concerns about these devices.

Other imaging technologies, such as PET, scintimammography, single photon emission tomography, tomosynthesis, and dedicated breast CT, are also being explored for use in breast cancer detection and diagnosis. Mammography continues to be the single best test for early detection of breast cancer; however, it is likely that in the coming years a more individualized approach based on risk and other factors will be used in breast cancer screening. Newer modalities will be incorporated when appropriate, likely as adjuncts to mammography.

EVALUATION OF THE SYMPTOMATIC PATIENT

Bilateral mammography should be the first imaging study performed in patients older than 30 years who present with breast masses that are suspicious for carcinoma. The mass should be indicated by placing a radiopaque marker over the site. This will assist the radiologist in a targeted mammographic evaluation of this area and will also ensure that the palpable abnormality corresponds to the mammographic abnormality, if one is visualized. Such correlation is important in assuring that the surgical biopsy of a palpable abnormality will encompass the mammographically suspicious area.

The primary reason for performing mammography in a patient with a suspicious palpable mass is to assess the affected breast for multifocal disease and the contralateral breast for suspicious abnormalities that should be biopsied concurrently. Mammography may also be helpful in definitively diagnosing the palpable abnormality as benign, thus avoiding biopsy.

Mammography should be performed before any intervention. A hematoma, resulting from percutaneous fine needle aspiration biopsy, can look similar to a small carcinoma. When such procedures have been performed prior to mammography, it is best to perform a follow-up mammogram 4 to 6 weeks later.

If mammography is negative in a patient with a clinically evident mass and dense breasts, US is often suggested as a subsequent imaging study. US can determine whether the mass represents a simple cyst. Simple cysts are virtually never malignant and do not require aspiration unless the patient has pain related to the cyst. US cannot provide a specific diagnosis for a solid or complex mass.

Alternatively, definitive diagnosis of a palpable mass can usually be made by performing a fine needle aspiration of the mass with a 22-gauge needle. When a simple cyst is present, the aspiration is both diagnostic and therapeutic, as all of the fluid can be withdrawn. In solid or complex masses, a cytologic examination of the cells removed at aspiration will yield the diagnosis.

In younger patients who present with breast masses, mammography must be used more judiciously. This more cautious approach is based on data from the atomic bomb survivors in Japan showing an excess risk of breast cancer in younger women exposed to high doses of radiation. These data combined with the low incidence of breast cancer in young women (less than 1% of breast cancer occurs in women younger than 30 years) suggest that a restricted use of mammography is prudent. Some experts also believe that dense breast tissue, which is more common in younger women, limits the sensitivity of mammography, but studies have shown that mammography can demonstrate up to 90% of cancers in women younger than 35 years (21).

Women younger than 30 years who have a focal suspicious palpable abnormality are frequently first evaluated with US. If the US is negative and the patient is older than 25 years, a single oblique view of the affected breast may be performed to assess for suspicious microcalcifications, which would not be visualized by US. Women younger than 25 years should not undergo mammography.

If fine needle aspiration is available, it may be used in lieu of imaging studies when young patients have suspicious palpable masses. In the extremely rare circumstance of a diagnosis of carcinoma, mammography can be performed subsequently. The radiologist should be aware that a previous needle aspiration may confound the mammographic assessment of the affected area, but it will not compromise assessment of surrounding or contralateral tissues.

Increased awareness of breast cancer has led many clinicians to request more imaging studies in young women. Breast imaging cannot replace careful clinical evaluation of the breasts. If there is no suspicious focal abnormality, imaging studies will not be helpful; they may subject the patient to unnecessary risk.

TECHNICAL CONSIDERATIONS IN BREAST IMAGING

Because both high-contrast and high-spatial resolution are needed for optimal mammography, standard radiographic equipment cannot be used for this examination. Mammography must be performed on a unit dedicated to this purpose. Mammographic equipment and technique differ from standard radiography in several ways. The anode material that is used to generate the x-rays in most dedicated film screen mammography units is molybdenum. This allows the production of lower energy x-rays, which in turn produces greater contrast between soft tissue structures. The structures of the breast do not differ greatly in their inherent contrast, so these low-kilovolt photons are extremely important in producing a high-contrast image. Some units also have rhodium anodes that can be used to increase the contrast in denser breasts, while keeping radiation dose and time of exposure low. Full-field digital mammography units often use tungsten anodes, which are more efficient, have better longevity, and can yield lower radiation doses than molybdenum anodes; the image processing possible with digital mammography allows high-quality mammograms utilizing tungsten anodes.

The radiologist must be able to discern tiny microcalcifications on mammograms; some of these calcifications may

be 0.1 mm or less in size. The small focal spot size used in mammography units and high-resolution digital radiographic detectors or high-resolution, single intensifying screens used with single emulsion film, contribute to the creation of images with high resolution.

All mammographic units are equipped with compression paddles that squeeze the breast against the image receptor or film holder. Good compression of the breast is essential to high-quality mammography for several reasons. Compression spreads overlapping breast structures so that true masses can be differentiated from summation shadows that occur because of overlapping soft tissues. The breast is immobilized during compression so motion unsharpness or blurring due to patient movement is minimized. Geometric unsharpness, caused by the finite focal spot dimension, is minimized by bringing the breast structures closer to the film. Compression renders the breast nearly uniform in thickness so the film density of tissues near the nipple will be similar to those near the chest wall. Radiation dose can be reduced by good compression; a thinner breast requires fewer photons for penetration. Beam attenuation is also reduced.

Some women find breast compression uncomfortable, but most can tolerate it once the benefits are explained. During routine mammography the breast is compressed for a few seconds while each film is taken. Many units are equipped with automated compression devices so the technologist can release the tension immediately after the film is exposed.

Other factors are also important to consider in the production of high-quality mammograms. These include other equipment features such as type of x-ray generator, beam filtration, grid use, as well as film-intensifying screen combinations and the film-processing system. All of these factors are interrelated and must be optimized to produce technically acceptable films of the breast.

Full-Field Digital Mammography

Full-field digital mammography (FFDM) units have been commercially available since 2000 and now account for the majority of mammography units in the United States. FFDM uses an electronic system for image capture and display. It has higher contrast resolution and better dynamic range than film screen mammography. Spatial resolution is lower with FFDM, but its greater contrast resolution still makes high-quality images possible. The radiation dose from FFDM is comparable to that of film screen mammography in smaller breasts; it may be lower in larger breasts. Advantages of FFDM over film screen mammography include a higher speed of image acquisition and thus increased throughput of patients, the ability to perform image processing (which may lead to fewer repeat films due to optimization of brightness and contrast), other image-processing algorithms (which may result in increased conspicuity of certain features including microcalcifications, integration of computer-aided detection, and diagnosis software programs), electronic storage thus eliminating lost films and the need for film storage, and the possibility of teleradiology.

The Digital Mammographic Imaging Screening Trial, a multicenter trial that enrolled more than 49,000 women in the United States and Canada, found no significant differences in the sensitivity of FFDM compared to film screen mammography for all women enrolled. However, FFDM performed significantly better than film screen mammography in premenopausal and perimenopausal women, in women younger than 50 years, and in women with dense breasts (22). These findings along with the technical advantages of FFDM have resulted in the steady replacement of film screen mammography with FFDM for breast cancer detection and diagnosis.

Quality Assurance

It is the responsibility of the radiologist to assure that highest quality of breast imaging is performed at his or her facility. All standards mandated by the Mammography Quality Standards Act (MQSA) must be met. These standards apply to both film screen and FFDM. MQSA was passed into law by Congress in 1992 to ensure that all women receive optimal mammography services. The law requires that every practice become accredited by the Food and Drug Administration (FDA). Specified standards for personnel (radiologists, technologist, and physicists), equipment used, radiation dose, and quality assurance practices are stipulated. Once FDA accreditation is granted, an annual survey by a physicist must be performed to ensure that the practice continues to meet quality control and equipment standards. All facilities performing mammography are inspected annually by an FDA inspector. Each radiologist who interprets mammograms must be fully informed of the MQSA regulations. Failure to comply with the law can result in sanctions or even closure of the mammography facility.

Mammographic Positioning for Screening

Mammography can be performed with the patient seated or standing. Most screening practices prefer the standing position because it allows faster throughput and is less cumbersome. Patients are able to lean into the unit to a greater degree when standing, thus allowing more of the posterior breast tissues to be imaged. Recumbent imaging is possible, but quite difficult; its use should be restricted to problem-solving situations.

In the United States, two views of each breast are generally taken for screening mammography. In some European countries, a single mediolateral oblique (MLO) view is taken for screening examinations, but studies have shown that one-view examinations miss 20% to 25% of breast cancers (23). Moreover single-view mammography would lead to an excessive number of patients being called back for additional views. Asking large numbers of patients to return for such views would result in unacceptable levels of patient anxiety and cost. The standard views for screening mammography are the MLO view and the craniocaudal (CC) view.

MLO View. The MLO view, when properly positioned, depicts the greatest amount of breast tissue. It is the most useful view in mammography. In countries using single-view screening, the MLO view is preferred. To perform an MLO view, the x-ray tube and image receptor, which are fixed with respect to one another, are moved to an angle that parallels the orientation of the patient's pectoralis major muscle. The technologist is given flexibility in choosing the angle so that the greatest amount of breast tissue possible can be imaged. The angle is generally between 40° and 60° from the horizontal.

The patient is asked to relax her arm and chest muscles and to lean into the machine. The breast is placed on the image receptor and compression is applied from the superomedial direction, the same direction from which the x-rays will be generated. The breast must be pulled anteriorly and spread in a superior-inferior direction as much as possible to minimize overlapping structures and to maximize the amount of tissue imaged. The nipple should be in profile. Compression must be applied vigorously (Fig. 20.1). By convention, in the MLO view a marker indicating the side (left or right) and type of view is placed near the axillary tissues of the breast.

A properly positioned MLO mammogram should show the pectoralis major muscle down to the level of a line drawn perpendicular to the muscle through the nipple (posterior nipple line). The nipple should be in profile so that the subareolar area can be adequately evaluated. The inframammary fold should be visible to ensure that the inferior portion of the breast has been imaged (Fig. 20.2).

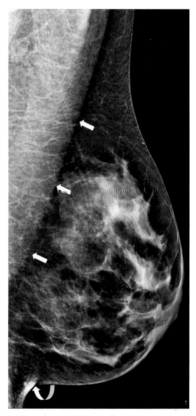

FIGURE 20.2. Normal Mediolateral Oblique View of Left Breast. The pectoralis muscle (*arrows*) is seen from the axilla to below the level of the posterior nipple line. The inframammary fold (*curved arrow*) is well seen and the nipple is in profile.

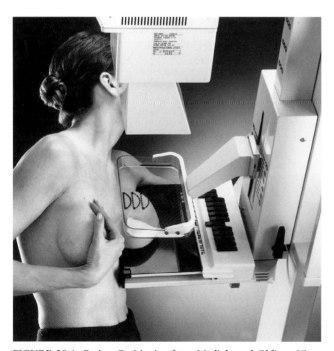

FIGURE 20.1. Patient Positioning for a Mediolateral Oblique View. (Courtesy of General Electric Medical Systems, Milwaukee, WI.)

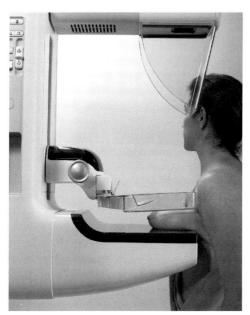

FIGURE 20.3. Patient Positioning for the Craniocaudal View. (Courtesy of Hologic Inc, Bedford, MA.)

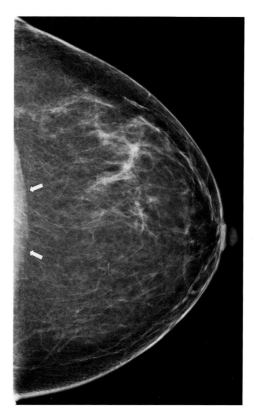

FIGURE 20.4. Normal Craniocaudal View of the Left Breast. Note that the nipple is in profile and the pectoralis muscle (*arrows*) is seen posteriorly indicating optimal visualization of breast tissue.

CC View. For the CC view, the unit is placed in the vertical position so that the x-ray tube is perpendicular to the floor. Photons will travel from the anode, located superior to the breast, to the image receptor underneath the breast. The breast is placed on the image receptor, pulled anteriorly, and spread horizontally before the compression plate is applied to the superior skin surface (Fig. 20.3). The nipple should again be in profile. The chest wall should rest against the image receptor. The markers indicating the side imaged and type of view should be placed near the skin close to the lateral aspect of the breast.

When evaluating a CC mammogram, optimal positioning can be assured when pectoralis muscle is seen centrally on the film and the nipple is in profile (Fig. 20.4). The pectoralis muscle can be visualized in about 30% of patients on the CC view. An alternative method of assuring appropriate visualization of posterior tissues is to measure the distance from the nipple to the edge of the film through the central axis of the breast; this distance should be within 1 cm of the length of the posterior nipple line as seen on the MLO view.

Interpreting the Mammogram

For interpretation, CC and MLO mammograms should each be viewed together in a mirror image configuration. This will allow the radiologist to scan the breasts for symmetry. Viewing conditions are extremely important for optimal interpretation. The room must be darkened. Computer workstations should be used for FFDM interpretation. High-resolution monitors with magnification capability are essential. If films are being interpreted, all adjacent view box light should be blocked out. Dedicated mammography film alternators and view boxes can do this automatically. If standard view boxes or alternators are used, exposed blackened film can be cut to mask out unwanted light. All visible breast parenchyma should be scanned systematically with magnification. This will allow visualization of tiny microcalcifications and will ensure that the radiologist has examined all parts of the breast in detail.

If previous mammograms are available, they should be compared to the current study so that the radiologist can eval-uate the examination for any changes in the mammographic appearance of the breasts. In turn, current questionable areas can be evaluated for their stability.

In most practices, patients are asked to complete a brief history form that includes questions relevant to breast health and cancer risk. Knowledge of the patient's history will be helpful in assessing the malignant potential and likely diagnosis of a particular mammographic finding. The risk of malignancy is much greater in a 60-year-old woman than in a 30-year-old woman. A woman with a personal or close family history of breast cancer is at greater risk for development of malignancy, and the interpretation of mammographic findings should be tailored accordingly. Other information such as previous surgical biopsies or hormone replacement intake must also be taken into account during interpretation of the mammogram.

Correlation with the physical examination is also extremely important so that false-negative reports can be minimized. All palpable lesions should be marked and assessed mammographically. Special views can image palpable lesions that occur in locations not included on standard mammography. The mammographer can also be certain that the mass felt corresponds to the mammographic abnormality. Areas of asymmetric tissue seen mammographically can be assessed for palpable abnormalities, which may render them more suspicious for malignancy.

Classic mammographic signs of malignancy are spiculated masses or pleomorphic clusters of microcalcifications; however, only about 40% of all occult breast carcinoma presents in these ways (24). In the remainder of cases, more subtle or indirect signs of malignancy are present. The radiologist must look at each mammogram with great care, utilizing all available diagnostic techniques so that false-negative diagnoses are

TABLE 20.2

DIAGNOSTIC MAMMOGRAPHIC VIEWS

■ VIEW	■ ABBREVIATION	■ PURPOSE
90° lateral	ML (mediolateral) or LM (lateral medial)	Localizing lesion seen in one view Demonstrate milk of calcium due to its gravity dependency
Spot compression	—	Determine whether lesion is real or is a summation shadow
Spot compression with magnification	M	Better definition of margins of masses and morphology of calcifications
Exaggerated craniocaudal	XCCL	Show lesions in outer aspect of breast and axillary tail not seen on CC view
Cleavage view	CV	Show lesions deep in posteromedial breast not seen in CC view
Tangential	TAN	Verify skin lesions Show palpable lesions obscured by dense tissue
Rolled views	RM (rolled medial) or RL (rolled lateral)	Verify true lesions Determine location of lesion seen in one view by seeing how location changes
Lateromedial oblique	LMO	Improved visualization of superomedial tissue Improved tissue visualization and comfort for women with pectus excavatum, recent sternotomy, prominent pacemaker
Implant displacement	ID	Improved visualization of native breast tissue in women with implants

minimized. This charge must be balanced against the need to minimize false-positive diagnoses. Each time a woman is subjected to a surgical biopsy, financial and emotional costs as well as risks are incurred.

Diagnostic Evaluation of the Indeterminate Mammogram

In the majority of cases, a two-view screening mammogram will provide a conclusive interpretation, but when the results of mammography are indeterminate, further evaluation is necessary; additional mammographic views (Table 20.2) (25), US and, infrequently, MR may be required for clarification. The workup must be tailored to the specific situation.

Projections other than the standard CC and MLO views may help to visualize a lesion that is seen only in one standard view or that is obscured by surrounding parenchyma. Tangential views of the skin can be used to establish a dermal location for calcifications or superficial masses. Dermal abnormalities do not represent breast cancer.

Further characterization of an abnormality can be accomplished with spot compression and magnification views. The compression plate used is much smaller than that used in standard views; therefore, greater force can be applied, which results both in further spreading of any overlying tissue and in bringing the abnormality closer to the film for increased detail. Magnification also produces finer detail, which allows more accurate assessment of the morphology of microcalcifications and the borders of masses.

Well-defined or partially obscured masses can be evaluated with US. A high-frequency (5 to 12 MHz), hand-held linear array transducer is most commonly used. A targeted evaluation of the mammographically visible abnormality is performed. Simple cysts are easily distinguishable from complex or solid masses. This differentiation is extremely important as simple cysts are always benign and require no further workup, whereas noncystic masses may represent cancers.

MR occasionally can be used as an adjunct to mammography and sonography when there continue to be equivocal findings. MR is not, however, a replacement for more conventional imaging.

ANALYZING THE MAMMOGRAM

Masses

Complete assessment of a mammographically visible, potentially malignant mass requires several steps. First, the radiologist must decide whether the mass is real. The left and right breasts must be compared in each view.

Most women have reasonably symmetric parenchyma; however, at least 3% of women have areas of asymmetric, but histologically normal breast tissue. When attempting to distinguish

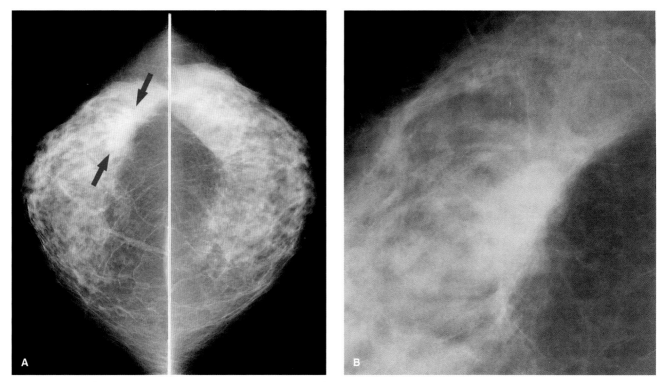

FIGURE 20.5. **Infiltrating Duct Carcinoma. A.** Craniocaudal views of both breasts, showing an asymmetric area of increased density in the outer aspect of the right breast (*arrows*). **B.** Magnification compression view shows this to be a true mass with defined, convex borders and increasing density toward its center.

asymmetric normal breast tissue from a true abnormality, the radiologist must look for the mammographic features of a mass. Masses have convex borders and become denser toward the center. They distort the normal breast architecture. True masses are seen in multiple projections and can still be visualized when focal compression is applied (Fig. 20.5).

Asymmetric breast parenchyma has an amorphous quality. On spot compression, the tissue spreads apart and fat can be seen interspersed with the denser breast structures in a pattern of normal architecture (Fig. 20.6). The appearance of asymmetric tissue varies significantly from one mammographic projection to another.

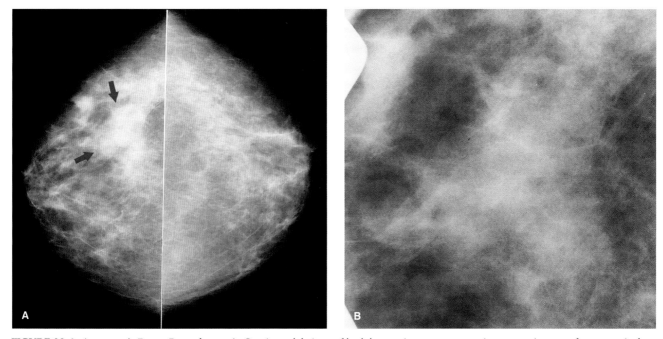

FIGURE 20.6. **Asymmetric Breast Parenchyma. A.** Craniocaudal views of both breasts in an asymptomatic woman. An area of asymmetric density is seen in the outer aspect of the right breast (*arrows*). **B.** Compression magnification view demonstrates normal breast architecture in the area of increased density. These findings are consistent with histologically normal, but asymmetric mammary parenchyma.

When evaluating the breast for a possible mass, it is important to correlate the mammographic findings with the physical examination. When a suspicious palpable abnormality corresponds to the area of asymmetry seen on mammography, a biopsy should be undertaken. In a study of 221 patients with mammographically visible asymmetries, only 3 patients had malignancies and all 3 had suspicious, palpable abnormalities corresponding to the visualized asymmetries (26).

Summation artifacts that resemble masses on mammography can be produced by overlapping breast tissue. They are visible in only one view and usually disappear when focal compression spreads the tissues apart.

Once the radiologist has concluded that a mass is present, its margins, density, location, and size should be assessed. The number of mammographically visible masses and their similarities or differences should be analyzed. Previous films should be compared with the current study to look for new masses or an increase in the size of a mass. It is impossible to evaluate one characteristic independent of the others.

Margins. The margins of a mass are probably the most important characteristics to be assessed. Overlying breast parenchyma often obscures margin analysis, but liberal use of magnification compression views, in multiple projections, will aid the radiologist.

Spiculated Margins. *Breast carcinoma* classically appears as a spiculated mass on mammography (Fig. 20.7); however, less than 20% of nonpalpable cancers present as such (24). Most spiculated-appearing breast cancers will be infiltrating ductal carcinoma; however, tubular and lobular carcinomas can present as such. Tubular carcinomas are more well-differentiated histologically and carry a better prognosis. Lobular carcinomas comprise about 10% of all invasive carcinomas. They are not mammographically distinguishable from invasive ductal carcinomas, although they are frequently more subtle. Single rows of lobular cancer cells can infiltrate surrounding tissues, so they generally cause less tissue distortion.

A very limited differential exists for a spiculated mass.

Fat necrosis from a previous surgical biopsy can appear spiculated (Fig. 20.8).

Scars from previous breast surgery should be carefully marked with radiopaque wires. Comparison should be made with previous films, both to determine the location of the abnormality that underwent biopsy and to assess for any increase in size of the

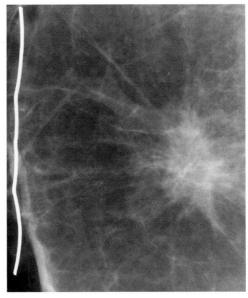

FIGURE 20.8. Postsurgical Fat Necrosis. This spiculated mass had been stable for 7 years. The radiopaque wire indicates the scar on the patient's skin from the previous lumpectomy.

presumed scar. Many scars will regress with time, but others will be stable in appearance and size. Any increase in size should be viewed with suspicion and biopsy should be undertaken.

Radial scar or complex sclerosing lesion can also present as a spiculated lesion. These are spontaneous lesions that are benign and consist histologically of central sclerosis and varying degrees of epithelial proliferation, represented by strands of fibrous connective tissue. Histologic differentiation of these lesions from carcinoma is mandatory.

Indistinct (Ill-Defined) Margins. Breast carcinoma can also present as a round mass with indistinct or ill-defined borders (Fig. 20.9). Benign lesions that can present as such include abscess, hematoma, and focal fibrosis.

Breast abscesses are most commonly seen in a subareolar location in lactating women (Fig. 20.10). Clinically, there is associated pain, swelling, and erythema.

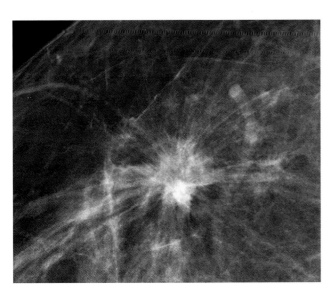

FIGURE 20.7. Classic Breast Carcinoma. This spiculated breast mass is an infiltrating duct carcinoma.

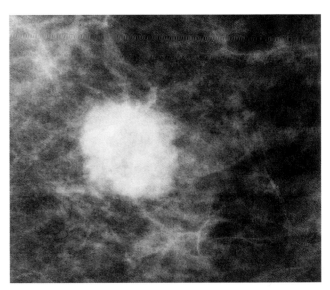

FIGURE 20.9. Infiltrating Duct Carcinoma. Lesion presenting as a round mass with indistinct, microlobulated borders.

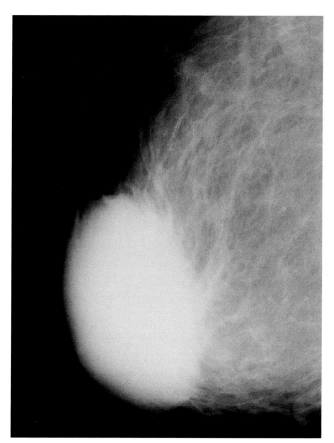

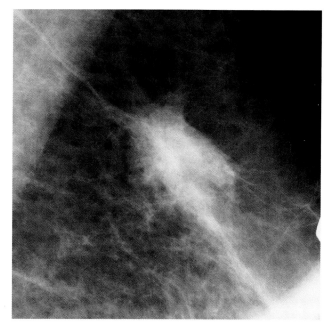

FIGURE 20.11. **Infiltrating Duct Carcinoma.** Magnification view of a palpable abnormality in the upper outer quadrant. The patient had undergone a negative fine-needle aspiration biopsy the previous day; the mammographic differential diagnosis included hematoma and carcinoma. Follow-up mammogram 6 weeks later demonstrated no resolution. Surgical biopsy showed infiltrating duct carcinoma.

FIGURE 20.10. **Large Subareolar Abscess.** The indistinct borders of the mass are the result of surrounding inflammation.

Spontaneous hematomas are seen in women on anticoagulant therapy or in those with blood dyscrasias. They can, of course, also be secondary to trauma, needle aspiration, or surgery. Correlation with the patient's history and physical examination will be helpful in discerning whether a lesion represents a hematoma. If doubt persists as to the nature of a possible hematoma, short-interval follow-up mammograms (4 to 6 weeks later) to demonstrate resolution will be helpful (Fig. 20.11).

Circumscribed (Well-Defined) Margins. Circumscribed masses are almost always benign; however, up to 5% of masses that appear well circumscribed on conventional mammograms may represent carcinomas (27). The "halo sign," which is a partial or complete radiolucent ring surrounding a mass, is not helpful in determining benignity. Sonography should be used to assess circumscribed masses prior to any additional mammographic views; if a simple cyst is diagnosed by US, no further imaging workup is required. Magnification compression views will be of great assistance in clarifying the nature of borders of an apparently well-circumscribed, solid mass. Masses that appear well circumscribed on conventional views may have indistinct or microlobulated margins on compression magnification views (28); such masses should undergo biopsy. If a solid mass appears circumscribed on magnification views and there are no previous mammograms available for comparison, the mass can generally be characterized as one that has a high probability of being benign. Such masses are frequently subjected to a course of follow-up mammography. The first of these surveillance mammograms should be performed 6 months following the original study.

Cysts are the most common well-circumscribed masses seen in women between the ages of 35 and 50 years (Fig. 20.12).

They are rare after menopause unless hormone replacement therapy has been instituted. Cysts can be accurately diagnosed by US and are virtually never malignant. A high-frequency (generally 5 to 12 MHz) US transducer is used in a targeted examination of the mass in question. On sonography, cysts are round or oval, smooth-walled, anechoic, and produce enhanced through transmission of sound. They can frequently be deformed with gentle pressure from the transducer. It is essential that the focal zone and gain of the US unit be optimally adjusted for the lesion so that cysts can be accurately diagnosed sonographically. The cyst must be thoroughly examined in two projections to rule out any irregularities or masses emanating from the walls.

Fibrosis is another manifestation of fibrocystic change that can be seen mammographically. It can be quite focal, giving it the appearance of a well-defined mass on the films. Such areas of focal fibrosis may also present with ill-defined borders, making them difficult to differentiate from carcinomas.

Fibroadenomas are the most common well-defined solid masses seen on mammography (Fig. 20.13). They are homogenous, but frequently show large, coarse calcifications. They may have a lobulated contour, but there are usually only a few large lobulations. If a fibroadenoma is not calcified, it cannot be distinguished from a cyst by mammography. Sonography will allow characterization of fibroadenomas as solid hypoechoic masses. The peak age of patients with clinically detected fibroadenomas is 20 to 30 years; however, fibroadenomas are seen into the eighth decade. They rarely appear or grow after menopause.

Primary breast malignancies to be considered when a well-defined density is visualized on mammography are infiltrating duct carcinoma, papillary carcinoma, mucinous carcinoma, and medullary carcinoma.

Lymphoma, either primary or metastatic, may also present as a well-circumscribed mass.

Metastatic disease to the breast from other sources may present as a well-circumscribed nodule. The most common primary cancer to produce breast metastases is melanoma, but a large variety of other primary sites have also been reported

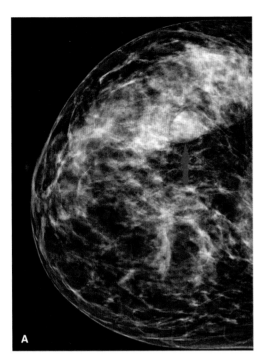
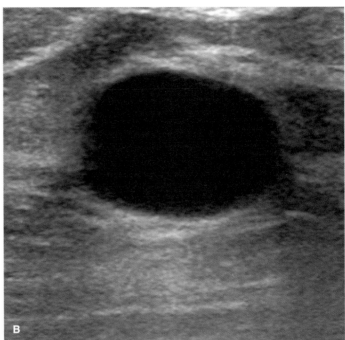

FIGURE 20.12. Simple Breast Cyst. A. Craniocaudal mammogram demonstrates a 1.5-cm mass in a 46-year-old woman (*arrow*). The mass is at least partially well circumscribed. B. US of the mass demonstrates a round, anechoic structure with well-defined margins and enhanced through transmission of sound. These features are diagnostic of a simple cyst.

to metastasize to the breast. When these malignancies are encountered, magnification compression views of the abnormality often demonstrate some irregularity to the contour of the mass (Fig. 20.14).

Density. Density is relevant to the analysis of mammographically detected masses when these masses contain lucent areas indicative of fat. Breast masses that clearly contain fat are benign. The assessment of density in homogeneous nonfatty

masses is not, however, useful in the prediction of benignity or malignancy.

Fat Density. Benign breast lesions that are purely fat density include oil cysts from fat necrosis, lipomas, and sometimes galactoceles. *Oil cysts* are generally the result of trauma (Fig. 20.15). They are round lucent lesions surrounded by a thin capsule; often they are multiple and can demonstrate rim calcifications. *Lipomas* are similar to oil cysts in appearance; they are also lucent with a surrounding capsule. The surrounding breast

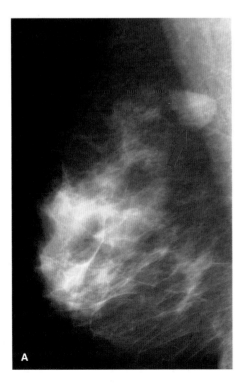
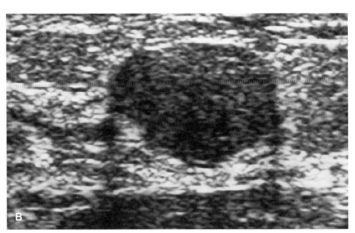

FIGURE 20.13. Fibroadenoma. A. Mediolateral oblique view of a 1.8-cm partially well-defined mass (*arrow*). B. US demonstrates a solid hypoechoic mass with a macrolobulated well-defined margin.

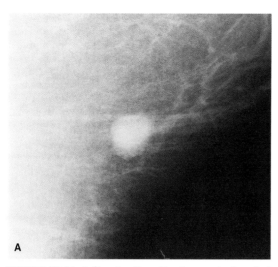 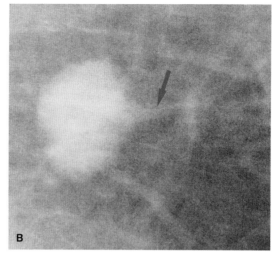

FIGURE 20.14. **Infiltrating Duct Carcinoma. A.** A well-circumscribed, 8-mm mass that had increased in size compared with a study done 1 year previously. **B.** Magnification view shows a spiculation anteriorly (*arrow*). Infiltrating duct carcinoma was proven at biopsy.

architecture may be distorted because of the mass effect of the lipoma. *Galactoceles* usually occur in lactating or recently lactating women and are probably the result of an obstructed duct. If the inspissated milk is of sufficient fat quantity, these lesions will appear lucent; however, they can also be of mixed or water density.

Mixed Fat and Water Density. Other benign masses that are mixed fat and water density are *hamartomas* (Fig. 20.16), which are rare benign tumors, and intramammary lymph nodes. *Intramammary lymph nodes* are frequently seen on mammograms. They are generally located in the upper outer quadrant in the posterior three-fourths of the breast parenchyma. They normally contain a fatty center or a lucent notch, representing fat in the hilus of the node (Fig. 20.17). Fat–fluid levels can occasionally be seen on MLO mammograms in galactoceles and postsurgical hematomas.

Location. Breast cancers can occur in any location within the breast. As such, the location of a lesion is helpful in mammographic diagnosis in only two situations. The first occurs when the mammographer is considering an intramammary lymph node in the differential. The second occurs when a lesion can be localized to the skin.

Intramammary nodes visualized on mammograms are almost always located in the upper outer quadrant of the breast. They have been noted in other locations in autopsy series, and there are rare case reports of visualization of such nodes by mammography in other locations in the breast.

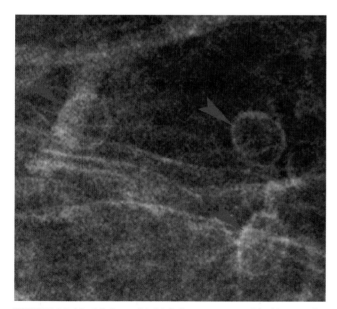

FIGURE 20.15. **Oil Cysts.** Multiple lucent masses with thin capsules (*arrowheads*) are characteristic of oil cysts. The patient had suffered trauma to the breast.

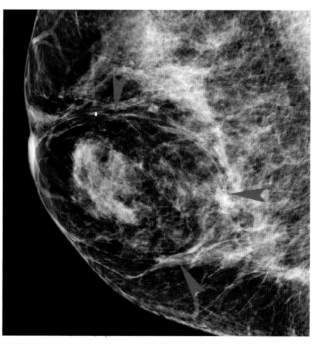

FIGURE 20.16. **Hamartoma.** Mediolateral oblique mammogram demonstrates a large mixed fat and water density mass with a thin capsule (*arrowheads*). The hamartoma had been stable for many years.

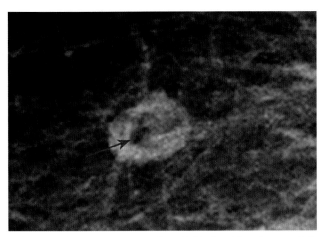

FIGURE 20.17. **Intramammary Lymph Node** with a characteristic lucent center (*arrow*) and well-circumscribed margins. The node was located in the upper outer quadrant.

Skin Lesions. If a lesion is located only on the skin, it does not represent a breast carcinoma. Frequently, however, skin lesions project over the parenchyma and can appear to be within the breast. Such lesions are usually recognizable by air trapping around the edges or in the interstices. This air trapping can produce a dark halo around one edge (Fig. 20.18). Air trapping will not, however, be evident with flat, pigmented skin lesions or sebaceous cysts.

It is helpful to examine the patient and place a radiopaque marker on any skin lesions or possible sebaceous cysts. The technologist can then perform a repeat film in the projection that the lesion was visualized. If necessary, this view can be followed by a tangential view to demonstrate that the lesion is located in the skin.

Size. By itself, the size of a mammographically discovered mass is not particularly helpful in determining its etiology. A spiculated or ill-defined mass should undergo biopsy no matter what

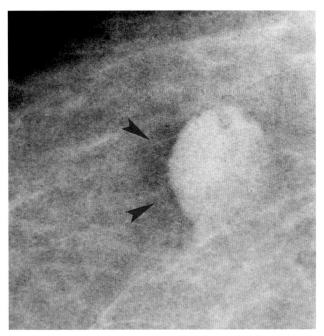

FIGURE 20.18. **Skin Nevus.** The dark halo produced around one edge is the result of air trapping (*arrowheads*).

its size. However, when the mammographer is dealing with a circumscribed mass that has a much lower chance of being malignant, size may play a role in determining the next step in the workup. US may not be helpful when lesions are less than about 3 to 5 mm in size, particularly in fatty breasts. Frequently, patients with such lesions will be asked to return in 6 months for a follow-up study to assess for interval growth. If the lesion increases in size, further investigation with US and possible biopsy can be performed. After the first 6-month follow-up, stable lesions should be followed at yearly intervals for a minimum of 3 years.

Larger, clinically occult masses require both US to prove they are solid and magnification views to prove they are circumscribed before surveillance mammography is suggested. Some experts advocate a size upper limit of 1 to 1.5 cm for masses that are to undergo follow-up, but research has shown that nonpalpable, circumscribed breast masses can be managed by periodic mammographic surveillance regardless of size (29). Generally, a 6-month follow-up of the affected breast is advocated; this is followed by a bilateral mammogram 6 months later and then annual mammography for at least 3 years to document stability.

Number of Masses. ***Multiple Masses.*** In many cases, multiple well-defined round masses will be seen on mammography. When evident, such masses are also frequently bilateral. Multiple, bilateral round masses are usually benign. They most often represent *cysts* or *fibroadenomas*, although *multiple papillomas* can also present in this way (Fig. 20.19). In patients with a history of previous malignancy, *metastasis* may also be considered, although metastatic disease is much more commonly unifocal.

All lesions should be evaluated carefully. Benign and malignant lesions can coexist in the same breast. A lesion with a different, suspicious morphology should prompt a biopsy.

When evaluating the patient with similar appearing multiple, bilateral, rounded breast masses, it is not generally advisable to perform US; the reason is that US is confusing and frequently demonstrates hypoechoic areas that, although disconcerting to the radiologist, do not prove to be malignant. *Multifocal primary breast cancers* generally present as obvious, ill-defined or stellate lesions that are suspicious in appearance (Fig. 20.20).

Calcifications

Clustered, pleomorphic microcalcifications, with or without an associated soft tissue mass, are a primary mammographic sign of breast cancer. Such calcifications are seen in more than half of all mammographically discovered cancers; about one-third of all nonpalpable cancers are manifest by calcifications alone, without an associated mass (24).

The calcifications associated with malignancy are dystrophic; they are the result of abnormalities in the tissues. Some malignant calcifications occur in necrotic tumor debris; others are the result of calcification of stagnant secretions that are trapped in the cancer (30).

Calcifications are a frequent finding on mammographic examinations. In the majority of cases, such calcifications will be benign and their origin, as such, will be easily identifiable. There is, however, a significant overlap in the appearance of benign and malignant calcifications. Only 25% to 35% of all calcifications that undergo biopsy will be malignant.

The importance of technically optimal mammography cannot be overstated when calcifications are being studied. The film exposure must be appropriate; an underexposed film can hide calcifications in a background of white breast tissue. Slight overpenetration of films is optimal for detection of calcifications.

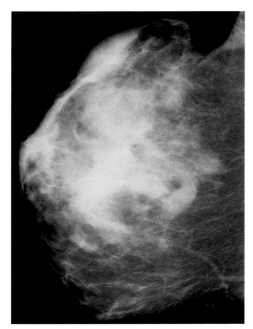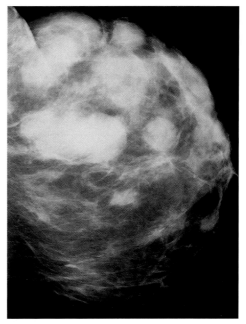

FIGURE 20.19. Multiple Benign Masses. Bilateral craniocaudal views show multiple large round masses in both breasts. The patient was asymptomatic. Differential diagnosis was cysts or fibroadenomas.

Magnification views will be extremely helpful for assessing the malignant potential of a group of calcifications.

Careful analysis of the form, size, distribution, and number of calcifications, as well as any association with other soft tissue structures, will allow the radiologist to determine which calcifications are unequivocally benign and which require biopsy or follow-up studies.

Form. *Benign Calcifications.* Some shapes of calcifications can be easily identified as benign. Any calcification with a lucent center should not cause concern. Calcifications with lucent centers arc often located in the skin. A skin marker can be placed over the calcifications and a subsequent tangential view taken to confirm their location in the skin (Fig. 20.21). Calcifications with lucent centers are also seen as a result of fat necrosis. Such calcifications can be smooth and round or they can be eggshell-type calcifications in the walls of an oil cyst (Fig. 20.22).

Calcifications that layer into a curvilinear or linear shape on 90° lateral films, yet appear as smudged clusters on CC views, are also representative of a benign process (Fig. 20.23). Such calcifications represent sedimented calcium ("milk of calcium") within the fluid of tiny breast cysts. Similar benign calcifications can also be seen within larger cysts and oil cysts. Sedimented calcium is a common finding in approximately 5% of women presenting for mammography.

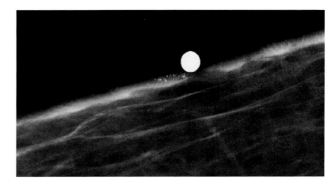

FIGURE 20.20. Multifocal Carcinoma. Craniocaudal view. The largest mass was palpable. The others were discovered by mammography (*arrowheads*). The more well-defined nodule (*curved arrow*) probably represented an intramammary lymph node.

FIGURE 20.21. Skin Calcifications. Tangential view showing calcifications to be in the skin. A radiopaque marker had been placed on the skin at the site of the calcifications. This was done to facilitate positioning for the tangential view.

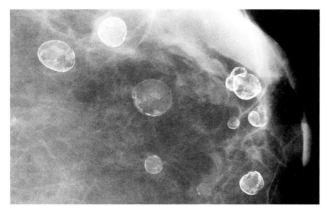

FIGURE 20.22. Eggshell Calcifications in Oil Cysts. These are large calcifications with lucent centers that are benign.

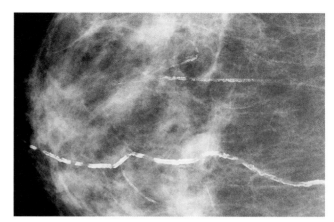

FIGURE 20.24. Arterial Calcifications. Arterial calcifications in the breast are identified by their location in the wall of a tortuous vessel.

Other benign calcifications that are easily recognizable by their form include arterial calcifications, the calcifications in a degenerating fibroadenoma, and calcifications associated with secretory disease. Arterial calcifications generally present as tubular parallel lines of calcium (Fig. 20.24). Occasionally, early arterial calcification can present a diagnostic problem, but this can usually be resolved by looking for soft tissue of the vessel in association with the calcification. Magnification in multiple projections can be helpful (Fig. 20.25).

Fibroadenomas can calcify in various patterns. Sometimes the calcifications are indeterminate, but the classic calcifications, associated with an atrophic fibroadenoma, are large, coarse, and irregular in shape (Fig. 20.26).

Secretory Disease. The calcifications associated with secretory disease are smooth, long, thick linear calcifications that radiate toward the nipple in a generally orderly pattern (Fig. 20.27). These calcifications are located in ectatic ducts. When periductal inflammation has occurred, these calcifications may appear more lucent centrally since calcium is deposited in the tissues adjacent to the ducts.

Malignant calcifications vary in shape and size (Fig. 20.28). The margins of the calcifications are jagged and irregular. Malignant calcifications are often branching. Ductal carcinoma in situ (DCIS), or noninvasive breast cancer, is most often detected mammographically as a result of such calcifications. Groups of pleomorphic calcifications that are more linear or

"dot-dash" in appearance are more commonly associated with high–nuclear-grade intraductal carcinomas that have luminal necrosis (comedocarcinomas) (Fig. 20.29). The lower-grade (cribriform and micropapillary) types are often manifest by more punctate or granular appearing calcifications. The morphology of the calcification cannot, however, be used to predict the subtype of DCIS since there is considerable overlap in the forms of the calcification associated with each subtype; frequently multiple DCIS subtypes exist together in the same lesion. In the high-grade (comedo) subtype, the calcifications can be an approximate indication of the size of the tumor, although the extent of disease is often greater than mammographically predicted. In the lower-grade varieties, correlation is even poorer. The biological behavior of these subtypes also differs; high-grade types are the most likely to recur (31).

Pleomorphic microcalcifications in association with a malignant soft tissue mass can also indicate areas of extensive intraductal component within or adjacent to the invasive tumor. It is especially important to recognize malignant calcifications occurring in tissues surrounding invasive cancers so they can be excised with the invasive tumor. Such extensive intraductal component-positive cancers also have a greater tendency to recur.

Indeterminate Calcifications. Morphologically, indeterminate calcifications account for the majority of mammographically generated biopsies of calcifications (Fig. 20.30). Such calcifications are most often associated with fibrocystic

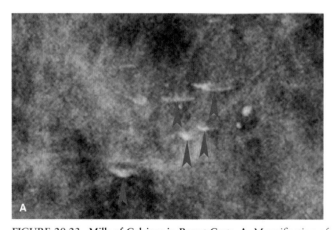

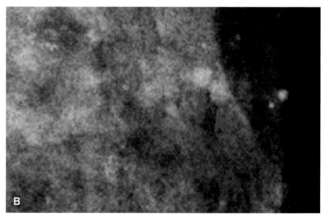

FIGURE 20.23. Milk of Calcium in Breast Cysts. A. Magnification of a 90° lateral mammogram showing diffuse linear calcifications (*arrowheads*). **B.** Craniocaudal magnification view of the same area showing smudged, rounded calcifications (*arrowheads*). This change in configuration between views is typical of sedimented calcium. The calcium is layering in the bottom of microcysts and so it appears as a line or meniscus when viewed from the side in the lateral projection. When viewed from the top, these calcifications simply appear smudged and rounded.

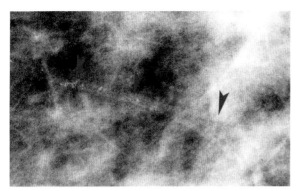

FIGURE 20.25. Early Arterial Calcification. Magnification view. The calcification can be seen clearly in the walls of an artery (*arrowheads*). The soft tissue of the artery was difficult to appreciate on the conventional views.

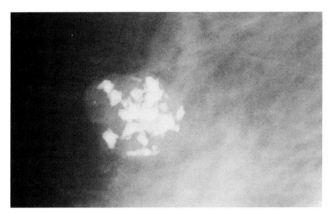

FIGURE 20.26. Degenerated Fibroadenoma. Typical large, coarse, irregular calcifications are seen in a fibroadenoma.

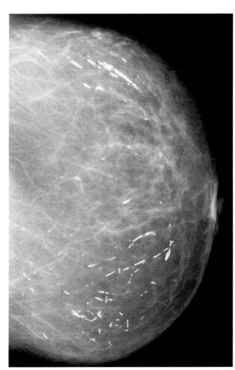

FIGURE 20.27. Secretory Calcifications. Craniocaudal view demonstrates long and thick calcifications in ectatic ducts that radiate toward the nipple.

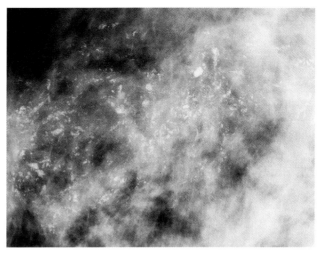

FIGURE 20.28. Malignant Calcifications. Magnification view of infiltrating ductal carcinoma. Note the irregular forms as well as the variety of sizes and shapes.

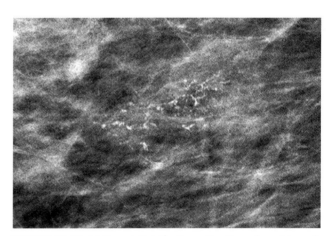

FIGURE 20.29. Malignant Calcifications. Fine-linear branching calcifications of high–nuclear-grade ductal carcinoma in situ (comedocarcinoma). Note the pleomorphism in the size and shape of the calcifications.

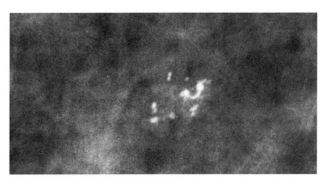

FIGURE 20.30. Indeterminate Calcifications. Magnification view of cluster of calcifications. There is some irregularity in shape and variation in size, but these calcifications were benign. They were associated with fibrocystic change.

change. Diagnoses included under the general category of fibrocystic disease are fibrosis adenosis, sclerosing adenosis, epithelial hyperplasia, cysts, apocrine metaplasia, and atypical hyperplasia. Occasionally, biopsy of indeterminate calcification will yield a diagnosis of lobular carcinoma in situ (LCIS), also called lobular neoplasia. Although not an invasive cancer, LCIS places a woman at higher risk for development of invasive breast cancer. Mammographically, LCIS has no distinct features. If it is clinically occult, it is most often found serendipitously adjacent to a focus of mammographically indeterminate, but histologically benign, calcifications.

Distribution. Calcifications that are diffuse or widely scattered and seen bilaterally are usually indicative of a benign process, such as sclerosing adenosis or adenosis. Multiple, bilateral clusters of calcifications that appear morphologically similar are also generally benign. Careful analysis with magnification is essential in these cases so that a morphologically dissimilar cluster is not overlooked. Such calcifications should be thoroughly examined with magnification views.

Malignant calcifications usually occur in groups or clusters within a small volume of tissue; they can also occur in a linear distribution suggesting cancerous tissue within a duct. DCIS can occasionally produce calcifications that encompass large areas of the breast. Calcifications that are morphologically suspicious or indeterminate and occupy a segment of the breast should undergo biopsy.

Size. Malignant calcifications are generally less than 0.5 mm in size. Because the calcifications associated with carcinoma are so small, they are frequently referred to as microcalcifications. Within a cluster, there will be a variety of sizes.

Benign calcifications are often larger. When benign disease produces clusters of calcifications, the size of these calcifications is usually similar.

Number. Calcifications associated with malignancy are generally quite numerous. The greater the number of calcifications, the more likely they are associated with malignant disease. Establishing the lower limit of the number of calcifications in a cluster that would require biopsy is extremely difficult. Assessment of the morphology of these calcifications by magnification views will influence this decision more than the actual number of calcifications.

Architectural Distortion

Breast cancer is occasionally heralded by distortion in the normal architecture of the breast (Fig. 20.31). Differential diagnosis includes fat necrosis related to scarring from previous surgery and a complex sclerosing lesion, also known as radial scar. On close inspection, fat may be seen interspersed with fibrous elements in the center of fat necrosis or complex sclerosing lesions, but this appearance is not specific for benignity. Similar findings can be seen in malignant lesions.

Biopsy is necessary for differentiation.

Increased Density of Breast Tissue

Hormone Therapy. Increasing parenchymal density of breast tissue can be bilateral or unilateral. Bilateral increased density is usually the result of estrogen replacement therapy in postmenopausal women. Such hormone therapy can give the breasts a more glandular, premenopausal appearance. Intrinsic hormonal fluctuations in premenopausal, pregnant, or lactating women may cause similar changes in the density of the breasts. Hormonally related changes in breast density are not associated with skin thickening.

Inflammatory Carcinoma. A unilateral increase in breast density with associated skin thickening may result from several processes. The most ominous of these is inflammatory carcinoma of the breast (Fig. 20.32). Clinically, this disease is manifest by a warm, erythematous, firm, tender breast. Histologically, the dermal lymphatics are diffusely involved. Mammographically, a focal mass may be seen within the dense tissue, but often the breast appears homogeneously dense. Inflammatory carcinoma of the breast is a locally advanced disease that carries a poor prognosis.

Radiation Therapy. A unilateral increase in parenchymal density with skin thickening can also be seen in patients who have undergone radiation therapy to the breast. Radiation changes are most pronounced during the first 6 months following therapy. They usually resolve gradually over a period of years.

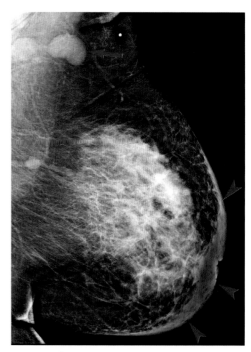

FIGURE 20.32. **Inflammatory Carcinoma.** Mediolateral oblique view demonstrates a diffuse increase in parenchymal density, along with skin thickening (*arrowheads*). An enlarged, dense lymph node (*arrow*) is seen in the axilla. The lymph node was palpable and was marked with a radiopaque skin marker. Pathology confirmed malignant adenopathy.

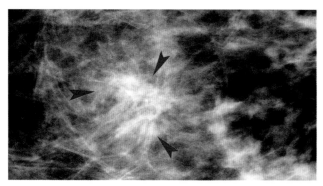

FIGURE 20.31. **Architectural Distortion Representing Breast Carcinoma.** Note how the cancer pulls the surrounding parenchyma toward it (*arrowheads*).

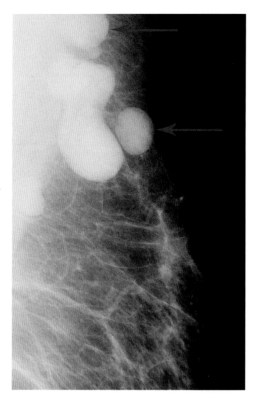

FIGURE 20.33. Lymphoma. Hodgkin disease involves the axillary lymph nodes. The nodes are homogeneous, dense, and enlarged (*arrows*).

Diffuse mastitis can produce a generalized skin thickening and increase in breast density. Clinical differentiation from inflammatory carcinoma is usually possible.

Obstruction to the lymphatic or venous drainage from metastatic disease, surgical removal, or thrombosis can produce a unilateral increase in breast density with skin thickening due to edema. The anasarca associated with congestive heart failure, renal failure, cirrhosis, or hypoalbuminemia most often presents as bilateral increased breast density with skin thickening; however, asymmetric involvement of the breasts can occur.

Correlation of physical examination findings and history will usually allow differentiation of the various causes of an increase in breast density.

Axillary Adenopathy

Axillary lymph nodes are frequently visualized on the MLO mammogram. Normally, they are less than 2 cm in size and have lucent centers or notches resulting from fat in the hilum. Fatty infiltration of the nodes themselves can cause lucent enlargement and replacement.

Mammographically, pathologic axillary nodes are homogeneously dense and enlarged. A variety of processes can result in replacement of normal nodal architecture. Malignant involvement of axillary nodes can be the result of primary breast cancer, metastatic disease, lymphoma, or leukemia (Fig. 20.33). Axillary nodes can also become pathologically enlarged because of inflammation. Patients with rheumatoid arthritis, systemic lupus erythematosus, scleroderma, and psoriasis may also have axillary adenopathy.

Coarse calcifications in axillary nodes may reflect granulomatous disease. Microcalcifications are occasionally seen in nodes involved with metastatic breast cancer. Gold deposits, seen in patients being treated for rheumatoid arthritis, are occasionally seen in axillary nodes and may be confused with calcifications.

US can be used to assess the axillary nodes at the time of a new diagnosis of breast cancer. Nodes are evaluated based on the size, length-to-width ratio, or morphology. Benign or normal lymph nodes are hyperechoic with a thin hypoechoic cortical rim on US (32). Tumor cells can invade both the cortical rim and the hyperechoic hilum, resulting in asymmetric focal hypoechoic cortical lobulation or complete replacement of the lymph node thus leading to an enlarged hypoechoic node without visible hyperechoic hilum (Fig. 20.34). If suspicious nodes are identified, they can be biopsied under US guidance, yielding more accurate preoperative staging.

The Augmented Breast

More than 1.5 million women in the United States have undergone augmentation mammoplasty. Imaging of the augmented breast poses unique challenges. Special techniques must be employed both to screen for breast cancer and to evaluate the patient for possible complications related to the implant.

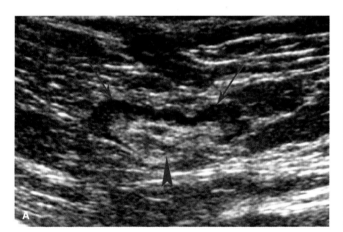
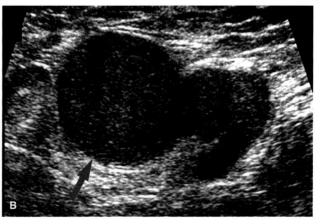

FIGURE 20.34. Axillary Lymph Nodes. A. US image of a normal axillary lymph node. The cortex is diffusely thin (*arrows*), while the hilum (*arrowhead*) is hyperechoic due to fat cells with areas of hyperechoic reflective interfaces from vessels and trabeculae. **B.** A 40-year-old woman with a new diagnosis of locally advanced right breast invasive ductal carcinoma. US of the right axilla showed enlarged hypoechoic lymph nodes (*arrow*) indicative of metastatic disease.

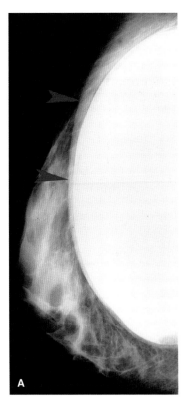
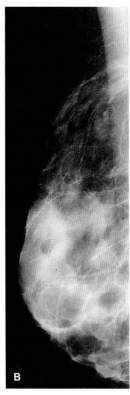

FIGURE 20.35. Breast Implants. A. Standard mediolateral oblique (MLO) view of a patient with a subpectoral silicone implant. Note the pectoralis muscle (*arrowheads*) anterior to the implant. B. MLO implant displacement view on the same patient. The implant has been displaced posteriorly, out of view, while the compression has been applied anteriorly.

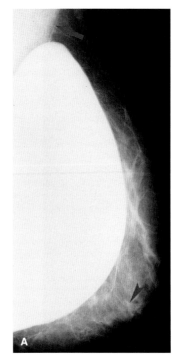
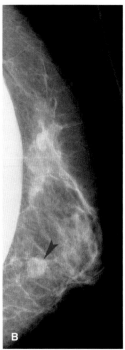

FIGURE 20.36. Infiltrating Duct Carcinoma. A. Standard mediolateral oblique (MLO) view in a patient with prepectoral silicone implants. Note the pectoralis muscle (*arrow*) extending posterior to the implant. A poorly defined 1-cm mass (*arrowhead*) was noted in the subareolar tissues. B. MLO implant displacement view in the same patient. The subareolar mass (*arrowhead*) is more clearly defined because of greater compression of the tissues anterior to the implant. Histologic examination of the mass showed infiltrating duct carcinoma.

Various types of implants have been used in augmentation procedures. They include silicone envelopes filled with saline or with viscous silicone gel, as well as double-lumen implants containing an inner core of silicone gel surrounded by an outer envelope filled with saline. Silicone is more radiopaque than saline, although neither allows adequate visualization of immediately surrounding tissue.

Implants can be placed either anterior (prepectoral) or posterior (subpectoral) to the pectoralis muscle. A fibrous capsule develops around the implant. Patients having prepectoral implants are subject to a greater risk of fibrous and calcific contractures around the implant. Such contractures are not only painful and deforming, but they also make mammography more difficult.

Screening mammography in the woman with implants requires the use of at least two extra views of each breast. Standard MLO and CC views are performed with moderate compression. Then the implants are displaced posteriorly against the chest wall, while the breast tissue is pulled anteriorly and more vigorously compressed (Fig. 20.35). The compression paddle keeps the implant from migrating into the field of view. Greater compression of anterior tissues allows more optimal imaging (Fig. 20.36). Both MLO and CC views are repeated using this technique. These modified views are called implant displacement views (33).

Implant displacement views are more difficult to accomplish in patients with prepectoral implants with associated capsular contractures around the implant. The implants are not easily displaced, and so less of the anterior breast tissue is depicted on the modified views. In such cases, a 90° lateral view may also be helpful in screening.

Although some breast tissue may be obscured in patients with implants, these women, when in the appropriate age groups, deserve the same careful screening examinations at the same intervals as patients without implants. The indeterminate mammogram in an implant patient should be evaluated in a manner similar to that in a patient without implants.

Women who have undergone augmentation mammoplasty may also present with abnormalities related to their implants. These include capsular contractures, herniations of the implant through rents in the capsules, implant rupture with free (extracapsular rupture) (Fig. 20.37) or contained (intracapsular rupture) silicone, and deflation of saline implants. Many patients will present for breast imaging subsequent to noticing a change in implant contour or size. Mammography is generally the first examination performed if the woman is older than 30 years; however, mammography is not useful in the detection of intracapsular silicone implant ruptures since the silicone is contained within the fibrous capsule that has developed around the implant. Extracapsular silicone implant ruptures can sometimes be detected by mammography, but often the free silicone is obscured by the overlying implant or is in an area of the breast or chest wall not imaged on the mammogram (34).

Other imaging modalities can be used for the assessment of implant complications. MR is the most accurate in identifying silicone implant rupture and in localizing free silicone (35). The protocol for breast implant evaluation consists of axial, sagittal, and/or coronal T2W sequences with and without water suppression and the inversion recovery (IR) sequences with water suppression. It is essential to use several projections in implant evaluation. The most effective sequence is the IR sequence, which suppresses the fat signal. The addition of water saturation results in a silicone only image. In the intracapsular silicone implant rupture, the implant shell

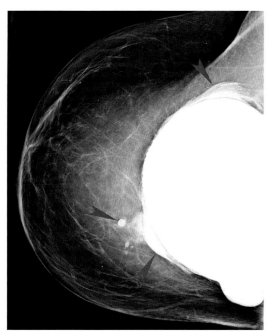

FIGURE 20.37. Ruptured Silicone Implant. Standard craniocaudal view of an asymptomatic patient with prepectoral silicone implants. The mammogram shows an extracapsular rupture of the implant with silicone outside the implant capsule (*arrows*).

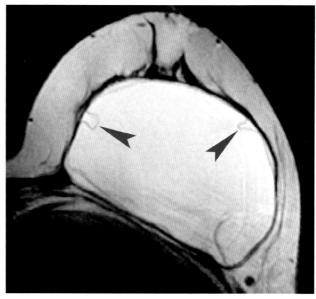

FIGURE 20.39. MR of Subtle Intracapsular Silicone Implant Rupture. Sagittal fast spin-echo T2-weighted image shows a focus of silicone gel trapped within a fold of the implant shell (*arrowheads*), known as "noose sign," "inverted teardrop sign," or "keyhole sign."

ruptures but the silicone remains within the fibrous capsule. Signs of intracapsular rupture on MR can be subtle. A linguine sign indicating intracapsular rupture occurs when the collapsed implant shell floats within the silicone gel contained in the fibrous capsule (Fig. 20.38). The noose, teardrop, or

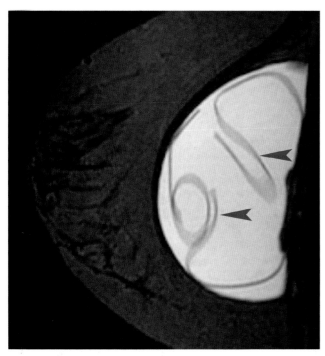

FIGURE 20.38. MR of Intracapsular Silicone Implant Rupture. Sagittal inversion-recovery T2-weighted images with water suppression shows multiple low-intensity curvilinear lines (*arrowheads*) contained within the fibrous capsule, representing the collapsed implant shell ("linguine sign"). There is no extracapsular silicone.

keyhole signs of intracapsular rupture indicate small amounts of silicone collected in a radial fold (Fig. 20.39). Over time, microscopic silicone can leak through the intact implant shell and collect at the implant shell surface, giving a subcapsular line sign. This can be difficult to differentiate from a small intracapsular rupture. In the extracapsular rupture, the envelope and fibrous capsule lose integrity resulting in free silicone gel extruding into breast tissue (Fig. 20.40). US is also used to detect implant rupture, but has a lower sensitivity (70%) compared to MR (94%) (36). Specificity with both US and MR are similar (92% to 97%). The success of US in the assessment of implant integrity is highly dependent on the operator; an experienced radiologist must scan the breasts in a methodical manner.

Neither US nor MR is indicated to evaluate rupture of saline implants since rupture of such implants will be evident both clinically and mammographically as implant deflation with resorption of the extruded saline.

The Male Breast

The most common indication for breast imaging in men is a palpable asymmetric thickening or mass. Gynecomastia is usually the cause. Breast cancer is rare, but can occur.

Normal male breast appears on mammography as a mound of subcutaneous fat without glandular tissue (Fig. 20.41). The nipple is small.

Gynecomastia generally appears as a triangular or flame-shaped area of subareolar glandular tissue that points toward the nipple. Fat is interspersed with parenchymal elements. A gradual merging of the more glandular elements with the fat occurs at the deep margin (Fig. 20.42). Gynecomastia can be unilateral or bilateral. When bilateral, it is most frequently asymmetric. Many causes have been reported, including ingestion of a variety of drugs, such as reserpine, cardiac glycosides, cimetidine, and thiazides, as well as marijuana. Testicular, adrenal, and pituitary tumors are associated with gynecomastia. Chronic hepatic disease, by virtue of reduced

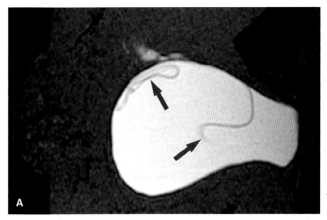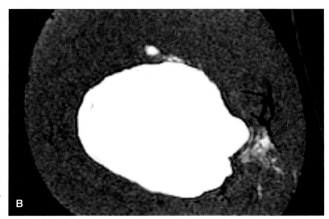

FIGURE 20.40. MR of an Extracapsular Silicone Implant Rupture. Sagittal (**A**) and coronal (**B**) inversion-recovery T2-weighted images with water suppression show extracapsular silicone (*arrowheads*) in the superior and lateral left breast. The partially collapsed implant shell (*arrows*) is seen within the silicone gel contained within the fibrous capsule that surrounds the implant.

ability to clear endogenous estrogens, can also cause male breast enlargement.

Male breast cancer is mammographically similar to that found in women. It can have a variety of appearances, including an ill-defined, spiculated, or circumscribed mass (Fig. 20.43). Microcalcifications can occur.

Comparison With Previous Films

The importance of comparing current mammograms with previous films cannot be overstated. In one series, developing densities accounted for 6% of nonpalpable breast carcinomas (24).

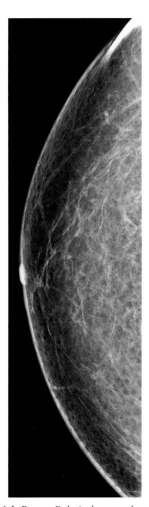

FIGURE 20.41. Male Breast. Relatively normal male breast, which is a mound of subcutaneous fat. Note the lack of glandular tissue.

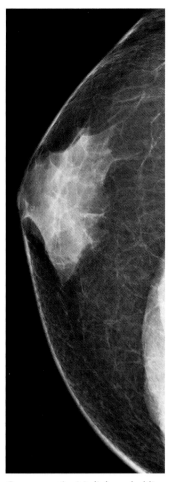

FIGURE 20.42. Gynecomastia. Mediolateral oblique view of a male with breast enlargement. Glandular tissue is seen in the subareolar area. This tissue gradually intersperses with the fat and does not appear as a mass.

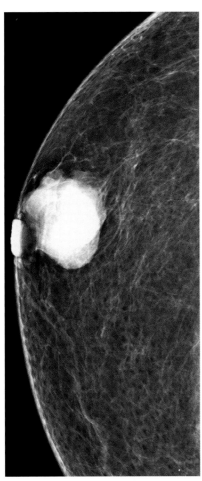

FIGURE 20.43. Male Breast Cancer. Mediolateral oblique view of the breast in a male. The mass has a defined interface with the surrounding fat.

Comparison with previous films will allow detection of subtle changes, in turn suggesting the need for further evaluation of such areas at an earlier time than might be possible if no comparison had been made (Fig. 20.44). It must, of course, be remembered that benign masses may appear or enlarge over time. In fact, in the majority of cases, interval change will be benign, but such changes should be fully evaluated by correlation with the history and physical examination as well as the use of ancillary testing methods such as US, aspiration, and biopsy.

Malignant masses that were stable in size for up to 4.5 years have been reported. Although such a long period of stability is unusual, these reports emphasize the need for suspicious appearing lesions to undergo biopsy regardless of their apparent lack of change in size on serial films. Such lesions may have been overlooked or misinterpreted on a previous study.

Any new microcalcifications or increase in a number of such calcifications deserve special consideration. Appropriate workup with magnification views will allow analysis of the morphology of such calcifications. Any calcifications that are not clearly benign deserve biopsy.

MAGNETIC RESONANCE IMAGING

Indications. In the last decade, MR of the breast has become an integral part of the routine breast imaging practice despite the lack of evidence regarding the impact on survival by the additional of this powerful imaging modality with conventional breast imaging tools such as mammography and sonography. Current common clinical applications of breast MR include screening of patients at high risk for developing breast cancer, preoperative staging of newly diagnosed breast cancer cases, detection of mammographically occult malignancy in patients with axillary nodal metastasis, and evaluation of response to neoadjuvant chemotherapy.

The American Cancer Society guidelines recommends MR as an adjunct to clinical breast examinations and annual mammography for women at risk for hereditary breast cancer, untested first-degree relatives of women with BRCA mutations, and any patient with a family history predictive of a lifetime cancer risk of at least 20% (14). This recommendation was based on a review of at least six prospective, nonrandomized studies of high-risk women, which reported significantly higher sensitivity for MR (range 77% to 100%) compared with mammography (25% to 40%), or with mammography plus US +/− clinical breast examinations (49% to 67%), despite substantial differences in patient populations and MR technique (37–43).

In the preoperative staging assessment of women with newly diagnosed breast cancer, MR is reported to be more accurate in assessing the tumor size and in detecting clinically and mammographically occult multicentric and contralateral disease (44–48). However, a recent meta-analysis of 2610 women in 19 studies confirmed that the additional MR detected lesions in 16% of these women did not result in improved surgical planning or reduction in local recurrence (49). Even though MR may be more accurate in visualization of the primary tumor lesions and in the detection of additional tumor foci, the tendency of MR to overestimate lesion size, multicentricity, and contralateral involvement can potentially eliminate some patients from breast conservation surgery toward more invasive surgery or mastectomy. The full impact of MR for this indication still needs further evaluation with randomized multi-institutional trials.

In women who present with axillary nodal disease and without a clinical or mammographically detectable breast lesion, MR is the imaging of choice to detect a primary breast lesion (50). The detection of a primary breast lesion would not only allow proper staging of these patients, but also may enable more appropriate choice of chemotherapy and radiation therapy. Some of these patients may be able to have breast conservation surgery as opposed to mastectomy after neoadjuvant chemotherapy.

The role of MR in assessing response to neoadjuvant chemotherapy remains controversial, despite multiple published studies with small sample sizes (51). The addition of functional imaging such as diffusion-weighted imaging, spectroscopy, and other advanced MR technology to the routine breast MR examination may offer prognostic indicator of early response to therapy. However, randomized multi-institutional trials are needed (18).

Technique. Breast MR should be performed on scanners operating at 1.5 Tesla (T) or higher field strengths. The patient is scanned in prone position with the breasts hanging into a dedicated receiver breast coil. Body coils should not be used for breast MR examinations. Ideally, imaging should be done between days 6 and 17 of the menstrual cycle. Bilateral studies should be performed.

The breast should be imaged in axial or sagittal planes or a combination of the two. Core pulse sequences when evaluating the breast for cancer include a three plane localizer, T1-weighted (T1W) images, T2-weighted (T2W) images with fat suppression, three-dimensional fat-suppressed gradient echo series precontrast administration, and three or more postcontrast acquisitions for approximately 6 to 8 minutes after the contrast agent injection. Thin-image slices of 3 mm

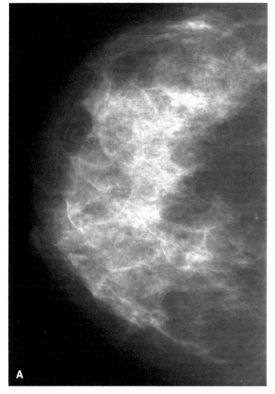
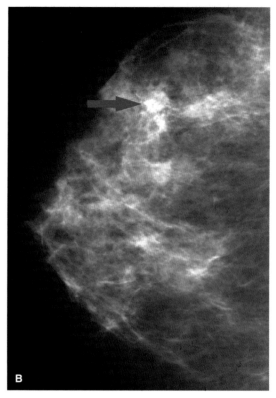

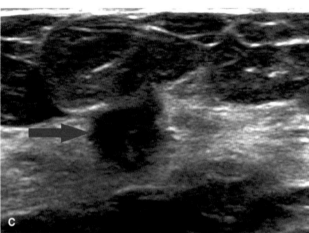

FIGURE 20.44. Infiltrating Duct Carcinoma.
A. Craniocaudal mammogram shows dense
mammary parenchyma, but no evidence of
malignancy. B. Mammogram 1 year later
shows development of a subtle new mass
(*arrow*). C. US shows an irregular solid mass
(*arrow*) with indistinct margins. Biopsy demonstrated infiltrating duct carcinoma.

or less is recommended, with pixel sizes of 1 mm or less in each in-phase direction (52). The T1W images allow clear differentiation of adipose tissue from glandular tissue. T2W fat-suppressed images allow identification of fluid-filled structures such as cysts. Dynamic images obtained prior to and after IV gadolinium enhancement help to identify potential malignancies on the basis of morphology and enhancement kinetics. The IV gadolinium DTPA dose ranges from 0.1 to 0.2 mmol/kg body weight.

Fat suppression can be accomplished before gadolinium administration by using chemical-selective fat saturation or water-only excitation techniques. After IV contrast administration, passive fat suppression can be accomplished with postprocessing image subtraction, but patient movement between pre- and postcontrast-enhanced images can degrade the images due to misregistration. Kinetic curves can be performed on enhancing lesions.

Interpretation. Each lesion should be evaluated for its shape, margin, internal architecture, precontrast T1 and T2 signal characteristic, enhancement characteristics, and change from prior studies. Predictors of benignity include smooth margins, nonenhancing internal septations, minimal or no enhancement, and diffuse patchy enhancement. Features suggestive of malignancy include spiculated or irregular borders (Fig. 20.46), peripheral or rim enhancement, segmental or regional enhancement (Fig. 20.47), and ductal enhancement. On the precontrast T1W fat-suppressed images, bright T1 signal intensity is suggestive of benign etiologies such as a complicated or hemorrhagic cyst, fresh fat necrosis, or the fatty hilum of an intramammary lymph node. Simple cysts have high T2 signal intensity, whereas most invasive carcinomas have low T2 signal intensity. Medullary or mucinous carcinoma can have high T2 signal intensity and look similar to cysts on MR.

Kinetic curves improve the specificity of breast MR. These curves can be evaluated qualitatively according to the curve shape and classified as a persistent pattern of enhancement, a plateau of enhancement, or washout of signal intensity

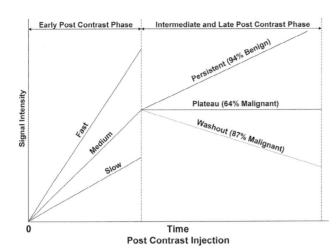

FIGURE 20.45. **Breast MR Kinetic Curves.** Schematic drawing of kinetic curves showing hypothetical signal intensities of a lesion after contrast injection. The shape of the curve aids in differentiating benign from malignant lesions. Rapid enhancement in the early postcontrast phase is more likely associated with malignant lesions. Washout of contrast in the immediate and late postcontrast phases also has a higher likelihood of malignancy.

(Fig. 20.45) (53). Most invasive carcinomas demonstrate rapid initial enhancement with a plateau or washout on delayed imaging. Some malignant lesions such as DICS, invasive lobular carcinoma, tubular carcinoma, and mucinous carcinoma may demonstrate slow initial enhancement. A curve showing a persistent increase in signal intensity after the first 2 minutes is more suggestive of a benign etiology, although some malignancies may show such enhancement. Kinetic curves are helpful for lesions that are indeterminate or benign in morphology and may influence the decision to biopsy. Any morphologically suspicious lesion, however, requires biopsy regardless of its enhancement kinetics.

THE RADIOLOGIC REPORT

The radiologic report should be clear and concise. The American College of Radiology has developed a standardized format and terminology called the Breast Imaging Reporting and Data System (BI-RADS) (54) for mammograms, breast US, and breast MR. All reports should begin with description of the overall breast composition. With mammography, this description of breast density will allow the clinician to gauge the sensitivity of the examination. The breast should be characterized as (1) composed almost entirely of fat,

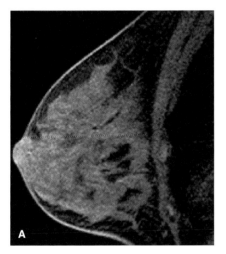

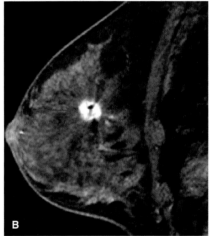

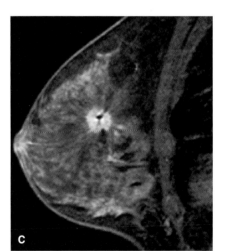

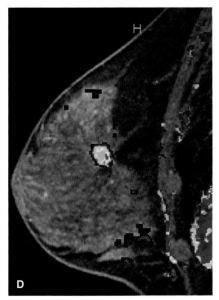

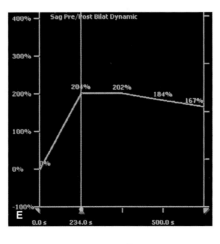

FIGURE 20.46. **MR of Infiltrating Ductal Carcinoma.** Precontrast (**A**), early (**B**) and late (**C**) post-IV contrast, fat-suppressed, T1-weighted, fast spoiled gradient-echo, sagittal MR images of the left breast show a round spiculated 16-mm enhancing mass (*arrow*) at 1-o'clock position with a central biopsy clip artifact. **D.** Computer-aided detection color map MR image shows areas of enhancement in color shades. **E.** The mass demonstrates rapid initial enhancement with delayed washout, as shown in the kinetic curve.

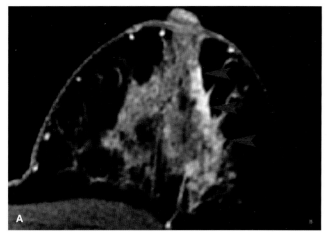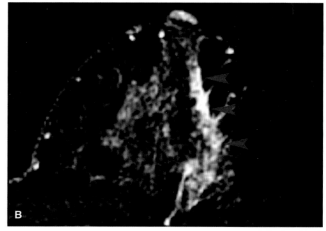

FIGURE 20.47. MR of Ductal Carcinoma In Situ (DCIS). Contrast-enhanced fat-suppressed T1-weighted fast spoiled gradient-echo (**A**) and subtraction (**B**) axial MR images of the left breast show a segmental area of non–mass-like heterogeneous enhancement (*arrowheads*) laterally. MR-guided biopsy showed low-grade DCIS.

(2) containing scattered fibroglandular densitie, (3) heterogeneously dense, which may obscure detection of small masses, or (4) extremely dense breast tissue, which lowers the sensitivity of mammography. A description of the significant findings on the mammogram, US, or MR should follow, and there should be comparison to any previous available examinations. The most important part of the breast imaging report is the assessment category, which should fall into one of the following six categories:

BI-RADS Category (0): **Need Additional Imaging Evaluation and/or Prior Mammograms for Comparison.** This category is reserved for screening examinations that require further imaging workup or comparison films in order to fully characterize a potential abnormality. The suggested additional studies such as US or additional mammographic views should be specified in the report. Prior mammograms are always helpful in the interpretation of a screening study. Category 0 should, however, be used for film comparison only in cases where the radiologist feels that such films are essential to the final assessment for the patient.

BI-RADS Category (1): **Negative.** No significant findings are present on a negative mammogram. The patient should return for routine screening.

BI-RADS Category (2): **Benign Finding.** There is a benign finding such as a lipoma, oil cyst, galactocele, intramammary lymph node, hamartoma, fibroadenoma, cyst, scattered round calcifications of adenosis, arterial calcifications, sedimented calcium within microcysts, secretory calcifications, duct ectasia, skin calcifications, or multiple bilateral well-circumscribed masses representing cysts or fibroadenomas. These patients should return for routine screening.

BI-RADS Category (3): **Probably Benign—Initial Short Interval Follow-Up Suggested.** The findings that should be included in this category are circumscribed masses, asymmetrical parenchymal densities that are not associated with palpable masses, and, occasionally, clusters of smooth round similar appearing microcalcifications. The probability that such abnormalities represent cancer is less than 2% (39); therefore, most mammographers recommend a plan of careful follow-up (55). The first follow-up mammogram of the affected breast should be performed 6 months following discovery of the abnormality. If the abnormality is stable, a bilateral study should be performed 6 months later and then a follow-up should occur at yearly intervals for a period of at least 3 years. Progression of a cancerous lesion depends on tumor biology and doubling time; hence the necessity of a lengthy follow-up. Some cancers may grow slowly and others may change rapidly.

BI-RADS Category (4): **Suspicious Abnormality—Biopsy Should Be Considered.** Included in this category are lesions that are not classically malignant but are suspicious enough to warrant biopsy. The probability that such a lesion will represent malignancy is approximately 25% to 35% in most practices in the United States. Category 4 lesions can be divided into three subdivisions (4A, 4B, and 4C with 4A the lowest suspicion for malignancy and 4C the highest); this division is optional, but may allow more meaningful correlation with biopsy results.

BI-RADS Category (5): **Highly Suggestive of Malignancy—Appropriate Action Should Be Taken.** These are lesions that have a very high probability of being malignant and should undergo biopsy. Spiculated masses and pleomorphic clusters of calcifications are included in this category.

BI-RADS Category (6): **Known Biopsy-Proven Malignancy—Appropriate Action Should Be Taken.** These are lesions that are already known to be malignant, but have not undergone definitive therapy. For example, this category should be used for proven cancers that are being imaged to assess their response to neoadjuvant chemotherapy prior to definitive surgery.

Clinicians must be cautioned that 9% to 16% of palpable malignancies are not seen mammographically; therefore, a negative mammogram should not preclude biopsy of a clinically suspicious mass.

INTERVENTIONAL PROCEDURES FOR THE BREAST

Mammographically suspicious abnormalities require histologic or cytologic examination for definitive diagnosis. Percutaneous, image-directed core biopsy or aspiration performed in the radiology department is the standard of care.

Needle localization followed by surgical excision is reserved for cases in which the percutaneous biopsy is inconclusive or for definitive surgery after percutaneous biopsy yields a malignant diagnosis.

Percutaneous Biopsy

Increasing use of mammographic screening has led to the discovery of greater numbers of potentially malignant but clinically occult breast lesions. Nearly all suspicious lesions are amenable to core biopsy either with stereotactic, US, or MR guidance.

Core biopsy is superior to fine needle aspiration biopsy for the following reasons:

1. Histologic evaluation of core biopsy specimens can be performed by all pathologists, whereas cytologic diagnosis of fine needle aspirates requires that the pathologist have special expertise and training.
2. The amount of tissue obtained from core biopsies is usually sufficient for diagnosis, whereas insufficient material for diagnosis is a frequent problem with fine needle aspiration.
3. Differentiation of invasive from noninvasive carcinomas is usually possible with core biopsy, whereas it is not possible with fine needle aspiration cytology.

Indications for core biopsy are similar to those for surgical biopsy. A full breast imaging workup must be completed before core biopsy is recommended. Core biopsy should not be substituted for short-interval follow-up of probably benign lesions as this approach is not cost-effective and may induce increased anxiety in some women. Technical difficulties such as inadequate visualization of the lesion may occasionally preclude the use of a core biopsy.

Core biopsies can be guided by stereotactic images, US, or MR (56). Currently, there are two types of stereotactic units available. One can be added onto a standard mammography machine but has limited working space and is generally used with the patient seated. The other is a prone dedicated unit that is more costly but offers the advantages of having the patient in a prone position so as to minimize movement and vasovagal reactions (Fig. 20.48). A stereotactic unit allows the x-ray tube to move independent of the compressed breast. The lesion is centered in the aperture within the compression plate and images at negative and positive 15° are obtained.

Calculation of the amount of deviation of the lesion in these two views allows the exact determination of the depth of the lesion. The needle guide is adjusted for exact positioning of the needle in three dimensions to the center of the lesion. After the injection of local anesthetic, a small skin incision is made to permit needle entry into the breast. Positioning of the needle is verified with stereotactic views and biopsies are taken (Fig. 20.49).

When US is used, the needle can be observed in real time as the biopsy is performed (Fig. 20.50). Adequate sonographic visualization of the lesion is essential if core biopsy is to be performed with US guidance. Most microcalcifications and some masses, particularly those in fatty replaced breasts, cannot be visualized, and hence, cannot be biopsied using US. Aspiration of fluid cannot be performed through a core biopsy needle. Some lesions chosen for US-guided biopsy will be atypical cysts; in such cases, it is prudent to attempt aspiration with a 22-gauge needle. If fluid is not obtained, a core biopsy can be performed.

Lesions that are seen only on MR can be biopsied in the magnet by using a grid system specifically designed to fit on the breast coil. There are several MR-compatible biopsy devices that allow vacuum-assisted biopsies under MR guidance. Contrast enhancement is required to ensure appropriate targeting. A marking clip can be placed following an MR-guided biopsy. The clip can then be used as the target for a mammographic needle localization procedure should that be necessary.

Either a 14-gauge automated biopsy gun or a 9- to 12-gauge vacuum-assisted needle can be used for a core biopsy. The standard 14-gauge gun works by a spring action mechanism that fires the needle through the lesion. The inner cannula containing the tissue notch is projected through the lesion first and then the cutting cannula is fired over it so that a small core of tissue is retained within the specimen notch. With the vacuum-assisted devices, suction is used to bring the tissue into the specimen notch of the needle, which is then cut by an inner rotating cannula. Vacuum-assisted devices generally require only a single-needle pass to obtain multiple specimens, whereas standard core biopsy requires multiple passes, one for each specimen. The vacuum-assisted needle offers improved ability to adequately sample microcalcifications when compared with the standard biopsy gun (57). Vacuum-assisted devices are also preferred for small lesions (5 mm or less in diameter).

The accuracy of core biopsy in diagnosing breast carcinoma approaches that of surgical biopsy with reported sensitivities of

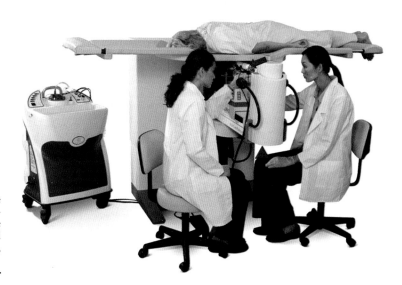

FIGURE 20.48. Dedicated Stereotactic Biopsy Unit. The x-ray tube (red arrowhead) moves independent of the compressed breast so stereoimages can be obtained. The needle guide is adjusted so that the biopsy needle (red arrow) will be centered in the lesion. (Courtesy of Hologic Inc, Bedford, MA.)

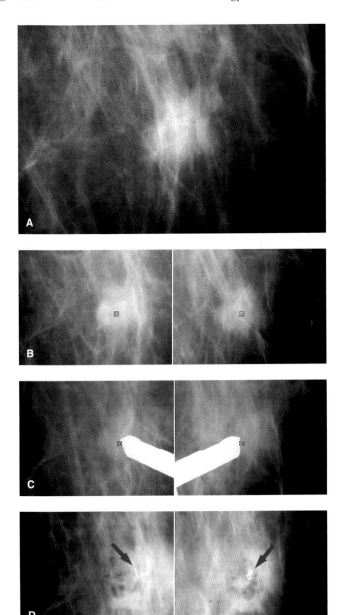

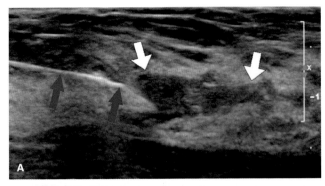

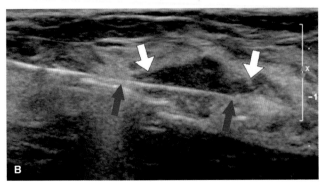

FIGURE 20.50. US-Guided Core Biopsy. A. Prefire longitudinal US showing a 14-gauge core biopsy needle (*red arrows*) at the edge of a solid hypoechoic mass (*white arrows*). **B.** The postfire image shows the lesion (*white arrows*) pierced by the needle (*red arrows*).

FIGURE 20.49. Stereotactic Core Biopsy. A. On the scout view, the lesion is centered in the aperture of the compression paddle. **B.** Stereoviews at −15° and +15° are obtained and the center of the lesion is marked in both views with the square target mark. **C.** After injection of local anesthetic, an 11-gauge vacuum-assisted core biopsy needle is inserted and prefire stereoimages are obtained to verify appropriate positioning of the needle; the needle should be inserted to a depth that is 5 mm short of the targeted center of the lesion. The vacuum-assisted device is then fired into the lesion and multiple biopsy samples are obtained. **D.** After the biopsy is performed, a marking clip (*arrows*) is inserted and stereoimages are obtained to verify appropriate positioning of the clip. Note air within the lesion where the biopsy specimens were obtained. In this case, the histologic diagnosis was invasive lobular carcinoma.

85% to 100% and specificities of 96% to 100% (58). In order to achieve such high sensitivities and specificities, it is essential that the mammographic, sonographic, and MR appearance of the lesion be correlated with the pathologic diagnosis. If there is discordance, repeat core biopsy or excisional biopsy should be performed. In cases where atypical ductal or lobular hyperplasia is diagnosed by core biopsy, excisional biopsy should be performed as 10% to 48% of these lesions will ultimately prove to be carcinoma (41). Post core biopsy management of papillary lesions, mucin-containing lesions, LCIS, and radial scars is controversial.

Localization of Occult Breast Lesions

If surgical excision of a nonpalpable, abnormality is to be performed, a localization will be required so that the surgeon is accurately directed to the lesion. Localizations are generally performed using needle-wire systems, which allow placement of a wire through an introducing needle that has been positioned in the breast at the site of the abnormality. The commercially available wires differ mainly in the configuration of the anchoring end.

Most mammographic units are equipped with a compression paddle that contains either one large hole marked on the edge with a grid or a series of smaller holes marked with letters or numbers. The seated patient is placed in the mammographic unit so that the lesion or marking clip to be localized is located under a hole in the compression plate. The skin surface closest to the lesion should be used for needle placement. For example, if the lesion is located at 12-o'clock position, a craniocaudal approach should be used. The breast is then filmed to determine the exact location of the abnormality. A needle is inserted parallel to the x-ray beam and through the abnormal area. The position of the needle with respect to the lesion is then checked by taking another film. If the needle position is satisfactory, the patient, with needle in place, is carefully removed from the mammography unit so that the tube can be rotated 90°. The patient is then positioned in the unit and compressed along an axis parallel to the needle. A film is taken to assess the depth of the needle tip with respect to the lesion. The needle must

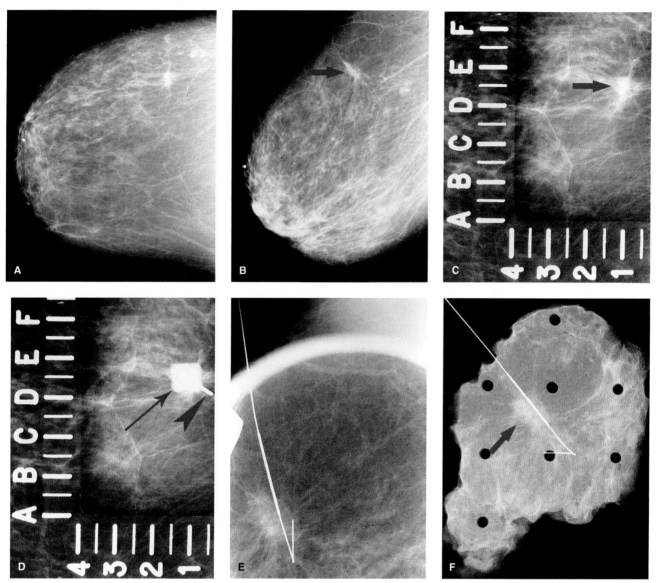

FIGURE 20.51. Needle Localization. Craniocaudal (**A**) and mediolateral (**B**) mammograms show a highly suspicious spiculated mass (*arrows*) in the upper outer quadrant. **C.** Localization was performed by placing the fenestrated compression plate over the lesion (*arrow*) and then placing a needle parallel to the x-ray beam through the lesion. **D.** The hub of the needle (*long arrow*) is superimposed on the lesion; the tip of the needle (*arrowhead*) is at the posterior edge. A film is then taken in the 90° orthogonal projection and, once the depth is adjusted, the hook wire is passed through the needle. **E.** A film in the same projection demonstrates the final depth of the wire. **F.** The excised tissue is sent for specimen x-ray to confirm that the mass (*arrow*) has been removed. Histologic examination in this case revealed invasive lobular carcinoma.

be beyond the lesion in order to proceed. This assures a fixed relationship between the localizer and the lesion. Optimally, the tip of the needle for a wire localization should be 1 to 2 cm beyond the lesion. Once the depth of the needle tip is satisfactory, the wire can be inserted through the needle and the needle withdrawn, leaving the wire in place (Fig. 20.51). The patient is then sent to the operating room for surgical excision (59).

Bracketed localization is advocated for nonpalpable lesions over 2 cm in size. More than one localization wire is placed to demarcate the extent of the lesion. This technique is particularly helpful for areas of microcalcifications over 2 cm in diameter; it promotes complete removal of such lesions.

Once the surgical excision has been performed, the excised tissue should be sent for x-ray. This assures that the mammographic abnormality and/or the marking clip has been removed. In a small number of cases (1.5%), localization will fail and the lesion or clip will not be removed. In most of these cases, the localization will have to be repeated.

Most localizations are performed under mammographic guidance, but US and MR can also be used to guide such procedures. The technique used in US is similar to that used for US-guided percutaneous biopsy. A high-frequency transducer is placed over the lesion and the needle is introduced obliquely under real time monitoring. When the tip is seen beyond the lesion, the wire can be inserted. Wire position should be confirmed by mammography.

US is most useful in guiding a localization when the abnormality is seen well in one projection, but is obscured by dense tissue in the second. It may also be useful when lesions are located in areas of the breast that are difficult to position within the hole in the localized compression paddle. US can only be used when the lesion can be visualized. Microcalcifications, in general, cannot be imaged, and not all soft tissue masses are well delineated by US.

Lesions seen only on MR can be localized by using the grid system that is used for MR-guided core biopsy. Contrast enhancement is generally required to confirm the location of the lesion prior to needle placement. X-ray specimen radiography may not identify the lesion as the contrast is no longer in the tissues. MR and pathologic correlation is, thus, extremely important. Discordant cases require postoperative MR to ensure removal of the lesion.

Other Interventional Procedures

Aspiration of sonographically atypical cysts can be performed for confirmation of the diagnosis by using either US or mammographic guidance. The majority of such lesions will be smooth-walled masses that are atypical either because they lack through transmission or because the fluid within them is not anechoic. In such cases, a 22-gauge needle can be inserted using a technique similar to that used for core biopsy. If fluid is withdrawn, the lesion should be totally aspirated. If fluid cannot be withdrawn, the lesion is presumably solid and core biopsy can be performed.

In cases where there is irregularity or nodularity of the cyst wall by sonography, core biopsy should be undertaken. Vacuum-assisted devices are preferable for biopsy of these types of lesions since only one-needle pass is required for sampling. It is likely that the fluid surrounding such lesions will leak into the surrounding tissues at biopsy, thus rendering the lesion difficult to visualize for multiple passes. Cytologic evaluation of fluid surrounding an intracystic lesion is unreliable for diagnosis.

Ductography can be used to investigate the cause of a spontaneous nipple discharge. The procedure involves injecting a contrast material into a duct, after which films are taken to look for intraductal tumors. These are most frequently papillomas and, less commonly, carcinomas. The utility of this study is controversial. If the patient has a bloody discharge, some surgeons prefer to inject the discharging duct with blue dye in the operating room before dissecting along it. Others prefer preoperative ductography to evaluate bloody discharge, and feel that if the ductogram is negative, the patient can be observed. The use of ductography in the evaluation of a unilateral, spontaneous serous discharge is similarly controversial since both bloody and serous fluid can be associated with small cancers that may not be visible mammographically. MR is receiving increased use for preoperative evaluation of suspicious nipple discharge as an alternative to ductography.

CONCLUSION

Breast cancer represents a significant public health problem. Over 180,000 new cases are diagnosed and nearly 45,000 women die of the disease each year in the United States. Early detection with screening mammography is the only proven way to lower mortality from breast cancer. Diagnostic accuracy can be increased with the use of special mammographic views, US, MR, and percutaneous biopsy techniques. Other modalities, such as PET, tomosynthesis, and dedicated breast CT are under study to determine their potential utility in detection and diagnosis of breast diseases. The use of breast imaging has increased over the last several decades, and mortality from breast cancer is declining. Our challenge, as radiologists, is to maintain the highest standards of quality in performance and interpretation of breast imaging studies; it is also to encourage all women to take regular advantage of these life-saving techniques.

References

1. Shapiro S. Evidence on screening for breast cancer from a randomized trial. Cancer 1977;39:2772–2782.
2. Nyström L, Rutqvist LE, Wall S, et al. Breast cancer screening with mammography: overview of Swedish randomized trials. Lancet 1993;341:973–978.
3. Hendrick RE, Smith RA, Rutledge JH, Smart CR. Benefit of screening mammography in women ages 40–49: a meta-analysis of new randomized controlled trial results. In: NIH Consensus Development Conference: Breast Cancer Screening for Women Ages 40–49. NIH Consensus Statement Online 1997 Jan 21–23;15(1): 1–35.
4. Paci E, Duffy SW, Giorgi D, et al. Quantification of the effect of mammographic screening on fatal breast cancers: the Florence Programme: 1990–1996. Br J Cancer 2002;87:65–69.
5. Tabar L, Vitak B, Chen HHT, et al. Beyond randomized controlled trials. Organized mammographic screening substantially reduces breast carcinoma mortality. Cancer 2001;92:1724–1731.
6. Smith RA, Saslow D, Sawyer KA, et al. American Cancer Society guidelines for breast cancer screening: update 2003. CA Cancer J Clin 2003;53:141–169.
7. U.S. Preventive Service Task Force. Screening for breast cancer: U.S. preventive service task force recommendation statement. Ann Intern Med 2009;151:716–726.
8. National Cancer Institute Fact Sheet: Mammograms. Available at: http://www.cancer.gov/cancertopics/factsheet/detection/mammograms. Accessed on June 25, 2010.
9. White E, Miglioretti DL, Yankaskas BC, et. al. Biennial versus annual mammography and the risk of late-stage breast cancer. J Natl Cancer Inst 2004;96:1832–1839.
10. Tabar L, Larsson LG, Andersson I, et al. Breast-cancer screening with mammography in women aged 40–49 years. Int J Cancer 1996;68:693–699.
11. Tabar L, Fagerberg G, Day NE, Holmberg L. What is the optimum interval between mammographic screening examinations? An analysis based on the latest results of the Swedish two-county breast cancer screening trial. Br J Cancer 1987;55:547–551.
12. Kerlikowske K, Grady D, Barclay J, et al. Effect of age, breast density, and family history on the sensitivity of first screening mammography. JAMA 1996;276:33–38.
13. Lee C, Dershaw D, Kopans D, et al. Breast cancer screening with imaging: recommendations from the society of breast imaging and the ACR on the use of mammography, breast MRI, breast ultrasound, and other technologies for the detection of clinically occult breast cancer. J Am Coll Radiol 2010;7:18–27.
14. Sasloe D, Boetes C, Burke W, et al. American Cancer Society guidelines for breast screening with MRI as an adjunct to mammography. CA Cancer J Clin 2007;57:75–89.
15. Curpen BN, Sickles EA, Sollitto RA, et al. The comparative value of mammographic screening for women 40–49 years old versus women 50–64 years old. Am J Radiol 1995;164:1099–1103.
16. Linver MN. Mammography outcomes in a practice setting by age: prognostic factors, sensitivity, and positive biopsy rate. National Institutes of Health Consensus Development Conference Syllabus, Breast Cancer Screening for Women Ages 40–49. Bethesda, MD: National Institutes of Health, 1997.
17. Feig SA, Ehrlich SM. Estimation of radiation risk from screening mammography: recent trends and comparison with expected benefits. Radiology 1990;174:638–647.
18. Berg W. Tailored supplemental screening for breast cancer: what now and what next? Am J Radiol 2009;192:390–399.
19. Kolb TM, Lichy J, Newhouse JH. Comparison of the performance of screening mammography, physical examination, and breast US and evaluation of factors that influence them: an analysis of 27,825 patient evaluations. Radiology 2002;225:165–175.
20. Berg W, Blume J, Cormack J, et al. Combined screening with ultrasound and mammography alone in women at elevated risk of breast cancer: results of the first-year screen in ACRIN 6666. JAMA 2008; 299:2151–2163.
21. de Paredes ES, Marsteller LP, Eden BV. Breast cancers in women 35 years of age and younger: mammographic findings. Radiology 1990;177:117–119.
22. Pisano E, Gatsonis C, Hendrick E, et al. Diagnostic performance of digital versus film mammography for breast cancer screening. N Eng J Med 2005;353:1773–1783.
23. Wald N, Murphy P, Major P, et al. UKCCCR multicentre randomized controlled trail of one and two view mammography in breast cancer screening. BMJ 1995;311:1189–1193.
24. Sickles EA. Mammographic features of 300 consecutive nonpalpable breast cancers. Am J Radiol 1986;146:661–663.
25. U.S. Department of Health and Human Services. Clinical Practice Guideline, Quality Determinants of Mammography, Screening and Diagnostic Views, AHCPR Publication No. 95-0632. Washington, CD: U.S. Department of Health and Human Services, 1994, pp. 25–31.
26. Kopans DB, Swann CA, White G, et al. Asymmetric breast tissue. Radiology 1989;171:639–643.
27. Marsteller LP, de Paredes ES. Well defined masses in the breast. Radiographics 1989;9:13–37.
28. Sickles EA. Breast masses: mammographic evaluation. Radiology 1989;173:297–303.
29. Sickles EA. Nonpalpable, circumscribed, noncalcified solid breast masses: likelihood of malignancy based on lesion size and age of patient. Radiology 1994;192:439–442.
30. Bassett LW. Mammographic analysis of calcifications. Radiol Clin North Am 1992;30:93–105.

31. Harris JR, Lippman ME, Veronesi U, Willet W. Breast cancer (second of three parts). N Engl J Med 1992;327:390–398.
32. Krishamurthy S. Current applications and future prospects of fine-needle aspiration biopsy of locoregional lymph nodes in the management of breast cancer. Cancer 2009;117:451–462.
33. Eklund GW, Busby RC, Miller SH, Job JS. Improved imaging of the augmented breast. Am J Radiol 1988;151:469–473.
34. Destouet JM, Monsees BS, Oser RF, et al. Screening mammography in 350 women with breast implants: prevalence and findings of implant complications. Am J Radiol 1992;159:973–978.
35. Gorczyca DP, Schneider E, DeBruhl ND, et al. Silicone breast implant rupture: comparison between three-point Dixon and fast spin-echo MR imaging. Am J Radiol 1994;162:305–310.
36. DeBruhl ND, Gorczyca DP, Ahn CY, et al. Silicone breast implants: US evaluation. Radiology 1993;189:95–98.
37. Warner E, Plewes DB, Shumak RS, et al. Comparison of breast magnetic resonance imaging, mammography, and ultrasound for surveillance of women at high risk for hereditary breast cancer. J Clin Oncol 2001;19:3524–3531.
38. Stoutjesdijk MJ, Boetes C, Jager GJ, et al. Magnetic resonance imaging and mammography in women with a hereditary risk of breast cancer. J Natl Cancer Inst 2001;93:1095–1102.
39. Lehman CD, Isaacs C, Schnall MD, et al. Cancer yield of mammography, MR, and US in high-risk women: prospective multi-institution breast cancer screening study. Radiology 2007;244:381–388.
40. Kriege M, Cecile TM, Brekelmans MD, et al. Efficacy of MRI and mammography for breast-cancer screening in women with a familial or genetic predisposition. N Engl J Med 2004;351:427–437.
41. Warner E, Plewes DB, Hill KA, et al. Surveillance of BRCA1 and BRCA2 mutation carriers with magnetic resonance imaging, ultrasound, mammography, and clinical breast examination. JAMA 2004;292:1317–1325.
42. Schrading S, Kuhl CK. Mammographic, US, and MR imaging phenotypes of familial breast cancer. Radiology. 2008;246:58–70.
43. Kuhl CK, Schrading S, Leutner CC, et al. Mammography, breast ultrasound, and magnetic resonance imaging for surveillance of women at high familial risk for breast cancer. J Clin Oncol. 2005;23:8469–8476.
44. Kuhl C. The current status of breast MR imaging. Part I. Choice of technique, image interpretation, diagnostic accuracy, and transfer to clinical practice. Radiology 2007;244:356–378.
45. Mann RM, Hoogeveen YL, Blickman JG, Boetes C. MRI compared to conventional diagnostic work-up in the detection and evaluation of invasive lobular carcinoma of the breast: a review of existing literature. Breast Cancer Res Treat 2008;107:1–14.
46. Harms SE, Flamig DP, Hesley KL, et al. MR imaging of the breast with rotating delivery of excitation off resonance: clinical experience with pathologic correlation. Radiology 1993;187:493–501.
47. Vallow L, Mclaughlin S, Hines S, et al. The ability of preoperative magnetic resonance imaging to predict actual pathologic tumor size in women with newly diagnosed breast cancer [abstract 4018]. Cancer Res 2008;69(suppl):262s.
48. Boetes C, Mus RD, Holland R, et al. Breast tumors: comparative accuracy of MR imaging relative to mammography and US for demonstrating extent. Radiology 1995;197:743–747.
49. Houssami N, Ciatto S, Macaskill P, et al. Accuracy and surgical impact of magnetic resonance imaging in breast cancer staging: systematic review and meta-analysis in detection of multifocal and multicentric cancer. J Clin Oncol 2008;26:3248–3258.
50. Singletary E, Middleton L, Le-Petross H. Unknown primary presenting with axillary lymphadenopathy. In: Bland K, Copeland E, eds. The Breast: Comprehensive Management of Benign and Malignant Disease. 4th ed. Philadelphia: Elsevier, 2009:1373–1381.
51. Le-Petross H, Hylton N. Role of breast MRI in neoadjuvant chemotherapy. Magn Reson Imaging Clin N Am 2010;18:249–258.
52. Rausch DR, Hendrick RE. How to optimize clinical breast MR imaging practices and techniques on your 1.5-T system. Radiographics 2006;26:1469–1484.
53. Kuhl CK, Mielcareck P, Klaschik S, et al. Dynamic breast MR imaging: are signal intensity time course data useful for differential diagnosis of enhancing lesions? Radiology 1999;211:101–110.
54. American College of Radiology. ACR Breast Imaging Reporting and Data System, Breast Imaging Atlas. Reston, VA: American College of Radiology, 2003.
55. Sickles EA. Periodic mammographic follow-up of probably benign lesions: results in 3,184 consecutive cases. Radiology 1991;179:463–468.
56. Berg WA. Image-guided breast biopsy and management of high-risk lesions. Radiol Clin North Am 2004;24:935–946.
57. Meyer JE, Smith DN, DiPiro PJ, et al. Stereotactic breast biopsy of clustered microcalcifications with a directional, vacuum-assisted device. Radiology 1997;204:575–576.
58. Bassett L, Winchester DP, Caplan RB, et al. Stereotactic core-needle biopsy of the breast: a report of the joint task force of the American College of Radiology, American College of Surgeons, and College of American Pathologists. Cancer 1997;47:171–190.
59. Kopans DB, Lindfors K, McCarthy KA, Meyer JE. Spring hookwire breast lesion localizer: use with rigid-compression mammographic systems. Radiology 1985;157:537–538.

SECTION V

■ CARDIAC RADIOLOGY

SECTION EDITOR: David K. Shelton

CHAPTER 21 ■ CARDIAC ANATOMY, PHYSIOLGY, AND IMAGING MODALITIES

DAVID K. SHELTON

IMAGING METHODS

Thorough knowledge of cardiac anatomy and physiology is important as a basis for cardiac imaging. Comprehensive knowledge of cardiac imaging also requires consideration of virtually all the available imaging modalities. Chest radiography provides the initial evaluation of most cardiac patients. A barium esophagram can provide additional information because of the close relationship of the esophagus to cardiac structures. Fluoroscopy increases the detectability of coronary and valvular calcification as well as provides dynamic and positional information. Transthoracic echocardiography, including pulse wave and color flow Doppler, and transesophageal echocardiography provide additional detailed imaging of internal cardiac anatomy and function. Nuclear cardiology, PET, and pharmacologic testing provide key functional, perfusion, and physiologic information. Cardiac and coronary angiography, although invasive, can provide detailed anatomic information that can lead directly to interventional or surgical therapy. CT, MDCT, CT angiography (CTA), and ultrafast CT with the use of IV iodinated contrast material are capable of providing critical information, particularly for pericardial or intracardiac disease. Recent technological advances in the latter also allow detection of premature coronary calcification, which may have prognostic implications. MR adds three-dimensional (3D) tomographic and motion studies of the myocardium, valves, and chambers without using ionizing radiation or intravascular contrast. Cardiac imaging requires familiarity with all imaging techniques and their associated physics, 3D cardiac anatomy, cardiac physiology, and cardiac disease processes.

ANATOMY

The four-chambered heart lies primarily in the anterior left hemithorax with the LV lying on the left hemidiaphragm (Figs. 21.1, 21.2). The RA extends to the right of the midline as it receives systemic blood from the superior vena cava (SVC), inferior vena cava (IVC), and coronary sinus. The RA and RV lie primarily anterior to the planes of the LA and LV. The RV is the most anterior chamber and abuts the sternum (Fig. 21.3). The LA is subcarinal and midline in the thorax, being supplied by the right and left superior and inferior pulmonary veins.

Frontal Projection. The right border of the cardiac silhouette is formed primarily by the RA, with the SVC entering superiorly and the IVC often seen at its lower margin (Figs. 21.1, 21.3). The left border of the heart is created primarily by the LV and LA appendage. The PA, aortopulmonary window, and aortic knob extend superiorly.

Lateral Projection. The RV is border forming anteriorly adjacent to the sternum, with its outflow tract extending superiorly and posteriorly (Fig. 21.2). The LA is border forming in the high posterior, subcarinal region. The LV is border forming inferiorly and posteriorly.

Right Atrium. The RA is divided into two portions. The smooth posterior wall develops from the sinus venosus, with the attached SVC and IVC in continuity posteriorly (Fig. 21.4). The trabeculated anterior wall is derived from the embryonic RA. The RA appendage extends superiorly and medially from the SVC opening. The crista terminalis is a muscular ridge that runs from the mouth of the SVC and fades inferiorly to the mouth of the IVC. It divides the two portions of the atrium

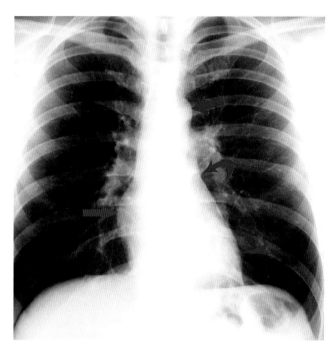

FIGURE 21.1. Normal Posteroanterior Chest Radiograph. Frontal view of the chest demonstrates normal heart size, contours, and chamber size. The hila and pulmonary vascularity are normal. The LV (*arrowhead*) is border forming on the left. The RA (*curved arrow*) is border forming on the right. The aortic knob (*red arrow*) is of normal contour, and the PA (*blue arrow*) is concave.

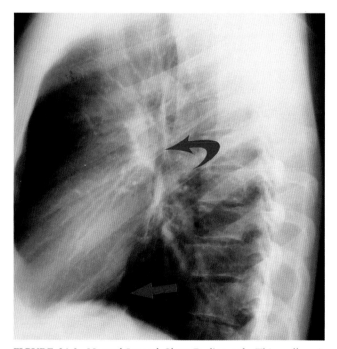

FIGURE 21.2. Normal Lateral Chest Radiograph. This well-positioned left lateral chest radiograph demonstrates the right ribs projected posterior to the left ribs because of divergence of the x-ray beam. The right and left bronchi are overlapped, and the sternum is seen in the lateral view. The true lateral projection allows evaluation of the inferior vena cava intersection (*arrow*) with the LV. There is no evidence of posterior displacement of the left bronchus (*curved arrow*) to indicate left atrial enlargement. There is no evidence of right ventricular encroachment into the retrosternal clear space.

and corresponds to an external sulcus terminalis. The medial or posterior wall of the RA is the interatrial septum, which contains a smooth, central dimpled area called the fossa ovalis. Inflow from the SVC, IVC, and coronary sinus enters the smooth posterior portion of the RA. The SVC has a free opening, whereas the IVC is partially guarded by a thin eustachian valve, which is occasionally absent or perforated (network of Chiari). The large draining coronary vein or coronary sinus enters the RA anterior and medial to the IVC. Its opening is guarded by the thebesian valve between the orifice of the IVC and the tricuspid valve.

Right Ventricle. The RV (Figs. 21.4, 21.5) lies anterior to the left ventricular outflow tract and wraps around it and to the left. The right ventricular outflow is directed superiorly, posteriorly, and to the left. The RV is divided into a posterior or inferior portion (inflow or sinus portion), which is heavily trabeculated, and a less trabeculated anterior or superior portion (outflow tract or pulmonary conus). The two portions of the RV are divided by the crista supraventricularis, which is a muscular ridge with a septal band called the moderator band. This band is present in more than 40% of patients, connects the interventricular septum to the anterior papillary muscle, and contains the right bundle branch. The infundibulum (conus arteriosus) is the smooth cephalic portion of the RV that leads to the pulmonary trunk.

Pulmonary Arteries. The muscular pulmonary conus extends to the semilunar, tricuspid pulmonary valve, with the pulmonary trunk extending superiorly and to the left. The left PA extends posteriorly as a continuation of the main PA, coursing over the top of the left main stem bronchus, then descending posteriorly. The right PA extends horizontally to the right, bifurcates within the pericardial sac, and exits the right hilum as the truncus anterior and interlobar arteries. The left main stem bronchus is hyparterial, meaning that it lies below the PA. The right bronchus is eparterial, meaning that it lies next to the right PA.

The ligamentum arteriosum arises from the superior, proximal left PA and crosses through the aorticopulmonary window to the floor of the aorta. The ligamentum arteriosum is the remnant of the ductus arteriosus, which closes functionally in the first 24 hours and closes anatomically by 10 days. Desaturated blood from the right heart circulates through the lungs and returns as oxygenated blood through the right and left superior and inferior pulmonary veins into the LA.

Left Atrium. The LA is the highest and most posterior chamber (Fig. 21.6). Its smooth walls are nestled between the right and left bronchi, and its posterior wall abuts the anterior wall of the esophagus. The left atrial appendage is a small pouch that projects superiorly and to the left and is smoother and longer than the right atrial appendage. The left atrial appendage extends anterior to the left superior pulmonary veins and is readily seen on MR and CT scans. The foramen ovale within the interatrial septum remains nominally patent in up to 25% of adults. Its inferior margin is a remnant of the septum primum and may be somewhat scalloped. The mitral valve is located anterior and inferior to the body of the LA, with the mitral valve leaflets extending into the LV.

Left Ventricle. The mitral valve is the conduit for blood flow from the LA to the LV and is in the high posterior "valve plane" of the LV (Figs. 21.5, 21.6). The anterior or septal leaflet of the mitral valve lies near the interventricular septum and extends to the posterior (noncoronary) cusp of the aortic valve. The smaller posterior mitral leaflet lies posteriorly and to the left. The chordae tendineae are strong fibrous cords that extend from the mitral leaflets to the papillary muscles of the LV. The inflow portion of the LV is posterior to the anterior leaflet of the mitral valve. The outflow portion of the LV is anterior and superior to the anterior mitral leaflet. The interventricular septum has a high membranous portion that is contiguous with

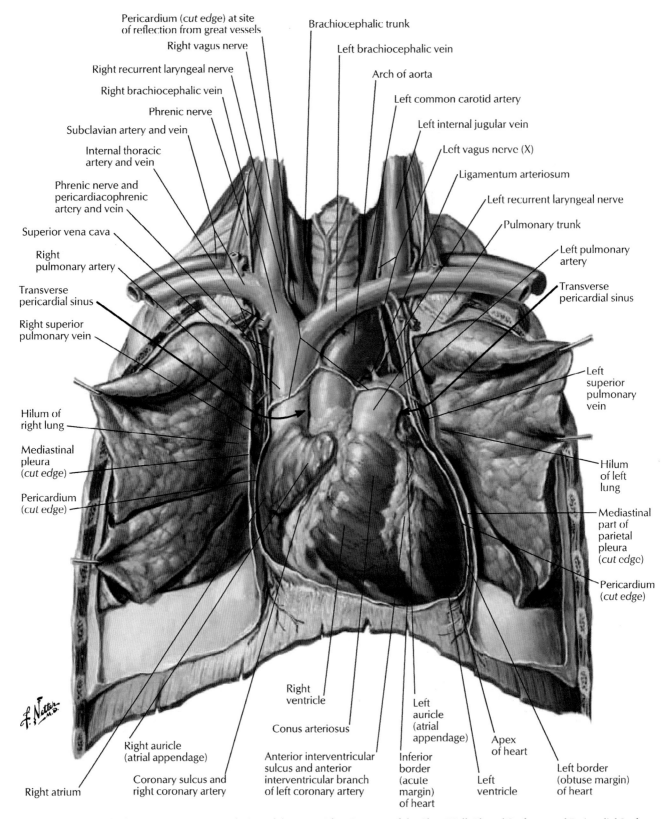

FIGURE 21.3. **Cardiothoracic Anatomy: Frontal View of the Heart After Cutaway of the Chest Wall, Pleural Surfaces, and Pericardial Surface.** Note the relationship of the RA, RV, left atrial appendage, and LV to the great vessels. (Reproduced with permission. Drawing by Netter FH. Atlas of Human Anatomy. The CIBA Collection of Medical Illustrations, Clinical Symposia. West Caldwell, NJ: CIBA-Geigy Corp, 1989.)

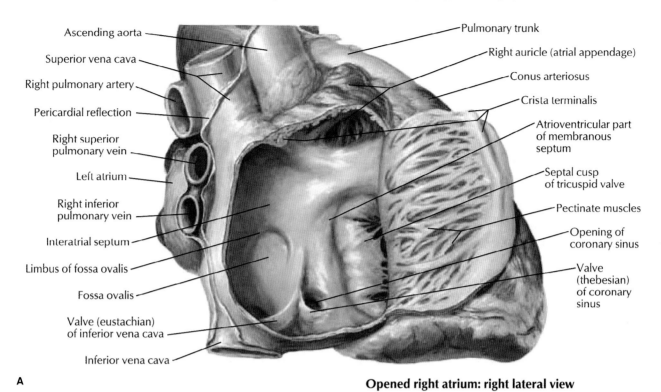

Ascending aorta

Superior vena cava

Right pulmonary artery

Pericardial reflection

Right superior pulmonary vein

Left atrium

Right inferior pulmonary vein

Interatrial septum

Limbus of fossa ovalis

Fossa ovalis

Valve (eustachian) of inferior vena cava

Inferior vena cava

Pulmonary trunk

Right auricle (atrial appendage)

Conus arteriosus

Crista terminalis

Atrioventricular part of membranous septum

Septal cusp of tricuspid valve

Pectinate muscles

Opening of coronary sinus

Valve (thebesian) of coronary sinus

A

Opened right atrium: right lateral view

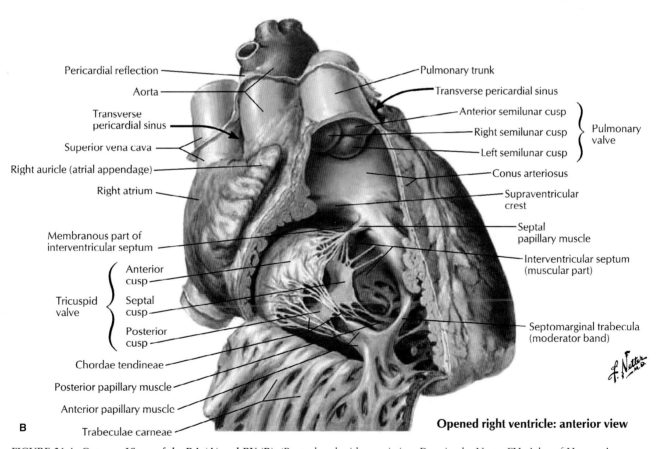

Pericardial reflection

Aorta

Transverse pericardial sinus

Superior vena cava

Right auricle (atrial appendage)

Right atrium

Membranous part of interventricular septum

Anterior cusp

Tricuspid valve   Septal cusp

Posterior cusp

Chordae tendineae

Posterior papillary muscle

Anterior papillary muscle

Trabeculae carneae

Pulmonary trunk

Transverse pericardial sinus

Anterior semilunar cusp

Right semilunar cusp   Pulmonary valve

Left semilunar cusp

Conus arteriosus

Supraventricular crest

Septal papillary muscle

Interventricular septum (muscular part)

Septomarginal trabecula (moderator band)

B

Opened right ventricle: anterior view

FIGURE 21.4. **Cutaway Views of the RA (A) and RV (B).** (Reproduced with permission. Drawing by Netter FH. Atlas of Human Anatomy. The CIBA Collection of Medical Illustrations, Clinical Symposia, West Caldwell, NJ: CIBA-Geigy Corp, 1989.)

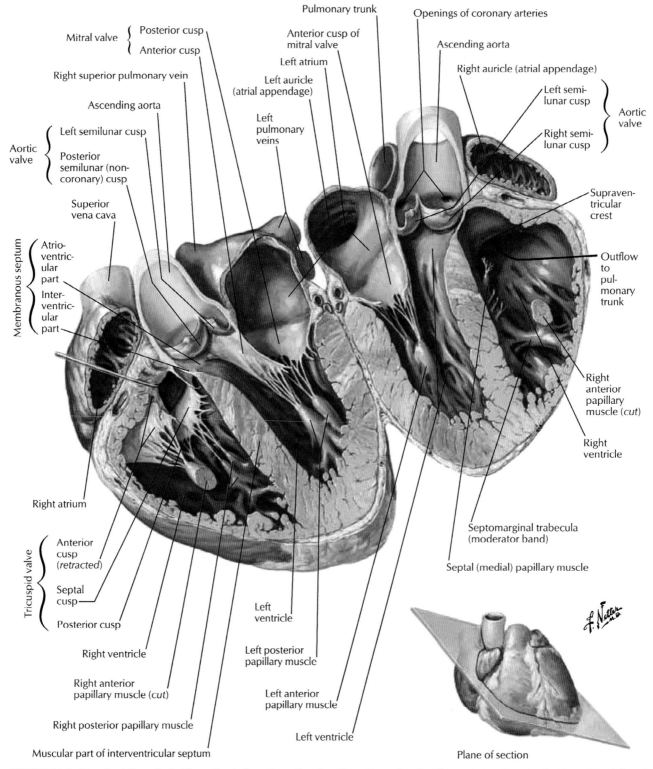

FIGURE 21.5. **Bisection Through the Heart Simulating a Four-Chamber View.** (Reproduced with permission. Drawing by Netter FH. Atlas of Human Anatomy. The CIBA Collection of Medical Illustrations, Clinical Symposia, West Caldwell, NJ: CIBA-Geigy Corp, 1989.)

the aortic root. The more muscular inferior portion of the septum extends to the left ventricular apex. The esophagus passes immediately posterior and is in contact with the muscular wall of the LV.

Aorta. The outflow tract of the LV leads into the aortic root through the aortic valve which is composed of right, left, and posterior (noncoronary) cusps. The sinuses of Valsalva are the reservoirs created by the closure of the aortic valve and from which the right and left coronary arteries arise. The posterior wall of the aorta is continuous with the anterior leaflet of the mitral valve and more superiorly abuts the anterior wall of the LA. The anterior wall of the aorta is continuous with the interventricular

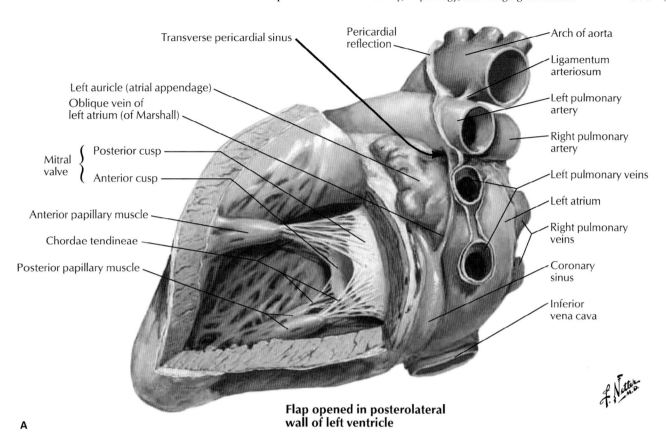

Flap opened in posterolateral wall of left ventricle

A

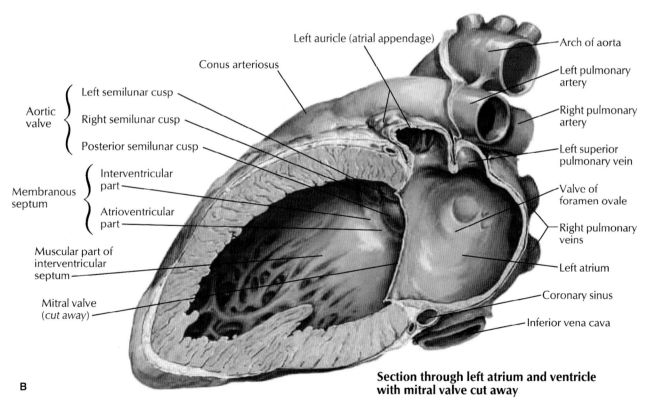

Section through left atrium and ventricle with mitral valve cut away

B

FIGURE 21.6. **Cutaway Views of the LV (A) and LA (B).** (Reproduced with permission. Drawing by Netter FH. Atlas of Human Anatomy. The CIBA Collection of Medical Illustrations, Clinical Symposia, West Caldwell, NJ: CIBA-Geigy Corp, 1989.)

septum. After coursing superiorly and then to the left, the aorta gives off the right innominate artery, left common carotid artery, and left subclavian artery. The aortic arch is the transverse portion of the aorta that abuts the left wall of the trachea, causing a characteristic indentation.

Conduction System. The sinoatrial node consists of specialized neuromuscular tissue that measures approximately 5 to 20 mm and is located on the anterior endocardial surface of the RA just above the SVC and right atrial appendage junction, near the crista terminalis. Electrical propagation spreads to both atria via Purkinje-like fibers and is recorded as the P wave on an electrocardiogram. The atrioventricular node is a 2 × 5 mm region of neuromuscular tissue on the endocardial surface, along the right side of the interatrial septum, just inferior to the ostium of the coronary sinus. The impulse is collected and delayed approximately 0.7 seconds in the atrioventricular node before passing into the bundle of His. The bundle of His is a 20-mm-long tract which extends down the right side of the membranous interventricular septum. The bundle of His bifurcates into a right and left bundle before arborizing through the two ventricles via the Purkinje system. The interventricular septum activates from superior to inferior, with the anterior or septal RV being the first to activate and the posterior or basal LV being the last to activate. This information is particularly useful when evaluating phase analysis or phase propagation in gated cardiac scintigraphy.

CARDIAC CATHETERIZATION

Left-sided catheterization is normally accomplished via arterial puncture in the femoral or brachial artery (Fig. 21.7). It is typically used for aortography, coronary and coronary bypass graft angiography, ventriculography, and evaluation for patent ductus arteriosus. Right-sided catheterization is typically accomplished by venous puncture in the femoral or brachiocephalic vein (Fig. 21.8). It is used for pulmonary angiography, catheterization of the RA and RV, or evaluation of shunt lesions such as an atrial septal defect.

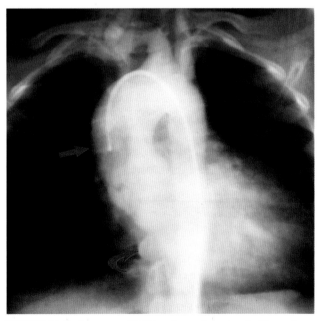

FIGURE 21.7. Aortogram Via Transfemoral Approach. The catheter is placed in the mildly dilated ascending aorta (*straight arrow*). Notice the reflux of contrast from the aortic valve into the LV (*curved arrow*) in this patient with aortic insufficiency.

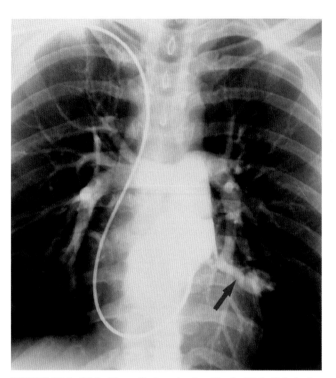

FIGURE 21.8. Right Heart Catheterization Via the Right Subclavian Vein. The catheter is positioned in the pulmonary conus. Contrast fills the main, right, and left pulmonary arteries. Note the arteriovenous malformation with a large feeding artery (*arrow*).

Important considerations include determination of the catheter course to help diagnose atrial septal defects (ASDs), ventricular septal defects (VSDs), patent ductus arteriosus, or persistent left SVC. During catheterization, oxygen saturation percentages are commonly determined, along with pressure measurements and pressure gradients (Table 21.1). Contrast is injected to demonstrate additional details of anatomy, as well as to evaluate for valvular lesions, chamber size, ventricular function, and wall motion.

Right atrial pressures are normally 2 to 5 mm Hg and oxygen saturation is 65% to 75%. Elevated right atrial pressures are seen with right heart failure, decreased compliance, and tricuspid valve disease. A 7% or greater increase in saturation from the IVC to the RA is considered evidence of a left-to-right shunt (ASD).

Right ventricular pressures are typically 25 systolic and 0 to 5 diastolic mm Hg. Elevated systolic pressures are seen with

TABLE 21.1

NORMAL VALUES FOR CARDIAC CATHETERIZATION

■ SITE	■ PRESSURE (mm Hg)	■ SATURATION (%)
Vena cava	5	60–65
Right atrium	2–5	65–75
Right ventricle	25/0	70
Pulmonary artery	25/10	73
Left atrium	2–8	94–98
Left ventricle	120/0–5	94–98
Aorta	120/80	94–98

TABLE 21.2

AVERAGE PHYSIOLOGIC DATA FOR CARDIAC CHAMBERS

■ PARAMETER	■ LEFT CHAMBERS	■ RIGHT CHAMBERS
Atrial end diastolic volume	50 mL	57 mL
Ventricular end diastolic volume	125–150 mL	165 mL
Ejection fraction	50%–75%	45%–55%
Stroke volume	70 mL	70 mL
Cardiac output	4–5 L/min	4–5 L/min
Cardiac index	2.8–4 L/min/m^2	2.8–4 L/min/m^2

pulmonary hypertension, pulmonic valve stenosis, and congenital heart lesions such as transposition and truncus arteriosus. Diastolic pressures increase with right heart failure. Saturations should be nearly the same as right atrial saturations. A 5% increase in saturation from RA to RV suggests a VSD.

Pulmonary arterial pressures are normally 25 systolic and 10 diastolic mm Hg, with a mean PA pressure of 15 mm Hg. A significant pressure gradient (>10 mm Hg) across the valve implies pulmonic valve stenosis. Increased pressures are seen with shunt lesions, pulmonary vascular disease, and pulmonary venous obstruction. Pulmonary arterial saturation should be approximately the same as right ventricular saturation, with a 3% difference considered significant for a shunt lesion.

Pulmonary capillary wedge pressure is typically 2 to 8 mm Hg and approximates the left atrial pressure unless there is evidence of pulmonary venous obstruction. Elevations in the left atrial or wedge pressure are usually seen with mitral stenosis and left-sided congestive heart failure. Normal left atrial saturation is approximately 94%, and a decrease greater than 5% implies a right-to-left shunt.

Left ventricular pressures are normally approximately 120 systolic and 0 to 5 diastolic mm Hg. Decreased systolic pressures are seen with shock and congestive heart failure. Elevated systolic pressures imply systemic hypertension or outlet obstruction. Increased diastolic pressure is seen with congestive heart failure. Decreased saturation at the left ventricular level would imply a right-to-left shunt. Aortic pressure is normally approximately 120 systolic and 80 diastolic, with a mean pressure of 70 to 100 mm Hg.

With each systolic contraction, the average stroke volume of each ventricle is 70 mL of blood (Table 21.2). End diastolic volume is normally 125 to 150 mL for the LV and 165 mL for the RV. A normal cardiac output is 4 to 5 L/min, with a normal cardiac index of 2.8 to 4.0 L/min/m^2 of body surface area. The normal ejection fraction is 50% to 75% for the LV and 45% to 55% for the RV. Typical end diastolic volumes are 57 mL for the RA and 50 mL for the LA. Coronary blood flow averages approximately 224 mL/min and increases up to sixfold during exercise.

Aortic Valve. The normal aortic valve orifice is 3 cm^2. Symptoms result from aortic stenosis usually when either the orifice is less than 0.7 cm^2 or when it is less than 1.5 cm^2 if there is aortic stenosis and insufficiency. Mild stenosis is indicated by a pressure gradient across the aortic valve greater than 25 mm Hg, moderate stenosis by a gradient greater than 40 to 50 mm Hg, and severe stenosis by a gradient exceeding 80 mm Hg.

Mitral Valve. The mitral valve orifice usually measures 4 to 6 cm^2. Mild mitral stenosis occurs with an orifice less than 1.5 cm^2, moderate mitral stenosis at less than 1.0 cm^2, and severe mitral stenosis at less than 0.5 cm^2.

Pulmonic stenosis is considered significant if the right ventricular systolic pressure exceeds 70 mm Hg.

PA hypertension is defined as a mean PA pressure of more than 25 mm Hg.

CHEST RADIOGRAPHY

The chest radiograph remains a mainstay for imaging of the heart and lungs. There are many approaches to reading the radiograph. Although most radiologists initiate the process with "global perception," it is important to develop a checklist scan technique. This discussion concerns adult posteroanterior and lateral radiographs.

Cardiac Silhouette

Size. The cardiothoracic ratio should not exceed 0.5 on a 72-in erect posteroanterior radiograph or 0.6 on a portable or anteroposterior (AP) examination. Other factors should be considered, such as fat pads and pectus deformity.

Shape. Various contour effects can be clues to underlying disease. "Water bottle" configuration occurs with pericardial effusion or generalized cardiomyopathy. Left ventricular or "Shmoo" configuration (after Al Capp's Shmoo) describes lengthening and rounding of the left heart border with a downward extension of the apex resulting from left ventricular enlargement. "Hypertrophy" configuration describes increased convexity of the left heart border and apex. Right ventricular hypertrophy and enlargement tends to lift the apex and create a more horizontal vector to the cardiac axis. Hypertrophy of either ventricle usually causes little enlargement of the silhouette unless dilatation is also present. Hypertrophy typically results from increased afterload, whereas dilatation occurs with failure or diastolic overload. "Straightening" of the left heart border is seen with rheumatic heart disease and mitral stenosis.

"Moguls of the Heart." Skiing the moguls of the heart refers to the left mediastinal outline beginning at the aortic knob. A prominent knob is a clue to ectasia, aneurysm, or hypertension. Notching or "figure 3" sign of the aorta suggests coarctation (Fig. 21.9). The second mogul is the main PA segment. Excessive convexity is seen with poststenotic dilatation, chronic obstructive pulmonary disease, PA hypertension, left-to-right shunts, and pericardial defects. Severe concavity suggests right-to-left shunts. The third mogul is a prominent left atrial appendage that in 90% of cases indicates prior rheumatic carditis (Fig. 21.10). It is not usually seen with other causes of left atrial enlargement. The fourth mogul is a bulge just above the cardiophrenic angle, seen with infarction or ventricular aneurysm. A fifth bulge at the cardiophrenic angle is caused by pericardial cysts, prominent fat pads, or adenopathy.

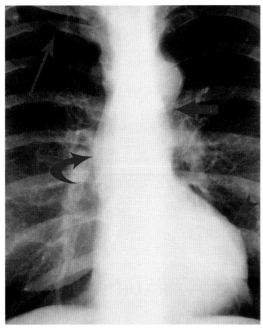

FIGURE 21.9. Aortic Coarctation. Notice the "figure 3 sign" or notching of the aorta near the aortic knob (*straight arrow*). The ascending aorta (*curved arrow*) is prominent, and the LV is excessively rounded (*arrowhead*). Rib notching is noted along the right fifth rib margin inferiorly (*long straight arrow*).

Chamber Enlargement

Left atrial enlargement is best confirmed by measuring the distance from the midinferior border of the left main stem bronchus to the right lateral border of the left atrial density (see Fig. 21.10). This distance is less than 7 cm in 90% of normal patients and is greater than 7 cm in 90% of patients with left atrial enlargement, as proven by echocardiography. This measurement can be approximated by placing one's right fifth finger under the left bronchus and while keeping the fingers closed, determining whether the LA is seen beyond one's four fingertips; if so, the LA is enlarged. Less sensitive signs of left atrial enlargement include splaying of the carinal angle, uplifting of the left main stem bronchus, and prominence of the left atrial appendage. On occasion, the enlarged LA will displace the descending aorta to the left. Massive left atrial enlargement can result in the LA becoming border forming on the right side, so-called "atrial escape." On lateral views, an enlarged LA will displace the left bronchus posteriorly, with the bronchi creating right and left legs for the "walking man sign." An enlarged LA also impresses against the esophagus.

Right atrial enlargement is more difficult to define on chest radiographs than left atrial enlargement, but fortunately, it is less common. Clues include a prominent atrial bulge too far to the right of the spine (more than 5.5 cm from the midline on a well-positioned posteroanterior radiograph). Another sign is elongation of the right atrial convexity to exceed 50% of the mediastinal or cardiovascular shadow. Right atrial enlargement usually accompanies right ventricular enlargement.

Left ventricular enlargement creates on the posteroanterior view an elongated left heart border with the apex pointing downward. Prominent rounding of the inferior left heart border is also seen (Fig. 21.11). The lateral view shows an enlarged LV extending behind the esophagus. The Hoffman–Rigler sign for left ventricular enlargement exists when the LV extends more than 1.8 cm posterior to the posterior border of the IVC at a level 2 cm cephalad to the intersection of the LV and IVC (Fig. 21.12). This sign requires a true lateral radiograph and can be false-positive if the lateral view is obliqued or there is volume loss in either lower lobe. This sign can be quickly applied by using one of the "2-cm fingertips" for a quick check without a ruler.

Right ventricular enlargement is not as easily detected as left-sided enlargement. If the heart is enlarged and Rigler sign does not show left ventricular enlargement, then consider right-sided enlargement. If the RV fills too much of the retrosternal clear space or "climbs" more than one-third of the sternal

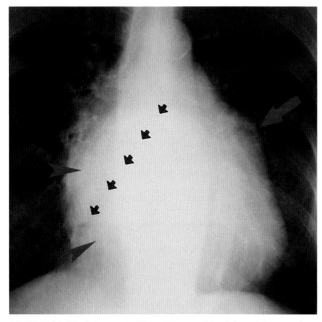

FIGURE 21.10. Rheumatic Heart Disease. The left atrial appendage is strikingly prominent (*arrow*). Splaying of the carina and a double density along the right heart border indicate left atrial enlargement (*arrowheads*). When the distance from the lateral margin of the LA to the midpoint on the undersurface of the left bronchus exceeds 7 cm, left atrial enlargement is likely (*black arrows*).

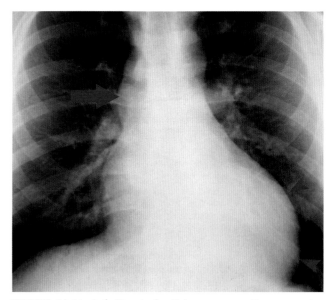

FIGURE 21.11. Left Ventricular Enlargement on Posteroanterior CXR. Prominence of the LV with rounding along the inferior heart border and an apex that is pointing downward (*arrowheads*) is indicative of "left ventricular configuration." The ascending aorta (*arrow*) is dilated because of aortic stenosis and insufficiency.

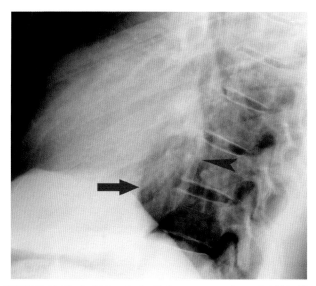

FIGURE 21.12. Left Ventricular Enlargement on Lateral CXR. The posterior margin of the LV (*arrowheads*) projects prominently behind the inferior vena cava (*arrow*) and overlaps the thoracic spine. The Hoffman–Rigler sign is positive.

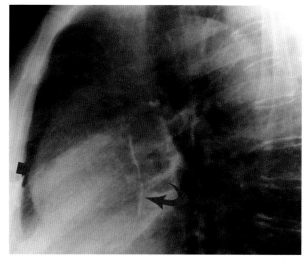

FIGURE 21.13. Calcified Aortic Aneurysm on Lateral CXR. The ascending aorta is enlarged in this patient with a syphilitic calcified aortic aneurysm. The anterior margin is identified by soft tissue prominence (*straight arrow*) overlapping the retrosternal clear space. The posterior margin is identified by calcification in the wall (*curved arrow*).

length, then right ventricular enlargement is likely. Indirect signs such as enlargement of the pulmonary outflow tract or hilar arteries add confidence.

Abnormal Mediastinal Contours

Aorta. Dilatation of the ascending aorta as a result of post-stenotic dilatation is seen in approximately 80% of patients with aortic stenosis (Fig. 21.11). It can also be seen in patients older than 50 years when there is tortuosity of the entire aorta or systemic hypertension. Ascending aortic aneurysm (calcific with syphilis, not calcified with Marfan syndrome) is another possibility (Fig. 21.13). A ductus bump adjacent to the aortic knob can be an indication of patent ductus arteriosus.

Azygos vein dilatation (>6 mm on upright PA or >1 cm on supine radiograph) is seen with intravascular volume expansion, elevated central venous pressure, and right heart failure (Fig. 21.21; see Fig. 22.16). Additional causes include the Valsalva maneuver, pregnancy, renal failure, vena cava obstruction, or azygos continuation of the IVC. Dilatation of the SVC often accompanies volume expansion or elevated central venous pressure but is more difficult to detect with certainty.

Cardiac Calcifications

Coronary Calcification. Radiographs commonly demonstrate coronary artery calcification in a 3-cm triangle along the upper left heart border, called the "CAC" (coronary artery calcification) triangle (see Fig. 22.1). If chest pain and coronary calcification are present, there is a 94% chance the patient will have occlusive coronary artery disease at angiography. Fluoroscopic detection of coronary calcification actually has higher sensitivity and specificity in screening asymptomatic individuals than does exercise tolerance testing. In symptomatic patients, the detection of coronary calcification approaches exercise tolerance testing in sensitivity and exceeds exercise tolerance testing in specificity. More than 82% of the patients with fluoroscopically demonstrated coronary artery calcification and positive exercise tolerance testing have significant coronary artery disease at angiography. Calcifications have more significance when seen in

patients younger than 60 years of age. Heavier and more extensive calcification correlates with more severe coronary disease. Detection of coronary calcification helps to differentiate patients with ischemic, from those with nonischemic, cardiomyopathy.

Valvular calcification is seen in 85% of patients with acquired valvular disease but is rarely detected in patients younger than 20 years of age. Aortic valve calcification is highly suggestive of valve disease. Calcific aortic stenosis is most often degenerative or atherosclerotic in origin and is usually seen in older males. Extensive aortic annulus calcification is atherosclerotic in nature and has been associated with conduction blocks.

Mitral valve calcification is highly suggestive of rheumatic valvular disease and is seen on chest radiograph in approximately 40% of patients with mitral stenosis. It is even more common in patients with stenosis and regurgitation. Atherosclerotic calcification of the mitral annulus occurs in approximately 10% of the elderly population (Fig. 21.14). It appears

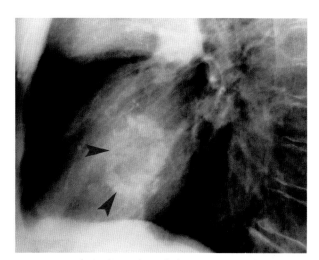

FIGURE 21.14. Mitral Annulus Calcification on Lateral CXR. Ovoid calcification of the mitral annulus (*arrowheads*) is secondary to atherosclerosis and is commonly associated with mitral insufficiency. Mitral calcification is best seen on a lateral radiograph.

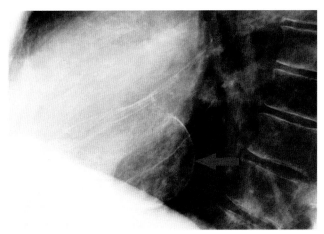

FIGURE 21.15. Calcified Ventricular Pseudoaneurysm on Lateral CXR. Thin, curvilinear calcification along the posterior wall of the LV (*arrow*) is indicative of a ventricular pseudoaneurysm.

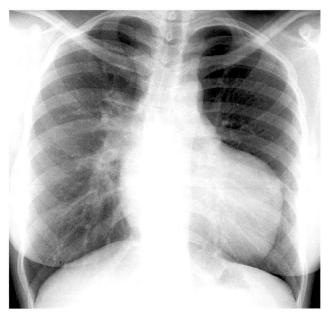

FIGURE 21.16. Chest Radiograph of Patient With Tetralogy of Fallot. Asymmetric pulmonary vasculature is evident with increased prominence of blood vessels on the right and decreased vascularity on the left. Note also right ventricular hypertrophy configuration and concave pulmonary artery segment.

as circular, ovoid, or C- or J-shaped calcification in the mitral annulus and can lead to mitral valve incompetence.

Sinus of Valsalva aneurysm calcification is seen as a curvilinear density anterior and lateral to the ascending aorta.

Calcified ligamentum arteriosum is seen as a linear calcification in the aortopulmonary window connecting the top of the left PA to the floor of the aortic arch.

Calcified LA. Thin curvilinear calcification in the wall of the LA is usually associated with mitral stenosis, left atrial enlargement, atrial fibrillation, and left atrial thrombus.

Calcified pericardium is typically anterior and inferior in location. It can be single or double layered and is associated with a high incidence of constrictive pericardial hemodynamics. Causes include viral, hemorrhagic, and tuberculous pericarditis as well as postsurgical scarring.

Calcified Infarct. Dystrophic calcification may occur in the myocardial wall from prior myocardial infarction.

Calcified Ventricular Aneurysm. Thin curvilinear calcification anterolaterally near the apex is most often seen with true aneurysms (see Figs. 22.10, 22.40). Posterior curvilinear calcification is usually seen in pseudoaneurysms (Fig. 21.15).

Calcified thrombus is seen as clumpy calcification in the LA or, less commonly, in the LV.

Calcified PAs. Thin eggshell-like calcification in the walls of the PAs is virtually diagnostic of long-standing pulmonary arterial hypertension (see Figs. 22.22, 22.23).

Tumors. Rounded or stippled calcifications are seen occasionally in atrial myxomas and rarely in other cardiac neoplasms (see Figs. 22.41 to 22.44).

Pulmonary Vascularity

The lungs have dual blood supply with PAs and systemic bronchial arteries.

Pulmonary Arteries. Increased circulation from left-to-right shunts results in enlargement of the main and hilar PAs with increased blood flow to the upper and lower lobes. Asymmetrical blood flow can be seen with pulmonary hypoplasia, Swyer–James syndrome, and congenital lesions such as pulmonary stenosis (increased to the left lung) or tetralogy of Fallot, which is increased to the right lung (Fig. 21.16).

Bronchial arteries arise from the aorta and penetrate into the lungs, traveling with the bronchi. Tetralogy of Fallot and pseudotruncus arteriosus result in a shift to bronchial circula-

tion. Bronchial arteries are also important in Rasmussen aneurysms from tuberculosis and systemic hypervascularity of any chronic infection.

Pulmonary arterial hypertension (Fig. 21.17) results in (*1*) dilated main PA, (*2*) right-sided cardiac enlargement, (*3*) central enlargement of left and right PAs, (*4*) rapid pruning of the peripheral PAs, (*5*) apparent decreased peripheral pulmonary circulation, (*6*) calcification of the central PAs (see Figs. 22.22, 22.23), and (*7*) secondary enlargement of the azygos vein.

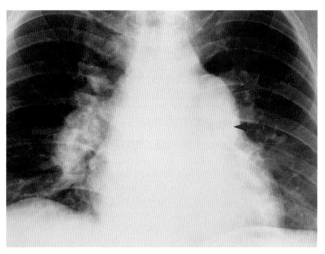

FIGURE 21.17. Idiopathic Pulmonary Hypertension. The main (*arrowhead*), right, and left (*arrows*) pulmonary arteries are dilated. The pulmonary arteries taper rapidly and peripheral pulmonary vascularity is decreased.

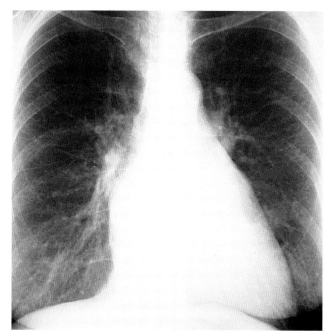

FIGURE 21.18. Pulmonary Venous Hypertension. Cephalization of blood flow is evident in this patient with mitral stenosis and enlarged left atrial appendage (*arrowhead*). The lower lobe vessels are constricted, and the upper lobe vessels are distended. Fullness in the hilar angle (*straight arrow*) is because of enlargement of the superior pulmonary veins crossing between the interlobar artery and the upper lobe artery.

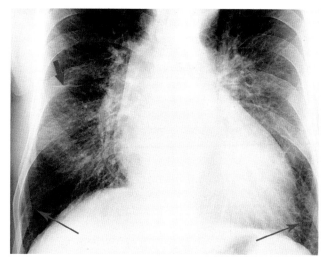

FIGURE 21.19. Interstitial Edema. The edema is indicated by prominent Kerley lines (*long arrows*). Thickening of the fissures (*fat arrow*) is also present, along with prominence of the LV and LA and cephalization of blood flow.

Pulmonary aneurysms and peripheral pulmonic stenosis can also cause unusual enlargements of the PAs and may be seen in Williams syndrome, Marfan syndrome, and collagen disorders.

Pulmonary venous hypertension (Fig. 21.18) results from mitral stenosis, mitral regurgitation, or elevated left ventricular pressure (aortic stenosis or congestive heart failure). The normal vessel caliber in the lower lobes is greater than that in the upper lobes by a 3:2 ratio because of hydrostatic pressure and the high compliance of the venous system. Elevated venous pressure causes progressive, edematous perivascular cuffing, which occurs first in the lower vessels, which have higher hydrostatic pressures. Perivascular edema in the lower lobes results in decreased compliance and progressive cephalization of blood flow. The chest radiograph shows decreased caliber of lower lobe vessels and increased caliber of upper lobe vessels. Cephalization of blood flow is the earliest radiographic sign of congestive heart failure and pulmonary venous hypertension. Cephalization begins at 10 to 13 mm Hg wedge pressure. Equalization of upper to lower pulmonary blood flow occurs at 14 to 16 mm Hg. Reversal of the normal distribution with the upper lobe vessels distended and the lower lobe vessels constricted occurs at 17 to 20 mm Hg. Hilar fullness, "Viking helmet sign" in the hila, and filling out of the right hilar angle commonly accompany reversed flow distribution.

Pulmonary Edema. Interstitial edema with Kerley A, B, and C lines and thickened pulmonary fissures occurs at 20 to 25 mm Hg wedge pressure (Fig. 21.19). Kerley lines represent thickened interlobular septa: A lines are long straight lines radiating toward the hila, B lines are horizontal lines connecting to the pleural surface near the costophrenic angle, and C lines are random reticular lines seen throughout the lungs. Alveolar edema begins at 25 to 30 mm Hg wedge pressure (Fig. 21.20). Chronic failure "toughens" the interstitium (often resulting in hemosiderosis and pulmonary ossification) and can add an additional 5 mm Hg protective zone prior to developing inter-

stitial or alveolar edema. These progressive signs of failure have been classified as stages 1 to 4 (Table 21.3).

Congestive Heart Failure. Radiographic findings include (*1*) cardiomegaly, (*2*) left ventricular and left atrial enlargement, (*3*) cephalization of blood flow, (*4*) azygos vein and SVC distension, (*5*) perivascular cuffing with haziness and unsharpness of the pulmonary vessels, (*6*) peribronchial cuffing with thickening of the bronchial walls seen as small "Cheerios" when viewed end on, (*7*) Kerley lines, (*8*) thickening of the pulmonary fissures, (*9*) subpleural edema, (*10*) pleural effusions, usually larger in the right hemithorax, and (*11*) alveolar edema in a "bat wing" or "butterfly" distribution, also often more pronounced on the right.

Right Heart Failure. The most common cause of right heart failure is left heart failure. Elevated left-sided pressures manifest in the pulmonary circuit and then in the right side of the heart. Long-standing venous hypertension leads to pulmonary arterial

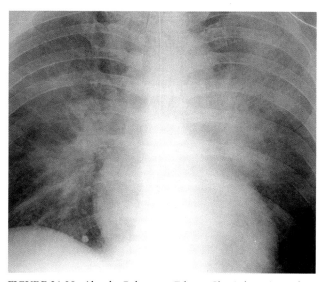

FIGURE 21.20. Alveolar Pulmonary Edema. Classic bat wing or butterfly perihilar alveolar infiltrates are present in a symmetrical cloud-like pattern.

TABLE 21.3

SIGNS OF PROGRESSIVE CARDIAC FAILURE

■ STAGE	■ SIGN	■ WEDGE PRESSURE (mm Hg)
1	Progressive cephalization	10–20
2	Interstitial edema and septal lines	20–25
3	Alveolar edema, often in bat wing perihilar distribution	>25–30
4	Chronic or severe pulmonary venous hypertension resulting in hemosiderosis, pulmonary ossification, and chronic interstitial disease such as from long-standing mitral stenosis	>30–35

hypertension. Elevated right-sided pressures cause right ventricular hypertrophy and dilatation, as well as systemic venous dilatation involving azygos vein, SVC, and jugular veins. Dilatation of the right heart can also cause tricuspid valve incompetence. Right heart failure protects the pulmonary circuit by accumulating edema and fluid outside the lungs, similar to the old therapeutic maneuver of rotating tourniquets.

Right heart failure may also occur with the dilated cardiomyopathies, including viral and alcoholic cardiomyopathy. When right heart failure is the result of a pulmonary disease such as chronic obstructive pulmonary disease, destructive lung disease, or primary pulmonary hypertension, the term *cor pulmonale* is used.

The Pericardium

The pericardium is composed of one continuous fibrous membrane that is folded back on itself, creating two layers. The inner layer of visceral pericardium or epicardium is closely attached to the myocardium and subepicardial fat. The outer layer or parietal pericardium is thicker and is often referred to simply as the pericardium.

Pericardial Effusion. Between the visceral and parietal layers is the pericardial space, which usually contains 20 mL of serous fluid. More than 50 mL of fluid is clearly abnormal, but 200 mL is required for detection by plain film radiography. Mediastinal and epicardial fat enable the pericardium to be visualized as a thin arcuate line paralleling the anterior heart border in the retrosternal region. A pericardial stripe exceeding 2 to 3 mm is indicative of pericardial thickening or effusion. Unfortunately, the thickened pericardial stripe can be seen on the lateral radiograph in only about 15% of patients with pericardial effusion. The "differential density sign" refers to a lucent margin along the left heart border on the PA radiograph or along the posterior cardiac border on the lateral radiograph. It is seen in up to 63% of patients with pericardial effusion but is less specific than the thickened pericardial stripe. Large pericardial effusions cause the heart to appear on frontal radiographs in the shape of a sac of water sitting on a tabletop (Fig. 21.21).

Pneumopericardium appears on plain films as radiolucency surrounding the heart and separated from the lung by a thin white line of pericardium (Fig. 21.22). Air may also be seen outlining the PAs or the undersurface of the heart.

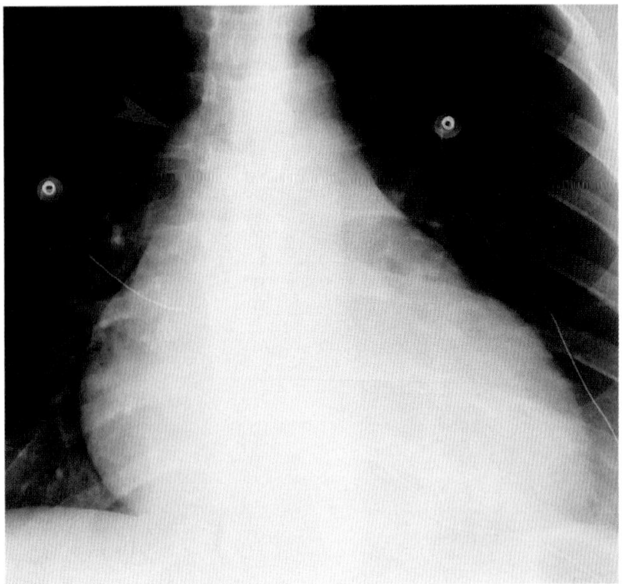

FIGURE 21.21. Pericardial Effusion. "Water-bottle configuration" of the cardiac silhouette is indicative of pericardial effusion or dilated cardiomyopathy. This patient with systemic lupus erythematosus has an enlarged azygos vein (*arrowhead*), decreased pulmonary vasculature, and clear lung parenchyma.

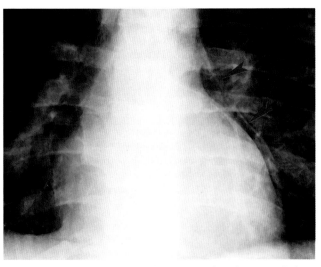

FIGURE 21.22. Pneumopericardium. Air within the pericardial sac enables visualization of the pericardium (*arrowheads*), seen as a thin white line paralleling the left heart border.

Pneumopericardium can be caused by trauma, infection, or pneumomediastinum. Firm attachment of the pericardium to the ascending aorta just above the main PA acts to contain the pneumopericardium.

Other Signs of Cardiac Disease

Situs Anomalies. Careful attention should be directed at the location of the aortic arch, gastric fundus, heart, pulmonary fissures, and the branching pattern of the bronchi. Normal anatomic positioning is termed *situs solitus*. *Situs inversus* means that the patient's entire anatomic arrangement is reversed in a right-to-left direction as a "mirror image." Situs inversus is associated with a 5% to 10% incidence of congenital heart disease, compared with less than 1% incidence for situs solitus. *Dextrocardia* indicates that the heart is in the right hemithorax. The apex of the heart lies to the right, with the long axis of the heart directed from left to right. *Kartagener syndrome* is a combination of situs inversus with dextrocardia, bronchiectasis, and sinusitis (Fig. 21.23). The latter findings are because of the abnormal mucosal cilia.

Dextroposition means the heart is shifted toward the right hemithorax. It is associated with hypoplastic right lung and an increased incidence of congenital heart disease, particularly left-to-right shunts. *Dextroversion* means the cardiac apex is to the right, but the stomach and aortic knob remain on the left. The LV remains on the left but lies anterior to the RV.

Dextrocardia with situs ambiguous and polysplenia is also called "bilateral left-sidedness." Each lung contains only two lobes and hyparterial bronchi. Bilateral SVCs are also common. The incidence of congenital heart disease is increased, most commonly that of ASD or anomalous pulmonary venous return. Dextrocardia with asplenia is referred to as "bilateral right-sidedness" because of bilateral minor fissures and three lobes in each lung. The cardiac anomalies are usually more complex and severe than in polysplenia.

Bony Abnormalities. Postoperative changes of sternotomy suggest prior cardiac surgery and the presence of cardiac disease. Sternal fractures from motor vehicle accidents are associated with a 50% incidence of cardiac contusion.

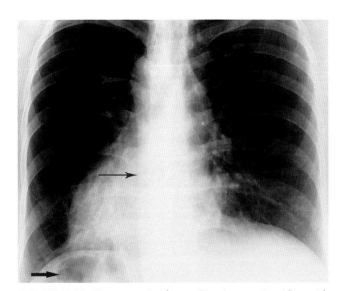

FIGURE 21.23. **Kartagener Syndrome.** Situs inversus is evident with dextrocardia, right-sided aortic arch (*arrowhead*), right-sided descending aorta (*long arrow*), and the gastric air bubble (*arrow*) on the patient's right. Evidence of bronchiectasis is present behind the heart and in the left lower lobe.

Hypersegmentation of the sternum (more than four to five segments) is present in 90% of patients with Down syndrome and offers a clue to the presence of endocardial cushion defect or complete atrioventricular canal. Wavy retrosternal linear opacities suggest dilated internal mammary arteries associated with coarctation of the aorta. Pectus excavatum is associated with an increased incidence of mitral valve prolapse and Marfan syndrome. A barrel-shaped chest with pectus carinatum is associated with VSDs and complete atrioventricular canal. Scoliosis with a "shield chest" is seen with Marfan syndrome, aortic valve disease, coarctation, and aortic dissection.

The presence of 11 or fewer ribs is highly associated with Down syndrome and atrioventricular canal. "Ribbon ribs" or bifurcated ribs and an overcirculation pattern suggest truncus arteriosus, whereas their association with an undercirculation pattern suggests tetralogy of Fallot. Rib notching and inferior rib sclerosis indicate collateral circulation through intercostal arteries and occurs with coarctation of the aorta and Blalock–Taussig operations. The third through the eighth ribs are most commonly involved. Fractures of the first and second ribs indicate high-velocity blunt trauma has occurred, and there is an increased risk of aortic injury.

The spine offers clues to the presence of aortic valve disease when changes of ankylosing spondylitis, neurofibromatosis, or rheumatoid arthritis are present. Scoliosis is associated with an increased incidence of congenital heart disease.

NUCLEAR CARDIOLOGY

Cardiac nuclear medicine is a central modality in cardiac imaging and is covered in detail in Chapter 56. Perfusion scans with thallium or new technetium agents are useful for diagnosing coronary ischemia and myocardial infarcts. Normal perfusion scans appear in the shape of a horseshoe in the vertical and long axes and in the shape of a doughnut in the short axis (see Fig. 56.2). The scans are accomplished during rest, with controlled exercise or with pharmacologic stress with IV dipyridamole. The stress and redistribution or rest images appear identical in normal patients. Hypoperfused segments on stress images, which fill in on rest, are indicative of ischemia. Hypoperfused segments on both rest and stress images are usually infarcts or scars. Myocardial infarction scanning can be accomplished using rest perfusion agents for "cold spot" imaging or technetium pyrophosphate for "hot spot" imaging (see Figs. 22.11, 22.12). Antimyosin antibody scans have also been used for diagnosing and sizing myocardial infarction.

Electrocardiogram-gated myocardial blood pool studies examine wall motion and allow left ventricular ejection fraction calculations (see Figs. 56.12, 56.13, 56.14). Ventricular function, aneurysms, and valvular disease may be studied with volume curves and functional images. Right ventricular ejection fraction calculations require first-pass examinations because of anatomic overlap of the RV with the atria in the left anterior oblique projection. First-pass cardiac studies can also diagnose SVC obstruction and left-to-right cardiac shunts (see Figs. 56.19, 56.20). Right-to-left cardiac shunts can be evaluated and quantified with technetium macroaggregated albumin or microspheres (see Fig. 56.21).

SPECT imaging has greatly improved the diagnostic capabilities of myocardial perfusion imaging and infarct scans. ECG-gated SPECT is readily accomplished and adds wall motion evaluation, ventricular volumes, and ejection fraction information to the study as well. PET is a newer technology with increased resolution compared to SPECT imaging. PET can assess cardiac metabolism as well as perfusion, enhancing its ability to evaluate cardiomyopathies, ischemia, infarction, and "hibernating" or viable myocardium.

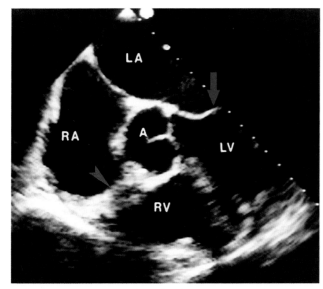

FIGURE 21.24. Transesophageal Echocardiogram. A five-chamber view of the heart is provided by a US probe within the esophagus. The probe is behind the LA and is depicted at the top of the image. All four chambers and the aortic valve are seen in one plane, the "five-chamber view." The LA and RA are separated by the interatrial septum. The aortic valve (*A*) is readily identified in the midplane. The RV and LV are separated by the interventricular septum. The closed tricuspid valve (*arrowhead*) is seen between the RA and RV, and a portion of the mitral valve (*arrow*) is seen between the LA and LV.

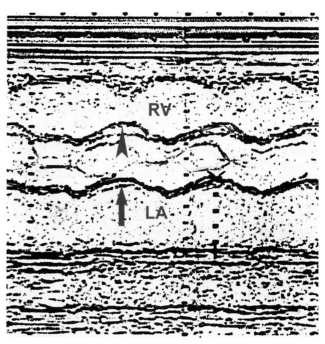

FIGURE 21.26. Aortic Root. An M-mode echocardiogram demonstrates anterior movement of the anterior (*arrowhead*) and posterior (*straight arrow*) walls of the aortic root during systole. The RV is seen anterior to the aortic root and the LA is seen posterior to the aortic root. Aortic valve motion can be seen within the aortic root.

ECHOCARDIOGRAPHY

Echocardiography includes M-mode, real-time 2D US, range-gated and color flow Doppler, and transesophageal US. Transesophageal echocardiography uses a nasogastric probe with a steerable ultrasonic beam that views the heart and aorta

from the close posterior position provided by the esophagus (Fig. 21.24). M-mode echocardiograms are produced by a narrow ultrasonic beam that is directed at cardiac structures and observed over time or is swept across an area of anatomy (Figs. 21.25 to 21.27). The returning echoes produce a time–motion study of cardiac structures. With a transthoracic technique,

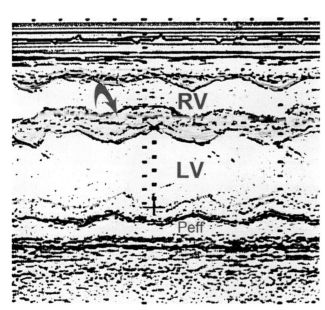

FIGURE 21.25. Pericardial Effusion. An M-mode echocardiogram with the ultrasonic probe at the top of the image demonstrates the RV, interventricular septum (*curved arrow*), and LV. Note the normal myocardial contractility with the interventricular septum contracting toward the posterior left ventricular wall during systole. A pericardial effusion (*Peff*) is seen as an echolucent space posterior to the left ventricular wall.

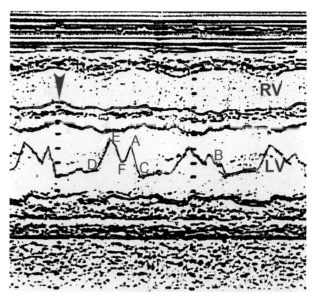

FIGURE 21.27. Normal Mitral Valve. An M-mode echocardiogram demonstrates the right ventricular cavity (RV) and left ventricular cavity (LV) separated by a band of echoes representing the interventricular septum (*arrowhead*). The moving mitral valve can be seen within the left ventricular cavity. Because of plane of section, the full systolic motion of the myocardium is not well visualized. The points of the mitral waveform are labeled with letters (see text).

anterior structures are usually displayed at the top of the image. The thickness and motion of the myocardium can be evaluated throughout the cardiac cycle. Pericardial effusions are shown as an echo-free space adjacent to the myocardium (Fig. 21.25). Large pleural effusions create an echolucent space posterior to the LV and pericardium.

The interventricular septum appears as a band of echoes near the midplane. It normally thickens and moves toward the posterior wall of the LV during systole (Fig. 21.25). Paradoxic septal motion may be seen in pericardial effusion, with cardiac tamponade, chronic obstructive pulmonary disease, asthma, ASDs, pulmonary hypertension, left bundle branch block, and septal ischemia. The interventricular septum measures less than 10 to 11 mm at end diastole and is compared with the thickness of the posterior wall of the LV for asymmetric or concentric hypertrophy.

The aortic root lies immediately posterior to the RV and measures 8 to 12 mm in neonates and 20 to 40 mm in adults (Fig. 21.26). The thin parallel aortic walls move anteriorly during systole. The aortic root is dilated with aortic stenosis, aortic insufficiency, tetralogy of Fallot, and aortic aneurysm. The thin aortic cusps seen within the aortic root should open widely during systole and should not reverberate.

The LA is seen posterior to the aortic root (Fig. 21.26). The normal size is no larger than 40 mm during diastole in adults. The LA is free of internal echoes and has a thin posterior wall that merges with the thicker left ventricular wall.

The LV lies inferior and lateral to the LA and is an echo-free space except for the thin chordae tendineae and the echogenic projections of the papillary muscles. The left ventricular posterior wall thickens during systole and contracts anteriorly. The transverse diameter of the LV does not normally exceed 5.7 cm during diastole. The wall measures approximately the same as the ventricular septum (10 to 11 mm).

The mitral valve produces a saw-toothed or M-shaped pattern posterior to the interventricular septum (Fig. 21.27). The anterior leaflet is the dominant echo and is continuous with the posterior wall of the aortic root. Immediately posterior to the anterior leaflet is the W-shaped pattern of the posterior leaflet. The two leaflets close during systole. The echo pattern of the anterior leaflet should be carefully scrutinized for evidence of thickening, delay in closure (seen with mitral stenosis), vegetations, prolapse, myxoma, or high-frequency vibration secondary to aortic regurgitation (Austin Flint phenomena). The specific points of the mitral waveform (Fig. 21.27) are the following:

A point: **A**trial contraction with peak anterior opening motion

B point: notch **B**etween the A and C points representing elevated left ventricular end-diastolic pressure

C point: **C**losure of the mitral valve occurs with contraction of the LV during systole

D point: early **D**iastole when mitral valve begins to open

E point: maximal **E**xcursion of the valve opening (this is the peak of early diastolic opening and the most anterior position of the valve during diastole)

F point: most posterior point of early diastolic **F**illing prior to atrial contraction

The E–F slope is a function of left atrial emptying rate and should be steep. With mitral stenosis, the slope will be flattened and look more squared off than M-shaped. With valve thickening and calcification, the squared-off part appears thickened.

The tricuspid valve is identified by locating the mitral valve and rotating the transducer medially. It has an M-shaped echo pattern similar to that of the mitral valve. The E–F slope is decreased with tricuspid stenosis and is increased with Ebstein anomaly, tricuspid regurgitation, and ASD.

The pulmonic valve is rather difficult to evaluate by M-mode echocardiography. The diameter of the pulmonary trunk is similar to that of the aortic root. Pulmonary valve motion is similar to aortic valve motion, except that only the posterior leaflet is well seen and there may be a small "A wave" because of atrial contraction.

CORONARY ANGIOGRAPHY

While CT coronary angiography (CTCA) is playing an increasingly important role, true coronary angiography will remain vitally important especially in preparation for coronary intervention. Selective catheterization of the coronary arteries was first accomplished in 1959 by Sones with the use of a flexible, tapered tip catheter using a cut-down procedure on the brachial artery. In 1966, Amplatz used J-shaped, preformed catheters with better torque control from a transfemoral approach. In 1968, Judkins used separate preformed catheters for the right and left coronary arteries. After selective catheterization of the coronary artery, hand injections of contrast verify the size and flow of the artery. The left coronary artery (LCA) generally requires 7 to 9 mL of contrast at 4 to 6 mL/s, whereas 6 to 8 mL at 3 to 5 mL/s is sufficient for the smaller right coronary artery (RCA). Pressure limits for power injectors should be set at less than 150 psi. The catheter tip should not be left wedged in the coronary ostium, as this might occlude blood flow.

Complications of coronary angiography include hematoma, pseudoaneurysm, and fistula formation at the puncture site, arrhythmias including premature ventricular contractions, heart block and asystole, myocardial infarction, stroke, emboli, and death. Indications for coronary arteriography include (*1*) confirmation of an anatomic cause for angina, (*2*) identification of high-risk lesions, (*3*) evaluation of asymptomatic patients with abnormal exercise tolerance test or occupational risk, (*4*) preoperative evaluation for cardiac surgery, (*5*) evaluation of patients with coronary artery bypass grafts for stenosis or occlusion, and (*6*) after myocardial infarction, for evaluation of interventional therapy.

Coronary Anatomy

The RCA arises from the right coronary cusp, and the LCA arises from the left coronary cusp. Approximately 85% of patients are right-dominant, meaning that the RCA supplies the posterior descending artery and the posterior and inferior surface of the myocardium. In 10% to 12% of patients, the LCA is dominant and supplies the inferior and posterior surface. Approximately 4% to 5% of patients are codominant. The LCA measures 0.5 to 1.5 cm in length before it divides beneath the left atrial appendage (Figs. 21.28, 21.29). The left anterior descending (LAD) artery extends anteriorly in the interventricular groove. The circumflex artery extends laterally and posteriorly under the left atrial appendage to the atrioventricular groove. An occasional third branch is the ramus intermedius, which extends as a first diagonal branch (d1) or a first marginal branch (m1).

The LAD gives off several septal branches that penetrate into the septum. One or more diagonal branches extend toward the anterolateral wall. Occasionally, a conus branch comes off after the first septal branch and extends to the right ventricular infundibulum. The circumflex artery gives off one or more obtuse marginal branches that supply the lateral wall of the LV.

The RCA passes anterior and to the right between the PA and the RA (Figs. 21.30, 21.31). Its first branch is a conus branch to the pulmonary outflow tract. The second branch is the sinus node branch with a smaller branch to the RA. Muscular branches

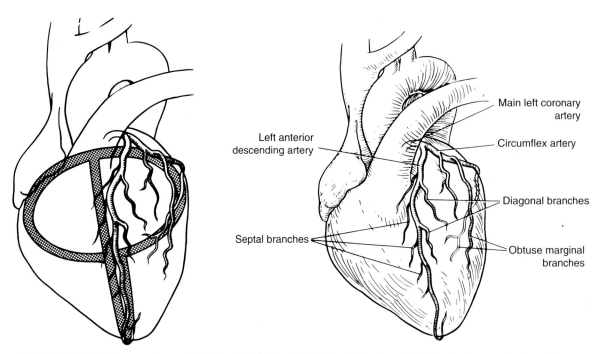

FIGURE 21.28. Left Coronary Artery (LCA) in the Left Anterior Oblique Projection. The LCA divides into the circumflex artery that makes up the *left side of the circle*, and the left anterior descending artery that makes up the *anterior portion of the loop*. Obtuse marginal branches extend from the circumflex artery; diagonal and septal branches extend from the left anterior descending artery. (Reproduced with permission from Kubicka RA, Smith C. How to interpret coronary arteriograms. Radiographics 1986;6:661–701.)

extend into the right ventricular myocardium. At the posterior turn, a large acute marginal branch is often given off anteriorly toward the diaphragmatic surface of the RV. The RCA then extends posteriorly in the atrioventricular sulcus and makes a 90° turn toward the apex in right-dominant systems. As the posterior descending artery, it supplies branches to the diaphragmatic myocardium and the posterior one-third of the interventricular septum. The distal RCA may also give off a variable number of posterolateral ventricular branches.

The coronary arteries can be visualized as a circle and loop, with the atrioventricular groove being the circle and the interventricular septum being the attached loop (Figs. 21.28 to 21.31). In the right anterior oblique projection, the circle is superimposed on itself and the loop is in profile. In the left anterior projection, the circle is more open and the loop is foreshortened. In the left anterior craniad view, there is a better, elongated view of the left main coronary artery, LAD, and ramus intermedius.

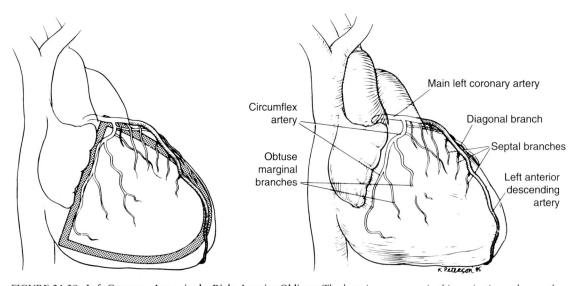

FIGURE 21.29. Left Coronary Artery in the Right Anterior Oblique. The *loop* is more open in this projection, whereas the *circle* is superimposed. The left anterior descending artery makes up the *anterior portion of the loop*. The circumflex artery and its obtuse marginal branches make up the *left side of the circle*. (Reproduced with permission from Kubicka RA, Smith C. How to interpret coronary arteriograms. Radiographics 1986;6:661–701.)

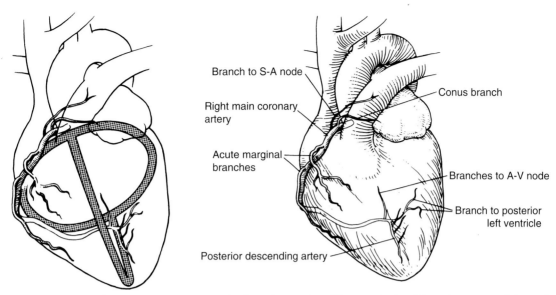

FIGURE 21.30. **Right Coronary Artery (RCA) in the Left Anterior Oblique Projection.** The *right portion of the circle* represents the RCA and the *posterior portion of the loop* represents the posterior descending artery. S-A, sinoatrial; A-V, atrioventricular. (Reproduced with permission from Kubicka RA, Smith C. How to interpret coronary arteriograms. Radiographics 1986;6:661–701.)

Coronary Pathology

Fixed Coronary Stenosis. A 75% reduction in cross-sectional area is required to cause a significant reduction in blood flow (see Figs. 22.4, 22.5). A 50% reduction in diameter corresponds to a 75% reduction in cross-sectional area. In general, stenoses >50% are considered clinically significant and will demonstrate decreased perfusion on stress myocardial perfusion imaging.

Other significant findings include coronary calcification, ulcerative plaques, and aneurysm formation. Collateral flow typically develops when there is greater than 85% stenosis.

Catheter-induced spasm is most often seen in the RCA as a smooth transient narrowing, 1 to 2 mm distal to the catheter tip. The patient usually remains asymptomatic.

Prinzmetal variant angina is angina secondary to prolonged coronary spasm. IV ergonovine may be used in a provocative test to incite coronary spasm, typical symptoms, and electrocardiographic changes. Prinzmetal angina is usually treated medically.

Kawasaki syndrome is an inflammatory condition of the coronary arteries, probably attributable to a prior viral syndrome, which results in coronary stenosis and coronary aneurysms, occasionally persisting into adulthood.

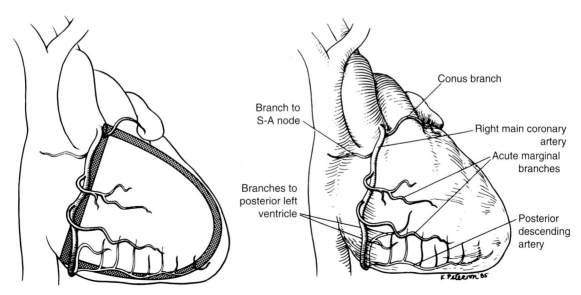

FIGURE 21.31. **Right Coronary Artery (RCA) in the Right Anterior Oblique Projection.** The RCA forms the atrioventricular *circle.* The *loop* is more opened in this projection with the posterior descending artery making up its inferior margin. S-A, sinoatrial. (Reproduced with permission from Kubicka RA, Smith C. How to interpret coronary arteriograms. Radiographics 1986;6:661–701.)

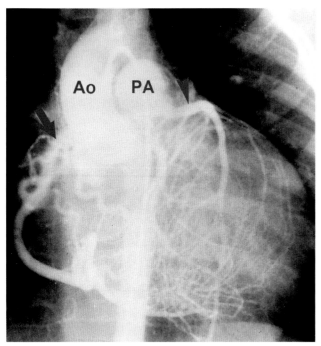

FIGURE 21.32. Aberrant Left Coronary Artery (LCA). The catheter in the ascending aorta (Ao) opacifies a dilated right coronary artery (RCA) (*arrow*). The LCA (*arrowhead*) arises from the pulmonary artery (PA) and is filled in a retrograde fashion via collateral flow from the RCA.

Myocardial bridging describes a normal variant in which the coronary arteries penetrate and then emerge from the myocardium rather than running along the surface of the epicardium. This causes arterial constriction during systole, which reverts to normal flow during diastole.

Anomalies of the coronary arteries include multiple coronary ostia with more than one coronary artery arising directly from one coronary cusp, a single coronary artery, and origination of the LCA from the PA (Fig. 21.32). This is an excellent area for evaluation by CTCA.

Therapeutic Considerations

The primary modes of therapy for coronary artery disease include many efficacious medical regimens, percutaneous coronary angioplasty and stenting, and coronary artery bypass graft surgery. Coronary artery bypass grafting usually uses saphenous vein grafts or native internal mammary arteries. Surgical bypass has been shown to prolong life in left main coronary artery disease and three-vessel disease. Percutaneous coronary angioplasty (see Fig. 22.5) is considered useful for both single-vessel and multivessel disease and has an 85% to 90% initial success rate. Restenosis remains a significant problem in up to 50% of cases, typically occurring within the first 6 months. Restenosis is less frequent with newer stents. Angioplasty is typically accomplished by balloon dilatation of the stenotic lesion over a guidewire. Angioplasty is considered successful when the stenosis is reduced to less than 50% of diameter narrowing, although long-term prognosis is better when there is less than a 30% residual stenosis. Directional and rotational atherectomy and atherectomy with the transluminal extraction catheter and laser angioplasty are additional percutaneous techniques that are currently used in specific situations.

CARDIAC ANGIOGRAPHY

Angiography of the heart in adults most often involves left-sided catheterization via arterial puncture with retrograde examination of the aorta, LV, and LA. Selective catheterization of the coronary arteries is also accomplished from the arterial side. Right heart angiography uses puncture of a neck or femoral vein with catheter placement in the RA, RV, pulmonary outflow tract, or PA. Additionally, the LA or LV may be seen on delayed or "levo-phase" views from a right-sided injection. It is also possible to access the left side during right heart catheterization by puncturing the atrial septum. End-hole catheters are used for pressure measurements, and pigtail or multiple side-hole catheters are used for intracardiac injections to avoid contrast injection into the myocardium itself. Blood flow is estimated with standard oximetry, thermodilution, and indicator dilution techniques.

Wall motion is evaluated globally and regionally. *Hypokinesia* describes diminished contractility or less systolic motion than normal. *Akinesia* means no systolic wall motion. *Dyskinesia* means there is paradoxical wall motion during systole. *Tardikinesia* refers to delayed contractility. *Asynchrony* refers to cardiac motion that is out of phase with the remainder of the myocardium.

Ventricular aneurysms appear as a bulge in the wall that moves paradoxically compared with other areas of the LV (Fig. 21.33). True aneurysms are lined by thinned, scarred myocardium and

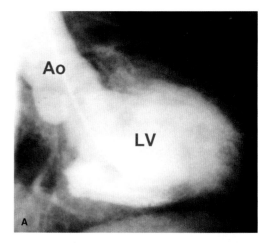

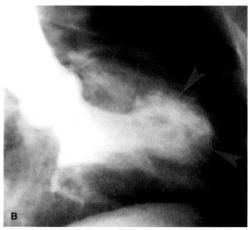

FIGURE 21.33. Left Ventricular Aneurysm. Diastole (**A**) and end systole (**B**). The left ventriculogram is accomplished with the pigtail catheter entering the LV from the aortic root (Ao). A paradoxical bulge near the apex (*arrowheads*) indicates a left ventricular aneurysm.

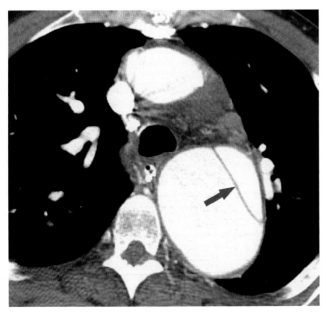

FIGURE 21.34. Type B Aortic Dissection. Contrast-enhanced MDCT scan demonstrates descending aortic aneurysm with intimal flap (*arrow*). The ascending aorta is normal.

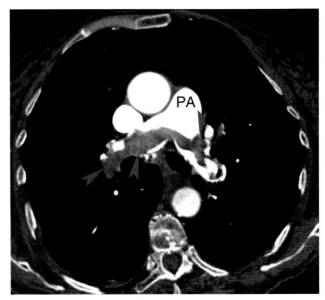

FIGURE 21.36. Pulmonary Artery (PA) Embolus. Contrast-enhanced CT examination shows a large filling defect (*arrowheads*) extending from the main PA into the main right and left PAs. This constitutes a "saddle embolus." The patient died in this case.

are typically located near the apex or anterolateral wall. Pseudoaneurysms are focal, contained ruptures that are often larger but have narrower ostia, and are most commonly located at the inferior and posterior aspect of the LV. Intramural thrombi may be seen in up to 50% of ventricular aneurysms.

CARDIAC CT

MDCT is useful in evaluating aortic aneurysms, aortic dissections (Fig. 21.34), aortic injuries, vascular anomalies (Fig. 21.35),

central pulmonary emboli (Fig. 21.36), intracardiac masses and thrombi (Fig. 21.37), pericardial thickening, fluid collections, and pericardial calcifications (see Fig. 22.47). Optimal contrast enhancement, ECG gating, and breath hold technique are required for optimal studies. Initially, ultrafast CT, or electron beam CT (EBCT), offered the advantage of high-speed scanning to better stop action and eliminate motion artifact, but has been replaced by new high-speed MDCT. Angled couch views supplement standard axial imaging. With cardiac gating, cine CT can provide wall motion studies, ejection fraction, and valve evaluation.

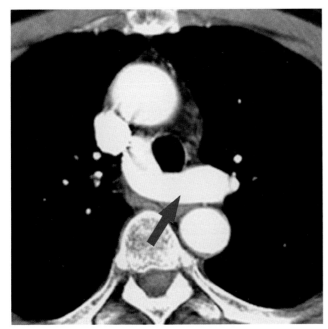

FIGURE 21.35. Aberrant Left Pulmonary Artery (PA). Contrast-enhanced MDCT demonstrates anomalous origin of left PA (*arrow*) from right PA, crossing posterior to the trachea, creating a pulmonary sling.

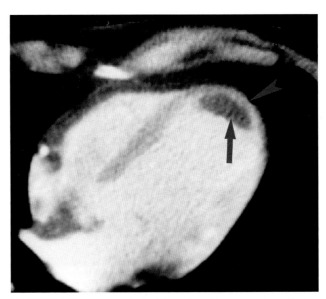

FIGURE 21.37. Intraventricular Thrombus. Contrast-enhanced, electron beam CT shows intraventricular clot (*arrow*), thinned myocardium (*arrowhead*), and akinesis, secondary to anteroapical infarct.

Coronary Artery Calcium Screening

As previously described, coronary artery calcification with chest x-ray (CXR) and fluoroscopy has been studied extensively. CXR has a sensitivity of 42% and fluoroscopy has a sensitivity of 40% to 79% and a specificity of 52% to 95% for detecting coronary calcification as an indicator of coronary stenosis. Coronary calcification is a significant marker for underlying atherosclerosis. EBCT has been studied thoroughly since the early 1990s as a coronary calcification screening modality and has a sensitivity of 70% to 74%, a specificity of 70% to 91%, and a negative predictive value of 97% when compared to coronary angiography (see Fig 22.2). Now MDCT has been shown to be equivalent to EBCT for coronary calcification detection and scoring.

EBCT allows 1.5- to 3.0-mm sections with an exposure time of 100 msec, 40 to 60 sections, with single breath hold acquisition, and ECG gated to end diastole. New 64-slice, and now even 320–slice, MDCTs have rotation speeds now down to 300 msec, temporal resolution of 42 msec, and spatial resolution to 0.33 mm. MDCT coronary calcium screening is also done with ECG gating, single breath hold, and arms up.

One method of scoring utilizes the Agatston method where coronary calcification is defined as an area with greater than 130 HU and larger than 2 mm². A score of 1 is given for 130 to 200 HU, 2 for 201 to 299 HU, 3 for 300 to 399 HU, and 4 for 400 HU or greater. This factor is assigned and multiplied by the area of the lesion for each coronary artery territory. This score is then summed for a total coronary calcification score or *Agatston score* (Fig. 21.38). A score of 0 to 10 is very low to low risk, 11 to 100 is moderate, 101 to 400 is moderately high, and greater than 400 is high risk for underlying stenosis and future cardiac events. However, the specific calcified area or artery may not correlate with specific stenoses.

The utility of coronary calcium screening lies in (1) early detection of calcium in asymptomatic patients for risk stratification and risk factor modification, (2) evaluation of progression or even regression of calcification as an indicator of atherosclerotic coronary disease, and (3) demonstration of the absence of calcification, thereby essentially ruling out significant underlying coronary stenosis.

CT Coronary Angiography

EBCT and now MDCT have been also shown to be efficacious for noninvasive CT coronary angiography (CTCA). Many laboratories are using 64-slice MDCT and now up to 320-slice MDCT for CTCA. Spatial resolution is now down to 0.33 mm with rotation speeds to 300 msec and temporal resolution to 42 msec. An entire heart can be scanned in 250 msec, less than half a heart beat. Because faster heart rates can lead to motion artifact, slowing the heart rate to 60 or 70 bpm with oral and IV beta-blockers is sometimes necessary. Contrast is delivered using a peripheral or jugular vein, 18 to 20 gauge needle, and 100 to 150 mL of iso-osmolar contrast at 4 mL/s. The study is acquired with arms up, single breath hold (10 to 30 sec), and ECG gating (prospective or retrospective). The contrast bolus is immediately followed by a 25 to 40 mL saline flush. The scan timing can be judged with a test bolus or can begin at the end of contrast injection. Optimal image quality has peak opacification in the LV and coronary arteries with less dense concentration in the RV and PAs.

ECG "pulsing" can reduce tube current during systole and increase it during diastole where the target images are usually constructed. This can reduce the radiation dose by up to 50%. Reconstruction is done to 0.5-mm slice thickness and a medium smooth reconstruction algorithm. Past processing is very important and is often done by the radiologist, especially for 3D reconstruction.

The coronaries can be evaluated for congenital abnormalities, presurgical anatomy, coronary calcifications and coronary plaque, or stenosis utilizing volume rendered 3D (Fig. 21.39), 2D, multiplanar (Fig. 21.40), maximal intensity projections (MIP) and coronary "straightening" views (Fig. 21.41). Stenoses greater than 50% are considered hemodynamically significant and those greater than 75% are considered high

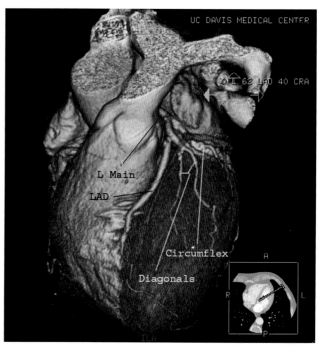

FIGURE 21.39. **Three-Dimensional Volume Rendered CT Coronary Angiogram.** The left anterior descending (LAD), branching diagonals, and circumflex coronary arteries are well seen in this left anterior oblique projection from MDCT. The left main coronary artery is partially seen under the left atrial appendage.

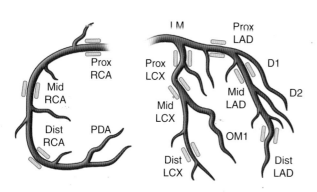

OM1 is Obtuse Marginal 1

D1 and D2 are Diagonal 1 and Diagonal 2

FIGURE 21.38. **Coronary Calcification Scoring From MDCT.** The report shows the score for each coronary artery and location. The summed score is over 1100, placing the patient in the very high-risk category.

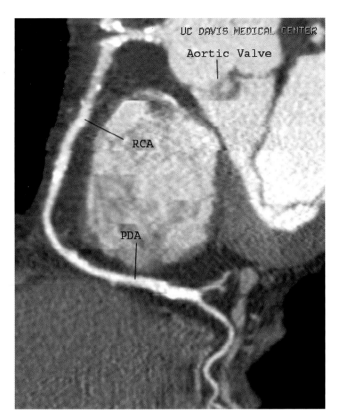

FIGURE 21.40. Maximum Intensity Projection (MIP) CT Coronary Angiogram. The aortic valve, right coronary artery (RCA), and posterior descending artery (PDA) are well seen in this left anterior oblique MIP projection from 16-slice MDCT.

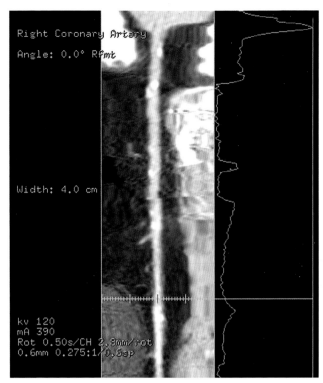

FIGURE 21.41. Right Coronary Artery in "Straightened" Maximum Intensity Projection View. This computer-reconstructed view effectively takes out the curves and makes it easier to see that, while there are atherosclerotic irregularities, there is no significant stenosis.

grade. Problems occur in grading stenoses with heavy coronary calcification and with stents. Patency, however, can be determined by evaluating coronary enhancement downstream. CTCA has also been shown to be useful and accurate for the follow-up of coronary artery bypass graft patency.

CARDIAC MR

Cardiac MR (CMR) combines many of the capabilities of the other imaging modalities into one examination. These include excellent static anatomic images and dynamic motion studies for function. CMR applications include congenital heart disease, aortic and PA disease, pericardial disease, ventricular function, valvular function, cardiomyopathies, and cardiac masses. *Cardiac pacemakers are considered contraindications,* but most prosthetic valves can be safely studied.

The best anatomic depiction is accomplished on spin-echo T1WI in which the moving blood produces a signal void or "black blood" appearance (Fig. 21.42). Gradient-echo or fast-field echo images impart bright signal to coherently flowing blood, creating a "white blood" appearance similar to contrast studies (Fig. 21.43). Electrocardiographic gating can be used similarly as gated cardiac SPECT and gated cardiac blood pool scintigraphy. Slice-specific information is acquired with reference to specific phases within the cardiac cycle. With gradient recalled echo technique, motion studies can show flowing blood as well as myocardial contractility.

Steady-state free precession (SSFP) cine imaging is another excellent technique for visually assessing LV function. SSFP, in contrast to older gradient-echo cine techniques, does not rely on the inflow of unsaturated spins to create contrast between the LV cavity and the endocardium. Because SSFP images are flow-independent, endocardial border detection is significantly enhanced. Furthermore, SSFP provides excellent spatial and temporal resolution and a high signal-to-noise ratio, and it requires relatively short breath-holding times.

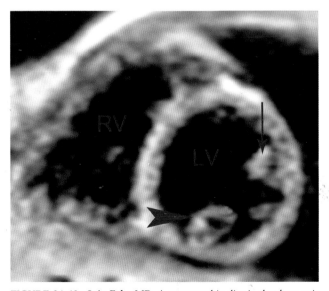

FIGURE 21.42. Spin-Echo MR. A tomographic slice in the short-axis projection demonstrates the RV, interventricular septum, and the LV. The anterior (*arrowhead*) and posterior (*arrow*) papillary muscles are seen within the left ventricular cavity. The spin-echo technique creates a "black blood" appearance because of the signal void of moving blood.

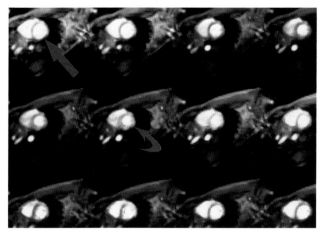

FIGURE 21.43. Fast-Field Echo MR. The fast-field echo technique creates a "white blood" depiction that shows wall motion, flowing blood, and turbulence during motion studies. The end diastole image (*straight arrow*) has the largest ventricular size. The end systole image (*curved arrow*) has the smallest ventricular cavity and the thickest wall.

Because of its high spatial resolution, reproducibility, and 3D data that require the operator to make no geometric assumptions, CMR has evolved into the reference standard for measuring mass, chamber volumes, and ejection fraction. Because of the exceptional contrast generated between the myocardium and blood pool (Fig. 21.44), CMR enables the

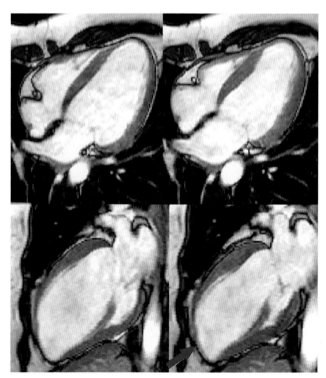

FIGURE 21.44. Left Ventricular Function MR. Steady-state free precession images in two standard planes at different phases in the cardiac cycle in a patient with a prior anterior myocardial infarction. The upper panels demonstrate a four-chamber long-axis image of the heart at end diastole on the left and end systole on the right. Note the thinned, distal anterior wall and apex (*arrow*) with reduced wall thickening during systole, which are suggestive of prior myocardial infarction in that region.

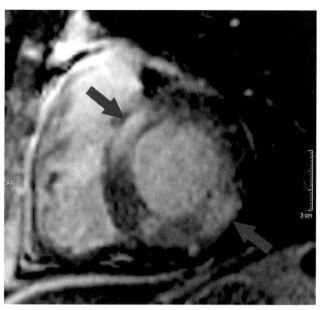

FIGURE 21.45. Infiltrative Cardiomyopathy: Amyloidosis. Short-axis late contrast-enhanced inversion-recovery gradient-echo MR image obtained 10 minutes following gadolinium infusion at 0.2 mM/kg in a patient with a plasma cell dyscrasia and evidence of amyloidosis on a bone marrow biopsy. There are focal regions of late gadolinium enhancement seen in the septum (*red arrow*) and inferolateral walls (*blue arrow*).

operator to precisely delineate both the endocardial and epicardial borders. SSFP is the favored technique for assessing ventricular dimensions. The flow-independent contrast facilitates the accurate demarcation of border contours around the papillary muscles and ventricular trabeculations, where blood pooling typically occurs, particularly in patients with low-flow states such as congestive heart failure.

MR images are acquired as tomographic slices through any selected plane. The planes may be angled to match cardiac (e.g., short-axis, four-chamber) or vascular (e.g., left anterior oblique aorta) anatomy. Tissue characterization of the myocardium is accomplished using T1WI and T2WI, contrast enhancement, and spectroscopy. This may be useful for neoplastic, inflammatory, or infiltrative conditions of the myocardium (Fig. 21.45).

CMR motion studies provide functional information including wall motion analysis, systolic wall thickening, chamber volumes, stroke volumes, right and left ventricular ejection fractions (Fig. 21.46), and valve evaluation (Fig. 21.47). Flowing blood becomes turbulent and loses its coherence when it passes through stenotic or regurgitant valves. The high-velocity stenotic jet or regurgitant flow is displayed as a wedge-shaped puff of dark turbulent flow readily identified on the white blood background with the gradient-echo technique (see Figs. 22.31, 22.32). Visual and region-of-interest grading can be accomplished for stenotic or regurgitant flow based on distance, area, or regurgitant volume. The regurgitant fraction can be calculated by comparing the right and left stroke volumes. Velocity-encoded cine MR techniques, using phase analysis, can calculate flow velocities and flow volumes in addition to the regurgitant volumes (Fig. 21.48). These techniques can be used in lieu of angiography for many cases.

Regional Myocardial Function. Conventional techniques for assessing ventricular motion rely primarily on evaluating motion of the endocardial service. These methods are insensitive to the deformation within the myocardium as well as to translation and torsion during contraction and relaxation.

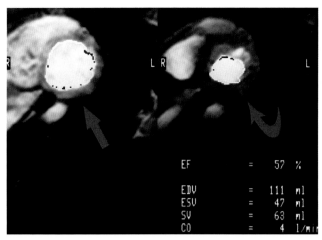

FIGURE 21.46. **MR Ejection Fraction Technique.** Regions of interest are drawn on the diastolic image (*straight arrow*) and the end systolic image (*curved arrow*) of each slice. An area ejection fraction (EF) is then calculated for each slice. Volume ejection fraction calculations are calculated using sequential slices that include the entire ventricular volume, end diastolic volume (EDV), end systolic volume (ESV), stroke volume (SV), cardiac output (CO), end diastole, and end systole.

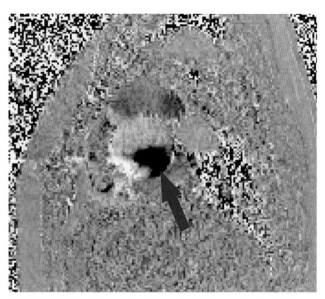

FIGURE 21.48. **Velocity Encoding, Aortic Regurgitation.** A phase-velocity, gradient-echo MR image set in the short axis of the LV demonstrates regurgitant flow (*arrow*) from the aortic valve during diastole.

Early efforts to characterize this dynamic 3D geometry provided insight into the complexities of cardiac motion but required implantation of radiopaque markers within the myocardium. *Myocardial tagging* (Fig. 21.49) places virtual markers within the heart through the manipulation of the magnetic field to facilitate visualization and quantification of regional function, including the rotational and translational motion that has been previously difficult to analyze. CMR is currently the *only* noninvasive technique with this capability. To generate a tagged sequence, a grid consisting of nulled orthogonal lines is applied to the heart at end diastole by altering the local magnetization with narrow and radiofrequency pulses.

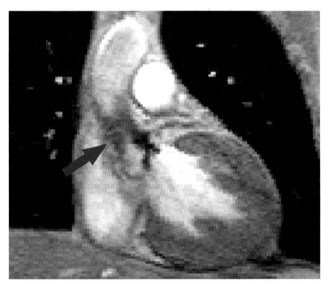

FIGURE 21.47. **Aortic Stenosis.** A midsystolic frame from a gradient-echo cine MR image set in a coronal view shows a calcified valve (low signal in leaflets) (*arrow*) and aortic stenosis. Note the turbulence in the ascending aorta caused by dephasing of spins with high-velocity flow distal to the stenotic orifice.

Because saturated rows of protons comprise this grid structure, the tagging is "embedded" in the tissue and its motion can be reliably tracked throughout the cardiac cycle. Intramural deformation can be visualized and the strain quantified at various sites within the myocardium.

Strain analysis is more accurate than planar wall thickening for detecting regional myocardial dysfunction, as this technique takes into account the motion of a selected segment in all directions simultaneously. Quantification of strain with tagged CMR can be performed with a high degree of precision, allowing for separation of the subendocardial, midmyocardial, and subepicardial layers. Although a precise assessment of 3D LV function can be achieved with this technique, the data analysis remains cumbersome and time-consuming. New methods of image acquisition and postprocessing analysis are currently under investigation, such as HARP (harmonic phase) and DENSE (displacement encoding with stimulated echoes), both of which allow more rapid analysis. Although it is not ready for routine clinical application, CMR strain imaging may become the diagnostic reference standard of the future, one that will enhance our ability to identify subtle abnormalities in function during stress testing and allow for earlier detection of disease states.

Myocardial tagging techniques have already enabled researchers to achieve a better understanding of cardiac function in both normal and diseased states. Tagging has characterized regional myocardial dysfunction in acute and chronic myocardial infarction, hypertrophic cardiomyopathy, valvular heart disease, and pulmonary hypertension. Furthermore, tagging has facilitated the detailed analysis of the local functional response of the myocardium to a number of therapies for congestive heart failure, including pharmacologic agents and surgical reduction treatments.

Coronary Magnetic Resonance Arteriography. Because about 35% of patients referred for their first invasive x-ray angiogram have normal epicardial coronary arteries, an appealing role for CMR in ischemic heart disease would be the noninvasive assessment of the coronary arteries with high temporal and spatial resolution, during relatively short acquisition times. Coronary magnetic resonance angiography (CMRA) has not matured to that point yet, but substantial

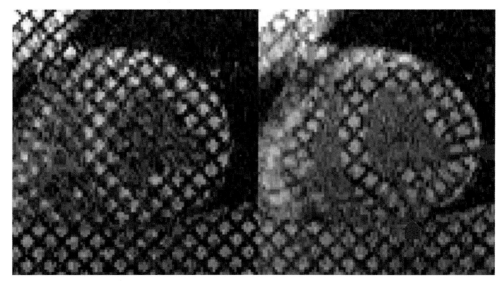

FIGURE 21.49. **Myocardial Tagging.** This technique is shown in a patient on day 3 after anterior myocardial infarction. The left panel represents a short-axis midventricular tagged image at end diastole, while the right panel depicts the end-systolic frame at the same location. Because the tags (*dark stripes*) remain embedded within the tissue throughout the cardiac cycle, deformation can be tracked and the strain quantified. Note the normal deformation in the posterolateral wall (3 to 6 o'clock position in the image) (*arrows*) and the reduced deformation in the anterior wall.

improvements have been achieved over the past few years. Given the small size, tortuous course, and motion of the coronary arteries, several technical challenges must be overcome to obtain images of diagnostic quality. Best in-plane resolution for CMRA is about 600 to 900 μm, which is still about twice the pixel size available in conventional angiography. Compensation for cardiac and coronary arterial motion is achieved by using short acquisition times and optimizing the timing of acquisition in mid diastole, when cardiac motion is least. Respiratory motion correction can be achieved by several different techniques. The advantages of conventional breath-holding techniques are shorter acquisition times and the freedom to repeat the acquisition if the images are subopti-

mal, but the shorter acquisition time results in lower signal-to-noise ratio. The signal-to-noise ratio can be greatly improved upon by longer acquisition times, but this requires respiratory compensation to avoid blurring of the images. The most commonly used techniques rely on diaphragmatic navigators, in which the lung-diaphragm interface is tracked and is used to predict the motion and position of the coronary arteries. Using this method, each acquisition takes about 5 to 10 minutes, with the current navigator efficiency of 30% to 50% during free breathing.

The advent of high-field (3T) coronary imaging offers enhanced image quality and resolution (Fig. 21.50) that may allow improved accuracy for detection of coronary artery

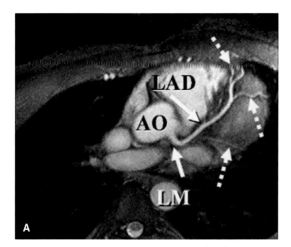
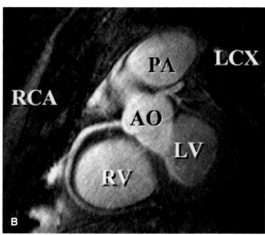

FIGURE 21.50. **Coronary MR Angiography.** Shown are curved multiplanar reformats of a three-dimensional, navigator-gated, T2-prepared gradient-echo coronary MR angiogram performed at 3.0 Tesla in a healthy volunteer. The image (**A**) on the left demonstrates normal left main artery (LM, *arrow*) and left anterior descending artery (LAD, *arrow*) at high spatial resolution (0.6 × 0.6 × 3 mm voxel size) that allows visualization of diagonal and septal branches (*broken arrows*). The image (**B**) on the right demonstrates the right coronary artery (RCA). AO, aorta; RV, right ventricle; LV, left ventricle; PA, pulmonary artery; LCX, left circumflex coronary artery. (From Flamm SD, Muthupillai R. Coronary artery magnetic resonance angiography. J Magn Reson Imaging 2004;19:686–709; reprinted with permission.)

disease, although large patient studies have not been performed to date using these higher field strengths. Because of the significant radiation dose associated with CTCA (especially to the breast), continued advancement of clinically applicable, noninvasive CMRA is expected.

Congenital Heart Disease. The versatility of CMR makes it an ideal tool for analysis of simple and complex congenital heart disease (CHD). In-depth discussion of each of the types of CHD is beyond the scope of this chapter and is covered in other chapters in this book. Structural assessment is enhanced by the ability to create 3D displays from image acquisitions. Morphologic assessment of atrial and ventricular situs and atrioventricular and ventriculoarterial connections is critical in the assessment of CHD. LV and RV volumes and mass are accurately measured in complex CHD and in the postoperative state. Valvular abnormalities can be evaluated with cine acquisitions. Shunt calculations are readily and accurately performed with phase velocity mapping of flow in the ascending aorta and main PA. Methods for measuring intramyocardial function, such as myocardial tissue tagging, offer insight into ventricular mechanics in disease states such as single ventricles. Preoperative sizing and anatomic mapping of the central PAs often aid with surgical planning. Assessment of congenital great vessel disease is straightforward. CMR has also become the modality of choice for postoperative assessment in this patient population.

Common congenital heart lesions include the intracardiac shunts, such as ASD and VSD (Fig. 21.51). CMR is complementary to echocardiography in straightforward CHD. The exception is anomalous pulmonary venous return with the often-associated sinus venosus ASD, where CMR is more accurate than echocardiography because of its 3D coverage of the chest. In addition to cine imaging demonstrating flow, velocity-encoded imaging is useful for both sizing defects and determining shunt ratios.

Complex CHD often requires the complementary use of echocardiography. CMR has the advantage of its 3D coverage and ability to easily image the great vessels and PA branches, a limitation of echocardiography. One example is tetralogy of Fallot, which is characterized by RV hypertrophy, membranous VSD, overriding aorta, and pulmonic or infundibular RV

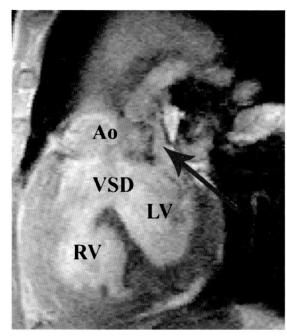

FIGURE 21.52. **Tetralogy of Fallot.** A parasagittal gradient-echo cine image in a patient with unrepaired tetralogy of Fallot. All of the findings of tetralogy are seen in this image: right ventricular (RV) hypertrophy, a membranous ventricular septal defect (VSD), overriding aorta (Ao), and infundibular stenosis (*arrow*). LV, left ventricle.

stenosis. CMR can easily demonstrate all aspects of this disease (Fig. 21.52), which often include systemic-to-pulmonary arterial collaterals; postoperatively, CMR can delineate residual shunting or the common finding of RV outflow tract aneurysm and pulmonic regurgitation. Other complex lesions, such as truncus arteriosus and L-transposition of the great arteries, are diseases where CMR is well suited to demonstrate arteriovenous connections and the presence and location of collateral vessels. Single ventricular hearts is another diagnosis that is well suited to CMR, because CMR can demonstrate morphology of the single ventricle and the relationship between the aortic valve and semilunar valves, and postoperatively CMR can evaluate shunt patency and effect on underlying chambers.

Understanding MR signal characteristics and details of 3D cardiac anatomy displayed in different tomographic planes is critical to the accurate utilization of CMR. It is easy to see why many have referred to CMR as the "one stop shop" because it really has the potential to provide a complete cardiac evaluation, short of interventional procedures. While there are still limitations at this point, CMR potential, and the fact that it does not use ionizing radiation, makes it a very powerful technique to evaluate the heart.

Suggested Readings

Armstrong WF, Ryan T. Feigenbaum's Echocardiography. 7th ed. Philadelphia: Lippincott Williams and Wilkins, 2009.

Bogaert J. Handbook of Clinical Cardiac MRI. New York: Springer-Verlag, 2005.

Boliga RR. An Introductory Guide to Cardiac CT Imaging. Philadelphia: Lippincott Williams and Wilkins, 2009.

Bonow RO, Mann DL, Zipes DP, Libby P, eds. Braunwald's Heart Disease: A Textbook of Cardiovascular Medicine. 9th ed. Philadelphia: W.B. Saunders Co., 2011.

Budoff MJ, Achenbach S, Duerinckx A. Clinical utility of computed tomography and magnetic resonance techniques for noninvasive coronary angiography. J Am Coll Cardiol 2003;42:1867–1878.

Budoff MJ, Shinbane JS. Cardiac CT Imaging: Diagnosis of Cardiovascular Disease. London: Springer-Verlag, 2010.

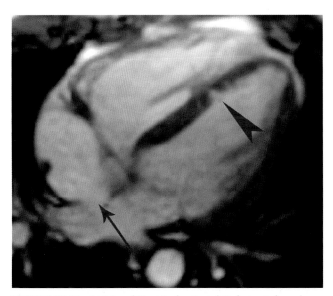

FIGURE 21.51. **Atrial and Ventricular Septal Defects.** A four-chamber long-axis steady-state free precession image in a patient with a secundum atrial septal defect (*arrow*) as well as a muscular ventricular septal defect (*arrowhead*).

Dodd JD, Kalva S, Pena A, et al. Emergency cardiac CT for suspected acute coronary syndrome: qualitative and quantitative assessment of coronary, pulmonary, and aortic image quality. Am J Roentgenol 2008;191:870–877.

Halpern EJ, Savage MP, Fischman DL, Levin DC. Cost-effectiveness of coronary CT angiography in evaluation of patients without symptoms who have positive stress test results. Am J Roentgenol 2010;194:1257–1262.

Ho V, Reddy GP. Imaging of the Cardiovascular System. Philadelphia: Saunders Elsevier, 2010.

Johnson PT, Pannu HK, Fishman EK. IV contrast infusion for coronary artery CT angiography: literature review and results of a nationwide survey. Am J Roentgenol 2009;192:W214–W221.

Kelley MJ, ed. Chest Radiography for the Cardiologist. Cardiology Clinics. Vol. 1. Philadelphia: W.B. Saunders, 1983:543–750.

Kelly JL, Thickman D, Abramson SD, et al. Coronary CT angiography findings in patients without coronary calcification. Am J Roentgenol 2008;191:50–55.

Kubicka RA, Smith C. How to interpret coronary arteriograms. Radiographics 1986; 6:661–701.

Leschka S, Alkadhi H, Plass A, et al. Accuracy of MSCT coronary angiography with 64-slice technology: first experience. Eur Heart J 2005;26:1482–1487.

Lipton MJ, Boxt LM, eds. Cardiac imaging. Radiol Clin North Am 2004;42:487–697.

Manning WJ, Pennell DJ. Cardiovascular Magnetic Resonance. 2nd ed. Philadelphia: Saunders Elsevier, 2010.

Matt D, Scheffel H, Leschka S, et al. Dual-source CT coronary angiography: image quality, mean heart rate, and heart rate variability. Am J Roentgenol 2007;189:567–573.

McGee KP, Williamson EE, Julsrud P. Mayo Clinic Guide to Cardiac Magnetic Resonance Imaging. Cary, NC: Oxford University/Mayo Clinic Scientific Press, 2008.

Miller SW, Abarra S, Boxt LB, et al. Cardiac Imaging: The Requisites. 3rd ed. Philadelphia: Mosby Elsevier, 2009.

Mohesh M, Cody DD. Physics of cardiac imaging with multi-row detector CT. Radiographics 2007;27:1495–1509.

Netter FH. Atlas of human anatomy. The CIBA collection of medical illustrations. West Caldwell, NJ: CIBA-Geigy Corp, 1989.

Oudkerk M. Coronary Radiology. New York: Springer-Verlag, 2004.

Pelberg R, Mazur W, Cardiac CT. Angiography Manual. New York: Springer, 2007.

Pohost GM, Nayak KS. Handbook of Cardiovascular Magnetic Resonance Imaging. New York: Informa Healthcare, 2006.

Schoenhagen P, Halliburton SS, Stillman AE, et al. Noninvasive imaging of coronary arteries: current and future role of multi-detector row CT. Radiology 2004;232:7–17.

Schoepf UJ, Becker CR, Ohnesorge BM, Yucel EK. CT of coronary artery disease. Radiology 2004;232:18–37.

Schoepf UJ, Schoepf UJ. CT of the Heart: Principles and Applications. Totowa, NJ: Human Press, 2005.

Stanford W, Thompson BH, Burns TL, et al. Coronary artery calcium quantification at multi-detector row helical CT versus electron-beam CT. Radiology 2004;230:397–402.

Thelen M, Erbel R, Kreitner KF, Barkhausen J. Cardiac Imaging: A Multimodality Approach. New York: Thieme, 2009.

Webb RB, Higgins CB. Thoracic Imaging: Pulmonary and Cardiovascular Radiology. Philadelphia: Lippincott Williams and Wilkins, 2005.

Zaret BL, Beller GA. Clinical Nuclear Cardiology. 4th ed. Philadelphia: Mosby Elsevier, 2010.

CHAPTER 22 ■ CARDIAC IMAGING IN ACQUIRED DISEASES

DAVID K. SHELTON AND GARY CAPUTO

Cardiac disease remains among the most common problems affecting patient morbidity and mortality today, despite many important dietary, pharmaceutical, interventional, and surgical advances. Most acquired cardiac diseases can be classified under six general categories: ischemic heart disease, cardiomyopathies, pulmonary vascular disease, acquired valvular disease, cardiac masses, and pericardial disease. Use of plain film, fluoroscopy, US, CT, MR, nuclear imaging, and angiocardiography must be integrated with the knowledge of specific disease processes.

ISCHEMIC HEART DISEASE

Coronary Artery Disease

Coronary artery disease is the most common cause of mortality in the United States, with approximately one American dying every minute. Six million to seven million Americans have active symptoms related to ischemic heart disease. Approximately 300,000 coronary artery bypass graft (CABG) surgeries are performed per year in the United States, with a similar number of percutaneous transluminal coronary angioplasties (PTCAs). There were 1.83 million cardiac catheterizations in the United States in 1999, and it has been estimated to reach 3 million by 2010.

Clinical presentations include (1) stable angina, (2) unstable angina (often preinfarction), (3) acute myocardial infarction, (4) congestive heart failure secondary to chronic ischemia or prior infarction sequelae, (5) arrhythmias, and (6) sudden death. Clinical symptoms are caused by luminal abnormalities of the coronary arteries including (1) atheromatous disease, (2) coronary thrombosis, (3) intraluminal ulceration and hemorrhage, (4) vasoconstriction, and (5) coronary ectasia and aneurysm. *Vulnerable plaque* is initiated by lipoprotein deposition into susceptible areas of the coronary walls and other arteries. Chronic inflammation elsewhere in the body, as well as in this developing plaque, is associated with cytokine and macrophage activity. A thin fibrous cap develops over the lipid core, and mechanical stress can lead to the exposure of the blood products which can then trigger the thrombotic cascade. Vulnerable plaque development, sudden rupture, and

thrombosis are now known to be the leading cause of myocardial infarction.

Risk factors for the development of atherosclerotic coronary artery disease include elevated serum cholesterol and C-reactive protein, tobacco smoking, diabetes, hypertension, sedentary lifestyle, obesity, age, male gender, chronic inflammation, and heredity. Aggravating conditions include aortic stenosis ventricular hypertrophy, cardiomyopathy, coronary embolism, congenital anomalies, Kawasaki syndrome, and anemia. Noninvasive imaging is often used as a screening test. Selective coronary angiography with ventriculography and now CT coronary angiography can be utilized to determine coronary anatomy and to direct the specific therapy.

A typical imaging workup includes chest radiography, nuclear medicine myocardial perfusion scans, and consideration for coronary angiography. Indications for coronary angiography include angina refractory to medical therapy, unstable angina, high-risk occupation such as pilot, and abnormal electrocardiograms or stress perfusion tests. Coronary angiography is considered following myocardial infarction when PTCA or intracoronary thrombolysis is being deliberated. Additional indications include development of mechanical dysfunction, progressive congestive failure, refractory ventricular arrhythmias, and follow-up of IV thrombolytic agents.

Coronary artery calcification occurs in the intima and is directly related to advanced atheromatous disease and coronary narrowing (Fig. 22.1). Coronary calcification is detected at angiography in 75% of patients with 50% diameter stenosis. Only 11% of men without significant coronary artery disease have coronary calcification. In the asymptomatic population, the detection of coronary calcification has a predictive accuracy of 86%. In symptomatic patients, coronary calcification is seen in 50% of patients with single-vessel disease, 77% of those with two-vessel disease, and 86% of those with three-vessel disease. Fluoroscopically detected coronary calcification in the presence of angina-like chest pain is associated with coronary stenosis 94% of the time. Overall, fluoroscopic detection of coronary artery calcification has a 73% sensitivity and 84% specificity for symptomatic patients. Exercise tolerance testing has a sensitivity of 76% to 88% and a specificity of 43% to 77%. Exercise testing with planar thallium imaging has a sensitivity and a specificity of approximately 85%.

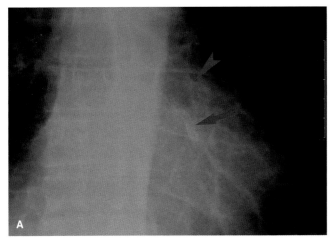

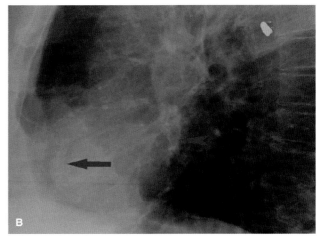

FIGURE 22.1. Coronary Artery Calcification—CXR. Frontal (A) and lateral (B) chest radiographs show atherosclerotic calcification in the left anterior descending (*arrows*) and left circumflex (*arrowheads*) coronary arteries. The patient had a retained bullet from a war wound in his chest.

Use of electron-beam CT (EBCT) and MDCT has improved the sensitivity for detecting coronary artery calcification to approximately 95% (Fig. 22.2). Importantly, CT also allows the grading of the severity of coronary calcification and thus can establish scores and risk scores which can help risk stratify the patient and allow follow-up after medical intervention. The absence of coronary calcification is associated with a very low risk of significant coronary disease. On the other hand, the younger the patient and the higher the calcification score implies the higher associated risk of underlying coronary artery disease and future cardiac events. The negative predictive value of a zero calcification score is 94% to 100%. For a summed coronary score or *Agatston score* (see Fig. 21.38): 0 to 10 is very low to low risk, 11 to 100 is moderate, 101 to 400 is moderately high, and greater than 400 is high risk for underlying stenosis and future cardiac events. With scores greater than 400, there is a sensitivity of 82% and a specificity of 62% for predicting an abnormal myocardial perfusion SPECT scan (Table 22.1).

Myocardial perfusion scanning, using thallium, Tc-99m-sestamibi, Tc-99m-tetrofosmin, or Tc-99m-teboroxime, is one of the primary imaging modalities for detecting myocardial ischemia. Stress images are obtained with exercise or pharmacologic agents such as adenosine dipyridamole. SPECT has increased the sensitivity of 90% to 94% and a specificity of 90% to 95%. The hallmark for segmental ischemia is a perfusion defect on stress testing that fills in during rest examination (Fig. 22.3). A defect that appears stable during both stress and rest examinations is usually an infarction. "Hibernating" regions of viable myocardium associated with tight coronary stenosis may appear as fixed defects on sestamibi or tetrofosmin images or on redistribution thallium images obtained 4 hours after stress.

Stress echocardiography using either exercise or pharmacologic stress modalities has also become a widely accepted method to detect significant (>50% to 70%) coronary artery stenosis. With the advent of digital image acquisition and cine-loop playback, prestress echocardiographic views can be

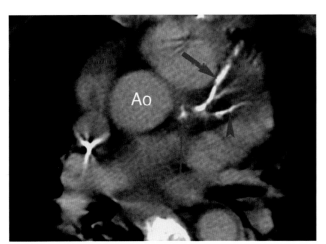

FIGURE 22.2. CT Coronary Calcification. MDCT of the thorax reveals calcification of the left main (*skinny arrow*), left anterior descending (*fat arrow*), and diagonal branch (*arrowhead*) coronary arteries. Detection and reporting of coronary artery calcification even on nongated noncoronary chest CT may lead to the opportunity to treat potentially serious heart disease before a myocardial infarction occurs. Ao, root of the aorta.

TABLE 22.1

CORONARY CALCIUM SCORING

■ CALCIUM SCORE	■ INTERPRETATION
0	No identifiable atherosclerotic plaque. Very low cardiovascular disease. Less than 5% chance of presence of coronary artery disease A negative examination.
1–10	Minimal plaque burden Significant coronary artery disease very unlikely
11–100	Mild plaque burden Likely mild or minimal coronary stenosis
101–400	Moderate plaque burden Moderate nonobstructive coronary artery disease highly likely
Over 400	Extensive plaque burden High likelihood of at least one significant coronary stenosis (>50% diameter)

The summed coronary calcification score, known as the *Agatston score*, can be assigned a percentile ranking for sex and age as well as a risk statement. The appropriate clinical utility depends upon other risk factors as well.

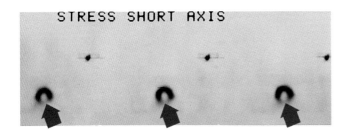

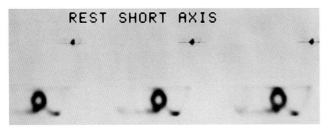

FIGURE 22.3. Myocardial Perfusion Scan—Scintigraphy. SPECT images of the left ventricle in short-axis projection demonstrate a defect (*arrows*) in the inferior wall of the left ventricle during stress, which is well perfused on the rest images. This is strong evidence of ischemic heart disease utilizing Tc-99m-sestamibi as the radionuclide and pharmacologic stress testing with dipyridamole.

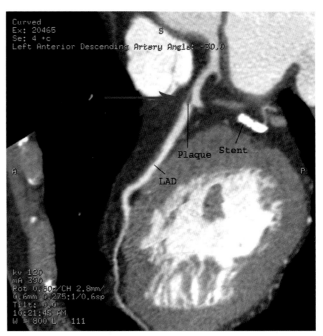

FIGURE 22.4. CT Coronary Angiogram of Left Anterior Descending. Left anterior oblique view of maximum intensity projection from MDCT, CT coronary angiogram demonstrates focal soft plaque in the proximal left anterior descending (*LAD*) coronary artery causing 70% stenosis. Percutaneous transluminal angioplasty was subsequently performed.

simultaneously compared with views taken either immediately postexercise or at peak pharmacologic doses. Development of new segmental wall motion abnormalities or worsening of resting abnormalities suggests stress-induced ischemia. One advantage of these techniques is that they also allow prior assessment of resting wall motion abnormalities that are consistent with either profoundly ischemic, stunned, hibernating, or infarcted myocardium.

The overall sensitivity of exercise echocardiography is 76% to 97% using pharmacologic stress agents; the sensitivity is 72% to 96% with dobutamine, approximately 85% with adenosine, and 52% to 56% with standard dose dipyridamole. The sensitivities for these tests are lowest for single-vessel disease and improve incrementally for two- and three-vessel disease. Stress echocardiography has a specificity of 66% to 100%.

Gated blood pool scintigraphy will demonstrate exercise-induced wall motion abnormalities in 63% of patients with significant coronary artery disease. With exercise, the ejection

fractions normally increase by at least 5%. Failure of ejection fraction to increase with exercise is an indication of myocardial dysfunction. Using these two findings, exercise-gated blood pool scintigraphy has a sensitivity of 87% to 95% and a specificity of 92% for coronary artery disease.

Coronary angiograms and CT coronary angiograms (Fig. 22.4) should be evaluated for the percent of stenosis, the number of vessels involved, focal versus diffuse disease, coronary anatomy, ectasia or aneurysm, coronary calcification, and collateral flow (Fig. 22.5). Collaterals may include epicardial, intramyocardial, atrioventricular, intercoronary, or intracoronary vessels (i.e., "bridging collateral"). The angiographer must count the number of major epicardial vessels with

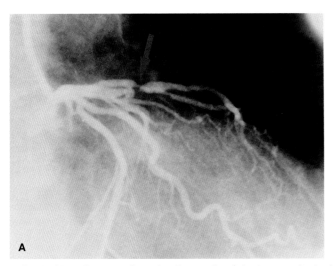

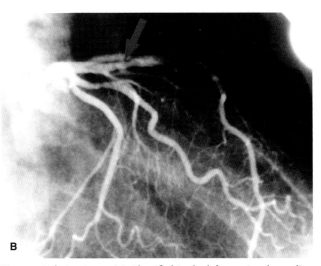

FIGURE 22.5. Coronary Stenosis—Conventional Angiogram. A. An 80% stenotic lesion (*arrow*) is identified in the left anterior descending artery (LAD) on conventional coronary angiography. The patient was experiencing classic angina. **B.** Marked improvement in the LAD lesion (*arrow*) is evident following percutaneous transluminal angioplasty. The angina symptoms resolved.

greater than 50% diameter narrowing. Patients are divided into one-vessel, two-vessel, or three-vessel disease on the basis of involvement of the right or left main coronary artery, left anterior descending (LAD) artery, and left circumflex artery. A 50% diameter narrowing roughly predicts a 75% cross-sectional area reduction, which is the physiologic point at which flow is restricted enough to result in ischemia under stress conditions. Reliability for estimating the percent diameter narrowing depends on the observer, projection, resolution, and presence of coronary calcification or ectasia. The degree of coronary disease may be assessed using percent stenosis of each individual coronary artery or of 5-mm segments of the coronary arteries. The right coronary artery is 10-cm long, the left main coronary artery is 1-cm long, the LAD is 10-cm long, and the left circumflex is 6-cm long for a total of 27 cm. These may be divided into fifty-four 5-mm segments. This scoring system allows the interpreter to quantify the number of 5-mm segments with stenoses in the 0% to 25%, 25% to 50%, 50% to 75%, and 75% to 100% ranges. The significance of 30% to 70% lesions is often clarified by correlation with stress-induced myocardial perfusion scintigraphy.

Percutaneous transluminal angioplasty has traditionally been reserved for localized lesions in one- or two-vessel disease (Fig. 22.5), but recent published series comparing PTCA with CABG in multivessel disease reveals no difference in the end-points of death and myocardial infarction. The PTCA group, however, requires a significantly higher number of repeat procedures during follow-up, although this has improved with more frequent use of stents. CABG, with the use of saphenous vein grafts or internal mammary arteries, is usually reserved for more complex or longer-segment disease. CABG markers are usually placed at the anastomotic site to help the angiographer during future selective angiography. Use of the internal mammary artery has better long-term results than saphenous vein grafts and has been correlated with increased survival. Recurrence of symptoms after CABG may be because of occlusion, graft stenosis, or progression of native vessel disease. Graft stenoses and acute occlusions may be amenable to percutaneous interventional techniques. Grafts and occasionally stents can be noninvasively evaluated with CTCA (Fig. 22.6), although metallic stents can cause imaging problems.

Echocardiography is useful in detecting some of the long-term complications of ischemic disease, including ventricular aneurysm, thinning of myocardium, akinesia, or dyskinesia. Aneurysms are best seen at the apex and septum. Mural thrombi may also be diagnosed but are difficult to visualize at the apex. Stress echocardiography with either exercise or pharmacologic stress techniques is increasingly used to evaluate for ischemia.

CT coronary angiography is capable of establishing the patency of CABGs. Ultrafast CT (EBCT) and now MDCT has a 93% sensitivity, 89% specificity, and 92% accuracy for establishing patency of the CABG grafts. EBCT and MDCT have also shown to be extremely sensitive for detecting coronary calcification. EBCT and MDCT with contrast can also evaluate wall motion, thrombi, old infarcts, aneurysm, and pericardial abnormalities.

MR can be used (*1*) to define the location and size of previous myocardial infarctions, (*2*) to demonstrate complications of previous infarctions, (*3*) to establish the presence of viable myocardium for possible revascularization, (*4*) to differentiate acute versus chronic myocardial infarction, (*5*) to evaluate regional myocardial wall motion and systolic wall thickening (Fig. 22.7), (*6*) to demonstrate global myocardial function with right ventricular and left ventricular ejection fractions, (*7*) to evaluate papillary muscle and valvular abnormalities, and (*8*) to evaluate regional myocardial perfusion (Fig. 22.8). Gadolinium-enhanced T1WI demonstrate areas of ischemia and reperfusion after myocardial infarction. MR with spectroscopy

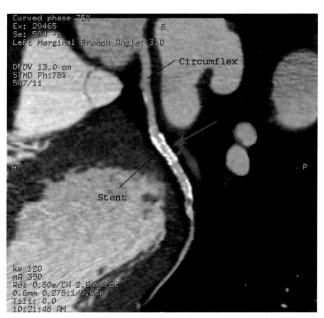

FIGURE 22.6. CT Coronary Angiogram (CTCA) of Left Circumflex. Left anterior oblique projection from MDCT. CTCA maximum intensity projection shows patent coronary stent (*arrow*) with good flow and no evidence of obstruction. Coronary calcification is also evident downstream. Metallic stents and dense calcification are often problematic because of the artifacts they may cause.

targeting myocardial phosphate metabolism can distinguish acute from chronic ischemia and reperfused, infarcted myocardium from reperfused, viable myocardium. With spin-echo imaging, MR has a 78% accuracy for establishing the patency of CABGs. Cine MR with gradient echo has a sensitivity of 88% to 93%, a specificity of 86% to 100%, and an overall accuracy of 89% to 91% for patency of CABGs. Similar to

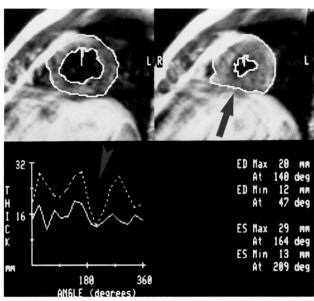

FIGURE 22.7. Wall Motion Evaluation—MR. Short-axis tomographic views of the LV are used for evaluation of systolic wall thickening. Regions of interest are drawn around the myocardium in diastole (*left*) and systole (*right*). The inferior wall (*arrow*) demonstrates hypokinesia and poor systolic wall thickening. The functional graph (*below*) confirms the findings (*arrowhead*). The patient had a previous inferior wall myocardial infarction.

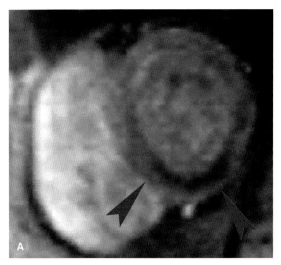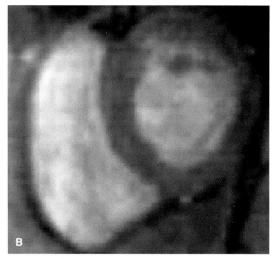

FIGURE 22.8. First-Pass Perfusion—MR. First-pass gadolinium-enhanced hybrid gradient-echo/echo planar perfusion images in a basal short-axis plane following adenosine stress (**A**) and at rest (**B**) demonstrate a reversible perfusion defect in the inferior wall (5:00 to 7:00 in the image) (*arrowheads*). The patient was later shown to have a 99% distal right coronary artery stenosis at cardiac catheterization.

dobutamine stress echocardiography, dobutamine stress cardiac MR can also be accomplished (Fig. 22.9).

Myocardial Infarction

After acute infarction, the chest radiograph will initially show a normal heart size in 90% of cases. Cardiomegaly and congestive failure will eventually develop in 60% to 70%, more frequently with anterior wall infarction, multivessel disease, or left ventricular aneurysm. Increasing stages of pulmonary venous hypertension, particularly alveolar edema, are associated with worsened prognosis.

Complications of myocardial infarction include the following:

Cardiogenic shock implies that systolic pressure is less than 90 mm Hg and is typically associated with acute pulmonary edema and worsened prognosis.

Atrioventricular block is common especially after inferior wall infarcts resulting from either ischemia or injury to the atrioventricular nodal branch of the right coronary artery or increased vagal tone. Complete heart block occurs with larger infarcts and has a worse prognosis.

Right ventricular infarction occurs in approximately 33% of inferior wall infarctions. Symptoms are caused by the reduction in right ventricular ejection fraction, which returns to normal within 10 days in approximately 50% of cases. The diagnosis may be established using technetium pyrophosphate (PYP) radionuclide scans. Complications include cardiogenic shock, elevated right atrial pressure, and decreased PA pressure. Right precordial EKG leads can also assist in making the diagnosis.

Myocardial rupture (3.3% of infarcts) may occur 3 to 14 days after infarction. The mortality rate approaches 100% and accounts for 13% of myocardial infarction deaths.

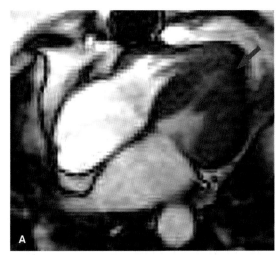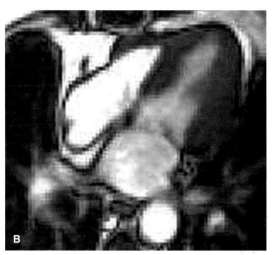

FIGURE 22.9. Dobutamine Cardiac Stress Test—MR. Two end-systolic steady-state free precession four-chamber long-axis image frames from a dobutamine cardiac MR stress test in a patient with chest pain 10 years following left internal mammary bypass graft to the left anterior descending artery. **A.** Image obtained at a low dose of dobutamine (10 μg/kg/min) and demonstrates ventricular cavity obliteration (*arrow*) at end-systole, implying normal systolic function. **B.** Image obtained during peak dobutamine dose (40 μg/kg/min) at a heart rate of 150 beats/min. At peak dobutamine, note the lack of wall thickening in the apical septum consistent with disease in the bypass graft that was proven at subsequent catheterization.

The chest radiograph shows acute cardiac enlargement secondary to leakage of blood into the pericardium. Rupture of the interventricular septum (1%) typically occurs between days 4 and 21, usually as a complication of anterior myocardial infarction and LAD disease. Mortality is 24% within 24 hours and 90% within 1 year. Swan–Ganz catheter measurements show an acute increase in saturation in the RV, although the wedge pressures may be normal. Chest radiographs show acute pulmonary vascular engorgement and right-sided cardiac enlargement because of left-to-right shunt. Pulmonary edema is not a typical feature. Echocardiography readily demonstrates the septal defect.

Papillary muscle rupture (1%) is suggested by abrupt onset of mitral regurgitation, with acute pulmonary edema on the radiograph. Typically, the left ventricle (LV) is only minimally enlarged, whereas the LA enlarges quickly. Inferior infarcts are associated with posteromedial papillary rupture. Anterior infarcts less commonly affect the anterolateral papillary muscle. Mortality is 70% within 24 hours and 90% within 1 year. Echocardiography confirms the diagnosis.

Ventricular aneurysm develops in approximately 12% of survivors from myocardial infarction. Ventricular aneurysms may also be caused by Chagas' disease or trauma and are rarely congenital—usually seen in young black males. Aneurysms present with congestive failure, arrhythmias, and systemic emboli. *True aneurysms* are broad-mouthed, localized outpouchings that do not contract during systole (see Fig. 21.34). They are typically anterior or apical and result from LAD disease. The chest radiograph shows a localized bulge along the left cardiac border and may show rim-like calcification in the wall (Fig. 22.10). Fluoroscopy detects up to 50%, whereas 96% are detected by radionuclide ventriculography or myocardial perfusion scan. Echocardiography, contrast-enhanced CT, and MR are also accurate at detecting true aneurysms.

Pseudoaneurysms are contained myocardial ruptures, consisting of a localized hematoma surrounded by adherent pericardium. Causes include infarction and trauma. Patients are at high risk for delayed rupture. Pseudoaneurysms are typically posterolateral or retrocardiac in location and have smaller mouths than true aneurysms (see Fig. 21.16). MR is most accurate at detecting pseudoaneurysms, but they can also be seen with echocardiography.

Dressler syndrome (4% to 7% of infarcts) is also known as the postmyocardial infarction syndrome and is similar to the postpericardiotomy syndrome complicating cardiac surgery. Onset is typically 1 week to 3 months postinjury (peak at 2 to 3 weeks), but relapses occur up to 2 years later. Presentation includes fever, chest pain, pericarditis, pericardial effusion, and pleuritis with pleural effusion usually more prominent on the left. Dressler syndrome is considered an autoimmune reaction and responds well to anti-inflammatory medications.

Infarct Imaging

The indications for myocardial infarct imaging include late admission, equivocal enzymes, equivocal electrocardiogram, recent cardiac surgery or trauma, and suspicion of right ventricular infarction.

Radionuclide Imaging. "Cold spot" imaging is accomplished with thallium or technetium perfusion agents (Fig. 22.11). Sensitivity is more than 96% within 6 to 12 hours, but only 59% for remote infarction. Acute infarction cannot be distinguished from remote infarction on cold spot imaging. "Hot spot" infarct imaging is positive in acute infarction and uses Tc-PYP (Fig. 22.12), Tc-tetracycline, Tc-glucoheptonate, indium-111 antimyosin antibodies, or F-18 sodium fluorine. Pyrophosphate (PYP) uptake occurs in myocardial necrosis as a result of PYP complexing with calcium deposits. The Tc-PYP scans turn positive at 12 hours, have peak sensitivity at 48 to 72 hours, and revert to normal by 14 days. Persistent abnormal uptake implies a poor prognosis or developing aneurysm. Cardiomyopathies and diffuse myocarditis show diffuse increased uptake. Contusions and radiation myocarditis show increased regional uptake of Tc-PYP.

EBCT and MDCT with contrast demonstrate poor perfusion of the infarcted segment immediately after administration of contrast. After a delay of 10 to 15 minutes, the

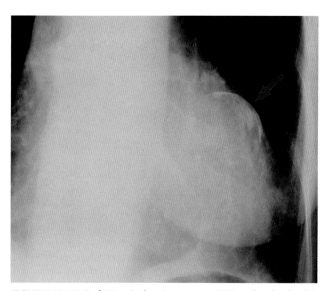

FIGURE 22.10. Left Ventricular Aneurysm—CXR. A localized calcified bulge (*arrow*) is seen along the left heart border, secondary to prior myocardial infarction complicated by left ventricular aneurysm.

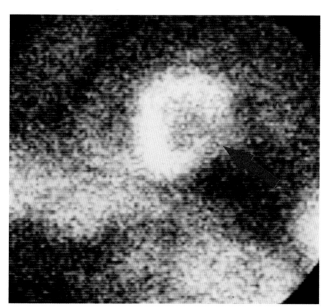

FIGURE 22.11. Myocardial Infarction—Scintigraphy. Resting, planar thallium image in the left anterior oblique projection demonstrates a defect in the inferoposterior wall (*arrow*), consistent with a myocardial infarction. Cold spot imaging can be accomplished almost immediately after the acute event.

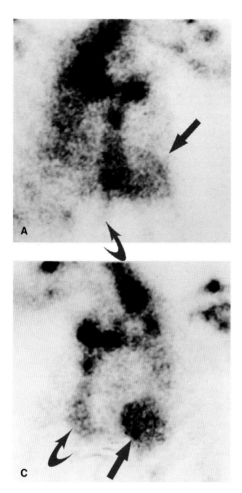

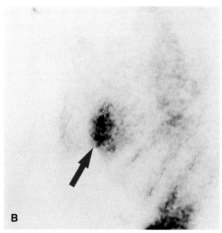

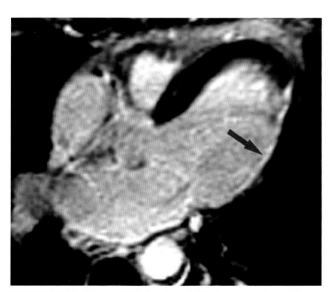

FIGURE 22.12. Myocardial Infarct Scan—Scintigraphy. Hot spot imaging was accomplished using pyrophosphate. Images are obtained in right anterior oblique (**A**), left lateral (**B**), and left anterior oblique (**C**) projections. Notice the uptake in the anterolateral wall of the myocardium (*arrows*), which is "hotter" than the sternum (*curved arrow*).

normal myocardium washes out, leaving a contrast-enhanced periphery of the infarcted zone.

MR demonstrates prolongation of T1 and T2 times secondary to edema of the acutely infarcted segment. Edema occurs within 1 hour after infarct and may be associated with myocardial hemorrhage. MR has a 93% sensitivity, 80% specificity, and 87% accuracy for acute myocardial infarction. The infarcted region is best delineated by high signal on T2WI; however, surrounding edema tends to overestimate the size of the infarct. T1WI with gadolinium demonstrates the acutely ischemic region and will help to differentiate reperfusion from occlusive myocardial infarction (Fig. 22.13). Regional wall thinning and lack of systolic thickening are good evidence of the size of the infarcted segment (Fig. 22.14). Scar tissue

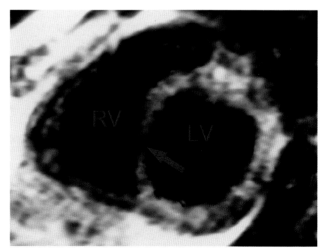

FIGURE 22.13. Myocardial Infarction—MR. Contrast-enhanced inversion-recovery gradient-echo image in a four-chamber long-axis plane 10 minutes following gadolinium infusion at 0.2 mM/kg in a patient with a prior lateral wall infarction. Note the area of bright enhancement (*arrow*) in the lateral wall that subtends the inner 50% of the wall.

FIGURE 22.14. Old Septal Infarction—MR. Spin-echo image demonstrates fixed thinning of the myocardial wall (*arrow*) attributable to prior myocardial infarction. *RV,* right ventricle; *LV,* left ventricle.

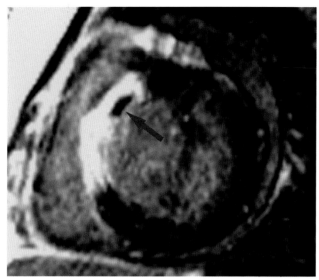

FIGURE 22.15. Microvascular Obstruction—MR. Short-axis late contrast-enhanced image using an inversion-recovery gradient-echo sequence 10 minutes following gadolinium infusion at 0.2 mM/kg shows infarct scar in the septum with a small hypoenhanced zone, which is consistent with microvascular obstruction (*arrow*). This region would be deemed nonviable based on the transmural extent of hyperenhancement and presence of microvascular obstruction.

will not contract, whereas viable myocardium (except when hibernating) will contract and thicken by at least 2 mm. Very high-grade stenotic coronary lesions may result in chronically ischemic myocardium with altered metabolism. This *hibernating myocardium* may act like postinfarction scar, but it remains viable and may improve in function with revascularization (Fig. 22.15). Unfortunately, it also remains at risk for acute infarction. "Stunned myocardium" describes postischemic, dysfunctional myocardium without complete necrosis, which is potentially salvageable.

Echocardiography demonstrates hypokinesis, akinesis, or dyskinesis in previously infarcted myocardial segments; however, this cannot be distinguished from stunned or hibernating myocardium. Global hypokinesis can also be seen with cardiomyopathic processes. Thinned, hyperechoic walls with resting wall motion abnormalities suggest transmural scar. Use of echocardiographic microbubble contrast can enhance the infarcted region by highlighting perfused areas, resulting in a negative contrast effect at the site of the infarct.

CARDIOMYOPATHIES

The prevalence of cardiomyopathies is approximately eight cases per 100,000 population in developed countries. One percent of cardiac deaths in the United States is attributable to

TABLE 22.2
CAUSES OF CONGESTIVE HEART FAILURE

Myocardial
  Cardiomyopathy (dilated, restrictive, hypertrophic)
  Myocarditis
  Postpartum cardiomyopathy

Coronary
  Transient ischemia
  Chronic ischemic cardiomyopathy
  Prior infarct or aneurysm

Endocardial
  Fibrosis
  Löffler syndrome

Valvular
  Stenosis
  Regurgitation

Pericardial
  Effusion
  Constrictive

Vascular
  Hypertension
  Pulmonary emboli
  Arteriovenous fistula
  Vasculitis

Extracardiac
  Endocrinopathy (thyroid, adrenal)
  Toxic
  Anemic
  Metabolic

cardiomyopathy. The mortality rate in males is twice that in females, and in blacks is twice that of whites. In developing countries and in the tropics, the prevalence and mortality rates are much higher, probably because of nutritional deficiency, genetic factors, physical stress, untreated hypertension, and infection, especially Chagas' disease.

The cardiomyopathies are a group of anomalies with three basic features: (*1*) failure of the heart to maintain its architecture, (*2*) failure of the heart to maintain normal electrical activity, and (*3*) failure of the heart to maintain cardiac output. General features of cardiomyopathies include cardiomegaly; congestive heart failure, often with relatively clear lungs; dilated LV and RV with elevated end-diastolic pressures and decreased contractility; and decreased ejection fractions. These findings are only seen in the later stages of hypertrophic and restrictive cardiomyopathies. Causes of congestive heart failure are listed in Table 22.2.

The cardiomyopathies may also be divided into dilated, hypertrophic, restrictive, and right ventricular types (Table 22.3).

TABLE 22.3
TYPES OF CARDIOMYOPATHIES

■ TYPE	■ VENTRICULAR WALL	■ VENTRICULAR CAVITY	■ CONTRACTILITY	■ COMPLIANCE
Dilated	LV thin	LV dilated	Decreased	Normal to decreased
Hypertrophic	LV thick	LV normal to decreased	Increased	Decreased
Restrictive	Normal	Normal	Normal to decreased	Severely decreased
Uhl anomaly	RV thin	RV dilated	Decreased	Normal to decreased

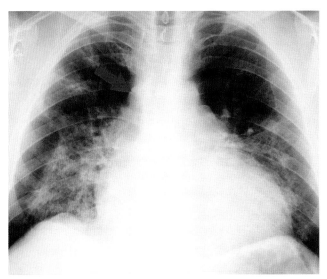

FIGURE 22.16. **Dilated Cardiomyopathy—CXR.** Chest radiograph shows the typical appearance of a dilated cardiomyopathy demonstrated with a water-bottle configuration of the heart and dilatation of the azygos vein (*arrow*). Pulmonary infiltrates are the result of pulmonary edema and capillary leak in this patient with viral myocarditis.

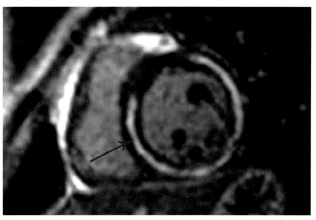

FIGURE 22.17. **Myocarditis—MR.** Short-axis late contrast-enhanced inversion-recovery gradient-echo image obtained 10 minutes following gadolinium infusion at 0.2 mM/kg in a 10-year-old with a history of myocarditis 6 months previously. Note the band of late gadolinium enhancement in the mid-myocardium (*arrow*) that can be seen in chronic or healed myocarditis.

Dilated Cardiomyopathy

In the western world, dilated cardiomyopathy accounts for 90% of all cardiomyopathies (Fig. 22.16). The term "congestive cardiomyopathy" should be reserved for a subgroup of the dilated cardiomyopathies, for which the etiology is unknown. Specific causes for dilated cardiomyopathies should be pursued as the specific therapy may vary: (*1*) ischemic cardiomyopathy (the most common cause) because of chronic ischemia, prior infarction, or anomalous coronary arteries; (*2*) acute myocarditis (Coxsackie virus most commonly) or long-term sequelae of myocarditis (Fig. 22.17); (*3*) toxins (ethanol and doxorubicin [Adriamycin]); (*4*) metabolic (mucolipidosis, mucopolysaccharidosis, glycogen storage disease); (*5*) nutritional deficiencies (thiamin and selenium); (*6*) infants of diabetic mothers; and (*7*) muscular dystrophies.

Clinical presentation is related to congestive heart failure, although the initial presentation may include cardiac arrhythmias, conduction disturbances, thromboembolic phenomena, or sudden death. Presentation may also differ, depending on left-sided dominance, right-sided dominance, or biventricular involvement.

Chest radiograph commonly demonstrates global cardiomegaly. Larger heart sizes are associated with worse prognosis. Coronary artery calcification may be a clue to ischemic cardiomyopathy. Gated myocardial scintigraphy shows decreased left ventricular ejection fraction, prolonged pre-ejection period, shortened left ventricular ejection time, and a decreased rate of ejection. Echocardiography shows a dilated LV with global hypokinesia, thinning of the left ventricular wall and interventricular septum, decreased myocardial thickening, left atrial enlargement, and often right ventricular hypokinesia. MR shows dilatation of the specific chambers, decreased thickness of the myocardium with nonuniformity seen in prior infarctions, pericardial effusions, right and left ventricular ejection fractions, stroke volumes, wall-stress physiology, and quality of systolic wall thickening.

Hypertrophic Cardiomyopathy

Hypertrophic cardiomyopathy may be familial (60%), autosomal dominant with variable penetrance, associated with neurofibromatosis and Noonan syndrome, or secondary to pressure overload. The hypertrophic cardiomyopathies are divided into two basic types: (*1*) *concentric hypertrophy*, which may be diffuse, midventricular, or apical in distribution and (*2*) *asymmetrical septal hypertrophy (ASH)*, also known as *idiopathic hypertrophic subaortic stenosis* (IHSS) (Fig. 22.18,

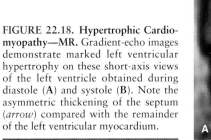

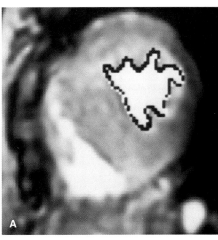

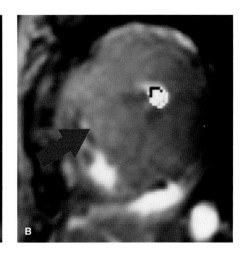

FIGURE 22.18. **Hypertrophic Cardiomyopathy—MR.** Gradient-echo images demonstrate marked left ventricular hypertrophy on these short-axis views of the left ventricle obtained during diastole (**A**) and systole (**B**). Note the asymmetric thickening of the septum (*arrow*) compared with the remainder of the left ventricular myocardium.

see Fig. 22.33). Either form may cause some degree of muscular outflow obstruction with a systolic pressure gradient. Systemic hypertension may cause left ventricular hypertrophy followed by dilation, pulmonary venous hypertension, and increased risk of coronary artery disease.

The clinical presentation includes angina, syncope, arrhythmias, and congestive heart failure. Sudden death occurs in up to 50% of patients. The overall mortality rate is 2% to 3% per year.

On chest radiography, 50% of patients with hypertrophic cardiomyopathy will have a normal chest radiograph and 30% have left atrial enlargement, commonly because of mitral regurgitation. Echocardiographic features of ASH include (1) hypertrophy of the interventricular septum (>12 to 13 mm), (2) abnormal ratio of thickness of the interventricular septum to left ventricular posterior wall (>1.3:1), (3) systolic anterior motion of the mitral valve with mitral regurgitation, (4) narrowing of the left ventricular outflow tract during systole, (5) high velocity across the left ventricular outflow tract with delayed systolic peaks on Doppler examination, (6) midsystolic closure of the aortic valve, and (7) normal or hyperkinetic left ventricular function.

Restrictive Cardiomyopathy

Restrictive cardiomyopathy is the least frequent form of cardiomyopathy. Etiologies include infiltrative disorders such as amyloid (Fig. 22.19), glycogen storage disease, mucopolysaccharidosis, hemochromatosis, sarcoidosis, and myocardial tumor infiltration. In the tropics, endomyocardial fibrosis is highly prevalent. A rare form of endomyocardial fibrosis associated with eosinophilia is called Löffler endocardial fibrosis. Restrictive cardiomyopathy should be considered when patients present with symptoms of congestive failure without radiographic evidence of cardiomegaly or ventricular hypertrophy (Fig. 22.19). The primary differential diagnosis is constrictive pericardial disease that can be differentiated by CT or MR (see Fig. 22.47).

Signs and symptoms are related to congestive failure, arrhythmias, and heart block. In late stages, the electrocardiogram shows low voltage. Pathophysiology includes impaired diastolic function with decreased ventricular compliance, poor diastolic filling, and elevation of right and left ventricular filling pressures. Early in the progression of the disease, ventricular systolic function is normal or near normal. There may be a significant decline in later stages.

The chest radiograph often shows a normal-sized heart with pulmonary congestion. Left atrial enlargement and pulmonary venous hypertension may be present. The PYP nuclear scans demonstrate hot spots in abnormal areas of myocardium in 50% to 90% of patients. Echocardiography may show decreased systolic and diastolic function with normal to decreased ejection fractions. Mild left ventricular wall hypertrophy is often present with a granular or "snowstorm" appearance to the myocardium, especially noted in the case of cardiac amyloidosis. MR shows high signal in the myocardium on T2WI in patients with amyloidosis and sarcoidosis. The atria are enlarged because of elevated diastolic pressures, but ventricular volumes are often normal. Mitral regurgitation and tricuspid regurgitation are readily depicted with gradient-echo cine MR and Doppler echocardiography. The inferior vena cava and superior vena cava may be greatly dilated.

Right Ventricular Cardiomyopathies

Cor pulmonale is defined as right ventricular failure secondary to pulmonary parenchymal or pulmonary arterial disease. It may be considered a secondary form of right ventricular cardiomyopathy. Etiologies include (1) destructive pulmonary disease such as pulmonary fibrosis and chronic obstructive pulmonary disease; (2) hypoxic pulmonary vasoconstriction resulting from chronic bronchitis, asthma, CNS hypoxia, and upper airway obstruction; (3) acute and chronic pulmonary embolism; (4) idiopathic pulmonary hypertension; and (5) extrapulmonary diseases affecting pulmonary mechanics such as chest deformities, morbid obesity (*Pickwickian syndrome*), and neuromuscular diseases.

The end result is alveolar hypoxia leading to hypoxemia, pulmonary hypertension, elevated right ventricular pressures, right ventricular hypertrophy, right ventricular dilation, and right ventricular failure. Symptoms include marked dyspnea and decreased exercise endurance out of proportion to pulmonary function tests. Blood gases demonstrate hypoxemia and hypercapnia.

The chest radiograph shows a normal-sized heart, mild cardiomegaly, or even a small heart (Fig. 22.20). Right

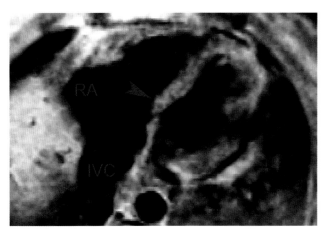

FIGURE 22.19. Restrictive Cardiomyopathy—MR. Spin-echo image demonstrates a variable high-density signal within the myocardium, a dilated right atrium (*RA*), and an enlarged inferior vena cava (*IVC*). The interventricular septum has an abnormal contour (*arrowhead*) because of high right ventricular pressures in this biopsy-proved case of amyloid cardiomyopathy.

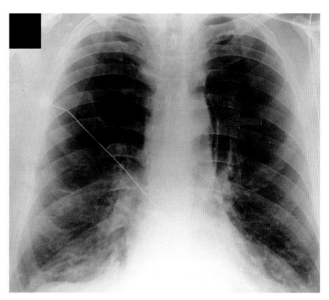

FIGURE 22.20. Cor Pulmonale—CXR. A posteroanterior chest radiograph demonstrates marked hyperinflation caused by chronic obstructive pulmonary disease. The anterior junction line (*arrow*) is herniated to the left of the aortic knob because of marked emphysema in the anterior segment of the right upper lobe.

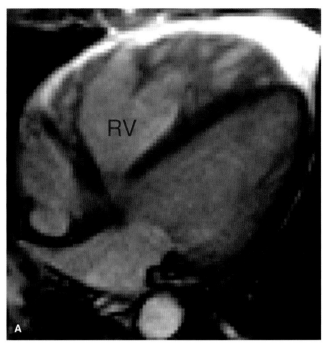
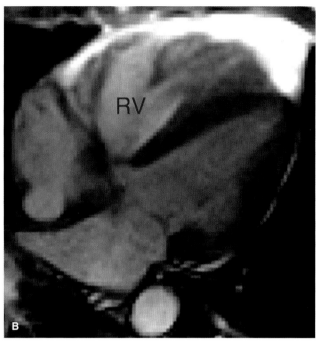

FIGURE 22.21. **Arrhythmogenic Right Ventricular Cardiomyopathy—MR.** End-diastolic (**A**) and end-systolic (**B**) frames from a four-chamber long-axis steady-state free precession cine acquisition in a patient with arrhythmogenic right ventricular cardiomyopathy. The right ventricle (*RV*) is dilated with severe global systolic dysfunction consistent with that diagnosis.

ventricular and right atrial enlargement may be present. The main and central PAs are prominent, and the periphery is oligemic. The interlobar artery typically measures more than 16 mm. The lungs show signs of chronic obstructive pulmonary disease, emphysema, or pulmonary fibrosis. Nuclear scintigraphy shows right ventricular enlargement with decrease in the right ventricular ejection fraction on first-pass examination. Echocardiography, CT, and MR show right ventricular and right atrial enlargement with thickening of the anterior right ventricular wall. M-mode echocardiography of the tricuspid valve shows a diminished A wave and flat E–F slope. Therapy is aimed at the underlying pulmonary disorder.

Uhl anomaly was initially described as a congenital disorder with "parchment-like thinning" of the RV. More recently, it has been described as an acquired disorder in infants or adults and is called "*arrhythmogenic right ventricular dysplasia*" (ARVD). This rare form of cardiomyopathy is limited to the RV with dilation of the RV chamber, marked thinning of the anterior right ventricular wall, and abnormal RV wall motion (Fig. 22.21). MR may also show fatty infiltration of the anterior RV-free wall (essentially diagnostic), dyskinesia, and even RV aneurysm. Clinical presentation includes syncope, recurrent ventricular tachycardia, and premature death from early congestive failure or arrhythmias. Familial occurrence has been reported, and males outnumber females by 3:1. Right ventricular ejection fractions are commonly reduced to less than half of normal, with mild reductions in the left ventricular ejection fraction. Treatment involves exercise restrictions and placement of an implantable cardioverter defibrillator (ICD).

PULMONARY VASCULAR DISEASE

Enlargement of the pulmonary outflow tract is seen in congenital heart disease with left-to-right shunts. Outflow tract prominence without evidence of a shunt lesion is usually the result of poststenotic dilatation secondary to pulmonary

stenosis, pulmonary arterial hypertension, Marfan syndrome, Takayasu arteritis, or idiopathic dilatation of the PA. Idiopathic dilatation of the PA demonstrates a dilated main PA; normal peripheral PAs; and normal, balanced circulation. This entity is much more common in females and is often associated with a mild systolic ejection murmur, but without evidence of pulmonary stenosis.

Pulmonary arterial hypertension should be considered whenever the main PA and left and right PAs are enlarged (Fig. 22.22). Signs of right atrial and ventricular enlargement or hypertrophy are often present. Systolic right ventricular and PA pressures exceed 30 mm Hg. Other findings include

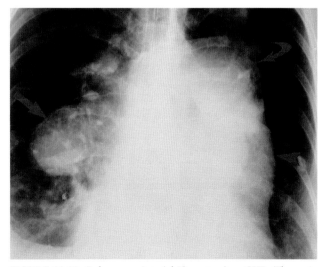

FIGURE 22.22. **Pulmonary Arterial Hypertension, CXR.** The main PA (*curved arrow*), left PA (*arrowhead*), and right PA (*straight arrow*) are extremely enlarged. Faint calcification is seen in the right PA. The patient had schistosomiasis with resultant vasculitis and pulmonary arterial hypertension.

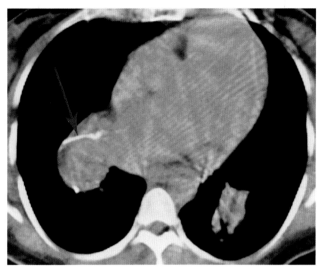

FIGURE 22.23. Pulmonary Arterial Hypertension—CT. Noncontrast CT demonstrates calcification in the wall of the right PA (*arrow*).

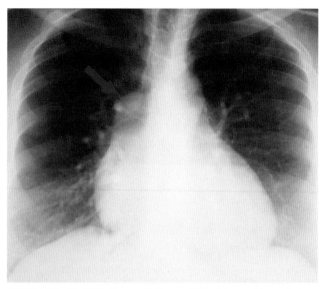

FIGURE 22.24. High Output Failure—CXR. Chest radiograph demonstrates cardiomegaly, vascular engorgement, and distension of the azygos vein in this pregnant patient with severe anemia. The azygos vein (*arrow*) is a good marker of intravascular volume expansion or elevated central venous pressures.

rapid tapering and tortuosity of the PAs. The peripheral lung zones appear clear. Calcification within the pulmonary arterial walls is virtually diagnostic of pulmonary arterial hypertension (Fig. 22.23).

The differential diagnosis for pulmonary arterial hypertension includes long-standing pulmonary venous hypertension (e.g., mitral stenosis), Eisenmenger physiology (from long-standing left-to-right shunts), pulmonary emboli, vasculitides (such as rheumatoid arthritis or polyarteritis nodosa), and primary pulmonary hypertension. Polyarteritis nodosa is a necrotizing vasculitis involving the medium-sized PAs. Radiographic findings include small pulmonary arterial aneurysms, focal stenoses, small infarctions, and signs of pulmonary hypertension. Primary pulmonary hypertension is most common in women in their third and fourth decades. Histologic examination reveals plexiform and angiomatoid lesions with no evidence of emboli or venous abnormalities. Symptoms include dyspnea, fatigue, hyperventilation, chest pain, and hemoptysis.

Increased pulmonary blood flow is caused by high output states and left-to-right shunts. High output states include volume loading, pregnancy, peripheral shunt lesions (arteriovenous malformations), hyperthyroidism, leukemia, and severe anemia (Fig. 22.24). The main and central PAs are enlarged with increased circulation to the lower lobes, upper lobes, and peripheral lung zones. Bronchovascular pairs show enlargement of the vascular component. The most common shunts in the adult are the acyanotic lesions including atrial septal defect, ventricular septal defect, patent ductus arteriosus, and partial anomalous pulmonary venous return. Cyanotic lesions with increased blood flow to the lungs include transposition of the great vessels, truncus arteriosus, total anomalous pulmonary venous return, and endocardial cushion defects. Ventricular septal defects with left-to-right shunting may occur acutely following myocardial infarction.

Decreased pulmonary blood flow with a small heart is caused by chronic obstructive pulmonary disease (see Fig. 22.20), hypovolemia, malnourishment, and Addison disease. When the cardiac silhouette is enlarged, the differential diagnosis includes cardiomyopathy, pericardial tamponade, Ebstein anomaly, and right-to-left shunts from congenital heart disease.

Asymmetrical pulmonary blood flow may be evident on chest radiography, angiography, or nuclear medicine pulmonary perfusion scans (Fig. 22.25). This may result from either decreased or increased blood flow to one lung. Pulmonary valvular stenosis often results in increased blood flow to the left lung. With resultant left PA dilatation, tetralogy of Fallot may

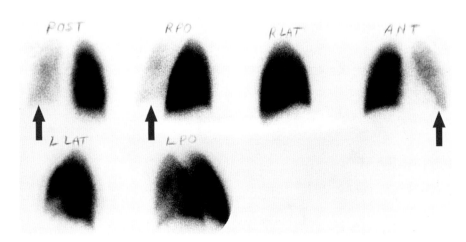

FIGURE 22.25. Asymmetrical Pulmonary Blood Flow. Multiple images from a ⁹⁹ᵐTc macroaggregated albumin pulmonary perfusion lung scan demonstrate marked reduction in the pulmonary blood flow to the left lung (*arrows*) in comparison with the right lung. A subtle left hilar mass was causing compression of the left PA. *POST*, posterior; *RPO*, right posterior oblique; *RLAT*, right lateral; *ANT*, anterior; *LLAT*, left lateral; *LPO*, left posterior oblique.

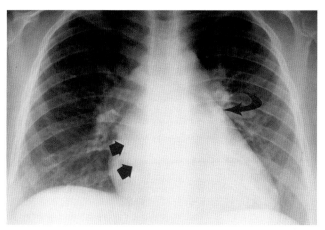

FIGURE 22.26. **Moderate Mitral Stenosis—CXR.** A chest radiograph demonstrates mild cardiomegaly with straightening of the left heart border, prominence of the left atrial appendage (*curved arrow*), and evidence of left atrial enlargement (*arrows*). Cephalization of blood flow and enlargement of the PAs indicate pulmonary venous and pulmonary arterial hypertension.

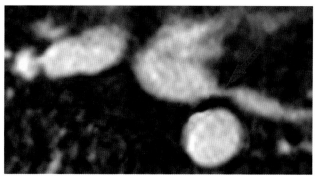

FIGURE 22.27. **Pulmonary Vein Stenosis—MR.** Axial image taken from a maximum intensity projection (MIP) of a three-dimensional gadolinium-enhanced MR angiogram demonstrating stenosis (*arrow*) of the left lower pulmonary vein in an asymptomatic patient status postradiofrequency ablation of the pulmonary veins for atrial fibrillation.

cause increased blood flow to the right lung (see Fig. 21.17). Surgical shunts, such as the Blalock–Taussig procedure, also increase blood flow to one lung. Decreased blood flow to one lung can occur with peripheral pulmonary stenosis (see Fig. 22.35), interruption of the PA, scimitar syndrome, pulmonary hypoplasia, Swyer–James syndrome, pulmonary emphysema, pulmonary embolism, fibrosing mediastinitis, or carcinoma affecting one artery (see Fig. 22.25). When examining a chest radiograph, one must be careful to exclude technical artifacts such as lateral decentering and soft tissue asymmetry such as mastectomy. The balance of circulation and size of the central PAs should be compared as well as the size of the bronchovascular pairs.

Pulmonary venous hypertension may be identified on radiographs, pulmonary angiograms, or nuclear medicine perfusion scans (Fig. 22.26, see Fig. 21.19). Pulmonary venous hypertension is considered mild with wedge pressures of 10 to 13 mm Hg, moderate with equalization of upper and lower lobe blood flow and wedge pressures of 14 to 16 mm Hg, or severe with the upper lobe vessels being distended more than the lower lobe vessels and wedge pressure 17 to 20 mm Hg. Progressive cephalization is accompanied by progressive secondary enlargement of the PAs and filling out of the hilar angles. The most common cause of pulmonary venous hypertension is elevation of left atrial pressures secondary to left ventricular failure (Table 22.4).

Pulmonary venous obstruction may occur due to congenital abnormality or atresia, tumoral involvement, or pulmonary venous stenosis, which is often iatrogenic (Fig. 22.27).

TABLE 22.4

CAUSES OF PULMONARY VENOUS HYPERTENSION

Left ventricular failure
Mitral stenosis
Mitral regurgitation
Aortic stenosis
Aortic regurgitation
Pulmonary venoocclusive disease
Congenital heart disease

ACQUIRED VALVULAR HEART DISEASE

Mitral stenosis in the adult is usually caused by rheumatic heart disease, with 50% of patients giving a history of rheumatic fever. Rarely, an atrial myxoma may mimic mitral stenosis on CXR. The incidence of mitral stenosis is higher in females by a ratio of 8:1. *Lutembacher syndrome* is a combination of mitral stenosis with a pre-existing atrial septal defect, resulting in marked right-sided enlargement.

The normal mitral valve area is 4 to 6 cm^2. With mild mitral stenosis (mitral valve area <1.5 cm^2), the chest radiograph may be normal and left atrial pressures will be elevated only during exercise. Moderate mitral stenosis (valve area <1.0 cm^2) produces signs of left atrial enlargement and pulmonary venous hypertension (see Fig. 22.26). Dyspnea on exertion is common. Severe mitral stenosis (valve area <0.5 cm^2) has marked left atrial enlargement, right ventricular enlargement, Kerley lines, pulmonary edema, and, occasionally, calcification in the left atrial wall. Patients are often dyspneic at rest, with resting left atrial pressure exceeding 35 mm Hg. Palpitations and atrial fibrillation with risk of atrial thrombi and systemic emboli are also common. Long-standing pulmonary venous hypertension leads to pulmonary arterial hypertension. Stages of progression of mitral stenosis are (*1*) stage 1: pulmonary venous hypertension with hilar angle loss; (*2*) stage 2: interstitial edema with Kerley lines; (*3*) stage 3: alveolar edema; and (*4*) stage 4: chronic, recurrent congestive failure, hemosiderin deposits, and ossification or calcifications in the lung.

The chest radiograph is often characteristic with a long, straight, left heart border, left atrial enlargement, prominence of the left atrial appendage, cephalization of blood flow indicating pulmonary venous hypertension, pulmonary arterial hypertension, left atrial calcification, mitral valve calcification, prominent main PA, right ventricular enlargement with filling of the retrosternal clear space, and dilatation of the inferior vena cava. Echocardiography shows a decreased E–F slope on M-mode, slow left ventricular filling, left atrial enlargement, thickened mitral valve, decreased excursion of the mitral valve with a narrow mitral orifice, parallel movement of the anterior and posterior leaflets, and atrial fibrillation. Gated nuclear angiograms are useful for following the left ventricular ejection fraction. MR grades the valvular disease and determines chamber volumes and ejection fractions. Velocity-encoded cine MR quantifies peak velocity and instantaneous blood flow. The peak gradient across the stenotic valve can be calculated when

TABLE 22.5

CAUSES OF MITRAL REGURGITATION

Rheumatic heart disease
Congenital heart disease
Mitral valve prolapse
Ruptured chordae tendineae
Infectious endocarditis
Papillary muscle rupture
Mitral annulus calcification

the echo times (TE) are less than 7 milliseconds, allowing measurements of velocities up to 6 m/s. Mitral commissurotomy or balloon valvuloplasty may be performed if the leaflets are pliable and not heavily calcified. Mitral valve replacement should be considered before left ventricular failure occurs.

Mitral regurgitation associated with rheumatic heart disease used to be the most common hemodynamically significant form of mitral regurgitation in adults. Today, mitral regurgitation is most commonly secondary to mitral valve prolapse, but is also by ischemia-related papillary muscle dysfunction and or infarct with papillary muscle rupture (Table 22.5).

The radiograph shows left atrial enlargement that is greater than that seen with pure mitral stenosis (Fig. 22.28). Left ventricular enlargement is also present. Pulmonary venous hypertension is less prominent than in mitral stenosis. The radiograph is near normal with mild mitral regurgitation; shows atrial enlargement and pulmonary venous hypertension with moderate disease; and shows progressive left atrial enlargement, left ventricular enlargement, pulmonary venous hypertension, and pulmonary edema with severe mitral regurgitation.

Echocardiography shows left atrial enlargement, left ventricular enlargement, and bulging of the atrial septum to the

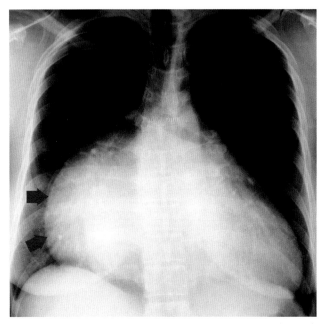

FIGURE 22.28. Mitral Regurgitation—CXR. A chest radiograph demonstrates marked left atrial enlargement with "atrial escape" where the LA (*arrows*) becomes the border forming along the right cardiac silhouette. Note the marked carinal splaying because of this massive left atrial enlargement.

right. Nuclear angiogram shows a dilated LV with an elevated left ventricular ejection fraction because of the hyperdynamic status. MR using gradient-echo and -gated cine mode shows the regurgitant jet projecting from the LV into the LA during systole. The regurgitant jet may be graded visually as mild, moderate, or severe based on the distance it extends toward the back wall. Grade 1 regurgitation is defined as turbulent flow extending less than one-third the distance to the back wall, grade 2 is less than two-thirds the distance to the back wall, and grade 3 is more than two-thirds of the distance to the back wall. The regurgitant fraction can be calculated by comparing the right and left ventricular stroke volumes, which are normally equal. The regurgitant fraction is equal to the right ventricular stroke volume minus the left ventricular stroke volume, divided by right ventricular stroke volume. Gated blood pool scintigraphy is used to follow the ejection fraction to optimize the timing of valve replacement. Echocardiography can be used to follow both the ejection fraction and left ventricular volumes.

Mitral valve prolapse is an interesting entity that has also been called "floppy mitral valve" or Barlow syndrome. It is seen in 2% to 6% of the general population and is more common in young women. It has an autosomal dominant transmission and is more common in patients with straight backs, pectus excavatum, and narrow anteroposterior diameters of the chest. Patients may be asymptomatic or have symptoms as a result of arrhythmias. A "honking" type of murmur or a murmur with midsystolic click is characteristic. The chest radiograph is usually normal, although occasionally patients will develop mitral regurgitation, left atrial enlargement, and pulmonary venous hypertension. Echocardiography demonstrates a characteristic bulging of the anterior or posterior leaflets usually beginning during midsystole when the valve should remain closed. This may also take the appearance of a pansystolic "hammock" type of leaflet bowing. Some patients develop myxomatous thickening of the mitral valve leaflets.

Aortic stenosis is caused by partial fusion of the commissures between the tricuspid aortic valve cusps. Alternatively, a *bicuspid aortic valve* is found in 1% to 2% of the population and is present in 95% of congenital aortic stenosis. Bicuspid aortic valve is most common in males and is present in 25% to 50% of patients with aortic coarctation. Of patients with a bicuspid aortic valve, 60% of those older than 24 years of age have calcification within the bicuspid valve. *Calcific or degenerative aortic stenosis*, on the other hand, is usually seen in older patients with systemic hypertension and is thought to be part of the atherosclerotic process. This type of aortic valve calcification tends to progress in association with coronary calcification, but may be associated with significant stenosis. Aortic valve calcification is best seen on the lateral or right anterior oblique chest radiographs. Noncalcific aortic stenosis is often a result of rheumatic heart disease and may coexist with mitral valve disease. The radiograph typically shows left ventricular hypertrophy and poststenotic dilatation of the aorta (Fig. 22.29). The ascending aorta is not normally seen on frontal chest radiographs in patients younger than 40 years and thus, in this setting, is suspicious. Echocardiography, CT, and MR may show dense or calcific aortic valve, a dilated aortic root, hyperdynamic function, and left ventricular hypertrophy. A bicuspid aortic valve, when present, can be directly visualized and evaluated by CT or MR (Fig. 22.30).

The aortic valve area is normally 2.5 to 3.5 cm². Symptoms typically occur when the valve area is less than 0.7 cm² or is less than 1.5 cm² if there is combined aortic stenosis and aortic insufficiency. Mild aortic stenosis is associated with a 13 to 14 mm orifice and greater than 25 mm Hg gradient. Moderate aortic stenosis has an 8 to 12 mm orifice and greater than 40 to 50 mm Hg gradient. Severe stenosis occurs at a less than 8-mm orifice with a gradient greater than 100 mm Hg. Cardiac MR

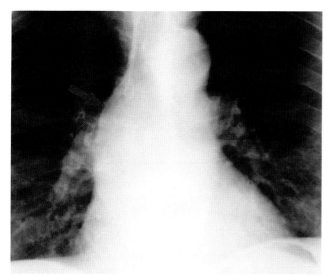

FIGURE 22.29. Aortic Stenosis—CXR. Note the enlarged ascending aorta (*arrow*), highly suggestive of poststenotic dilatation in this patient with aortic stenosis and normal heart size.

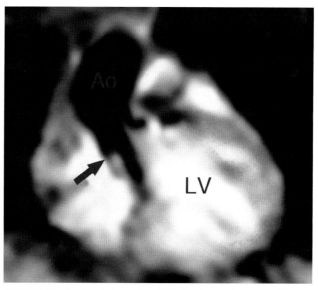

FIGURE 22.31. Aortic Stenosis—MR. Gradient-echo coronal image of the ascending aorta (*Ao*), aortic valve (*arrow*) and left ventricle (*LV*). Note the signal void in the entire ascending aorta as a result of marked turbulence caused by severe aortic stenosis.

and echocardiography show increased ventricular muscle mass with hypertrophy as well turbulent flow (Fig. 22.31, see Fig. 21.48). MR and blood pool scintigraphy may show increased or decreased left ventricular ejection fraction (depending on LV status), decreased rate of ejection, prolonged left ventricular emptying time, but a normal left ventricular filling rate.

Symptoms progress from angina to syncopal episodes to congestive failure with the possibility of sudden death with severe stenosis. Therapy is usually valve replacement, although some cases are amenable to valvuloplasty.

Aortic insufficiency is primary when it is attributable to aortic valve disease or is secondary when it is the result of aortic root disease (Table 22.6). Physical examination reveals a water-hammer pulse, a decrescendo diastolic murmur, and, occasion-

ally, an *Austin–Flint murmur,* caused by vibrations of the mitral valve from regurgitant flow.

Chest radiograph shows a dilated, calcified aortic root with a normal heart size in mild disease. With moderate disease, the LV and cardiac silhouette enlarge. With severe disease, left atrial enlargement and congestive heart failure develop. Symptoms include dyspnea on exertion, fatigue, and other symptoms of congestive failure.

Echocardiography and MR show the dilated aortic root, the regurgitant aortic flow (Fig. 22.32, see Fig. 21.49), diastolic flutter of the interventricular septum or anterior mitral leaflet (Austin-Flint phenomena), left ventricular dilation, increased wall motion, increased ejection fraction, and early mitral valve closure. The ratio of the regurgitant flow width to the aortic root is helpful for grading the severity. Ventricular function may be followed by echocardiography, nuclear scintigraphy, or MR. Once congestive failure begins to occur, the LV will dilate and the LVEF will fall.

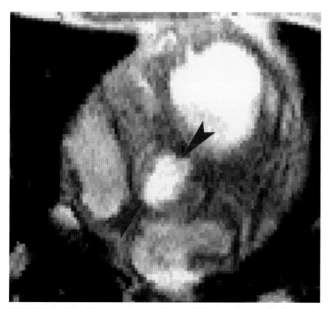

FIGURE 22.30. Bicuspid Aortic Valve—MR. A midsystolic frame of a gradient-echo image set in a double oblique orientation through the short axis of the aortic valve. Note the "fish-mouth" opening of the two leaflets (*arrowheads*) of the aortic valve, consistent with a bicuspid valve.

TABLE 22.6

CAUSES OF AORTIC INSUFFICIENCY

Valvular
  Congenital
  Rheumatic
  Infectious endocarditis
  Trauma

Aortic root
  Syphilis
  Dissecting aneurysm
  Marfan syndrome
  Rheumatoid arthritis
  Reiter syndrome
  Relapsing polychondritis
  Giant cell arteritis

Subvalvular
  Aneurysm of sinus of Valsalva
  Subaortic stenosis
  High ventricular septal defect

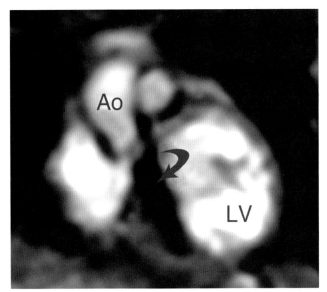

FIGURE 22.32. Aortic Regurgitation—MR. Gradient-echo coronal image through the ascending aorta (*Ao*) and left ventricle (*LV*) demonstrates regurgitant flow from the aortic valve into the left ventricle (*curved arrow*).

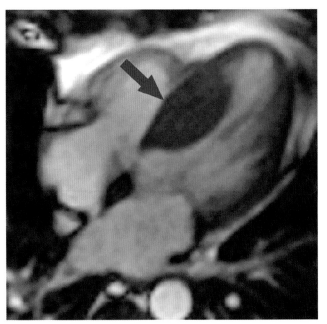

FIGURE 22.33. Hypertrophic Cardiomyopathy—MR. Four-chamber long-axis steady-state free precession end-systolic image in a patient with hypertrophic cardiomyopathy and marked asymmetric septal hypertrophy (*arrow*). Note the relatively normal wall thickness in the apex and lateral walls.

Supravalvular aortic stenosis is the result of a localized hourglass-type narrowing above the valve, a discrete fibrous-type membrane, or a diffuse hypoplastic tubular configuration of the ascending aorta. Supravalvular aortic stenosis is often associated with peripheral pulmonary stenosis and valvular or subvalvular aortic stenosis. This combination of findings can be seen in Marfan syndrome or Williams syndrome. The coronary arteries are dilated because of the elevated systolic pressure and narrowing of the aortic root (<20 mm). The aortic cusps themselves are normal.

Subvalvular/subaortic stenosis may be a fixed anatomic defect or a dynamic functional obstruction. Fixed subaortic stenosis is associated with congenital heart disease, especially ventricular septal defect, in 50% of cases. *Type 1* subaortic stenosis is a thin membrane located less than 2 cm below the valve. *Type 2* is a thick, collar-type constriction. *Type 3* subaortic stenosis is an irregular, fibromuscular type of narrowing. *Type 4* is a funnel-like constriction of the left ventricular outflow tract. The mitral valve is normal.

The functional type of subaortic stenosis has also been called ASH, IHSS, or hypertrophic obstructive cardiomyopathy. The appearances vary slightly. Findings may be evident with nuclear scintigraphy, but they are more obvious on echocardiography and MR (Fig. 22.33). The interventricular septum is significantly thicker than the left ventricular free wall in 95% of patients. The left and right ventricular cavities are normal or small in 95% of patients. Systolic anterior motion of the mitral valve is best seen on echocardiography but may also be identified with MR. ASH may partially obstruct outflow in systole. The aortic cusp may flutter or partially close during systole. Mitral regurgitation is a common secondary finding attributable to abnormal mitral valve position or papillary muscle attachment.

Pulmonic stenosis is seen in 8% of congenital heart disease and is uncommon as an acquired disease in adults. Symptoms may be secondary to cyanosis or heart failure. A systolic ejection murmur is heard over the left sternal border. The chest radiograph often shows dilatation of the main and left PAs with increased flow into the left lung (Fig. 22.34). Right ventricular hypertrophy or enlargement is seen on chest radiographs, MR, and echocardiography. Systolic doming of the pulmonic valve is secondary to incomplete opening and is best seen on echocardiography. Rarely, calcification may be identified in the pulmonic valve.

Valvular pulmonic stenosis is caused by partial commissural fusion in 95% of cases. Symptoms typically start in childhood and progress into adulthood. A pulmonic click is common, and the electrocardiogram often shows right ventricular hypertrophy. On angiography, a jet of contrast may be seen extending well into the left PA. In dysplastic pulmonic stenosis (5% of cases), the cusps are immobile, thick, and redundant. There is no click and typically no poststenotic dilatation.

Infundibular or subvalvular stenosis is common with tetralogy of Fallot and often occurs with ventricular septal defects. Because of the location of the stenosis, preferential flow goes to the right lung (see Fig. 21.17).

Peripheral pulmonary stenosis or supravalvular stenosis commonly (up to 60%) accompanies pulmonary valvular stenosis. Sites of narrowing include the main PA, bifurcation, lobar, and segmental arteries (Fig. 22.35). Associated syndromes include Williams syndrome, tetralogy of Fallot, Ehlers–Danlos syndrome, and postrubella syndrome. Postrubella syndrome is associated with intrauterine growth retardation, deafness, cataracts, mental retardation, and patent ductus arteriosus. Williams syndrome is associated with hypercalcemia, elfin facies, mental retardation, and supravalvular aortic stenosis. Ehlers–Danlos syndrome is a defect in collagen formation associated with joint laxity, skin stretchability, aneurysms, and mitral regurgitation.

Pulmonic insufficiency is very uncommon in adults and is usually the result of subacute bacterial endocarditis (SBE). Pulmonic insufficiency demonstrates regurgitant flow from the pulmonic valve into the RV on echocardiography or MR.

Bacterial Endocarditis. Patients predisposed to SBE include those with rheumatic heart disease, mitral valve prolapse, aortic stenosis, aortic regurgitation, bicuspid aortic valves (50% of aortic SBE), mitral stenosis, mitral regurgitation, congenital heart disease (especially ventricular septal defect and tetralogy of Fallot), or prosthetic valves (4% of SBE), and drug addicts. IV drug abusers are particularly at risk for tricuspid valve involvement. Tricuspid valve involvement is suspected when multiple septic pulmonary emboli are seen on chest radiography. *Streptococcus viridans* was previously reported as the most common bacterial etiology; however, *Staphylococcus*

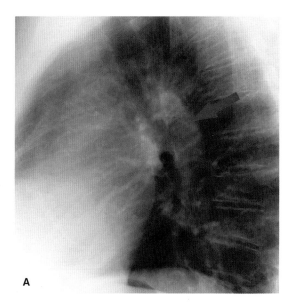

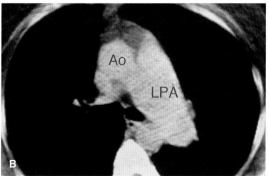

FIGURE 22.34. Pulmonary Stenosis—CXR. A. Lateral chest radiograph demonstrates marked poststenotic dilatation of the left PA (*arrow*). **B.** CT through the ascending aorta (*Ao*) demonstrates marked dilatation of the left pulmonary artery (*LPA*).

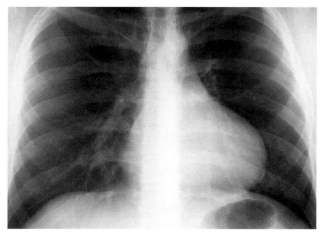

FIGURE 22.35. Peripheral Pulmonary Stenosis—CXR. A chest radiograph demonstrates classic right ventricular configuration indicative of RV hypertrophy. Asymmetric blood flow is noted with decreased markings in the left lung because of peripheral stenosis.

aureus has now become the most common bacterial agent. *Serratia* and *Pseudomonas* organisms are also common offenders, particularly in certain geographic locations. *Candida* is the most common fungal agent, followed by *Aspergillus.*

Valve vegetations can be detected in 50% to 90% of patients with known bacterial endocarditis. The vegetations cause excessive vibration of the valves during systole, and the leaflets may appear slightly thickened or fuzzy. The actual vegetations may be seen to prolapse when the valve is closed. The vegetations may cause valvular incompetence or acute valvular destruction. The vegetations, or chronic areas of thickening, may remain even after successful antibiotic therapy. It is difficult to discern acute infective vegetations from chronic changes. Infections of prosthetic valves result in exaggerated valve motion, partial valvular obstruction, loosening of the sutures, and perivalvular leak or frank dehiscence. MR and transesophageal echocardiography are quite good at detecting perivalvular or perisutural leaks. Noninfectious vegetations and focal valve thickenings may be seen with carcinoid syndrome (right heart valves), *Libman–Sack vegetations* of systemic lupus erythematosus, *Lambl excrescences* (focal benign thickening), and myxomatous degeneration.

Other forms of endocarditis include *Chagas' disease*, which is common in South America and Africa. Chagas' disease is a late sequelae of acute myocarditis involving the parasite *Trypanosoma cruzi*. This may result in cardiomyopathy or ventricular aneurysm. Patients with AIDS may also develop an endocarditis and cardiomyopathy, possibly because of viral infections. Indium-labeled white blood cell scans, PET-CT, or gallium scans may prove useful in patients for whom echocardiography is inconclusive or in whom secondary endocardial or aortic abscess is suspected (Fig. 22.36).

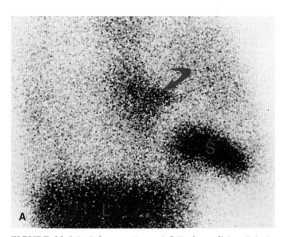

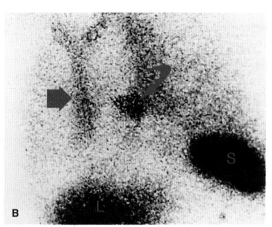

FIGURE 22.36. Subacute Bacterial Endocarditis—Scintigraphy. Anterior (**A**) and left anterior oblique (**B**) views of the chest from an indium-labeled white cell scan shows migration of indium-labeled white cells to the area of severe aortic endocarditis. Note the marked increased activity (*curved arrows*) in the heart to the left and posterior to the sternum (*fat arrow*). Marked uptake is normal in the liver (*L*) and spleen (*S*).

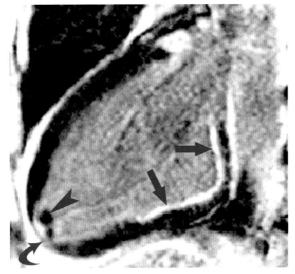

FIGURE 22.37. Thrombus in the Left Ventricle—MR. Late contrast-enhanced image in a two-chamber orientation using an inversion-recovery gradient-echo sequence 10 minutes following gadolinium infusion at 0.2 mM/kg. Note the subendocardial hyperenhancement in the basal inferior wall (*arrows*) and focal transmural hyperenhancement at the apex (*curved arrow*). The *arrowhead* identifies a thrombus at the apex that fails to take up contrast.

CARDIAC MASSES

Cardiac masses include thrombi, primary benign tumors, primary malignant tumors, and metastatic tumors. Lipomatous hypertrophy, moderator bands, and papillary muscles may simulate cardiac masses. Because most cardiac masses do not deform the outer contours of the heart, chest radiography is typically not useful, except for the occasional calcific mass. Nuclear scintigraphy, CT, and cardiac angiography identify intracardiac masses. Echocardiography is usually the initial mode of evaluation, and MR may be helpful when there is uncertainty.

Thrombi are the most frequent cause of an intracardiac mass and are most common in the LA and LV, where they present a risk of systemic emboli (Fig. 22.37). Intra-atrial thrombi

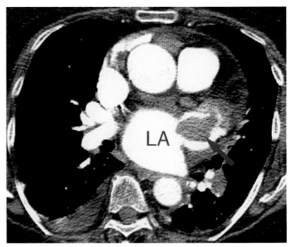

FIGURE 22.39. Left Atrial Thrombus—CT. Contrast-enhanced MDCT demonstrates large thrombus (*arrow*) in the appendage of the left atrium (*LA*).

are usually associated with atrial fibrillation, often secondary to rheumatic heart disease. Atrial thrombi commonly occur along the posterior wall of the LA. Clots within the left atrial appendage are difficult to detect on transthoracic echocardiography but are readily identified with transesophageal echo (Fig. 22.38), CT (Fig. 22.39), and MR. Left ventricular thrombi are usually secondary to recent infarction or ventricular aneurysm (Fig. 22.40). The differentiation of tumor versus clot is best done with MR using gradient-echo techniques. Clots typically have low signal, whereas tumors have intermediate signal. Clots will not enhance, whereas neoplasms will typically appear as enhancing masses on CT or MR.

Benign Tumors. Atrial myxoma makes up 50% of primary cardiac tumors and is the most common primary benign tumor (Figs. 22.41, 22.42). It occurs most frequently in patients in the 30- to 60-year age range and is often accompanied by fever, anemia, weight loss, embolic symptoms (27%), or syncope. Myxomas frequently calcify; most (75% to 80%) occur in the LA and they can mimic rheumatic valvular disease clinically. Cine-mode gradient-echo MR is useful for determining the morphology of the lesion. *Intracardiac lipomas* or *lipomatous hypertrophy* are readily identified on MDCT. MR is also

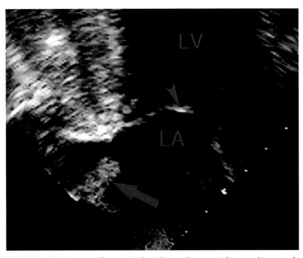

FIGURE 22.38. Left Atrial Thrombus—Echocardiography. Transesophageal echo shows echogenic thrombus (*arrow*) in the left atrium (*LA*). The mitral valve (*arrowhead*) and the left ventricle (*LV*) are shown.

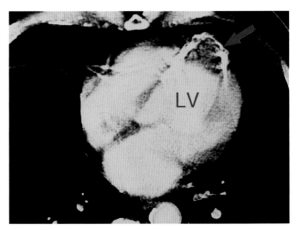

FIGURE 22.40. Left Ventricular Thrombus—CT. Axial contrast-enhanced CT through the left ventricle (*LV*) demonstrates calcification in an apical, left ventricular aneurysm (*arrow*). Note the nonenhancing low-density thrombus within the aneurysm.

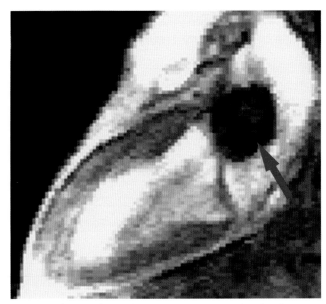

FIGURE 22.41. Left Atrial Myxoma—MR. Two-chamber, long-axis gradient-echo cine image shows a left atrial myxoma (*arrow*). The myxoma has very low signal on this gradient-echo image.

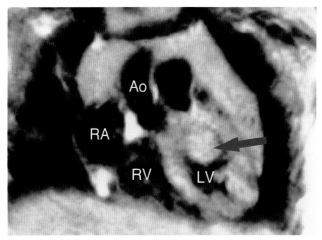

FIGURE 22.43. Left Ventricular Rhabdomyoma—MR. Coronal spin-echo image through the aorta (*Ao*) and left ventricle (*LV*) demonstrates a high-signal polypoid mass near the outflow tract of the LV (*arrow*). This young patient had tuberous sclerosis, and a presumptive diagnosis of ventricular rhabdomyoma was made. Note the delineation of the right atrium (*RA*) and right ventricle (*RV*).

useful and will demonstrate characteristic bright signal on T1WI and remain relatively bright on T2WI. Fat saturation sequences help to make the specific diagnosis of lipoma, which is the second most common benign cardiac tumor.

Cardiomegaly, left atrial enlargement, pulmonary venous hypertension, and ossific pulmonary nodules may be seen. Echocardiogram, MR, and CT show the atrial filling defect which may prolapse into the ventricle during diastole (Fig. 22.42). Atrial myxomas may be pedunculated and are usually lobulated. On M-mode echo, the E–F slope is typically decreased with numerous echoes seen behind the mitral valve.

Other benign tumors include fibromas (12% of which may calcify), lipomas, rhabdomyomas, and the rare teratoma. Rhabdomyomas (Fig. 22.43) are found in 50% to 85% of tuberous sclerosis patients. Hydatid cysts typically show a bulge along the left heart border, with associated curvilinear calcification, and are at risk for rupture into the pericardium or myocardium.

Malignant Tumors. Metastatic tumors are the most common malignant cardiac tumor and are 10 to 20 times more frequent than primary cardiac tumors. Breast, lung, melanoma, and lymphoma are the most common neoplasms to metastasize to the heart. MR is excellent for detecting intracardiac tumors (Fig. 22.44) and for evaluating direct tumor extension or pericardial involvement. Angiosarcoma is the most common primary malignant cardiac tumor, followed by rhabdosarcoma, liposarcoma, and other sarcomas.

PERICARDIAL DISEASE

Pericardial effusion is the most common abnormality of the pericardium. The normal pericardial stripe is 2 to 3 mm on chest radiograph and CT and less than 4 mm on MR. Plain films show thickening of the pericardial stripe or differential

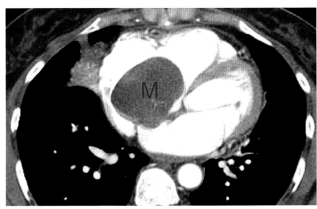

FIGURE 22.42. Right Atrial Myxoma—CT. Contrast-enhanced MDCT demonstrates a large right atrial myxoma (*M*), which was noted to prolapse through the tricuspid valve.

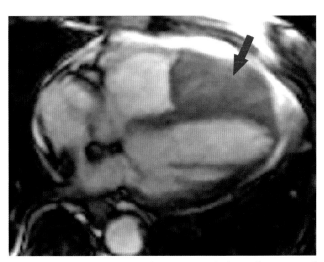

FIGURE 22.44. Metastasis to the Heart. Single frame from an axial steady-state free precession cine series in a patient with metastatic non–small cell lung carcinoma with tumor (*arrow*) visualized filling the RV apex.

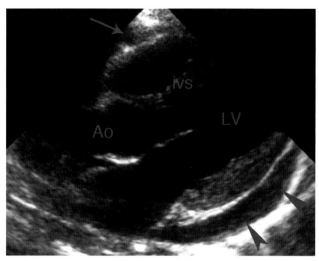

FIGURE 22.45. Pericardial Effusion—Echocardiography. Longitudinal image through the interventricular septum (*ivs*), aortic root (*Ao*), and left ventricle (*LV*) demonstrates a pericardial effusion (*arrowheads*). A smaller anterior component of the pericardial effusion is also noted (*arrow*).

density sign in up to 63% of patients with pericardial effusions. The water-bottle configuration is seen in chronic effusions. Fluoroscopy shows decreased cardiac pulsations. The normal pericardium contains approximately 20 mL of fluid, whereas it takes approximately 200 mL to be detectable by plain film. Echocardiography detects very small quantities (<50 mL) of pericardial fluid, usually as a posterior sonolucent collection (Fig. 22.45). Small effusions (<100 mL) will appear as anterior and posterior sonolucent regions. Moderate-sized effusions (>100 to 500 mL) demonstrate a sonolucent zone around the entire ventricle. Very large effusions (>500 mL) extend beyond the field of view and may be associated with the "swinging heart" inside the pericardium. Pericardial effusions are evident on chest CT performed for other reasons (Fig. 22.46). CT is useful in detecting loculated pericardial effusions. MR may characterize the fluid. Simple serous fluid appears dark on T1WI (probably because of fluid motion) and bright on gradient-echo images. Complicated or hemorrhagic effusions appear bright on T1WI and dark on

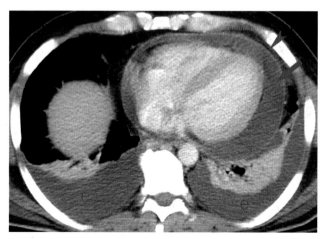

FIGURE 22.46. Pericardial Effusion—CT. Axial image from a CT of the thorax shows a large pericardial effusion (*arrow*) as well as bilateral pleural effusions (*e*). The pericardium (*arrowhead*) is seen as a thin high-attenuation line bounding the pericardial effusion.

TABLE 22.7

CAUSES OF PERICARDIAL EFFUSION

Idiopathic

Infectious
    Viral (Coxsackie, echovirus, adenovirus)
    Bacterial (Staphylococcus, Streptococcus, Haemophilus
      influenza)
    Fungal (Candida, Aspergillus, Nocardia)
    Mycobacterial

Autoimmune
    Systemic lupus erythematosus
    Rheumatoid arthritis
    Scleroderma
    Dressler and postpericardiotomy syndromes
    Radiation induced

Neoplastic   Lymphoma, lung, breast metastases
Drug induced   Procainamide, hydralazine, phenytoin

Metabolic
    Uremia
    Myxedema
    Cholesterol

Miscellaneous
    Congestive heart failure
    Aortic dissection
    Sarcoidosis
    Pancreatitis
    Trauma

gradient-echo imaging (probably because of susceptibility artifact). The differential diagnosis for pericardial effusions is listed in Table 22.7.

Cardiac tamponade refers to cardiac chamber compression by pericardial effusion under tension, compromising diastolic filling. *Pulsus paradoxus* describes an exaggeration of the usual drop in systolic pressure greater than 10 mm Hg during inspiration. This occurs as a result of septal shift and paradoxic septal motion during right ventricular filling. Clinical examination shows marked jugular venous distension, distant heart sounds, and a pericardial rub. The chest radiograph shows rapid enlargement of the cardiac silhouette with relatively normal-appearing vascularity. Echocardiography typically shows the septal shift, paradoxic septal motion, diastolic collapse of the RV, and cyclical collapse of the atria.

Constrictive pericardial disease is the result of fibrous or calcific thickening of the pericardium, which chronically compromises ventricular filling through restriction of cardiac motion. Age of onset is usually 30 to 50 years, and the incidence in men exceeds that in females by 3:1. The most common cause is postpericardiotomy. Other etiologies include virus (Coxsackie B), tuberculosis, chronic renal failure, rheumatoid arthritis, neoplastic involvement, and radiation pericarditis. Calcification is seen on radiographs in up to 50% of patients. Pleural effusions and ascites are common, and there may be an associated protein-losing enteropathy. Clinical findings include ankle edema, neck vein distension, pulsus paradoxus, pericardial diastolic knock, and ascites. Chest radiographs show normal to mildly enlarged cardiac silhouette with small atria, dilated superior and inferior vena cava and azygos vein, and a flat or straightened right heart border. Echocardiography shows thickened pericardium, abnormal septal motion, and increased

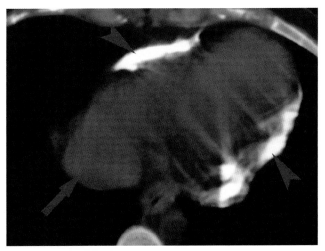

FIGURE 22.47. Constrictive Pericarditis—CT. Nonenhanced CT demonstrates pericardial calcification (*arrowheads*) and a dilated inferior vena cava (*arrow*). Note the distortion of the ventricles.

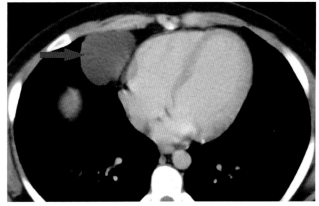

FIGURE 22.49. Pericardial Cyst—CT. Contrast-enhanced CT shows the typical findings of a pericardial cyst as a nonenhancing sharply defined mass (*arrow*) in the right cardiophrenic angle. CT attenuation is uniform throughout measuring 28 H.

left ventricular ejection fraction with small end-diastolic volume. Small effusions may be seen with "effusive constrictive pericarditis," which has both thickening and effusion.

CT is particularly good at demonstrating pericardial thickening (>3 mm) and pericardial calcification in difficult cases (Fig. 22.47). Reflux of contrast into the coronary sinus and IVC, a bowed interventricular septum, flattening of the RV, enlarged RA, ascites, and pleural effusions may also be seen. MR shows pericardial thickening (>4 mm); dilatation of the RA, inferior vena cava, and hepatic veins; sigmoid septal shift; and narrowing of the RV. Abnormal flow mechanics may also be seen in the vena cava and atria. The finding of an abnormally thick pericardium is important in differentiating constrictive pericardial disease from restrictive cardiomyopathy.

Pericardial cysts are most common in the cardiophrenic angles, right more common than left (Figs. 22.48, 22.49).

They are usually asymptomatic and are more frequent in males. The cysts are attached to the parietal pericardium, are lined with epithelial or mesothelial cells, contain clear fluid, and range in size from 3 to 8 cm. They occasionally communicate with the pericardial space. CT attenuation numbers are typically 4 up to 40 H and do not significantly increase with contrast enhancement. MR demonstrates characteristic low signal on T1WI, with no internal enhancement and bright signal on T2WI (Fig. 22.50). The differential diagnosis for a cardiophrenic angle mass includes pericardial cyst, fat pad, lipoma, enlarged lymph nodes, diaphragmatic hernia, and ventricular aneurysm.

Congenital absence of the pericardium (Fig. 22.51) is more common in males than females by 3:1. The age at diagnosis is infancy through age 81. Complete left-sided absence (55%) is more common than foraminal defects (35%) or total absence (10%). Associated conditions include bronchogenic cysts, ventricular septal defects, diaphragmatic hernias, and sequestrations. With complete absence, the heart is shifted toward the left with a prominent bulge of the right ventricular outflow tract, main PA, and left atrial appendage. Insinuation of the lung into the anteroposterior window and beneath the heart is characteristic. Decubitus views show a widely

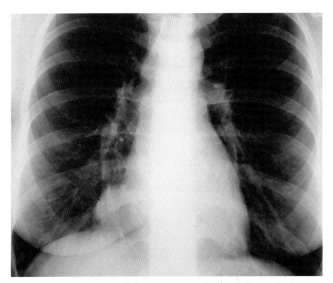

FIGURE 22.48. Pericardial Cyst—CXR. Chest radiograph demonstrates a soft tissue mass in the right costophrenic angle (*arrow*). Contrast-enhanced CT confirmed a pericardial cyst with no enhancement and CT attenuation of 8 H. Findings are indicative of a benign pericardial cyst.

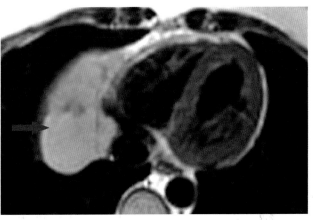

FIGURE 22.50. Pericardial Cyst—MR. Axial T2W spin-echo image demonstrates a pericardial cyst (*arrow*) in the classic right costophrenic angle location with homogeneous bright internal signal on T2WI. The cyst showed uniform low signal on T1WI, not shown.

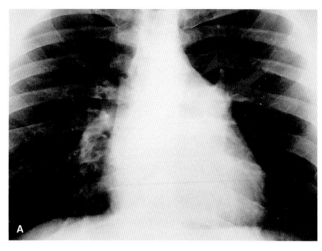

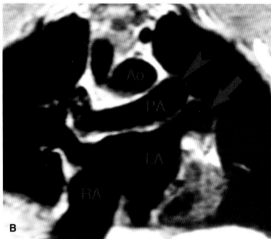

FIGURE 22.51. Partial Absence of the Pericardium. A. Chest radiograph demonstrates prominence (*arrowhead*) of the main pulmonary artery and an unusual bulge along the left heart border (*arrow*). **B.** Coronal plane spin-echo MR confirms enlargement of the main PA (*arrowhead*) and shows herniation of the left atrial appendage (*arrow*) caused by a defect in the pericardial sac. *Ao*, ascending aorta; *LA*, left atrium; *RA*, right atrium.

swinging cardiac silhouette. Partial absence of the pericardium risks strangulation of cardiac structures, with the possibility of sudden death. Surgical closure of partial defects is usually recommended.

Suggested Readings

Armstrong WF, Ryan T. Feigenbaum's Echocardiography. 7th ed. Philadelphia: Lippincott Williams & Wilkins, 2009.

Bogaert J. Handbook of Clinical Cardiac MRI. New York: Springer-Verlag, 2005.

Boliga RR. An Introductory Guide to Cardiac CT Imaging. Philadelphia: Lippincott Williams & Wilkins, 2009.

Bonow RO, Mann DL, Zipes DP, Libby P. Braunwald's Heart Disease: A Textbook of Cardiovascular Medicine. 9th ed. Philadelphia: W. B. Saunders Co., 2011

Budoff MJ, Achenbach S, Duerinckx A. Clinical utility of computed tomography and magnetic resonance techniques for noninvasive coronary angiography. J Am Coll Cardiol 2003;42;1867–1878.

Budoff MJ, Shinbane JS. Cardiac CT Imaging: Diagnosis of Cardiovascular Disease. London: Springer-Verlag, 2010.

Dodd JD, Kalva S, Pena A, et al. Emergency cardiac CT for suspected acute coronary syndrome: qualitative and quantitative assessment of coronary, pulmonary, and aortic image quality. AJR Am J Roentgenol 2008;191: 870–877.

Halpern EJ, Savage MP, Fischman DL, Levin DC. Cost-effectiveness of coronary CT angiography in evaluation of patients without symptoms who have positive stress test results. AJR Am J Roentgenol 2010;194: 1257–1262.

Ho V, Reddy GP. Imaging of the Cardiovascular System. Philadelphia: Saunders Elsevier, 2010.

Johnson PT, Pannu HK, Fishman EK. IV contrast infusion for coronary artery CT angiography: literature review and results of a nationwide survey. AJR Am J Roentgenol 2009;192:W214–W221.

Kelly JL, Thickman D, Abramson SD, et al. Coronary CT angiography findings in patients without coronary calcification. AJR Am J Roentgenol 2008;191:50–55.

Kelley MJ, ed. Chest Radiography for the Cardiologist. Cardiology Clinics. Philadelphia: WB Saunders, 1983;1:543–750.

Kubicka RA, Smith C. How to interpret coronary arteriograms. Radiographics 1986;6:661–701.

Leschka S, Alkadhi H, Plass A, et al. Accuracy of MSCT coronary angiography with 64-slice technology: first experience. Eur Heart J 2005;26:1482–1487.

Lipton MJ, Boxt LM, eds. Cardiac imaging. Radiol Clin North Am 2004; 42:487–697.

Manning WJ, Pennell DJ. Cardiovascular Magnetic Resonance. 2nd ed. Philadelphia: Saunders Elsevier, 2010.

Matt D, Scheffel H, Leschka S, et al. Dual-source CT coronary angiography: image quality, mean heart rate, and heart rate variability. AJR Am J Roentgenol 2007;189:567–573.

McGee KP, Williamson EE, Julsrud P. Mayo Clinic Guide to Cardiac Magnetic Resonance Imaging. Rochester: Mayo Clinic Scientific Press, 2008.

Miller SW, Abarra S, Boxt LB. Cardiac Imaging: The Requisites. 3rd ed. Philadelphia: Mosby Elsevier, 2009.

Min JK, Shaw LJ, Berman DS. The present state of coronary computed tomography angiography. J Am Coll Cardiol 2010;55:957–965.

Mohesh M, Cody DD. Physics of cardiac imaging with multi-row detector CT. Radiographics 2007;27:1495–1509.

Netter FH. Atlas of Human Anatomy. The CIBA Collection of Medical Illustrations. West Caldwell, NJ: CIBA-Geigy Corp, 1989.

Oudkerk M. Coronary Radiology. New York: Springer-Verlag, 2004.

Pelberg R, Mazur W. Cardiac CT Angiography Manual. New York: Springer, 2007.

Pohost GM, Nayak KS. Handbook of Cardiovascular Magnetic Resonance Imaging. New York: Informa Healthcare, 2006.

Schoepf UJ, Becker CR, Ohnesorge BM, Yucel EK. CT of coronary artery disease. Radiology 2004;232:18–37.

Schoepf UJ, Schoepf UJ. CT of the Heart: Principles and Applications. Totowa, NJ: Human Press, 2005.

Schoenhagen P, Halliburton SS, Stillman AE, et al. Noninvasive imaging of coronary arteries: Current and future role of multi-detector row CT. Radiology 2004;232:7–17.

Stanford W, Thompson BH, Burns TL, et al. Coronary artery calcium quantification at multi-detector row helical CT versus electron-beam CT. Radiology 2004;230:397–402.

Thelen M, Erbel R, Kreitner KF, Barkhausen J. Cardiac Imaging: A Multimodality Approach. New York: Thieme, 2009.

Webb RB, Higgins CB. Thoracic Imaging: Pulmonary and Cardiovascular Radiology. Philadelphia: Lippincott Williams & Wilkins, 2005.

Zaret BL, Beller GA. Clinical Nuclear Cardiology. 4th ed. Philadelphia: Mosby Elsevier, 2010.

Note: Page numbers followed by "*f*" indicate figures, respectively.